Pediatric Hand Surgery

Giorgio Pajardi
Editor

Pediatric Hand Surgery

Springer

Editor
Giorgio Pajardi
Department of Hand Surgery and Rehabilitation
S. Giuseppe MultiMedica Hospital, Milan University
Milano, Italy

ISBN 978-3-031-30983-0 ISBN 978-3-031-30984-7 (eBook)
https://doi.org/10.1007/978-3-031-30984-7

This Springer imprint is published by the registered company Springer Nature Switzerland AG
The registered company address is: Gewerbestrasse 11, 6330 Cham, Switzerland

To my grandchildren Beatrice, Tommaso and Alice,
who carry our projects and our dreams into their future.

Preface

When 8 years ago Elisa Geranio from Springer suggested that I should write this book, I asked her to have a few days of meditation before answering. I love challenges and I love overcoming them even more, but I imagined that selecting and coordinating so many colleagues on such a niche topic would have been a truly demanding undertaking right from the start. So it was, but I am happy to have accepted the proposal and I hope the readers of these pages are as well.

The theme is fascinating and always current. Congenital malformations of the hand can hardly be caged in rigid classifications and certainly do not respond to preordained reconstructive schemes.

Scientific rigour, experience and dexterity of the surgeon are useless if they are not spiced up with imagination, which allows us to project what we are building today into the dimension of growth, thinking of the dexterity of what will be a child and then a young adult.

A heartfelt thanks to all my Friends—who I hope will remain so in the future, despite my harassment - who have responded to my appeal by giving us the precious gift of their experience.

Thanks to my team, who contributed in every way to complete the work, transfusing years of coaching in my paediatric clinics and operating rooms. They are my future because unlike the other branches of hand surgery, the paediatric field requires at least fifteen years of experience to see the result in the young adult of what was decided during the first visit a few days after birth.

Special thanks to Chiara Novelli, who was able to support and solicit Colleagues from all over the world, avoiding that the effort and at times the disappointment for some delay could let them run out of enthusiasm. Thanks to the Publisher for the honour reserved for me and my country, offering me this unique and unrepeatable experience.

Last but not least, thanks to my wife and daughters who have always sustained and supported me actively in my human and professional choice, which is difficult and certainly not commercial, supporting the families with the “Associazione la Mano del Bambino” and during the tiring process of care, with a special dedication to my daughter Martina who has tenaciously chosen to follow me in the most rewarding profession that exists.

Milano, Italy Giorgio Pajardi

Contents

1 The Congenital Hand: Psychological Aspects

Daniela Pajardi and Alessandra Viano

Abstract

The hand is fundamental to human psychosensorial development and becomes a means and a symbol of autonomy because it can reach every area of the body. Furthermore, hands play a central role in social and emotional relationships because they express emotionality, they are protagonists in nonverbal communication, and they are also constantly visible to others as well as to their owner.

The relationship between patient and health specialists grows and is shaped in this difficult, emotionally intense context. Health personnel face a problem that requires joint and coordinated intervention from various professionals: surgeons, physiotherapists, and psychologists. Especially when the patient is a child there is a complex interaction between health workers, children, and their family system. The psychological and emotional aspects can have an impact in terms of compliance with the therapeutic plan, relationships, and quality of life.

Keywords

Hand congenital malformation · Hand disfigurement · Multiprofessional approach · Decision making · Parenting stress

The functionality and visibility of the hand make this body part full of emotional meaning. The team that deals with conditions and pathological conditions involving the hand needs to face the psychological aspects raised by such an important part of the body.

The hand is fundamental in human psychosensorial development and becomes a means and a symbol of autonomy as it can reach every part of the body. When people lose the possibility of carrying out these actions on their own, they markedly lose independence. Furthermore, it is important to remember that hands play a central role in social and emotional relationships because they express emotionality: we caress with the hand. The hand is the protagonist in nonverbal communication, but is also constantly visible to others as well as to its owner.

When a person is faced with traumatic or malformity problems, this latter aspect is important from a motivational point of view: the subject cannot avoid confronting his/her own difficulties and reactions raised in the social context. Therefore, visibility is an element that sustains and pushes toward the need to elaborate and accept one's own condition or the condition of

D. Pajardi
Department of Humanities, University of Urbino, Urbino, Italy
e-mail: daniela.pajardi@uniurb.it

A. Viano (✉)
Department of Hand Surgery and Rehabilitation, San Giuseppe Hospital IRCCS MultiMedica, Milan University, Milan, Italy

G. Pajardi (ed.), *Pediatric Hand Surgery*, https://doi.org/10.1007/978-3-031-30984-7_1

their child for the parents of a child with congenital pathological hand conditions.

Whether originating from malformation or traumatic injury, pathological conditions of the upper limb affect and modify many areas of individual life and requires significant psychological effort to accept and adapt.

The relationship between patient and health specialists grows and is shaped in this difficult context. Especially when the patient is a child there is a complex interaction among health workers, children, and their family system.

1.1 Psychological Aspects

Compared with other congenital problems with greater resonance and in-depth knowledge, the congenital hand anomaly is less well known. In those pathological conditions such as labio-palatoschisis or Down's syndrome congenital upper limb anomalies can easily be seen.

Considering that this topic is rarely exposed by the media and there is a lack of information and knowledge about it, it could be suspected that hand pathological conditions have less of a psychological impact than other congenital malformations or traumatic impairments. However, such a conclusion would underestimate the psychological and social problems raised by a disability involving a part of our body that is indispensable owing to the functional and relational roles it plays in everyone's life.

The psychological aspects related to the congenital upper limb or hand anomaly have long been considered secondary and undervalued compared with other malformations such as those affecting the face.

The peculiarity of the hand, however, was underlined not only by the health specialists directly involved in this field, but also by the importance attributed to the hand by those parents and by those children who face particularly serious and complex syndromic patterns [1]. Therefore, parents who face the congenital pathology of their child, may experience more difficulties in receiving information from the neonatology clinic where the child is born than if they consult specialized centers.

This difficulty, although bypassed by the possibility of checking the internet, highlights the low mediatic resonance that involves ordinary people as well as health professionals.

On the other hand, usually because of the presence of many different problems affecting the newborn, which can sometimes even affect body parts that are essential for survival, clinicians have great expectation for a solution to congenital problems.

Health personnel face a problem that requires a joint and coordinated intervention by various professionals: surgeons, physiotherapists, and psychologists.

The parent notes that there are different critical issues that will involve their child. Hypotheses and expectations are formulated considering the current problem, the future, and possible solutions at the same time.

It becomes important that parents understand aspects concerning any functional limitation, aesthetic dimension, as well as numerous personal and relational factors related to the characteristics and meanings that the hand assumes within the life of the individual and their family system.

Several observations proposed by psychologists, surgeons, and physiotherapists working on this topic highlight the need for a synergistic approach involving various professionals [2].

Parents will more easily accept and complete a therapeutic plan if they emotionally process and accept their child's hand.

If a parent is not even beginning to emotionally confront his/her child's hand, the therapeutic option will always be unacceptable and a source of frustration, although improving the quality of life and functionality. The proposal would be refused because it would be considered inadequate with respect to expectations, especially if the only acceptable proposal for the parent is an impossible "restitutio ad integrum."

Detecting parents' expectations, particularly unrealistic and impossible ones, represents a useful tool to identify early on the difficulties that could alter parents' ability to guide their child into the different phases of the therapeutic plan.

This first approach to parents' expectations and desires is very important as clinicians have the awareness that for young patients it is important to follow a therapeutic plan until the end. If the parents cannot complete the required steps, the child loses the possibility of improving his/her situation. Moreover, starting the therapy would mean more visits, surgeries, and physiotherapy sessions for the child without improving his/her functional and physical condition. Furthermore, patients' quality of life is equally important: if an appropriate re-elaboration of the hand is not achieved and the hand is not emotionally accepted by the owner and their family, it is likely that it will not be used because it is experienced as a source of psychological problems.

The interventional role of the psychologist within the team is therefore to support the patient and their relatives, as early as possible, in a re-elaboration process leading to the acceptance of re-elaboration and acceptance of the congenital hand.

In practical terms, it is essential that the psychologist attends the first visits and then, subsequently, is available to the family throughout the therapeutic protocol.

1.2 Patients, Hand, and Emotions

Parents attending the Hand Surgery department to find a solution for their child's hands experience intense emotions of anxiety, depression, fear, frustration, shame, anger, sadness, and for some children even total acceptance or a sense of pride [3].

Even when they are of high intensity, such emotional manifestations are common reactions to stressful events, and in most situations, the participants can find support and reach acceptance within the proposed therapeutic protocol.

However, if such emotions became stable and do not spontaneously evolve and resolve, it is essential to evaluate the duration and, intensity of these emotions and their impact on quality of life.

In the event of psychological problems that cannot be solved by counseling, patients should be switched to a psychotherapeutic approach.

The interview with the psychologist allows the patient to face emotional aspects, helping the parents to expose and understand his/her doubts and perplexities. Usually, parents' uncertainties concern aspects strictly related to the therapeutic options and protocol, but usually they are worried also about life situations involving social skills, general child development, and educational aspects.

Sometimes parents find it difficult to tell the difference between their child with a congenital hand malformation and somebody who has had an injury of a traumatic nature.

In the case of a child with a congenital hand there is no interruption of a psychological and neuropsychological continnum.

In terms of self-perception, the subject who is born with a congenital anomaly of the hand is, in fact, "perfect to himself."

Even if completely understandable, the fact that the child is experienced by parents as a "damaged child", because it is morphologically different, requires a prompt response. In fact, this parents' perception will inevitably affect the parent/child relationship and it will bias the development of the child's own self-image. It should not be forgotten that personal identity arises from the interaction of the individual with other significant individuals and with the social systems to which he/she belongs.

It goes without saying that we can affirm that the development and evolution of the self-identity is in all respects a development, because it is a making of meanings that develops during social interaction. For children, especially younger ones, parents represent "the other" by antonomasia. It is very important to start the early and timely processing of acceptance and management of emotions linked to hand malformation: it is a way of consolidating the construction of self and social identity and preventing psychological and psychopathological risks in adolescence [4].

If the parent accepts the hand anomaly of the child, then the child will be able to accept their hand, with a positive impact in terms of compliance with the therapeutic plan and in terms of quality of life.

The birth of a child with a congenital disease is often a situation for which the parents are not prepared, especially because it is usually an unexpected event.

The discovery that their baby has a congenital hand anomaly obscures a happy moment of parents' life, whether the parents learn of the child's congenital hand anomaly at birth or during prenatal diagnostics.

Most parents discover the congenital hand condition at childbirth because prenatal screening revealed that the child was healthy, and the anomaly had not been discovered earlier.

The parents must face a highly stressful situation, which can also be more distressing because the malformation is unexpected and sometimes totally ruled out by the prenatal screening. Prenatal screening is, in fact, commonly considered to be able to rule out any anomaly at all. This fallacy originates because parents do not consider that screening results have a statistical value, but they attribute to them fantastic and unrealistic powers. Prenatal screening is very important to allow parents to develop their acceptance of the malformation and to avoid trauma at the birth of their child [4].

When parents realize that their child has a hand anomaly, the request to clinicians is to fix the problem as soon as possible to reach a situation of normality: the parent would like to count a five-fingered hand. The intensity of the parents' emotional reaction to the child's congenital hand anomaly is independent of the gravity and vastness of the condition, but it is related to the visibility of the hand by others' eyes [5].

Parental emotional experiences need to be accepted in an appropriate professional context able to recognize the difficulty parents are facing and to support them. In this way, parents' emotions can become proactive and motivate them to improve their child's condition instead of remaining on an emotionally static level.

Initially, the feelings of guilt and the psychological experience of having generated an "incomplete" child experienced by parents can in fact in some cases freeze all possible parental ability to act, making it almost impossible for them to choose whether or not to follow the proposed plan. On the contrary, some parents are moved by the urgency to fix the problem as soon as possible without stopping to think about what they are willing to do. Both reactions highlight the difficulty in accepting the child's congenital hand condition and the perception of medicine as an omnipotent science. This belief, which is sometimes fed by the media, sustains parents' often unrealistic expectation of solutions.

When the real potential of surgery is explained, the parent with unrealistic expectations will inevitably be disappointed. This feeling usually interferes in the surgeon/parent relationship in the form of mistrust, distrust, or even rejection, because it disregards what parents expected and hoped for.

In these situations, even the best possible solution and the most successful intervention will easily disappoint and there will be less motivation to follow the therapeutic plan, consequently leading to a higher risk of drop-out.

The relationship between parents and the care team is a crucial element of medical care and the psychologist can have a "joint" function.

To fulfill this function, in our team the psychologists attend and observe the visit with the surgeon, perform interviews with parents after the visits, offer the possibility of the family meeting the psychologists and to be supported through the entire treatment phase. On the operational level, the possibility for the different professionals to compare their impressions becomes crucial to reciprocally activating interventions based on the patient's detected needs.

The probability of treatment drop-out is lower when parents accept the congenital hand condition and when the unrealistic expectations of the possible solution of the child's problem are detected and modified. This approach allows major compliance with the proposed plan, avoiding that child skipping scheduled surgical interventions or neglecting the physiotherapeutic protocol, which, for the patient, would mean losing a chance to improve their condition [1, 5]. The therapeutic protocol can have parts that can be unexpected, both in terms of surgical proposal and in terms of activities that the parent did not expect to continue.

As a matter of fact, some surgical suggestions are more difficult than others to accept for parents. Indeed, sometimes they fear the proposed surgery because they perceive the intervention as possible further damage to their child's body.

Proposals such as toe transfer and the removal of finger nubs increase fears and enhance the psychological perception of damage. In the case of the toe transfer, the parents report the fear that the foot, from which the toe is removed can be functionally and aesthetically damaged.

In the case of the removal of the finger nubs, parents may be doubtful about the nubs because the fact they can count five fingers can be more important than functional improvement. In the case of finger nubs, the segments are not fingers, neither in anatomical nor in functional terms.

Parents must face a difficult decision-making process to decide whether to proceed with an unexpected surgery. In this process, timing is also fundamental as, from a surgical point of view, it is essential to intervene when the child is about 1 year old to allow the child to develop the functionality of the hand. However, parents perceive the baby as fragile and delicate, too young and small to tolerate surgery and anesthesia.

In this view, parents' request to wait a few years before performing surgery is completely understandable. However, the idea that the surgical treatment can be postponed until school age is still too common and it is also an indications that is not very respectful of psychological, neuropsychological, functional, and rehabilitative findings. Actually the hand is important because not only it is involved at the beginning of child development, it also supports their adequate cognitive and emotional evolution.

The earlier the surgery is performed, the easier it will be for the child to accept their post-surgical hand. Parents must also face the difficulty of taking responsibility and deciding for another individual: their child. Parents often report doubts about how their child will evaluate their decision about surgery, once grown up. Kim et al. [6] pointed out that mothers of infants with hand and foot malformations have a similarly high level of stress to mothers with infants with other malformations. Stress must be analyzed by clinicians because it can influence the decision-making strategies of parents in adhering to or rejecting a certain surgical path.

These considerations should have highlighted the psychological issues involved in the congenital hand condition and in the relationship with the clinicians and staff, participating in improving the condition of the child.

To summarize, the decision-making process regarding the surgery and the subsequent treatment is particularly long and painful: parents face a problem that they had not ever considered possible and furthermore, for which they must make a choice on behalf of their child, basing their decision on unfamiliar and unknown medical notions.

The contact with the health care setting represents a moment that is particularly full of anxiety: the parents bring their own expectations, and they must face them to the limits of medical/surgical knowledge. On the one hand, the possibility of facing a diagnosis and the consequent proposal of a therapeutic plan uplift and reassure the parent. On the other hand, however, comparing their unrealistic expectations with the available possibilities is a difficult and emotional moment for parents who have to face a truth for which they are not ready and that is difficult to accept. Parents may be so involved in their feelings and expectations. Therefore, it is essential that the surgeon communicates using comprehensible language, avoiding at best the use of technical terms, to prevent increasing anxiety levels in the parents and overcoming their distress [7].

The gap between the professional assessment of the surgeon and the evaluation of the parents is sometimes intense and relevant. The surgeon values functionality the most, whereas the parents also value the aesthetic dimension, which also has high expectations invested in it. It is important that the surgeon is aware of the link between functional and aesthetic elements: a hand with unnatural movements, although morphologically normal, catches the eyes more than a hand that can be moved naturally, even if morphologically different from what is expected.

Hoping for success in giving their child a "five-fingered hand", the parents keep repeating the same question and asking for the same explanations, requesting unrealistic solutions: it is not due to a cognitive problem but to the emotional difficulty in complying on a psychological level.

Understanding means that they must leave behind their illusions and hopes of giving their child a "normal" hand. Parents' pain can be so intense that they try to propose unlikely solutions that do not have any scientific basis such as using stem cells or replacing their child's hand with their own. In the latter case it can be classified as "acting out" from a psychological point of view.

This attention to aesthetic aspects and the desire to remove the psychological distress caused by the hand of their child lead some parents to request the use of aesthetic prostheses, even for very small children. The request for the use of these safeguards must be carefully assessed and evaluated in relation to the specific case to avoid the prosthesis becoming a hiding place for the malformation and a way of not accepting the condition [8].

From a psychological point of view, the request for prosthetics should come directly from the person concerned. In order to allow the development of the sensitivity and functionality of the limb, the guidelines suggest not introducing aesthetic prostheses before adolescence. This would allow complete and optimal development of the limb. However, when talking of a request for early prosthesis, we refer to those that are asked for in children who are only a few months old: in these cases, the request expresses a parents' need.

The specialist can accept the prosthesis request when there is no risk of mystification of the parent's difficulties in accepting the child's congenital hand anomaly and the related difficulty in accepting the child entirely with his hand.

The prosthesis, in fact, does not replace a hand and does not eliminate the malformation, but it simply hides it. Furthermore, from a pragmatic point of view, the child grows quickly, and the prostheses must be replaced every 6 months which is unnecessary and harmful, as well as very onerous. The strong emotional involvement in every proposed treatment, especially surgery, aimed at improving a child's situation represent crucial moments for the parents.

For some parents, the possibility of identifying the optimal solution is closely related to the possibility of starting to accept the child and the malformation. It is not strange that each parent seeks a solution that can help to cope with the experiences raised by the hand anomaly of their child, depending on the emotional experiences and the extent of their acceptance of the situation.

The phase following surgery represents for some parents facing a situation that has been immediately experienced to be better than the starting one, whereas for others it is the clash with the limits of surgery and, therefore, the end of their unrealistic and miraculous expectations. After the surgery, the hand needs a new process of acceptance and re-elaboration of the situation of the child, which is sometimes as tiring and as intense at the emotional level as the time of the birth of the child.

Despite the difficulties during the decision-making process that lead to the decision to perform the surgery, it should be underlined that during follow-up parents confirm that they are satisfied with the results obtained, both from an aesthetical and from a functional point of view [9, 10]. Furthermore, it is easier to deal with surgery, even if experienced as aggressive and potentially damaging, rather than facing the impossibility of intervening in any way. Therefore, it is not correct to talk about a single event of re-elaboration and acceptance of the congenital hand anomaly, but it would be more appropriate to consider re-elaboration and acceptance as a process involving different moments of a family system's life related to the different steps of the clinical pathway.

1.3 Psychologist's Intervention: Timing Mode

The interview with the psychologist offers a space where the parent can reprocess the problem, gives the opportunity to express doubts and perplexities about the therapeutic pathway, supports parents in decision-making, highlighting realistic or even unrealistic expectations, and facilitates communication between the care team and the family. Sometimes in rare and specific situations the psychologist can veto, even if temporarily, the possibility of performing surgery.

It is important that the family that welcomes the newborn receives the psychological support as close as possible to the moment when the malformation is discovered.

The promptness of the psychological assistance has the aim of receiving the family's emotional experiences triggering the resources to support or activate the re-elaboration of the child's situation that are present within the family system. Franzblau et al. [11] underlined the risk that children live with stress that is unrecognized by parents and caregivers. Parents play a strategical role in promoting coping resources, self-esteem, social and emotional support: for this reason, it is very important that clinicians inform parents about potential stressors and help them to screen for signs of unmanaged emotional stress (e.g., anxiety, anger).

The presence of the psychologist during the first medical examination is useful to support the family because it allows us to observe relational aspects that are discussed and expanded in the interview following the meeting with the surgeon. It is advisable that this first medical examination takes place as soon as possible; it can even occur before the child's birth when a prenatal diagnosis is made.

In the presence of prenatal diagnosis, the parents can start the emotional process of accepting the child's condition before birth. On the contrary, parents who discover their child's problem at birth experience it as a particularly traumatic event especially because they have been reassured by prenatal screening. As mentioned above, prenatal screening is too often interpreted as absolute certainty regarding the health and integrity of the unborn child, instead of being considered a statistical probability, which it is.

From the viewpoint of offering support to the family system, it should not be surprising that the first medical examination is planned a long time before the surgical procedure: it is in fact crucial to allow the parents to have time and space to discuss the above-mentioned aspects. One of the advantages is the possibility of meeting the surgeon on many different occasions and at different stages of the re-elaboration process, which leads to the parents accepting the situation of the child. Sometimes the parent repeats the same question several times, not because they do not cognitively understand what has been explained to them, but because they must reprocess the difference between hopes and expectations and what can really be done by the surgeon.

The importance of parents' and children's emotional reactions requires all the clinicians involved to pay attention to the whole family, and, therefore, that the whole team are able to understand and give meaning to behaviors and attitudes of the family that are often incomprehensible to the health personnel: the role of the psychologist is also to help the whole team in this task by consulting together.

The presence of a psychologist as a stable figure in a surgical team is not yet common practice. The possibility of the patient being admitted for psychological consultation on the surgeon's indication as a common practice and as part of the standard protocol is essential; in fact, through this the family can be helped to accept the specialist and the team without feeling its emotions as pathological reactions.

Furthermore, the psychological consultation can help to better manage their child's condition, so that parents feel relieved and can shift their attention toward a process of elaboration and acceptance of the psychological support of the whole family system, thus considering not only the parents and the child but also any siblings. The latter are in fact involved in their sibling's problem as part of the family and it is important to understand how parents report to them about the condition because it is a meter indicating how parents are emotionally processing it. It is also important to notice if a sibling's role is correctly balanced or if they are excluded or hyper-responsible in their relative's condition.

The whole family is included in the therapeutic pathway starting from the psychological interview following the first medical examination with the surgeon and all the following access to medical care before and after surgery, and at follow-ups.

As expected, even the young patient must be involved, and it can be done in many different ways according to their age, because, based on it, the relevant main topics will be different. During the first years of the child's life, they do not compare themselves with the social environment nor are they aware of or emotionally challenged by their condition. Consequently, the interview will focus on parents' needs while taking care not to exclude the child from communication, to avoid feelings of exclusion and anxiety. In fact, even if very young, the baby pick up on the fact that much attention and focus are concentrated on excluding inadequate modality of processing experiences associated with their hand, and it can damage the relationship with the care team.

If at first all the members of the family are involved with respect to their cognitive and emotional resources, the child will have more opportunities to have an individual space to expose their own feelings and doubts in the future. In fact, at around 4/5 years of age the child is more competent and involved in the discussion both during the surgical visits and during the interviews. It is therefore essential that surgeon and clinicians explain their points using clear and concise language. They should also encourage parents to offer clarifications and information to their child in order to lead and reassure them during the steps of the therapeutic plan. As patients are followed up until complete physical development, the opportunity for individual interviews may also be evaluated. Some thematic nuclei are more typical of the first years, whereas others appear later, among them, it is important to underline the critical topic of the comparison with others and with the child's social environment.

Initially, parents report experiencing glances as intrusive, disturbing, and indelicate, capable of arousing feelings of shame and intense discomfort; they are afraid that the child might experience the same emotions. These fears become more intense and reappear at specific moments of the life cycle, and particularly when the child needs to be included in new social contexts such as school [3, 12].

The child perceives that they is different from others at about 2 years of age and sometimes people start asking them about it. Therefore, the child will start asking questions about what happened and the reasons for this difference.

During the interview between the psychologist and parents it is important to discuss this topic, in order to help parents to accept the child's questions and supporting him during the inclusion in new contexts, for example, by talking and explaining to teachers and educationalists.

It is also important to remember that even the surgery and its results need to be discussed, as after any surgery there is a change that requires parents and child to adapt to the new reality. Furthermore, after surgery it is always necessary to undergo physiotherapy treatment that is usually highly intense and challenging, even on the psychological side. Unlike the surgeon, who manages the surgical gesture inside the operating room, the physiotherapist involves the parents in a program that proceeds slowly and requires the direct involvement of the parent. The parent will be required to touch and manipulate the child's "hand" and therefore, to become aware of the results achieved, but also to confront the limits.

The attention of the psychologist must therefore always be directed to the whole family system and its subsystems: the individual, the couple, interpersonal, and the sibling systems.

Considering the complexity of the congenital hand condition, it is essentially a multidisciplinary approach that carefully and respectfully deals with the needs of the child and those of the family. This requires many professionals to integrate in order to provide a complete and adequate response to the child's problem and able to promote the harmonious development of the child and not only of their malformed hand.

Working in a multidisciplinary team, in a context in which the surgical gesture and the subsequent rehabilitation steps remain undoubtedly central, is fundamental when dealing with a traumatic event that has such a strong impact on daily living [2, 13].

References

1. Pajardi D, Martorana U, Pajardi G. Congenital malformations and compliance to the treatment: influence of parents' personal perception of the relationship with the medical team. Clin Exp Plast Surg. 2005;37(1):65–9.
2. Tedeschi M, Tondelli G. Problemi psicologici in chirurgia della mano. Psychological problem in hand surgery. Riv Chir Riab Mano Arto Sup. 1992;29(1, 2):205–11.
3. Carlsson IK, Dahlin LB, Rosberg H-E. Congenital thumb anomalies and the consequences for daily life: patients' long-term experience after corrective surgery. A qualitative study. Disabil Rehabil. 2018;40(1):69–75. https://doi.org/10.1080/09638288.2016.1243159.
4. Didierjean-Pillet A. The psychological approach of hand's congenital disparity [Approche psychologique de la malformation congénitale de la main. La malformation congénitale, le désir de savoir]. Ann Chir Plast Esthet. 2002;47(1):2–8. https://doi.org/10.1016/S0294-1260(01)00079-6.
5. Pajardi D, Viano A. Malformazioni congenite della mano: aspetti psicologici e supporto. In: Landi A, Catalano F, Luchetti R, editors. Trattato Italiano di Chirurgia della Mano. Roma: Verduci; 2007. p. 995–9.
6. Kim J, Gong HS, Kim HS, Seok HS, Oh S, Baek GH. Parenting stress in mothers of children with congenital hand or foot differences and its effect on the surgical decision-making for their children. J Orthopaed Surg. 2019;27(2):2309499019838900. https://doi.org/10.1177/2309499019838900.
7. Baek GH, Kim J. Improving understanding and outcomes in congenital hand differences. Plast Reconstruct Surg. 2021;148(5):769E–74E. https://doi.org/10.1097/PRS.0000000000008413.
8. Pilla G, Verni G. Protesi per amputazioni di arto superiore in età infantile. Artificial limbs for upper- extremity in children. Chirurgia della Mano. 1989;26(1):119–21.
9. Bellew M, Haworth J, Kay SP. Toe to hand transfer in children: ten year follow up of psychological aspects. J Plast Reconstr Aesthet Surg. 2011;64(6):766–75. https://doi.org/10.1016/j.bjps.2010.09.017.
10. Bradbury ET, Kay SPJ, Hewison J. The psychological impact of microvascular free toe transfer for children and their parents. J Hand Surg. 1994;19(6):689–95. https://doi.org/10.1016/0266-7681(94)90236-4.
11. Franzblau LE, Chung KC, Carlozzi N, Chin AYT, Nellans KW, Waljee JF. Coping with congenital hand differences. Plast Reconstr Surg. 2015;135(4):1067–75. https://doi.org/10.1097/PRS.0000000000001047.
12. Bradbury E. The psychological and social impact of disfigurement to the hand in children and adolescents. Dev Neurorehabil. 2007;10(2):143–8. https://doi.org/10.1080/17518420701281122.
13. Bradbury E. People with disfigurement. Leicester: BPS Books; 1996.

Babies Hand Imaging and X-ray

2

Gaetana A. Rispoli and Maurizio Zompatori

Abstract

Pediatric diagnostic imaging for hand pathology uses all the basic radiology exams such as X-ray, CT scan, MRI, ultrasound and colour Doppler US. The choice of the best diagnostic imaging technique depends on the specific disease and on the patient's collaboration.

Conventional X-ray is still today an invaluable diagnostic approach, notably for trauma and malformations. Radiography has many advantages in pediatric examinations: most importantly it does not need sedation and exposes the child to a very low radiation dose.

On the other hand, when required by the clinical assessment, the choice of a second-line investigation must be taken, considering the obstacle of a not-collaborating patient, in a long and static MRI examination, as well as the risk of a high dose radiation exposure, in CT-scan exams.

Ultrasound provides an excellent diagnostic potential in tendon, muscle and soft tissue injuries and diseases. Furthermore, US does not use radiations, and it is highly repeatable and undemanding. Therefore, when performed by experienced radiologists, US can provide complete clinical information.

Diagnostic imaging has a primary role in patient treatment and preoperative planning, and it can lead to significant changes in patient therapeutic pathways.

Keywords

Pediatric hand pathology · Diagnostic imaging approach · X-ray · Computed tomography · Ultrasound · Magnetic resonance

2.1 Traumatic Injuries

Hand traumatic injuries are extremely common in children. The growth and development of the skeletal system influence both the radiological aspect of a fracture and its remodelling characteristics during the healing process.

A child bone lesion may appear typical and thus easily detectable, yet it is often insidious; therefore, a correct interpretation of radiological imaging requires a thorough knowledge of the evolutionary anatomy of the skeleton.

Conventional radiography comprises two standard projections: antero-posterior (AP) and latero-lateral (LL), taken to investigate the fingers and the wrist; or AP and oblique, to investigate the hand. Additional oblique projections, such as the scaphoid projection, can complete the

G. A. Rispoli (✉) · M. Zompatori
Department of Radiology, San Giuseppe MultiMedica Hospital, IRCCS University of Milan, Milan, Italy
e-mail: gaetanaanna.rispoli@multimedica.it; maurizio.zompatori@unibo.it

G. Pajardi (ed.), *Pediatric Hand Surgery*, https://doi.org/10.1007/978-3-031-30984-7_2

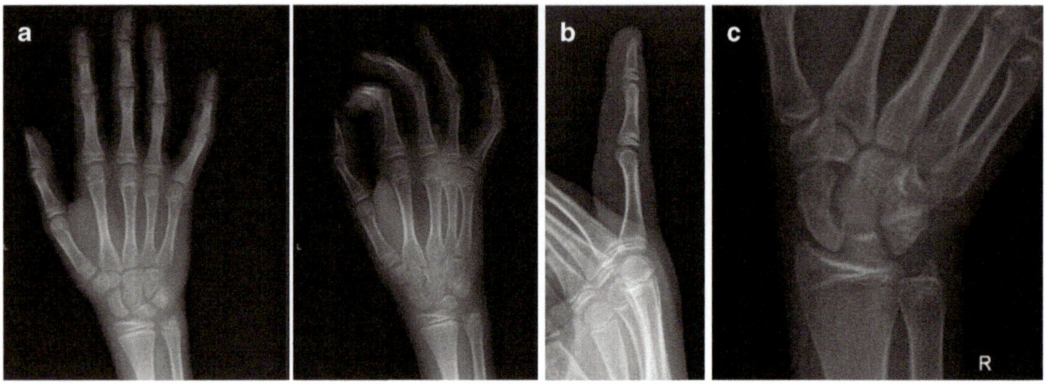

Fig. 2.1 Standard projections (**a**) AP e obl of the hand; (**b**) lateral projection for the fingers; (**c**) scaphoid projection

exam if indicated by the radiology specialist (Fig. 2.1).

In case of uncertain radiologic interpretation, notably in the physeal region traumas, a comparative radiograph of the contralateral limb may help resolve any doubts.

Pediatric diaphyseal finger fractures have aspects similar to the adult ones (simple or compound, displaced or undisplaced, transverse, oblique, spiral, etc.) (Fig. 2.2), but there is a peculiar diaphyseal injury, typical of the pediatric age: the *Greenstick fracture* (Fig. 2.3). In the upper limb, it usually concerns the forearm (radius and ulna): it is a transverse fracture of the cortex and the spongy bone, without disruption of the cortex and the periosteum on the opposite side, that appears simply bent.

Physeal fractures are very common in children, as the cartilage of the growth plate is fragile and porous, thus vulnerable in most traumas.

Physeal injuries are classified into five categories according to the Salter–Harris classification.

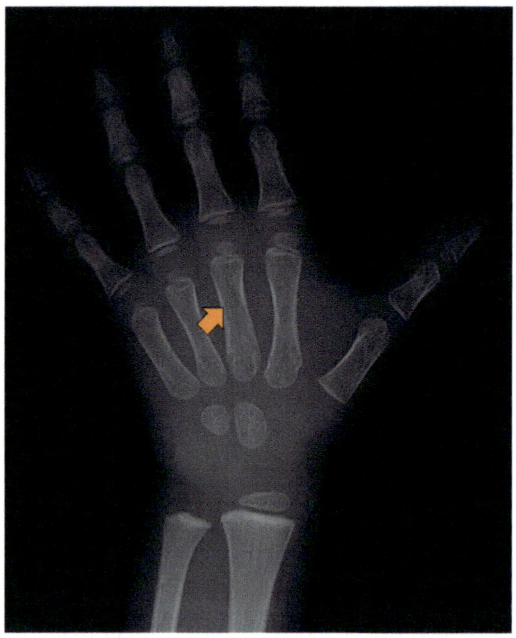

Fig. 2.2 Diaphyseal finger fractures (III metacarpal)

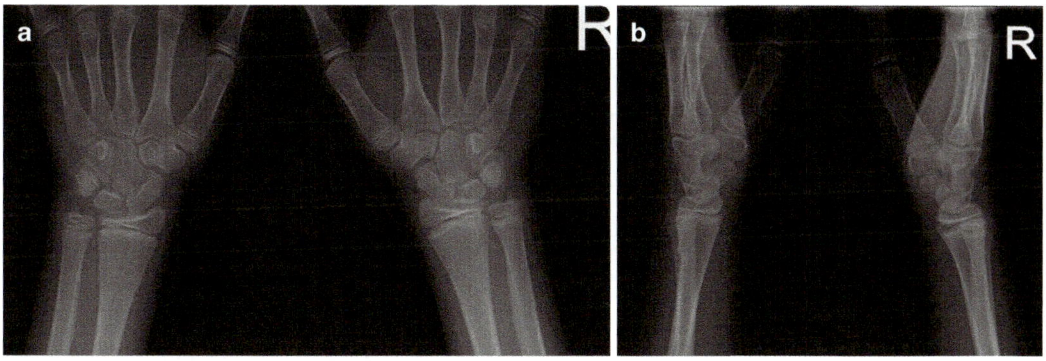

Fig. 2.3 (**a**, **b**) Greenstick fracture distal radius left, pr. Ap e lateral comparative

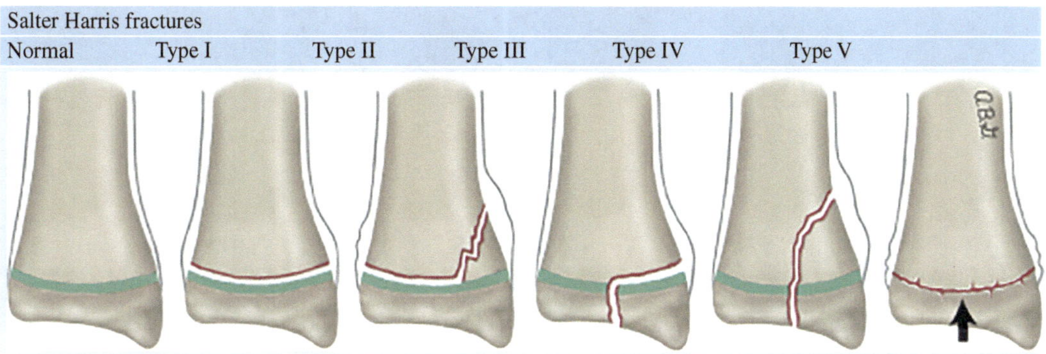

In Salter–Harris types I and II, a correct diagnosis can be obtained by using only the AP and lateral x-ray projections (Fig. 2.4).

In high-energy injuries (Salter–Harris types III and IV) that typically affect the articular profile, CT scan may be required to visualize in greater detail the comminuted fragments.

CT scans deliver a higher dose of radiation than standard X-rays, thus this method should be used according to clinical indication, respecting the ALARA principles (*as low as reasonably achievable*) (Fig. 2.5).

For its high resolution, CT scan remains an essential imaging technique for the settings of fractures where detection and treatment of subtle findings are vital to prevent subsequent complications, also thanks to modern multiplanar (MPR) and 3D volumetric reconstructions (Fig. 2.6a–c).

Finally, the Salter–Harris type V, which is hardly visualized on X-ray, is easily diagnosed with the help of MRI, as the bone injuries show high signal intensity on T2-weighted images. Besides, MRI does not deliver ionizing radiations (Fig. 2.7a, b).

Carpal bone injuries are rare in young children, where the ossification nuclei are still mainly cartilaginous, whereas they are quite common during adolescence. Carpal lesions are difficult to evaluate radiologically: both X-ray and CT scan often lead to misunderstanding, as cartilage is radiolucent.

When clinical assessment remains uncertain, in persistence of pain and in the absence of evident fracture, a bone bruise must be suspected and appropriately investigated using MRI. Bone bruises are not visible on conventional radiographs or CT scan images, whereas they can be well visualized with MRI on fluid-sensitive fat-suppressed sequences.

The bone contusion shows high T2 signal intensity, a finding that represents marrow oedema and haemorrhage. The distal radius and carpal bones are common locations for a bone contusion in the pediatric wrist (Fig. 2.8).

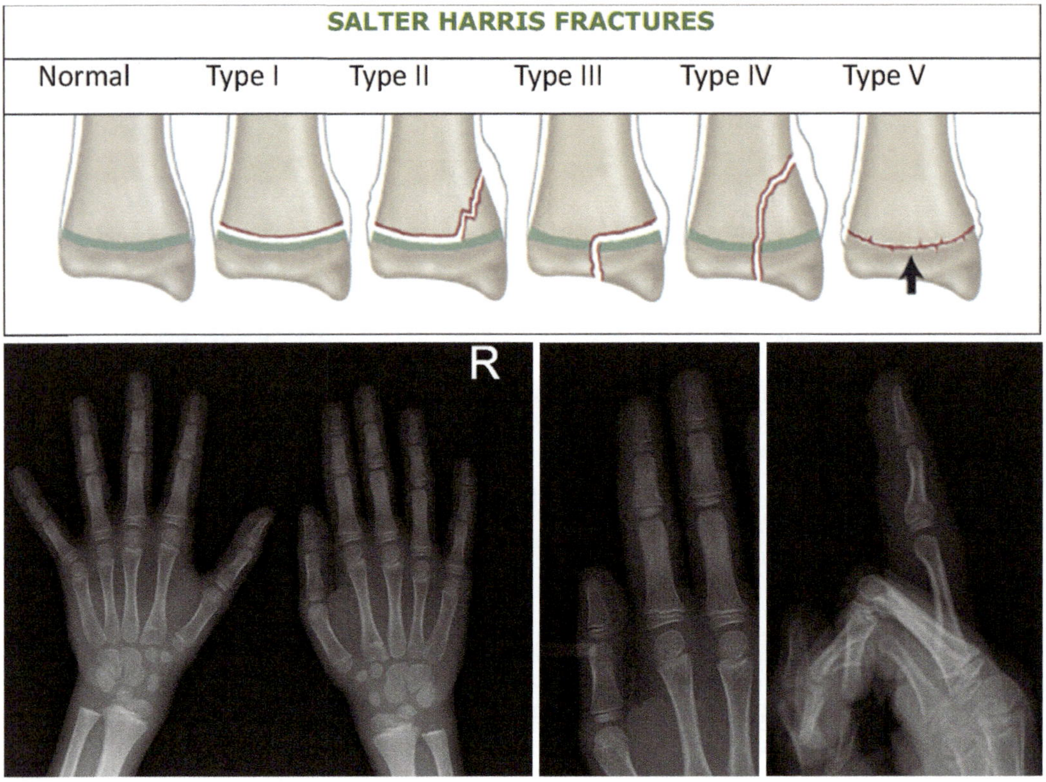

Fig. 2.4 Salter–Harris type II fracture (II finger right): comparative X-ray, particular AP e LL

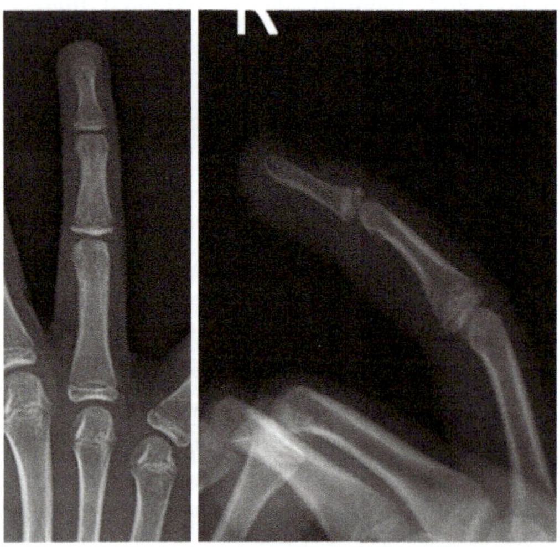

Fig. 2.5 Salter–Harris type III fracture (IV finger)

Among the carpal lesions, scaphoid fracture is the most frequent in children. Most pediatric scaphoid injuries result from falls onto an outstretched pronated hand, but any compressive force, such as a direct blow that causes a crush injury, can result in a scaphoid fracture.

Coexisting soft-tissue injuries are often occasional findings during MR imaging to evaluate suspected scaphoid fractures.

MR imaging is the best modality for diagnosis of radiographically occult scaphoid fractures in children. MR imaging has been shown to have an extremely high negative predictive value for scaphoid fracture when performed as early as 2 days after injury. Additionally, MR imaging can detect significant soft-tissue injuries, TFCC tear,

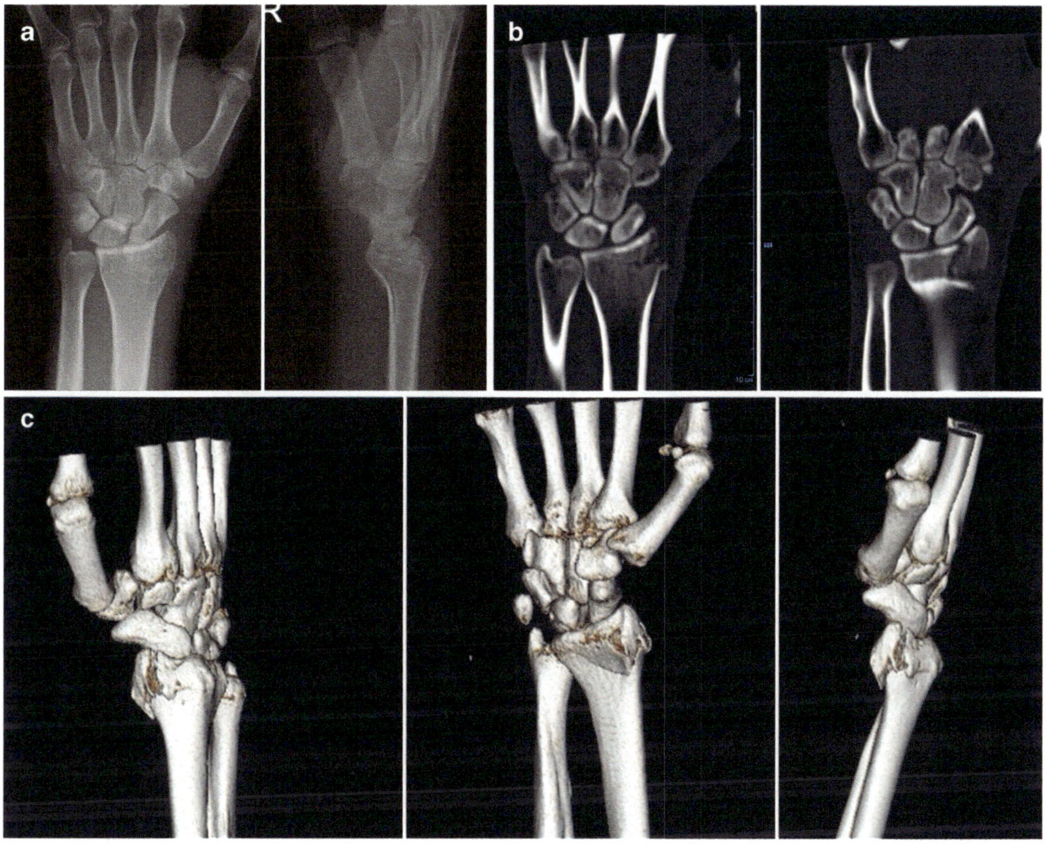

Fig. 2.6 Radial fracture: (**a**) ray; (**b**) Ct scan, MPR recontrusction; (**c**) 3d volumetric recostruction

intercarpal ligament injury and bone contusion with no distinct fracture (Fig. 2.9a–c).

Conventional X-ray has a primary role in post-traumatic follow-up, to evaluate fragments misalignments, bone healing and above all bone remodelling. Bone plasticity and great periosteal vascularization make these processes the faster, the younger the patient (Figs. 2.10, 2.11, and 2.12).

A careful radiological follow-up can quickly identify angular deformities of the fracture site, even before the clinical evidence, thus allowing a prompt surgical correction and a more favourable healing. Over a longer time, it is possible to assess if there are any vascular physeal damages that hesitated in longitudinal growth arrest, pseudarthrosis or residual joint stiffness.

Follow-up timing should thus depend on the type of trauma and, if necessary, it should be extended until the complete skeletal maturation.

Finally, US is the imaging technique of choice in pediatric patients: it doesn't use radiations, it is repeatable and it provides an excellent investigation of muscle and tendon injuries—which may be associated with fractures of the hand bones, especially in the physeal injuries (Fig. 2.11).

The high detail of US images—obtained at high-frequency probes (14–18 MHz), currently

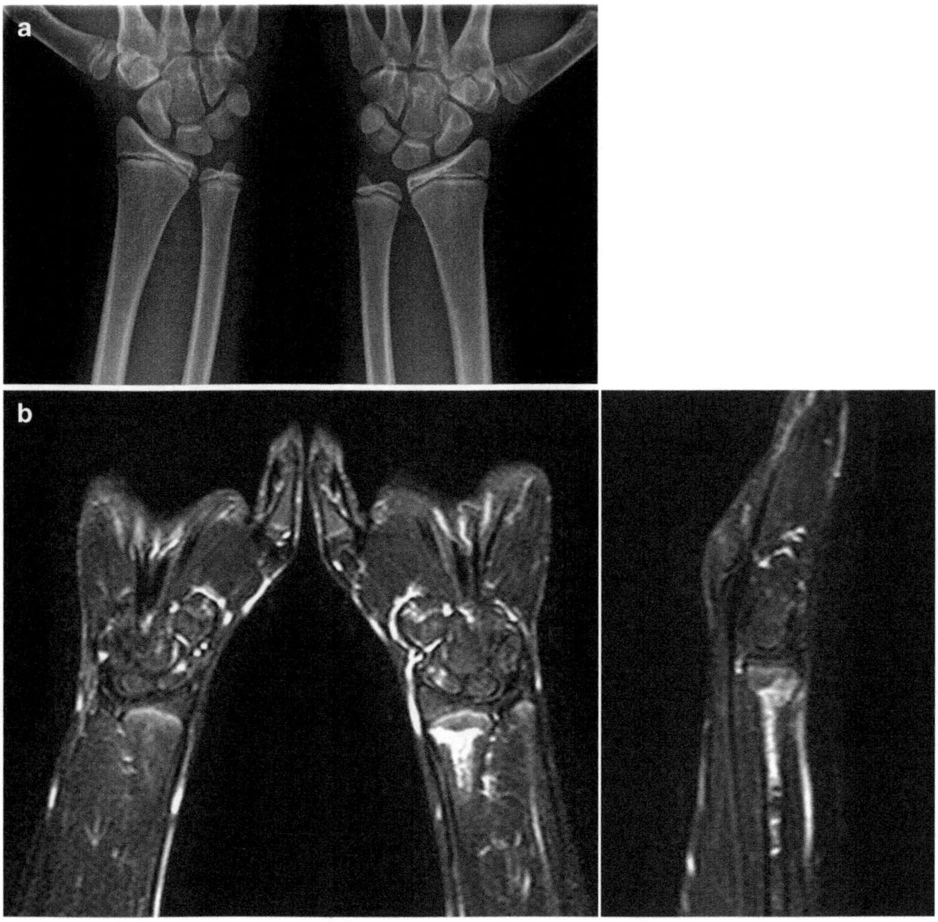

Fig. 2.7 (**a**) Frontal comparative X-ray in right wrist trauma shows normal findings. (**b**) Same day MRI: Coronal fluid-sensitive fat-suppressed MR image (STIR) of the distal forearm and wrist shows marrow oedema through the distal radius extending into both sides of the growth plate, a finding that is the imaging hallmark of unrecognised fracture

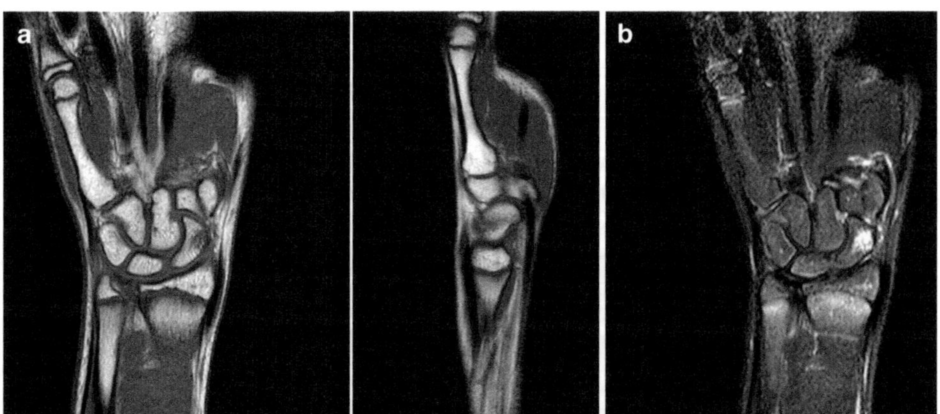

Fig. 2.8 Nine-year-old boy with bone scaphoid contusion—MR imaging 10 days after trauma in persistent pain wrist (normal findings X-ray): (**a**) MR image cor e sag T1 shows hypointensity in the scaphoid area; (**b**) Coronal fluid-sensitive fat-suppressed image (STIR) shows hyperintensity in the same scaphoid area, hallmark of marrow oedema due to bone contusion

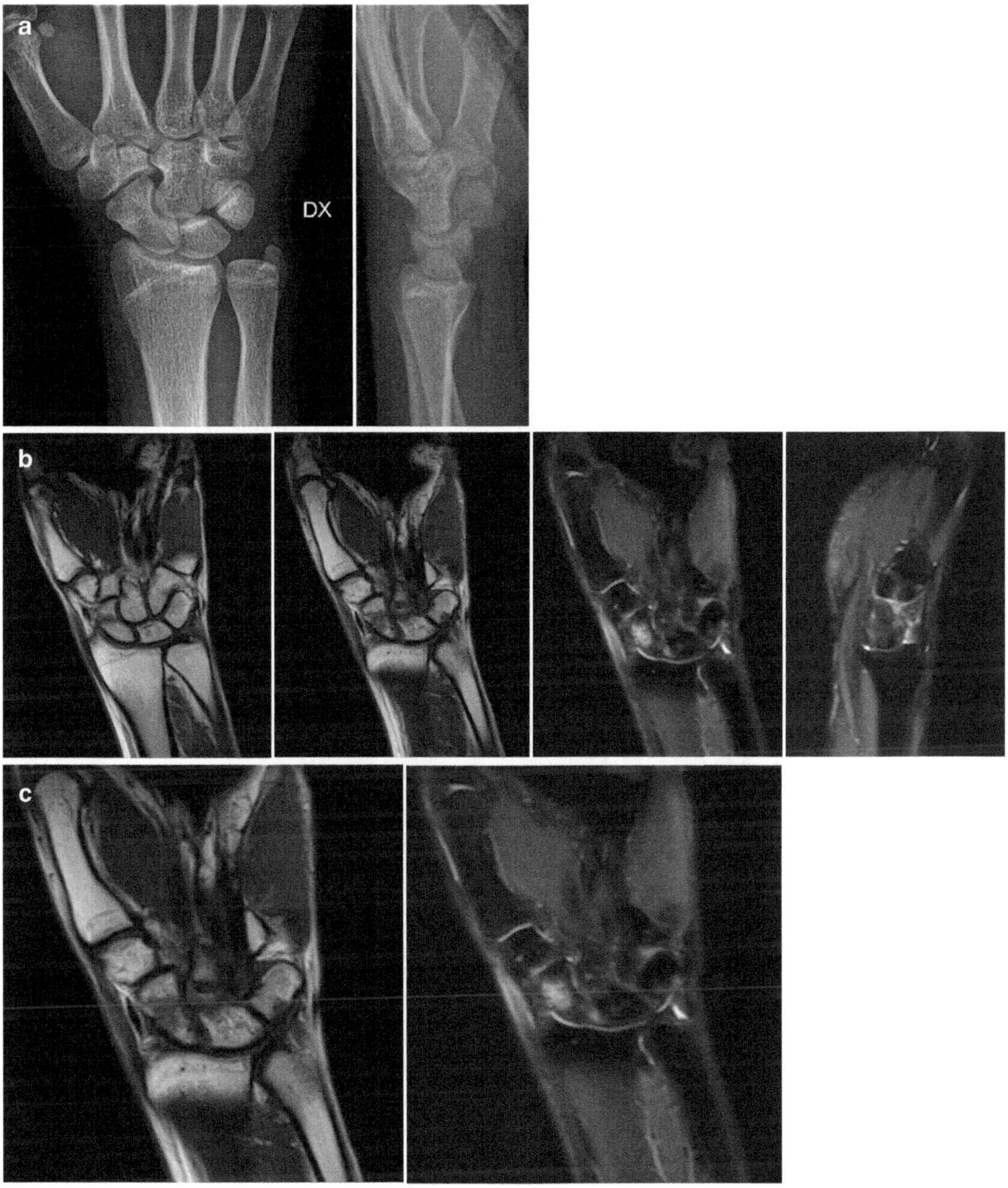

Fig. 2.9 (**a**) Suspected scaphoid fracture. (**b**) MRI-coronal T1 e T2-fluid-sensitive fat-suppressed image and fat-suppressed images show scaphoid fracture with articoular fluid effusion. (**c**) Coesisting TFCC tear

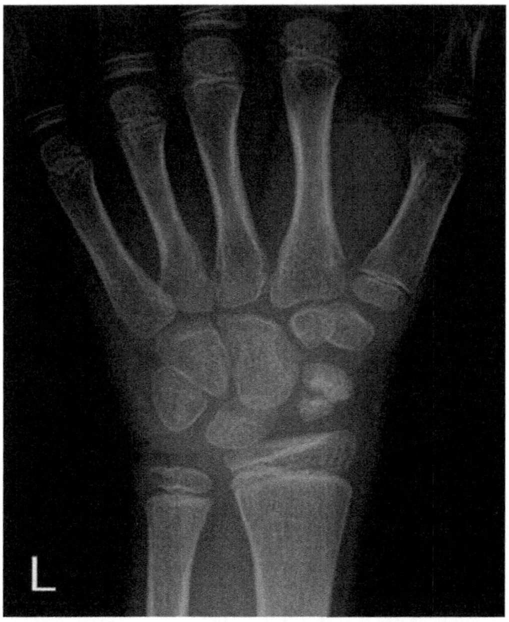

Fig. 2.10 X-ray scaphoid fracture (11 years old)

available—allows an expert operator to obtain excellent diagnostic results in the morphologic evaluation of muscle and tendon injuries. Radiography, CT scan and MRI are static, US has the advantage of dynamic image acquisitions (through both active and passive mobilization), thus providing more functional information.

In the very young child, whose tendon structures are so small that they are below the resolution power of the MRI (minimum layer of 3 mm), the US is the only exam that can provide useful information. It can show the presence of traumatic injuries of tendons, retinacula, ligaments, vessels, nerves and soft tissues—both in acute and old traumas. This applies to both micro-trauma (lesions of pulleys and tendons of the fingers) and macro-trauma (complex fractures involving large joints, such as the wrist).

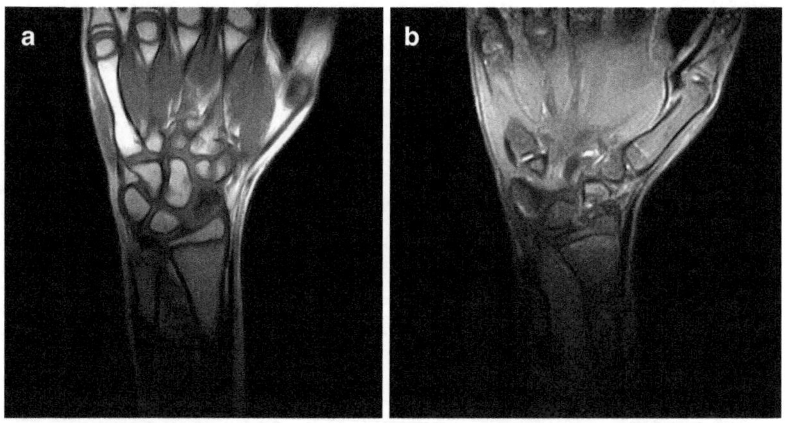

Fig. 2.11 Two months later—MRI T1-weight (**a**) and T2 weight (**b**): suspected evolution in osteonecrosis of the scaphoid

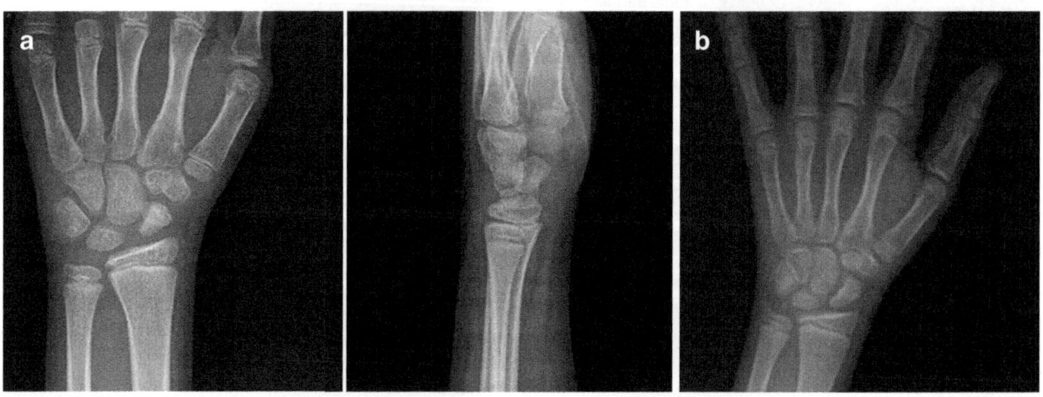

Fig. 2.12 X-ray scaphoid fracture: (**a**) 6 months later; (**b**) 30 months later

2.2 Congenital Hand Deformities and Syndromic Malformations with Prevalent Bone Involvement

Congenital hand malformations comprise a wide spectrum of congenital anomalies, which occur between the fourth and the eighth week of pregnancy. They are often associated with a congenital syndrome or they are a part of it.

Once again conventional X-ray is essential for an initial diagnosis, for its simplicity, low cost, high tolerability and low dose of radiation (Fig. 2.13).

X-ray investigation is indicated in all congenital malformation, differentiation defects (synostosis, symphalangism, syndactyly, arthrogryposis, camptodactyly and clinodactily), agenesis, duplications (polydactyly, triphalangism, and mirror hand syndrome), hyperplasia and hypoplasia, and finally in all dysplastic and dystrophic form, both if isolated or part of a more complex syndrome (Figs. 2.14a, b and 2.15).

The radiological indication includes a single AP radiograph, but a controlateral limb image may be useful, and it is thus suggested, to verify whether the malformation is present on both sides, and otherwise to compare the alteration to the normal anatomy (Fig. 2.16).

As the current therapeutic approach is aimed at timely surgical treatment, radiologic investigations are often repeated over time to evaluate the possible appearance of the ossification nuclei that are physiologically absent at birth. Thereby serial X-ray exams show the appearance of supernumerary bones as well as bone agenesis, thus providing to the surgeon critical information to plan

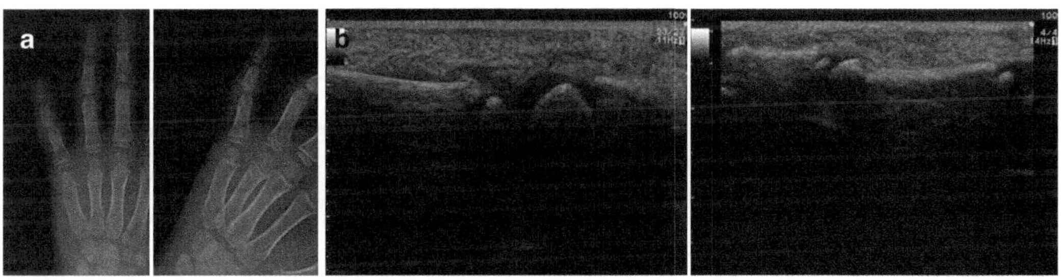

Fig. 2.13 Pacellar fracture proximal phalanx V finger: (**a**) X-ray; (**b**) US visualize the fragment of fracture and no tendon tears

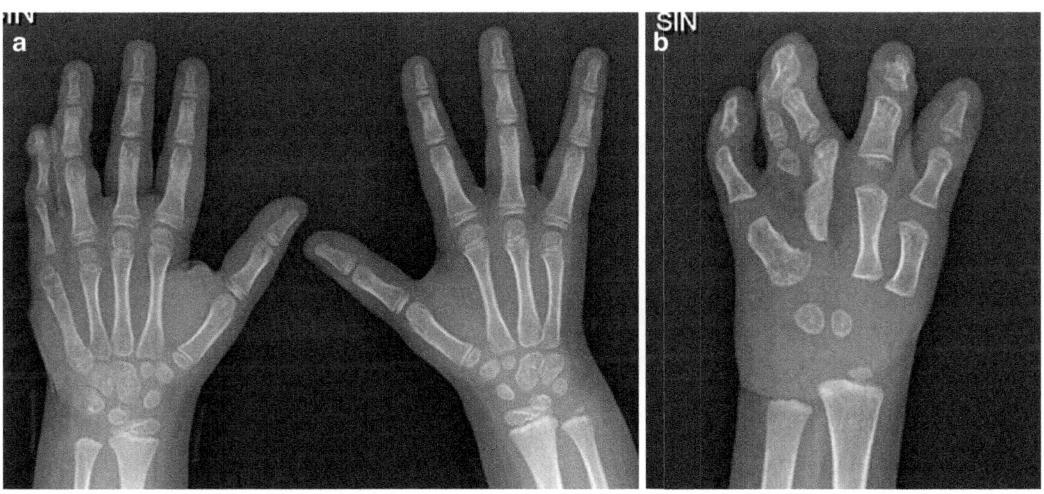

Fig. 2.14 (**a**) Hypodisplasia and agenesia; (**b**) duplication phalanx and agenesis

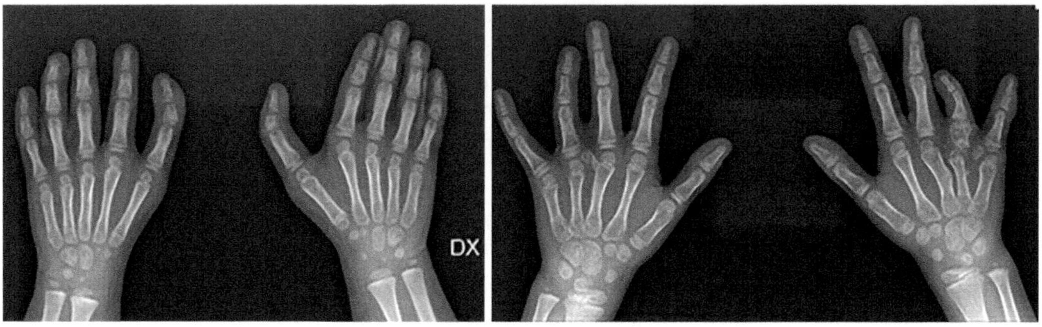

Fig. 2.15 Mirror hand syndrome and soprannuneraries bone sketch

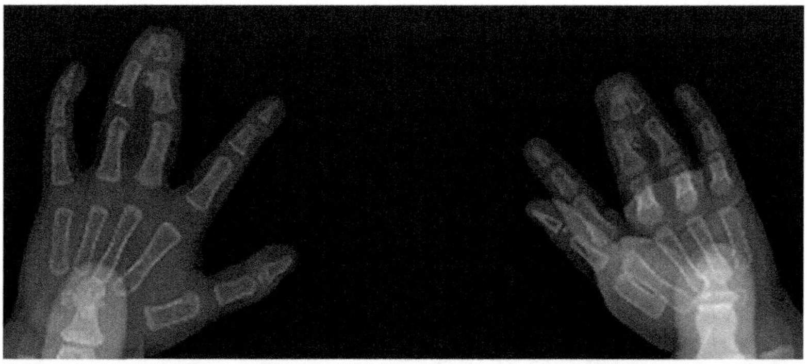

Fig. 2.16 Bilateral symmetric syndactyly bone

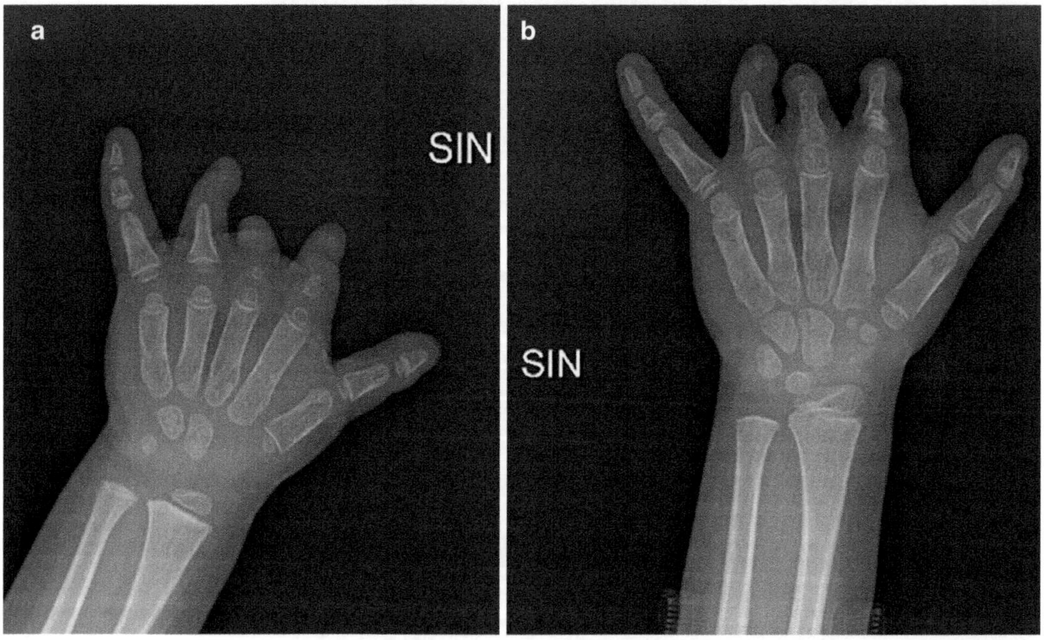

Fig. 2.17 (**a**) Agenesis fingers in 5 year old girl; (**b**) 5 years later phalanx ossification nuclei appear

and predefine the surgical intervention. Similarly, in complex syndromes, they are used in post-operative follow-up, to schedule further re-intervention (Fig. 2.17a, b).

In planning a therapeutic/surgical approach, conventional X-ray are supported by other techniques, such as US and MRI. US investigation, in addition to being cost-effective and well tolerated by children, is highly repeatable and provides dynamic images, which are optimal for the investigation of muscle and tendon alterations associated with hand malformations.

For example, in the pre-operative evaluation, US is used to assess whether the supernumerary bones are supported by a muscular-tendon structure or not. Or in the opposite case, to research muscles before the surgical correction of a major malformation with partial bone agenesis.

Moreover, US exams provide a dynamic study of joints, with particular attention to anatomical alterations of synovial structures and tendons; this permits to identify the congenital trigger thumb, with or without the characteristic Notta nodules (commonly found on the palmar side at the metacarpophalangeal joint).

MRI, despite showing both bone and muscle in greater anatomical detail, cannot be indicated in initial diagnostic preoperative approach because of the elevated cost and the need of sedation of children. For this reason, MRI is used for vascular and lymphatic malformations.

2.3 Congenital Vascular Malformations and Vascular Tumours

Diagnostic approach to vascular anomalies must provide a distinction between vascular tumours (haemangioma, haemangiopericytoma) and congenital vascular malformations (CVM).

Appropriate anamnesis and careful clinical examination are essential in the initial clinical approach, but, primarily in complex cases and preoperative evaluations, need to be supported by diagnostic imaging techniques.

The diagnostic imaging exams aim to identify and describe anatomical, pathological and haemodynamic characteristics of each lesion, as well as the secondary effects on surrounding tissues and the associated systemic manifestations.

The Doppler US is the first-line and essential diagnostic technique, which can be followed by further investigations with CT scan and MRI.

In CVM and vascular tumours, conventional X-ray has marginal usefulness, whereas it is often erroneously requested, as the first-line investigation, for focal pain or swelling. In such cases, the presence of calcified phleboliths could lead up to the discovery of unknown CVM. Sometimes X-ray is indicated in complex CVM, which is associated with bone-developing anomalies for excessive or poor blood supply to epiphyseal, metaphyseal or diaphyseal region (secondary bone hypertrophy and hypotrophy).

Colour Doppler US is the first-line investigation for CVM and vascular tumour: it allows to locate the lesion and define its haemodynamic characteristics: low flow in benign lesions, such as haemangioma; high flow in arteriovenous malformations (AVM); and extremely low flow in venous malformations (VM) and absence of flow in lymphatic malformations (lymphangioma—LM) (Fig. 2.18).

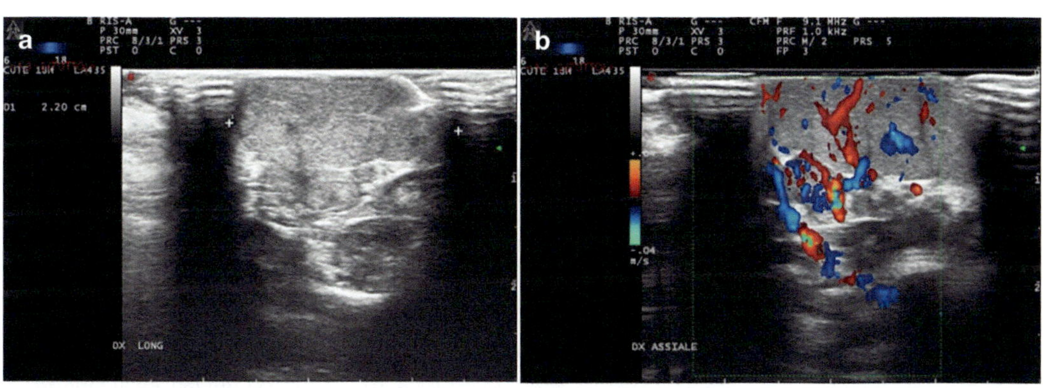

Fig. 2.18 US haemangioma hand: (**a**) B mode show soft echogenic mass; (**b**) colour Doppler image reveals a highly vascular mass consistent with capillary hemangioma

A possible diagnostic limitation of Doppler US exams may be encountered for lack of patient collaboration, which can result in different alterations, such as flow abnormalities induced by the Valsalva manoeuvre consequent to the baby's crying; or in movement artefacts. In the event of bulky or deep-located lesions, the exact definition of the lesion extension can be difficult. In such cases, the US exam has to be compared to a second-line investigation, such as MRI.

After the initial US investigation, MRI (with or without contrast medium) is the imaging technique of choice for all CMV. The great advantages of this method, in addition to the absence of radiation, are the high spatial resolution, the wide visual field (that is far larger than the US one) and the possibility of displaying simultaneously the blood flow distribution of the lesion and the surrounding soft and bone tissues.

Unfortunately, the long duration of the exam and the disturbing noise of the machine may frighten and irritate the babies, thus requiring the patient sedation.

The best study for vascular malformations needs a high-field MRI machine (at least 1.5 Tesla), so as to obtain the best contrast and spatial resolution for small lesions. By using different tissue "weighting" (T1, T2, STIR, generally with fat-suppression), CVM may be easily characterized in morphological and spatial terms (size, location and compartmentalization—limited to subcutaneous tissue or extended to sub-fascial, muscular or bone structures) (Figs. 2.19, 2.20, 2.21, and 2.22).

Finally, the MR angiography (MRA)—with contrast medium—allows to differentiate the CVM according to the type of blood flow (arterial, venous and absence of flow); and the post-processing reconstruction (MIP and 3D) provides the surgeon an optimal spatial representation.

In a few selected cases, despite the high dose of radiation, CT scan is indicated as an alterna-

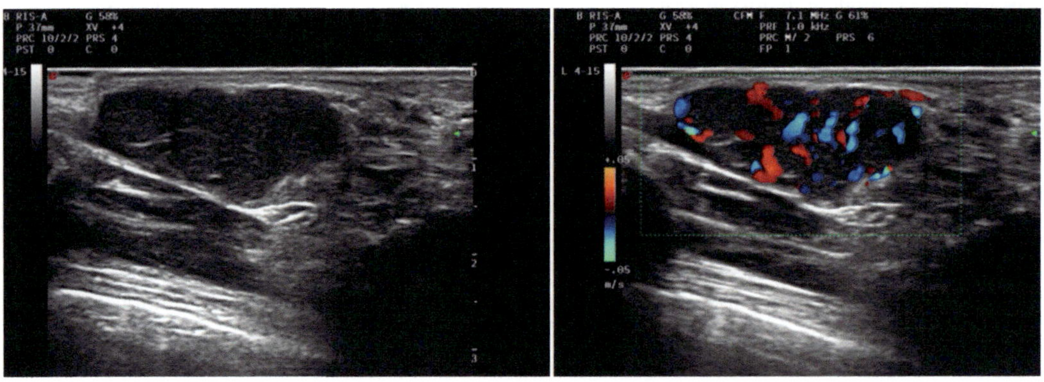

Fig. 2.19 B mode and colour Doppler US show soft echogenic mass highly vascular in intercarpal space like haemangioma

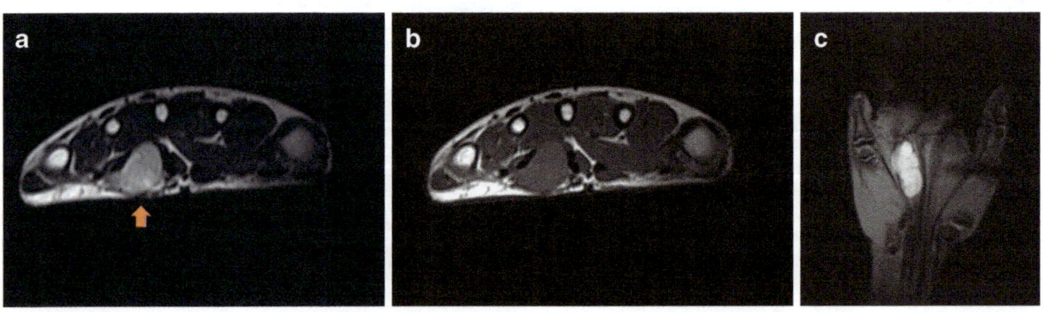

Fig. 2.20 Hand haemangioma MRI: sequence axial T2GE (**a**), T1 (**b**) and coronal T2-fat sat (**c**)

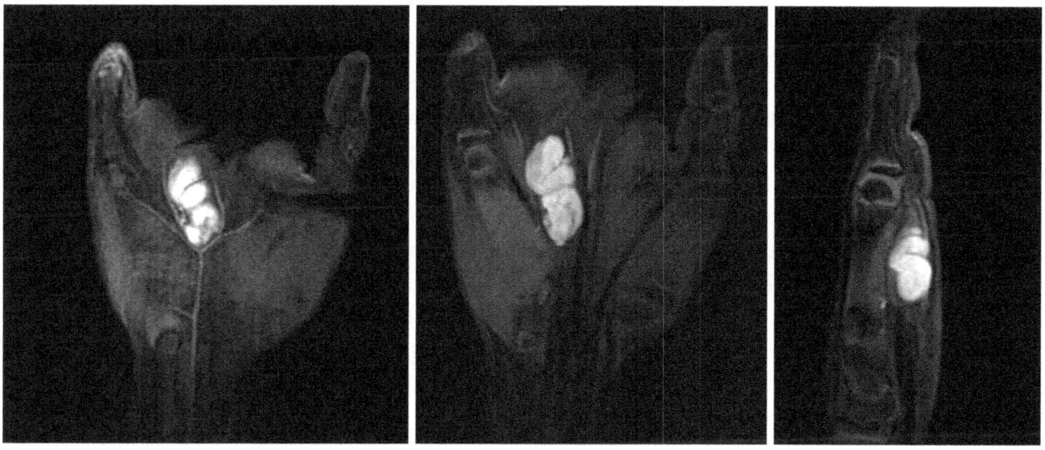

Fig. 2.21 Post contrast gadolinium T1 sequence coronal and sagittal: rapid omogenous capillar enhancement of the lesion

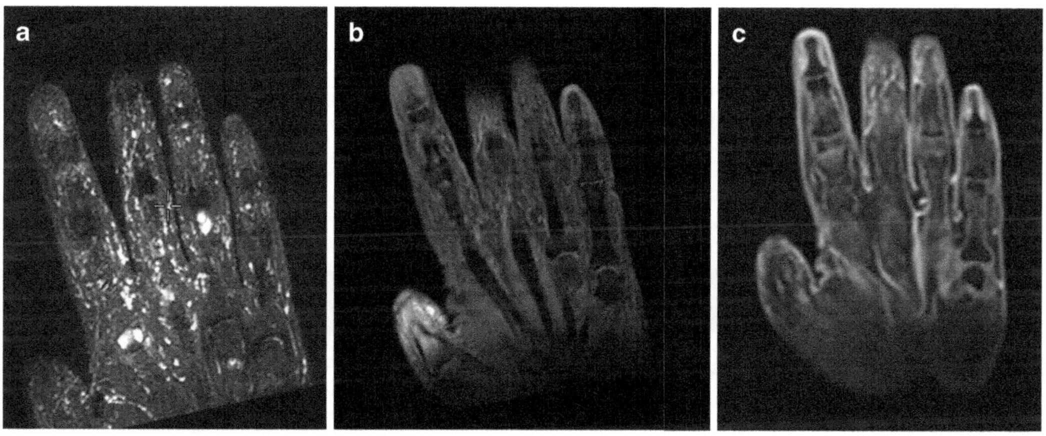

Fig. 2.22 MRI of a venolymphatic malformation. T2 fat sat sequence with MIP reconstruction shows a reticular micronodular pattern with hyperintensity in subcutaneous fat (**a**), T1 weight (**b**), T1 post mdc (**c**) absence of enhancement into the malformation

tive to MRI for patients who can't withstand sedation and thus need a faster exam. Furthermore, CT scan is indicated in the follow-up of extremely bulky AVM, which have been previously treated through embolization with spiral or metallic clips—as these materials determine relevant artefacts in MR images.

Currently, digital angiography is no more indicated as the diagnostic exam for studying the exact architecture and haemodynamics of CVM, the research of arterial afferent pedunculi, nidi and venous efferences—as all these elements are well displayed in MRI. Digital angiography has instead a therapeutic indication for voluminous AVM and other lesions that can be successfully treated through endovascular embolization.

2.4 Tumours, Post-traumatic or Post-surgical Inflammatory and Infectious Diseases

Diagnostic imaging of tumours is directly related to the lesion onset location.

Hand neoplastic lesions include: benign bone tumours (chondroma, aneurismatic bone cyst and solitary cyst), malign bone tumours (osteochondroma, Ewing tumours, etc.) and soft tissue neoplasm (rhabdomyosarcoma, synovial-sarcoma, etc.).

The diagnostic pathway in bone neoplastic lesions starts with a conventional X-ray exam in standard projections (Fig. 2.23a) and needs to be completed by MRI with contrast medium injection (Fig. 2.24). This is the diagnostic gold standard, as it allows a simultaneous evaluation of bone and surrounding soft tissues, as long as the exact extension, necessary for the preoperative planning.

The only real MRI limitation is the poor accuracy in the evaluation of bone erosion and cortex interruption, as they do not change in T1 and T2-weighted sequences. In this case, CT scan provides a greater accuracy, to study the bone structure (Figs. 2.23b and 2.24), identify small early lesions and evaluate the healing process and remodelling after the treatment. For all these advantages, the patients must still be exposed to a significant dose of radiation.

All benign and malign expansive lesions that originate from soft tissues are well visualized in US investigations: a simple, cost-effective, repeatable exam that, in expert hands, has high sensibility and accuracy.

US exams easily identify the solid or fluid nature of a lesion: thus allowing to diagnose benign lesions (lipoma, haemangioma and cyst), that have well-known characteristics, without the need of second-line investigations.

By using high-frequency probes and colour Doppler US in association with B-mode evaluation, a first differentiation between benign and malign lesions can guide the diagnostic pathway (Fig. 2.25).

However, when ultrasonography is not sufficient to provide a diagnostic certainty or the lesion is bulky and thus not entirely visible with a US probe, MRI, with and without contrast medium, is indicated, for an evaluation of local extension and spatial relationship with contiguous structures.

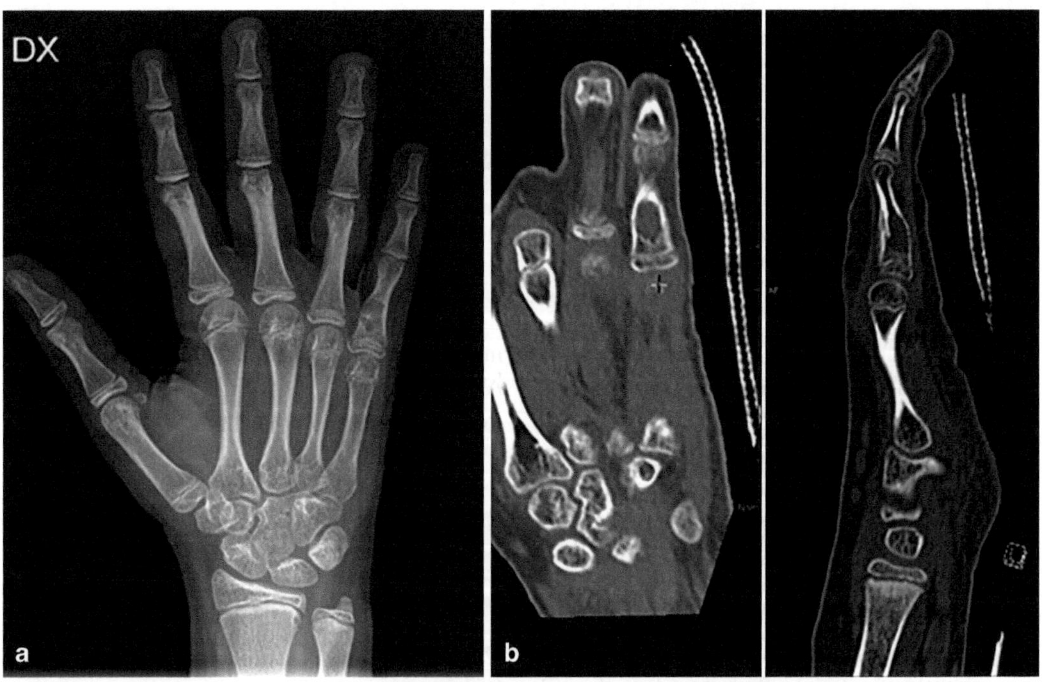

Fig. 2.23 Enchondroma V finger: (**a**) litic expansive lesion without cortical erosion in RX; (**b**) CT scan—MPR reconstruction—high resolution imaging for the study of bone and cortical structure

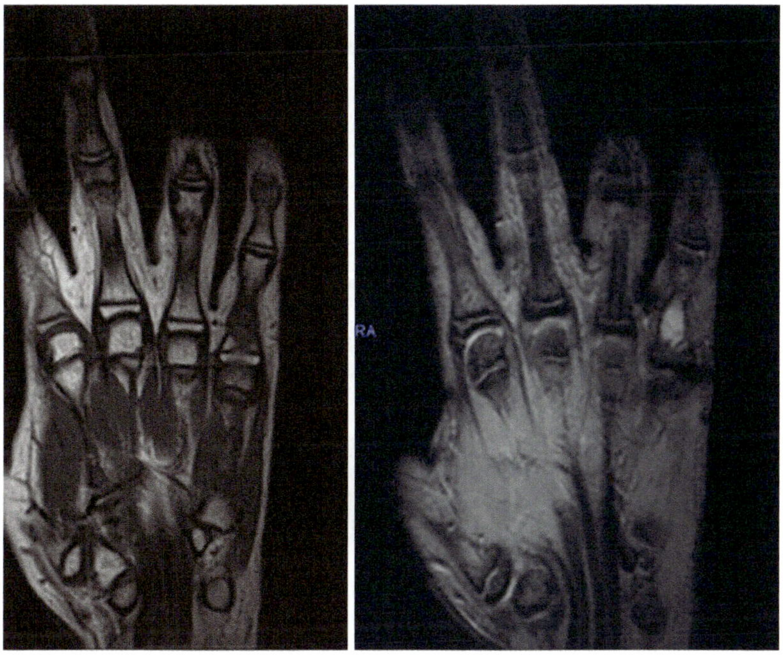

Fig. 2.24 MRI enchondroma V finger—T1 and T2 weight sequence

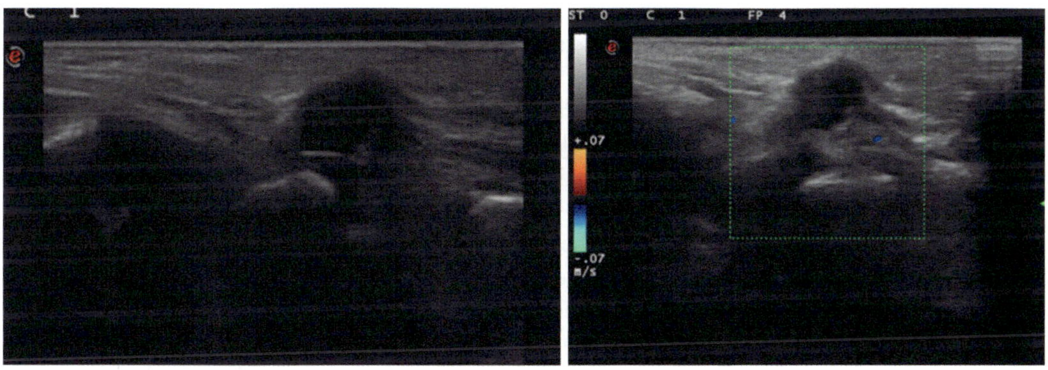

Fig. 2.25 US B-mode and colour Doppler in nodular mass III finger: Giant cell tumor of tendon sheath

In soft tissue neoplasms, follow-up MRI has a primary role, as it provides the greatest reliability in recognizing small nodular recurrences against a background of post-therapeutic inflammatory tissue (Fig. 2.26).

In soft tissue neoplasms, rather than for morphological characteristics and spatial location, CT scan is used for disease staging: research of distant metastasis, primarily to the lungs. It is therefore indicated in certain oncologic protocols.

Hand inflammatory diseases are frequent in pediatric patients. They can be primary (rheumatologic diseases) or secondary (post-traumatic or post-surgery); these lesions can involve superficial tissues (inflammation and peri-cicatricial abscesses) as well as deep structures, such as joints (synovial membrane, articular capsule, tendons, retinacula, etc.).

In all these cases US is once more the first-line exam.

In acute primary inflammatory disease, without involvement of joints and periarticular structures, US high frequency probes allow to visualize joint effusion, synovial hypertrophy and diffusion of the inflammatory process to

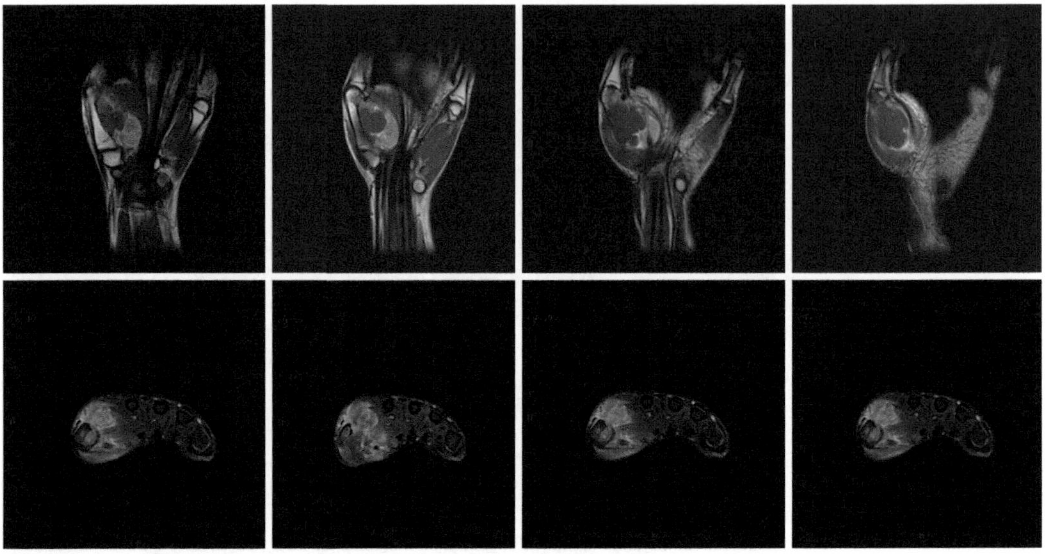

Fig. 2.26 MRI—expansive and infiltrating mass around I finger (Rabdomiosarcoma): T1 pre (coronal) e post (axial) gadolinium: aggressive tissue with infiltration of the bone and contiguous muscles with high and inhomogeneous enhancement

contiguous tendon structures (tenosynovitis and peri-tendinitis).

In chronic affections (such as in juvenile rheumatoid arthritis), US evaluates the evolution of erosions, cortex irregularities, synovial hyperplasia, calcifications and bone neo-apposition or reabsorption. Furthermore, in these patients, power Doppler (i.e. capable of detecting very low flow in hyperaemic areas) can assure a follow-up of the activity of rheumatological diseases.

In these patients, there is rarely necessary a second-line investigation, but when there is, MRI is the choice. This expensive and hardly tolerated method is reserved to those joints which are not entirely evaluable by US (coxo-femoral joint, vertebral joints, etc.).

Finally, US is an optimal method for studying the post-traumatic (open wound, compound fracture) and post-surgical complications: subcutaneous panniculus adiposus and its morphologic variations, as well as differentiation between lymphoedema and panniculitis, thanks to colour and power Doppler (panniculitis is highly hyperaemic); superficial extension and joint diffusion of inflammation. This allows a prompt patient orientation to the best therapy, so to assure the success of treatments.

Moreover, US is the exam of choice for the study of post-traumatic or post-surgical abscesses. US identifies location, margins, characteristics (fluid, with particulate matter; infectious or not-infectious nature according to colour Doppler examination of parietal hyperaemia) and possible presence of gas—that limits US reliability.

When inflammatory processes and collections are widely extended, involving surrounding bone structures that are not well evaluated by US method, MRI is indicated. In these cases, T2-weighted sequences with great fluid resolution can provide a complete evaluation of location and extension of the abscess, as well as of the involvement of contiguous bone structures. If bone is affected by the inflammatory process, it will show high signal intensity on T2-weighted images, so that a prompt therapeutic intervention may avoid osteomyelitis and other severe consequences.

Further Reading

Ballah D, Cahill AM, Fontalvo L, Yan A, et al. Vascular anomalies: what they are, how to diagnose them, and how to treat them. Curr Probl Diagn Radiol. 2011;40(6):233–47.

Battle J, Carmichael K. Incidence of pin track infections in children's fractures treated with Kirschner wire fixation. J Pediatr Orthop. 2007;27:154–7.

Brandon C, Caoili EM, Feng FY, Girish G, Jacobson JA, Wang G. Sonography of wrist ganglion cysts: variable and non-cystic appearances. J Ultrasound Med. 2006;26(10):1323–8.

Brisse H, Orbach D, Klijanienko J, Fréneaux P, Neuenschwander S. Imaging and diagnostic strategy of soft tissue tumors in children. Eur Radiol. 2006;16:1147–64.

Cardinal E, Bureau N, Aubin B. Role of the ultrasound in musculoskeletal infections. Radiol Clin N Am. 2001;39:191–201.

Cerezal L, del Piñal F, Abascal F, García-Valtuille R, Pereda T, Canga A. Imaging findings in ulnar-sided wrist impaction syndromes. Radiographics. 2002;22(1):105–21.

Chang GH, Paz DA, Dwek JR, Chung CB. Lower extremity overuse injuries in pediatric athletes: clinical presentation, imaging findings, and treatment. Clin Imaging. 2013;37:836–46.

Curtis DJ, Downey EF Jr, Brower AC, Cruess DF, Herrington WT, Ghaed N. Importance of soft-tissue evaluation in hand and wrist trauma: statistical evaluation. AJR Am J Roentgenol. 1984;142(4):781–8.

Davis KW. Imaging pediatric sports injuries: upper extremity. Radiol Clin N Am. 2010;48(6):1199–211.

Donnelly LF, Adams DM, Bisset GS 3rd. Vascular malformations and hemangiomas: a practical approach in a multidisciplinary clinic. AJR Am J Roentgenol. 2000;174(3):597–608.

Dubois J, Alison M. Vascular anomalies: what a radiologist needs to know. Pediatr Radiol. 2010;40(6):895–905.

Dubois J, Patriquin HB, Garel L, et al. Soft-tissue hemangiomas in infants and children: diagnosis using Doppler sonography. AJR. 1998;171:247–52.

Dwek JR. The periosteum: what is it, where is it, and what mimics it in its absence? Skelet Radiol. 2010;39(4):319–23.

Dwek JR, Cardoso F, Chung CB. MR imaging of overuse injuries in the skeletally immature gymnast: spectrum of soft-tissue and osseous lesions in the hand and wrist. Pediatr Radiol. 2009;39(12):1310–6.

Ecklund K, Jaramillo D. Patterns of premature physeal arrest: MR imaging of 111 children. AJR Am J Roentgenol. 2002;178(4):967–72.

Egol K, Koval KJ, Zuckerman JD. Handbook of fractures. 4th ed. Philadelphia, PA: Lippincott Williams & Wilkins; 2010. p. 660–80.

Flors L, Leiva-Salinas C, Maged IM, Norton PT, et al. MR imaging of soft-tissue vascular malformations: diagnosis, classification, and therapy follow-up. Radiographics. 2011;31(5):1321–40.

Fuller DJ, McCullough CJ. Malunited fractures of the forearm in children. J Bone Joint Surg Br. 1982;64(3):364–7.

Greulich WW, Pyle S. Radiographic atlas of skeletal development of the hand and wrist. 2nd ed. Stanford, Calif: Stanford University Press; 1959.

Jaimes C, Chauvin NA, Delgado J, Jaramillo D. MR imaging of normal epiphyseal development and common epiphyseal disorders. Radiographics. 2014;34:449–71.

Johari AN, Sinha M. Remodeling of forearm fractures in children. J Pediatr Orthop B. 1999;8(2):84–7.

Johnson KJ, Haigh SF, Symonds KE. MRI in the management of scaphoid fractures in skeletally immature patients. Pediatr Radiol. 2000;30:685–8.

Kaawach W, Ecklund K, Di Canzio J, Zurakowski D, Waters PM. Normal ranges of scapholunate distance in children 6 to 14 years old. J Pediatr Orthop. 2001;21(4):464–7.

Kaiser S, Rosenborg M. Early detection of subperiosteal abscesses by ultrasonography: a means for further successful treatment in pediatric osteomyelitis. Pediatr Radiol. 1994;24:336–9.

Kannikeswaran N, Sethuraman U. Lunate and perilunate dislocations. Pediatr Emerg Care. 2010;26(12):921–4.

Kaste SC, Hill A, Conley L, Shidler TJ, Rao BN, Neel MM. Magnetic resonance imaging after incomplete resection of soft tissue sarcoma. Clin Orthop Relat Res. 2002;397:204–11.

Legiehn GM, Heran MK. Venous malformations: classification, development, diagnosis, and interventional radiologic management. Radiol Clin N Am. 2008;46(3):545–97.

Lurie B, Koff MF, Shah P, et al. Three-dimensional magnetic resonance imaging of physeal injury: reliability and clinical utility. J Pediatr Orthop. 2014;34:239–45.

Mahnken AH, Bücker A, Adam G, Günther RW. MRI of osteomyelitis: sensitivity and specificity of STIR sequences in comparison with contrast-enhanced T1 spin echo sequences. Rofo. 2000;172:1016–9.

Narváez JA, Narváez J, Aguilera C, De Lama E, Portabella F. MR imaging of synovial tumors and tumor-like lesions. Eur Radiol. 2001;11(12):2549–60.

Navarro OM, Laffan EE, Ngan BY. Pediatric soft-tissue tumors and pseudo-tumors: MR imaging features with pathologic correlation: part 1. Imaging approach, pseudotumors, vascular lesions, and …. Radiographics. 2009;29(3):887–906.

Paltiel HJ, Burrows PE, Kozakewich HP, et al. Soft-tissue vascular anomalies: utility of US for diagnosis. Radiology. 2000;214:747–54.

Patil P, Dasgupta B. Role of diagnostic ultrasound in the assessment of musculoskeletal diseases. Ther Adv Musculoskelet Dis. 2012;4(5):341–55.

Pineda C, Espinosa R, Pena A. Radiographic imaging in osteomyelitis: the role of plain radiography, computed tomography, ultrasonography, magnetic resonance imaging, and scintigraphy. Semin Plast Surg. 2009;23:80–9.

Sanchez TR, Jadhav SP, Swischuk LE. MR imaging of pediatric trauma. Magn Reson Imag Clin North Am. 2009;17:439–50.

Shi DP, Zhu SC, Li Y, Zheng J. Epiphyseal and physeal injury: comparison of conventional radiography and magnetic resonance imaging. Clin Imaging. 2009;33(5):379–83.

Siegel MJ. Magnetic resonance imaging of musculoskeletal soft tissue masses. Radiol Clin N Am. 2001;39:701–20.

Teefey SA, Dahiya N, Middleton WD, Gelberman RH, Boyer MI. Ganglia of the hand and wrist: a sonographic analysis. AJR Am J Roentgenol. 2008;191(3):716–20.

Tibrewal S, Jayakumar P, Vaidya S, Ang SC. Role of MRI in the diagnosis and management of patients with clinical scaphoid fracture. Int Orthop. 2012;36(1):107–10.

Trevor W, Oren M, Jennifer M, Wolf MD. Soft-tissue complications associated with distal radius fractures. Oper Tech Orthop. 2009:100–6.

Tsai TS, Evans HA, Donnelly LF, Bisset GS 3rd, Emery KH. Fat necrosis after trauma: a benign cause of palpable lumps in children. AJR Am J Roentgenol. 1997;169:1623–6.

Hand Defects: An Isolated Anomaly Or a Syndromic Disease?

3

Angelo Selicorni, Paola Cianci, Silvia Tajè, and Massimo Agosti

Abstract

Patients with hand congenital defects are a very heterogeneous cohort. Like for any other major malformation, one of the goals of the clinical approach is to define if the anomaly is an isolated problem or if it's part of a more complex genetic disease. This definition sometimes it's not so easy, but it's crucial in order to define a correct prognosis for the child and a proper genetic counseling for parents, for their relatives and, in the future, for the patient itself. Tor achieves the aforementioned result, it's important to follow a specific methodologic approach that starts from a detailed clinical analysis of the patient and that can properly use the known genetic tests. In this field in recent years, new very powerful tests have become available (array CGH and NGS) greatly increasing the possibility of a correct framing also in front of very complex children, and so saving time and money.

A. Selicorni (✉) · P. Cianci · S. Tajè
Pediatric Department, Mariani Foundation Center for Fragile Child, "Sant'Anna" Hospital, ASST Lariana, Como, Italy

M. Agosti
Pediatric Department, "F. Del Ponte" Hospital, ASST Settelaghi, University of Insubria, Varese, Italy

Keywords

Major malformations · Hand anomalies · Syndromic diseases · Apert syndrome · Pfeiffer syndrome · Saethre–Chotzen syndrome · Crouzon syndrome · Freeman–Sheldon syndrome · Oro-facio-digital syndromes · EEC syndrome · Array CGH · Next Generation Sequencing (NGS)

3.1 Definitions

Like in other parts of the body, the hands can be an area in which different kind of congenital anomalies can be evident. Generally speaking, we can distinguish these defects into two different types. We can in fact observe *major malformations* that are congenital anomalies with relevant medical consequences (e.g., the loss of a thumb, the presence of a supernumerary finger, etc.) and which frequently deserve a surgical approach; or *minor anomalies* that refes to defects with no or very minimal clinical impact which can have only aesthetic consequences (e.g., a mild skin syndactyly or a clinodactyly of the fifth finger) [1]. These defects are due to an intrinsic embryological abnormal process. We know that organogenesis takes place during the first 10 weeks of gestation, so that these anomalies develop in the embryo only during that range of time.

G. Pajardi (ed.), *Pediatric Hand Surgery*, https://doi.org/10.1007/978-3-031-30984-7_3

Different combination of these possible areas of involvement

- Abnormal growth pattern (both poor or increased)
- Presence of major malformations (considering both the classical and the occasional one)
- Abnormal psychomotor development
- Peculiar minor anomalies (especially but not exclusively related to facial gestalt)

↓

Specific genetic defect

Fig. 3.1 Clinical features of a syndrome

Sometimes interpretation of these signals is not so easy. The example can be the evidence of a post-minimum skin appendix on the ulnar side of the hand. This little anomaly has no meaningful medical consequences but it's a very mild expression of a postaxial polydactyly which is a true major malformation.

Again together with malformations, a hand anomaly could also be the result of *deformation*. We define deformation as those congenital defects which are not related to an embryonal abnormal developmental process but that arise after a normal embryogenesis due to a damage to normally developed structures. The classic example of deformation is the consequences of amniotic band disruption process in which we can observe lesion at the hands/fingers of various severity, very often asymmetrical in clinical presentation between different fingers and different hands.

Similarly to every kind of congenital defects, also hand anomalies can be isolated or part of a broader disease named syndrome. In 2005, Biesecker discussing this point related to polydactyly stated that "… the problem of non syndromic polydactyly is formally insoluble…. So we define "*syndrome*" a clinical condition in which a child can have various medical/functional problems which are due to a single genetic anomaly". Figure 3.1 defines the areas of involvement of a syndrome [2]. A classical example is represented by Apert syndrome: a very common pattern of craniofacial anomalies is associated with an absolutely typical and severe syndactyly pattern of hands and feet, with possible associated anomalies in growth, psychomotor development; all these features are due to a specific mutation in FGFR2 gene.

3.2 Why a Proper Classification of Hand Malformations Is So Important?

The relevant question is what are the consequences of a correct classification of a hand congenital defect as isolated or syndromic. Table 3.1 analyzes the situation. It's obvious that in case the child is affected by a genetic syndrome, his prognosis, in the great majority of the situation, is more deeply influenced by the natural history of the syndrome itself, rather than by the specific functional prognosis of the hand defect. Survival, physical growth, psychomotor and intellectual development can be more or less severely conditioned by the natural evolution of the disease. The frequency, needs and type of medical follow-up can be extremely different in the two situations (isolated or syndromic defect) and the hand defect can often represent a minor problem to face in comparison with the others in a syndromic setting. Finally, the recurrence risk of the usually healthy parents and of the child himself as soon as he/she will be an adult will be very different according to the classification of the defect as isolated or syndromic.

Table 3.1 Consequences of a correct classification of a congenital hand anomalies

	Isolated defect	Syndromic defect
General health prognosis	Usually favorable	Potentially critical[a]
Survival	Normal	Potentially abnormal[a]
Growth pattern	Normal	Potentially abnormal[a]
Psychomotor and intellectual development	Normal	Potentially abnormal[a]
Follow-up needs	Only related to the hand malformation	Often need for a wider multidisciplinary approach[a]
Functional prognosis of the hand malformation	Only related to the type of malformation and the possibility of surgical correction	Strongly influenced also by the general functional prognosis of the syndrome
Recurrence risk for parents	Usually low (apart from specific monogenic isolated condition)	Potentially increased[b]
Recurrence risk for the child	Usually low (apart from specific monogenic isolated condition)	Potentially increased[b]

[a]Related to the natural history of the syndrome
[b]Related to the genetic basis of the syndrome

3.3 The Clinical-Genetic Diagnostic Process

The classification of a defect as isolated or syndromic could not be so easy and quick. Usually hand anomalies are diagnosed at birth, even if sometimes the ultrasound studies during pregnancy could have generated some doubts. It's important to state that a complete evaluation of the phenotype is possible only after birth; for this reason, prenatal counseling should always be very cautious because surprises are frequent.

In the neonatal period, we can have different scenarios. In some situations, the clinical data are already clear and absolutely convincing toward a syndromic condition. This is the case in which the newborn shows multiple congenital defects, clear dysmorphic features, abnormal birth auxological parameters, and/or abnormal neurologic status. In these cases, the question is whether it's possible to perform a "gestaltic diagnosis" or not. More often the hand anomaly seems at first glance to be an isolated problem. In this context, it's important to perform a proper clinical and instrumental evaluation, in order to search for possible associated major malformations, functional defects (e.g., audiological or visual deficiency), and dysmorphic minor anomalies. Family and pregnancy history is essential too in order to better classify the problem. It's well known the existence of an isolated hand defects which can have a mendelian segregation mostly according to autosomal dominant inheritance (e.g., pre- and postaxial polydactyly, triphalangeal thumb, and ectrodactyly). In addition, some genetic syndromes (like Pfeiffer syndrome, for example) have a dominant transmission too. It's always important to consider that in some situations the variability of expression of the disease and the absence of intellectual involvement can have prevented the recognition of the disease in a relative. For all these reasons, a three generations genealogic tree should always be performed and direct parents' evaluation could be useful, in order to deeply evaluate possible familiar pathological traits that can be crucial for the classification of the proband's defect.

If no associated anomalies are evident, it can be reassuring for the clinicians, but it must be kept in mind that the hypothesis of a syndromic condition needs to be confirmed by the evolution of the child. So a proper pediatric-genetic follow-up is strongly recommended in order to confirm the classification of the hand defect as isolated. Growth and developmental data and somatic and medical evolution are paramount in order to define the situation [2, 3].

As we have said before, sometimes the diagnosis could be made quite easily in the neonatal period, if the clinical data are enough expressed and the experience of the clinician related to that condition is high. Table 3.2 summarized some examples of syndromes that can be diagnosed at

Table 3.2 Possible gestaltic neonatal syndromic diagnosis

Syndrome	Hand defect	Associated anomalies	Genetic defect
Apert syndrome	Complete syndactyly	Craniostenosis dysmorphisms, possible growth and developmental anomalies	Autosomal dominant FGFR2 mutation
Cornelia de Lange syndrome	Limb reduction defects, missing fingers of ulnar side	Peculiar dysmorphisms, hirsutism pre- and postnatal growth retardation, psychomotor retardation, intellectual disability	Mutation in different gene of the cohesion family (NIPBL, SMC1A, SMC3, RAD 21, HDAC8, ANJRD11, BRD4) most genes follow an autosomal dominant inheritance, some others X linked inheritance
VATER association	Radial ray defect	Vertebral anomaly imperforate anus, esophageal athresia, trachea esophageal fistula, heart anomaly	Unknown
Rubinstein–Taybi syndrome	Large/bifid thumbs/hallux	Peculiar dysmorphisms, psychomotor delay, growth retardation	Microdeletion 16p13.3, autosomal dominant CREBP or EP300 gene mutation
Freeman–Sheldon syndrome	Hand contractures,	Whistling face, other joints contractures (as in patient with distal arthrogryposis)	Autosomal dominant MYH3 gene mutation
Holt–Oram syndrome	Monolateral radial ray defect	Heart congenital defects, ECG anomalies	Autosomal dominant TBX3 gene mutation
Meckel–Gruber syndrome	Postaxial polydactyly	Cystic renal disease, occipital encephalocele	Four different subtypes involving different genes with autosomal recessive inheritance
Fanconi anemia	Radial ray deficiency	Multiple congenital defects, increased risks to develop hematologic and non-hematologic neoplasia, bone marrow insufficiency	Heterogeneous disease with 19 genes involved with autosomal recessive inheritance Karyotype with DEB showing increased chromosome fragility

birth in front of a hand anomaly. In these situations, nowadays the clinical hypothesis can frequently be confirmed by specific genetic tests. Later the use and the limits of the genetic tests will be discussed more in to details.

3.4 Main Syndromic Conditions Associated with Hand Anomalies

The number of syndromes associated with hand anomalies, also limiting the discussion to major hand malformations, is extremely wide, so a detailed discussion is impossible to be performed in a short chapter. So we will briefly discuss some malformative/genetic conditions that must be known because of their frequency and clinical relevance.

3.4.1 Amniotic Band Sequence

Amniotic band sequence is a congenital limb disorder with an extremely variable clinical presentation. Its frequency is about 1 in 1200 live births. It is characterized by the presence of partial to complete, congenital, fibrous, circumferential, constriction bands/rings on any part of the body, with a particular predilection for the upper or lower extremities. Phenotypes range between a mild skin indentation to complete amputation of parts of the fetus (e.g. digits, distal limb); fusion of digits mimicking syndactyly can also be evident. Classically, the damage of the extremities is asymmetrical between different digits and different hands. This feature and constriction rings are the clues of the clinical diagnosis. The commonly accepted view is that amniotic band sequence occurs when the inner membrane (amnion) ruptures without injury to the outer membrane (chorion), this exposes the baby to fibrous sticky tissue (bands) from the ruptured amnion which can float in the water of the uterus; these fibrous tissues can entangle the baby, reducing blood supply and causing congenital abnormalities. In some cases, a complete "natural" amputation of a digit(s) or limb may occur before birth or the digit(s) or limbs may be necrotic and require surgical amputation following birth. No genetic test is indicated or required, because the diagnosis can be simply done by clinical evaluation. This a classical nongenetic condition in which the prognosis of the newborn regarding growth and psychomotor development is absolutely normal. Because of its environmental origin, the recurrence risk for the parents and for the child himself is not increased in comparison with general population [4].

3.4.2 Poland Syndrome

Poland syndrome has an incidence of 1/20–30,000 live births. Clinical diagnosis is made in neonatal period or later in patient with an asymmetrical hypoplasia of pectoral muscles with possible involvement of the rib cage, associated with ipsilateral anomalies of the upper limb; more rarely the limb involvement can be bilateral. In particular limb, anomalies can be variable and can be characterized by shortness of fingers, syndactyly of hypoplastic fingers, global hypoplasia of the hand and of the forearm. Both growth and psychomotor development are usually normal. Up to now, no molecular anomaly has been discovered as a cause of Poland syndrome whose diagnosis is still only clinically based [5].

3.4.3 Acrocephalosyndactylies

Acrocephalosyndactyly syndromes represent a group of inherited congenital malformation disorders characterized by craniosynostosis and fusion or webbing of the fingers or toes, often with other associated manifestations. Most of these conditions are due to the mutation of FGFRs' genes. The condition whose clinical diagnosis is easier is *Apert syndrome*. The patients affected with this disease show craniosynostosis frequently of the coronal sutures giving a acro-brachycephalic shape of the cranium. The facial features are influenced by the cranium anomalies. In particular, eyes are prominent due to shallow orbits, midface is flat, palate is high and arched, mandible is relatively prominent. The hands and feets show skin and osseus fusion that involves at minimum the second, third, and fourth ray but it can involve all the fingers. The patients have a growth in the lower part of normal curves. They can have some delays in psychomotor development; mean IQ is 70 with a range between 50 and 90. The children can manifest nutritional, respiratory and neurosurgery complications that should actively monitored and treated. The genetic defect is represented by autosomal dominant mutation of FGFR2 gene [6].

Pfeiffer syndrome is another common disease belonging to this group. The core anomaly is localized to the hands and feet in which thumbs and hallux are large and medially deviated and in which is evident skin syndactyly involving 2°–3° fingers and toes (less frequently 3° and 4°). According to the presence/severity of craniosynostosis are known three different subtypes: type 1 with mild expression, good prognosis, and normal intellectual development, type 2 with a more severe involvement, severe craniosynostosis and worse prognosis and type 3 quite similar to type 2, without evidence of clover leaf skull. Mutation of FRGFR1 (exon7) and FGFR2 (exons 8 and 10) are the biological markers of the disease [7].

Saethre–Chotzen syndrome is another disease of this group in which hand and feet anomalies are evident. In particular, patients affected have brachydactyly, because of shortness of terminal phalanges and partial skin syndactyly of 2–3° fingers less frequently 3–4°. Thumbs can be triphalangeal. The feet hallux is large and it's possible to see skin syndactyly of toes. Together with these anomalies, the patients show facial dysmorphisms with asymmetric face, ptosis, strabismus, downslanting of palpebral fissures, hypertelorism, hypoplastic maxilla, high arched palate, and peculiar ears. Craniosynostosis is not constantly present and can involve different sutures with variable severity. Physical growth and intellectual development are usually normal except for patients with chromosomal microdeletions that can show intellectual disability. Genetic defect involves autosomal dominant mutation or microdeletion of the TWIST gene on chromosome 7p21 [8].

Another common disease of this group is *Crouzon syndrome* in which classically no hands and feet anomalies are present.

3.4.4 Arthrogryposis Multiplex Congenita

Arthrogryposis multiplex congenital is a large and heterogeneous group of disorders characterized by congenital limb contractures. It manifests as a limitation of movement of multiple limb joints at birth that is usually nonprogressive and may include muscle weakness and fibrosis. Typically mothers of these children describe decreased intrauterine fetal movement which leads secondarily to the contractures. The reduced movements can have a neurologic basis (cerebral, spinal, or peripheral nerves involvement) a muscular basis (myasthenia gravis, muscular dystrophies, and mitochondrial diseases) or a connectival basis; a reduce intrauterine space can be responsible too. The incidence of the syndromes with multiple contractures is about 1/3000 live births. It's easy to understand that it would be very long and complex to go into details in this large chapter. Within this group, we identify a subgroup named distal arthrogryposis and in this category, we want to put our attention to one syndrome whose phenotype is so typical to be recognized at birth. This is the case of *Freeman–Sheldon syndrome* in which the newborns show joints' contractures as typical for distal arthrogryposis, associated with contractures of facial muscles causing a very little mouth (whistling face). In the skin under the mouth is classically evident an "H shape" skin fold. This combination of facial features is absolutely specific for this disease and permits a gestaltic diagnosis. Usually, the psychomotor development of these children is pretty normal while weight growth can be slow because of nutritional difficulties. Autosomal dominant mutations of MYH3 gene are responsible of about 90% of the cases [9].

3.4.5 Bardet–Biedl Syndrome

Bardet–Biedl is a genetic syndrome characterized by the association between obesity, retinal dystrophy, polydactyly, genital anomaly, hypogonadism, and renal defects.

Its prevalence is about 1/100,000–1/160,000 live births. The clinical diagnosis is made if a proper combination of primary (major) and secondary (minor) criteria are present: primary features are retinal dystrophy, polydactyly, obesity, learning disability, hypogonadism, renal and urinal tract anomalies. Secondary criteria are the following: language delay, ocular anomalies like cataracts strabismus, brachydactyly or syndactyly, ataxia, mild spasticity in particular at lower limbs, diabetes, hepatic fibrosis, and heart problems. Clinical diagnosis is possible when a patient shows four major criteria or three major criteria and two minors. As regards hand polydactyly is often the first manifestation evident at birth. Usually is a postaxial polydactyly and is evident in70–80% of the cases. The variability is wide; from one extremity to all four can be involved. The last chance regards about 21% of patients. Feet are more frequently interested. Apart from psychomotor problems, patients with Bardet Biedl syndrome can evolve toward severe impairment of visual ability from the age of 15. Usually, first visual symptoms can be evident from 6 to 8 years of age. The syndrome has an autosomal recessive inheritance and about 20 different genes can be involved, so molecular confirmation of a clinical diagnosis is hardworking and not always possible [10].

3.4.6 Fanconi Anemia

The disease is characterized by the association of progressive bone marrow insufficiency, increased risks of development of neoplasia, congenital defects and extreme toxicity to exposure to radiations and chemotherapy drugs. Its incidence is about 1/160,000. Between the various possible congenital defects, 50% of the patients have skeletal anomalies whose 70% involve upper limbs. In particular, the thumbs can be absent, little, bifid or triphalangeal. The radius can be short of absent too and, in this case, ulna is short and arched. The stature is short while psychomotor development can be delayed. As we have reported, there is an increased risk of hematologic and non-hematologic neoplasias. This means that patients need to be followed properly in order to early diagnose possible tumors. The syndrome has a genetic basis and an autosomal recessive etiology. That means that recurrence risk is 25% for an healthy couple of parents of an affected child. About 19 genes have been related to the syndrome. A screening test is represented by cytogenetic analysis with DEB exposure in order to show an increased chromosomal fragility [11].

3.4.7 Holt–Oram Syndrome

Holt–Oram is a rare syndrome characterized by the association of preaxial limb defect and heart anomalies. Its prevalence is 1/100,000 newborns. At upper limb, it's possible to diagnose various types of malformations: absent thumbs, triphalangeal thumbs, phocomelia, radial hypo/aplasia, carpal bone anomalies, abnormal elbow movements, possible anomalies at clavicles and scapula. In total, 75% of patients have heart problems; 60% of them show an interatrial defect, 30% have interventricular muscular defect. Other heart malformations have been described. In total, 40% of patients have an ECG anomaly also in absence of a cardiac malformation. Growth and psychomotor development are usually normal. In total, 70% of affected children show autosomal dominant mutation of TBX5 gene [12].

3.4.8 VATER/VACTERL Association

VATER association is a complex malformative condition characterized by a particular spectrum of anomalies including: vertebral defect, imperforate anus, tracheo-esophageal fistula, esophageal atresia and renal/radial dysplasia. Later, the observation of a high frequency of cardiac and limb anomalies in these patients permitted to modify the original acronym from VATER to VACTERL. Its prevalence is between 1/20,000 and 1/40,000 newborns As regard limb anomalies, they are present in 40–50% of the affected individuals. The most common defects are the following: radial hypo/aplasia, thumb hypo/aplasia preaxial polydactyly. VATER's patients grow normally and have a normal achievement of the common psychomotor milestones. Up to now, no specific genetic defect has been discovered as associated with the disease whose diagnosis is still now only clinical. No formally defined clinical criteria are available. Hall suggested that clinical diagnosis can be acceptable if the patient has an anomaly in all three regions of the body (limbs, thorax, and inferior abdominal region/ pelvis). Other authors believe that esophageal and anal defects are mandatory in order to consider this diagnosis [13].

3.4.9 Oro-Facio-Digital Syndromes

Oro-facio-digital syndromes refer to numerous conditions in which major or minor anomalies can be evident at the oral cavity (mouth, tongue, teeth, and jaw), facial structures (head, eyes, and nose), and digits (fingers and toes). Association with major problems in different organs or apparatus are described. The literature reports up to 17 types of oro-facio-digital syndrome, but research is necessary to confirm and clarify all of these types. Hands involvement is usually characterized by brachydactyly, syndactyly, or preaxial polydactyly. The prognosis and the severity of the disease are very variable between different types. For most of them the exact genetic basis of the condition is unknown; the pattern of inheritance is different in the various subtypes [14].

3.4.10 Cornelia de Lange Syndrome

Cornelia de Lange syndrome, or as recently stated Cornelia de Lange spectrum, refers to a phenotype characterized by quite typical facial dysmorphisms, hirsutism, intrauterine and postnatal growth retardation, psychomotor delay, and intellectual disability of different severity. The prevalence of the condition is from 1/10,000 to 1/30000 live births. About 1/3 of patients can show limb malformation mostly at upper limb. The defect is quite variable and can splurge from severe limb reduction anomalies toward the absence of various fingers typically of ulnar side. Some patients can show a combination of reduction defects in one hand and postaxial polydactyly in the contralateral hand. Genetic basis is very complex and heterogeneous and refers to possible mutations in genes of the cohesion complex. However, it's important to state that patients with major limb involvement usually show mutation in only one gene (NIPBL) which is responsible for about 60–65% of the genetic defects and correlates with the more classical phenotype. It should be remembered that in a significant amount of patients, also with a quite classical phenotype, the molecular defects cannot be evidenced on blood lymphocyte but it's necessary to test another tissue (usually cells obtained from oral mucosa brush). This phenomenon is named somatic mosaicism [15].

3.4.11 Rubinstein–Taybi Syndrome

Rubinstein–Taybi syndrome is characterized by the association of typical facial dysmorphisms, psychomotor delay/intellectual disability, and peculiar shape of thumbs and hallux. Its prevalence at birth is 1/100,000–1/125,000. The eyes and nasal region are the hallmarks of this condition regards facial dysmorphisms. Thumbs and halluxs are classically large and in 1/3 of patients deviated (varism or valgism). Sometimes they can be also bifid or duplicated (preaxial polydactyly). Occasionally, a postaxial polydactyly of feet can be observed.

As stated, patients with Rubinstein Taybi syndrome have a variable degree of intellectual disability; growth can be reduced, especially in the first years of life, also if some of these children can evolve toward overweight/obesity in preadolescent/adolescent age. The genetic basis of the syndrome is heterogeneous. Some patients can show a microdeletion of the short arm of chromosome 16 (16p11.2), the majority has an autosomal dominant mutation in CREBP gene (localized in the 16p11.2 region) and lastly a minority of individuals have an autosomal dominant mutation of EP300 gene. Somatic mosaicism has been observed in Rubinstein Taybi patients too [16].

3.4.12 Smith–Lemli–Opitz Syndrome

Smith–Lemli–Opitz syndrome is a disease of cholesterol metabolism associated with multiple congenital anomalies caused by a deficiency of 7-dehydro-cholesterol reductase enzyme (7DHC) which is important into conversion of 7DHC to cholesterol. Its prevalence is 1/20,000–1/40,000 live births. The main clinical problems are facial dysmorphisms, prenatal and postnatal growth retardation, microcephaly, psychomotor retardation and intellectual disability of moderate severe degree and multiple malformations (cleft palate, heart anomalies, central nervous system defects, ambiguous genitalia hypoplastic penis, and hypospadias). At the extremities, postaxial polydactyly and peculiar 2–3° toes syndactyly (Y shaped) are evident. Clinical hypothesis can be confirmed with the dosage of serum 7DHC or 8DHC which are abnormally high in front of a cholesterol concentration quite low. Molecular study of the gene coding for the defective enzyme is another way to confirm the diagnosis. The disease has an autosomal recessive pattern of inheritance, so diagnosis is extremely important for a proper genetic counseling for further pregnancies [17].

3.4.13 Greig Syndrome

Greig cephalopolysyndactyly syndrome is characterized by macrocephaly, preaxial polydactyly or mixed pre- and postaxial polydactyly, and widely spaced eyes. Mildly affected patients may have subtle craniofacial findings. Greig syndrome is part of a clinical spectrum whose mild spectrum is represented by preaxial polysyndactyly type IV and crossed polydactyly (preaxial polydactyly of the feet and postaxial polydactyly of the hands plus syndactyly of fingers 3–4 and toes 1–3). Individuals with classical form can have seizures, hydrocephalus, and intellectual disability, but this covers only 10% of patients. The diagnosis of Greig syndrome is based on clinical findings and family history. The molecular basis of the disease is represented by *GLI3* gene anomalies. They can be a deletion involving GLI3 gene (7p14.1 region) or a pathogenetic dominant mutation of the gene sequence itself. The detection rate of genetic tests is about 75% [18].

3.4.14 EEC Syndrome

EEC syndrome is an acronym for Ectrodactyly-Ectodermal Dysplasia-Cleft Lip/Palate. It is a rare form of ectodermal dysplasia. The symptoms can be variable and most commonly refers to hand/feet malformation (ectrodactyly or split hand/foot malformation), ectodermal dysplasia symptoms (with hair and glands anomalies), and cleft lip and/or palate. Other frequent features are distinctive facial features, eyes and urinary tract anomalies EEC syndrome is inherited with an autosomal dominant pattern. More than 90% of individuals have mutations in the TP63 gene (EEC type 3). Other individuals with EEC syndrome are thought to have a mutation in a region on chromosome 7 (EEC1) [19].

3.5 Differential Diagnosis According Types of Hand Defect

In Tables 3.3, 3.4, 3.5, 3.6, and 3.7 we summarize the main syndromes that should be considered in differential diagnosis in front of a particular major anomaly of the hands. Of course, the lists are not exhaustive but can be useful for a first approach. As it's well known it's now possible to use databases of free access (Orphanet) or affordable (Oxford Medical database, POSSUM) that can help clinicians to generate a list of possible diagnosis starting from clinical features (major and minor) of the patient [20].

Table 3.3 Syndromes with preaxial polydactyly

Biemond syndrome
Brachio-Oculo facial syndrome
Cranio Fronto nasal dysplasia
Fanconi anemia
Fetal-alcohol syndrome
Goltz syndrome
Greig syndrome
Hydrocephalus syndrome
Jeune syndrome
Kaufmann–Mckusick syndrome
Larsen syndrome
Meckel–Gruber syndrome
Nager syndrome
Oro-facio-digital syndrome
Short rib polydactyly syndrome
Robinow syndrome
VATER association

Table 3.4 Syndromes associated with postaxial polydactyly

Acro-callosal syndrome
Acrocephalopolysyndactyly
Bardet–Biedl syndrome
Biemond syndrome
Carpenter syndrome
Craniofrontonasal dysplasia
Ellis–Van Creveld syndrome
Fetal–Valproate syndrome
Goltz syndrome
Greig syndrome
Holt–Oram syndrome
Hydrolethalus syndrome
Jeune syndrome
Joubert syndrome
Kaufman–Mckusick syndrome
Pallister–Killian syndrome
Maternal diabetes syndrome
Orofaciodigital syndromes
Pallister–Hall syndrome
Schinzel–Giedion syndrome
Short rib polydactyly syndrome
Simpson–Golabi–Behmel syndrome
Smith–Lemli–Opitz syndrome
Young–Simpson syndrome

Table 3.6 Syndromes associated with absent/hypoplastic thumb

Aase syndrome
Acrorenal syndrome
Brachio-oculo-facial syndrome
Fanconi anemia
Feingold syndrome
Fetal alcohol syndrome
Holt–Oram syndrome
LADD syndrome
Lenz syndrome
Maternal diabetes syndrome
Nager syndrome
Rothmund–Thompsen syndrome
Smith–Lemli–Opitz syndrome
VATER association
Yunis–Varon syndrome

Table 3.5 Syndromes associated mesoaxial polydactyly

Ellis–van Creveld syndrome
Holt–Oram syndrome
Kaufman–Mckusick syndrome
Orofaciodigital syndromes
Robinow syndrome
Pallister–Hall syndrome

Table 3.7 Syndromes associated with triphalangeal thumb

Aase syndrome
Fanconi anemia
Fetal hydantoin syndrome
Holt–Oram syndrome
LADD syndrome
Nager syndrome
Townes syndrome

3.5.1 The New Genetic Tests and Their Use in the Diagnostic Process

Genetic tests are changing, increasing the possibility of testing and modifying the approach to the diagnosis. Up to 10 years ago, the geneticist had few opportunities to use genetic tests to confirm a clinical diagnosis. It was possible to evaluate the number of chromosomes and their general structure with the possibility of detecting deletion or duplication with 5–10 Mb of size. The next step was the discovery of *molecular cytogenetic* with FISH (fluorescent in situ hybridization) study. Thank to this approach, there was the possibility of showing more little deletions/duplications in specifically related chromosomal regions to confirm the suspicion of defined syndromes or, later on, to search for abnormalities in the terminal part of chromosomes (telomeres) in very complex children with a so-called "chromosomal phenotype." At gene level, it was growing the availability of tests able to identify mutation in single gene considered to be the cause of specific disease [21].

The first revolution was related to the introduction in clinical practice of the *array CGH* technology. Thank to this new approach, completely different from cytogenetics from a methodological point of view, it has become possible to detect deletion or duplication of very low size (hundreds of bases instead of millions of bases) extremely increasing the number of patients in whom an abnormality has been detected. This technology has now taken the place of the old standard karyotype as first-level cytogenetic approach. The side effect of array CGH implementation is the discovery of a great number of variants (both deletion or duplication) which are absolutely benign or for which is not possible to define for sure the real meaning (named VOUS = variant of unknown significance). This means that the correct interpretation of the results of an arrayCGH study needs a specific and very specialist competence [21].

At molecular level during the last few years, it has become clear that genetic basis of the great majority of the genetic syndromes is highly heterogeneous. For a lot of syndromes in fact, the number of genes, whose mutations were related to that phenotype, has been increasing months after months. This situation created difficulty in performing complete molecular study of patients suspected to be affected by a highly heterogeneous disease. The last revolution was so related to the introduction of a new approach in sequencing technology named NGS (next-generation sequencing) [21]. Thank to this approach it was possible to study at the same time hundreds and hundreds of genes selecting their really important part: the exons, the coding part of every gene. In this way, we are able to study in a single experiment all the genes related to a specific syndrome, all the known genes related to a specific problem (the so-called genetic panels), all the exons of the known genes (named clinical exome) all the exons of our genome (WES = Whole exome sequencing) [22]. Table 3.8 summarizes these definitions. Thank to this new approach the time necessary to study at the molecular level a single patient greatly decreased. In addition, this approach has improved tremendously the possibility to reach a diagnosis in very complex children affected by the so-called "ultra rare diseases"; a lot of papers describing the analysis of different cohorts of patients report a detection rate from 30% to 50%. Moreover, this technology demonstrated to be very cost-effective. Economic studies showed that the cost of this new analysis is absolutely lower than that of the various single genetic tests performed by patients without having a significant result [23, 24].

Table 3.8 the new various possibility available thank to NGS technology

Genetic panels	Analysis of the exons of all the genes related to an heterogeneous syndrome (e.g. Bardet–Biedl syndrome) or related to a specific clinical problem (epilepsy)
Clinical exome	Analysis of the exons of all the known genes
Whole-exome sequencing	Analysis of all the exons of our genome
Whole-genome sequencing	Analysis of all the exons and introns of our genome

For this reason, some authors suggested a new methodological approach to the child with multiple congenital defects which is shown in Fig. 3.2. If the clinician has a reasonable clinical hypothesis, it's important to search the confirmation with usual genetic tests. If a good hypothesis is lacking, it's better to use the new technology (array CGH and WES in sequence) instead of wasting time in performing genetic tests with few possibilities to reach the goal. As for array CGH, the more we know the more we can have doubts. Also a WES study can generate results with unknown or hardly interpretable meaning; for this reason, this kind of tests need to be managed by expert geneticists [25–27].

What is important to understand is that with this approach, the physician's role is no less important than in the past. A very deep and detailed clinical analysis is extremely important in order to accurately define the phenotype of the patient and in order to compare it with the pheno-

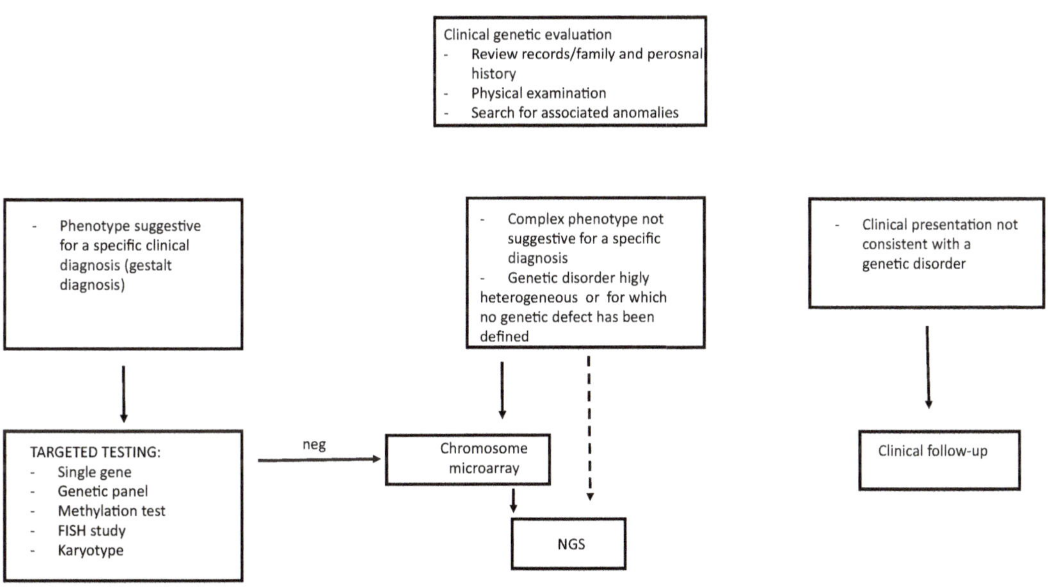

Fig. 3.2 New methodological approach to a child with multiple congenital defects

type of patients which show a specific genetic defect. Whereas in the past the clinician's task was only to suggest a possible clinical diagnosis and seek the confirmation with genetic testing, the new technology has added a new role: to confirm that a specific genotype suggested by array-CGH or WES may be the correct explanation for the patient's phenotype.

References

1. Rasmussen SA, Olney RS, Holmes LB, Lin AE, Keppler-Noreuil KM, Moore CA, National Birth Defects Prevention Study. Guidelines for case classification for the National Birth Defects Prevention Study. Birth Defects Res A Clin Mol Teratol. 2003;67:193–201.
2. Solomon BD, Muenke M. When to suspect a genetic syndrome. Am Fam Physician. 2012;86:826–33.
3. Dy CJ, Swarup I, Daluiski A. Embryology, diagnosis, and evaluation of congenital hand anomalies. Curr Rev Musculoskelet Med. 2014;7:60–7.
4. Durga R, Renukadevi TK. Amniotic band syndrome – a dreaded condition. J Clin Diagn Res. 2016;10:QD04–5.
5. Moir CR, Johnson CH. Poland's syndrome. Semin Pediatr Surg. 2008;17:161–6.
6. Kumar GR, Jyothsna M, Ahmed SB, Sree Lakshmi KR. Apert's Syndrome. Int J Clin Pediatr Dent. 2014;7:69–72.
7. Vogels A, Fryns JP. Pfeiffer syndrome. Orphanet J Rare Dis. 2006;1:19.
8. Kress W, Schropp C, Lieb G, Petersen B, Büsse-Ratzka M, Kunz J, Reinhart E, Schäfer WD, Sold J, Hoppe F, Pahnke J, Trusen A, Sörensen N, Krauss J, Collmann H. Saethre-Chotzen syndrome caused by TWIST 1 gene mutations: functional differentiation from Muenke coronal synostosis syndrome. Eur J Hum Genet. 2006;14:39–48.
9. Gurjar V, Parushetti A, Gurjar M. Freeman-sheldon syndrome presenting with microstomia: a case report and literature review. J Maxillofac Oral Surg. 2013;12(4):395–9.
10. Forsythe E, Beales PL. Bardet-Biedl syndrome. Eur J Hum Genet. 2013;21(1):8–13.
11. Mehta PA, Tolar J. Fanconi anemia. [updated 2018]. GeneReviews® [Internet]. Seattle, WA: University of Washington, Seattle; 2002. p. 1993–2018.
12. Krauser AF, Schury MP. Holt Oram syndrome StatPearls [Internet]. Treasure Island, FL: StatPearls Publishing; 2018.
13. Chen Y, Liu Z, Chen J, Zuo Y, Liu S, Chen W, Liu G, Qiu G, Giampietro PF, Wu N, Wu Z. The genetic landscape and clinical implications of vertebral anomalies in VACTERL association. J Med Genet. 2016;53:431–7.
14. Dave KV, Patel SC, Dudhia BB, Panja P. Orofacial digital syndrome. Indian J Dent Res. 2013;24(1):132–5.
15. Kline AD, Moss JF, Selicorni A, Bisgaard AM, Deardorff MA, Gillett PM, Ishman SL, Kerr LM, Levin AV, Mulder PA, Ramos FJ, Wierzba J, Ajmone PF, Axtell D, Blagowidow N, Cereda A, Costantino A, Cormier-Daire V, FitzPatrick D, Grados M, Groves L, Guthrie W, Huisman S, Kaiser FJ, Koekkoek G, Levis M, Mariani M, McCleery JP, Menke LA, Metrena A, O'Connor J, Oliver C, Pie J, Piening S, Potter CJ, Quaglio AL, Redeker E, Richman D, Rigamonti C, Shi A, Tümer Z, Van Balkom IDC, Hennekam RC. Diagnosis and management of Cornelia de Lange syndrome: first international consensus statement. Nat Rev Genet. 2018;19:649.
16. Hennekam RC. Rubinstein-Taybi syndrome. Eur J Hum Genet. 2009;14(9):981–5.
17. Nowaczyk MJ, Irons MB. Smith-Lemli-Opitz syndrome: phenotype, natural history, and epidemiology. Am J Med Genet C Semin Med Genet. 2012;160C(4):250–62.
18. Biesecker LG. The Greig cephalopolysyndactyly syndrome. Orphanet J Rare Dis. 2008;24:3–10.
19. Okamoto N. Ectodactyly-ectodermal dysplasia-clefting syndrome. Ryoikibetsu Shokogun Shirizu. 2001;33:615–7.
20. Ahmed H, Akbari H, Emami A, Akbari MR. Genetic overview of syndactyly and polydactyly. Plast Reconstr Surg Glob Open. 2017;5(11):e1549.
21. Durmaz AA, Karaca E, Demkow U, Toruner G, Schoumans J, Cogulu O. Evolution of genetic techniques: past, present, and beyond. Biomed Res Int. 2015;2015:461524.
22. Lee H, Deignan JL, Dorrani N, Strom SP, Kantarci S, Quintero-Rivera F, Das K, Toy T, Harry B, Yourshaw M, Fox M, Fogel BL, Martinez-Agosto JA, Wong DA, Chang VY, Shieh PB, Palmer CG, Dipple KM, Grody WW, Vilain E, Nelson SF. Clinical exome sequencing for genetic identification of rare Mendelian disorders. JAMA. 2014;312:1880–7.
23. Valencia CA, Husami A, Holle J, Johnson JA, Qian Y, Mathur A, Wei C, Indugula SR, Zou F, Meng H, Wang L, Li X, Fisher R, Tan T, Hogart Begtrup A, Collins K, Wusik KA, Neilson D, Burrow T, Schorry E, Hopkin R, Keddache M, Harley JB, Kaufman KM, Zhang K. Clinical impact and cost-effectiveness of whole-exome sequencing as a diagnostic tool: a pediatric center's experience. Front Pediatr. 2015;3:67.
24. Monroe GR, Frederix GW, Savelberg SM, de Vries TI, Duran KJ, van der Smagt JJ, Terhal PA, van Hasselt P, Kroes HY, Verhoeven-Duif NM, Nijman IJ, Carbo EC, van Gassen KL, Knoers NV, Hövels AM, van Haelst MM, Visser G, van Haaften G. Effectiveness of whole-exome sequencing and costs of the traditional diagnostic trajectory in children with intellectual disability. Genet Med. 2016;18:949–56.

25. Stark Z, Tan TY, Chong B, Brett GR, Yap P, Walsh M, Yeung A, Peters H, Mordaunt D, Cowie S, Amor DJ, Savarirayan R, McGillivray G, Downie L, Ekert PG, Theda C, James PA, Yaplito-Lee J, Ryan MM, Leventer RJ, Creed E, Macciocca I, Bell KM, Oshlack A, Sadedin S, Georgeson P, Anderson C, Thorne N, Melbourne Genomics Health Alliance, Gaff C, White SM. A prospective evaluation of whole-exome sequencing as a first-tier molecular test in infants with suspected monogenic disorders. Genet Med. 2016;18:1090–6.
26. Levenson D. Whole-exome sequencing strategy proposed as first-line test. Am J Med Genet. 2016:1387–8.
27. Thevenon J, Duffourd Y, Masurel-Paulet A. Diagnostic odyssey in severe neurodevelopmental disorders: toward clinical whole-exome sequencing as a first-line diagnostic test. Clin Genet. 2016;89:700–7.

4 Paediatric Trigger Finger

Chiara Novelli and Giorgio Pajardi

Abstract

Paediatric trigger thumb and trigger finger represent distinct conditions and should not be treated like adult-acquired trigger finger. Paediatric trigger thumb presents not at birth but early in childhood. Recently, our understanding of the pathophysiology of paediatric trigger thumb and paediatric trigger finger has improved leading to a better understanding of the problem and of its treatment. Paediatric trigger thumb may spontaneously resolve with splint, although in several years. Open surgical release of the A1 pulley of the thumb is an alternative option that nearly uniformly restores thumb interphalangeal joint motion. Paediatric trigger finger usually requires surgical approach; isolated release of the A1 pulley has been associated with high recurrence rates. Awareness of the anatomic factors that may contribute to triggering in the paediatric finger and willingness to explore and address other involved components of the flexor mechanism can prevent surgical failure.

Keywords

Congenital trigger · Trigger finger · Trigger thumb · Splinting

Trigger thumb is one of the most common paediatric hand conditions and responds universally to simple surgical release; however, trigger fingers are more complex, often owing to systemic conditions or anatomical abnormalities, and require consequently a wide and ample treatment.

Paediatric trigger thumb is a common condition. The reported specific incidence has increased from one in 2000 new-borns two decades ago to 3.3 in 1000 in a recent report [1]. It often presents in children at about 24 months, but can occur earlier, some times at about 6 months, or later. Reports of siblings and twins with trigger thumbs are common and some patients report a positive family history, which suggests a possible genetic predisposition [2, 3].

The aetiology of trigger thumb in children remains uncertain. The main accredited hypothesis is that there is an anatomical mismatch between the diameter of the tendon sheath and the diameter of the flexor pollicis longus (FPL) tendon.

Khoshhal et al. [4] examined specimens from the A1 pulley of children who had undergone trigger thumb release and found both myofibroblasts and cyto-contractile proteins (vimentin and a-smooth muscle actin). The authors suggested

C. Novelli (✉) · G. Pajardi
Department of Hand Surgery and Rehabilitation, S. Giuseppe Hospital IRCCS MultiMedica, Milan University, Milan, Italy
e-mail: chiara.novelli@multimedica.it; gpajardi@centrostudimano.it

G. Pajardi (ed.), *Pediatric Hand Surgery*, https://doi.org/10.1007/978-3-031-30984-7_4

from these findings that trigger thumbs result from a developmental fibrous tissue proliferation at the A1 pulley. A recent ultrasound study of children with trigger thumbs demonstrated no abnormalities of the FPL tendon or the A1 pulley, but confirm the size mismatch between the cross-sectional area of the tendon compared with that of the pulley [5].

The condition normally presents with a fixed flexed thumb interphalangeal joint (IPJ), with the presence of a small nodule on the volar face of the metacarpo-phalangeal joint (MPJ), Notta nodule (Fig. 4.1). Sometimes it is possible to find some cases in which thumb is fixed in extended position, with impossibility to reach IPJ flexion; normally these are cases in which, when the baby performs the full flexion, he feels discomfort so he avoids any movement.

The relatives find the condition accidentally because the triggering is painless. In the first phases often, babies resolve themselves the triggering, being able to play and to be completely autonomous; even later when the finger is fixed in flexion it does not produce any functional limitation, but babies show to relatives the 'strange condition'.

Sometimes it is supposed to be the result of a trauma or of a subluxation, but normal radiograms and ultrasound exclude it. Moreover, the presence of Notta nodule is diriment. But more often relatives discover the condition after a light trauma because they focus for the first time on their baby's thumb.

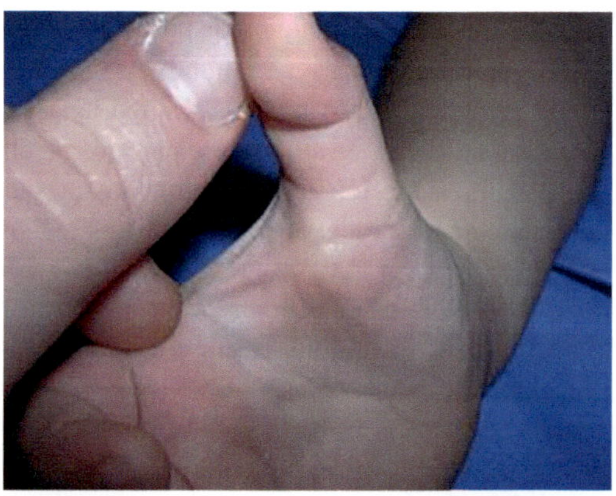

Fig. 4.1 "Notta's" nodule in paediatric trigger thumb

The differential diagnosis of trigger thumb includes congenital clasped thumb and thumb-in-palm deformity resulting from cerebral palsy or arthrogryposis, even if in expert eyes the clinical conditions are completely different. The single congenital condition that could really mimic trigger finger is congenital absence of extensor pollicis longus, condition that presents with a IPJ flexion, but this last case presents no dorsal crease in the IPJ, and no Notta nodule.

Regarding to treatment there's no uniqueness direction.

Normally instructions vary from a first period of 3 to 6 months of splinting to open surgical release in cases of splinting failure.

Exploring the literature [6] some authors suggested that all the therapeutic attitudes could be considered correct and could in some way lead to problem resolution. They analyze results of simple observation, versus stretching and exercises, versus night splinting with or without daily exercises versus open surgery, and find out that all the series lead in some way to different percentage of clinical resolution, evidently in different periods of time treatment.

Anyway investigating correctly the data, it is evident that splinting or observations or stretching leads to a complete resolution preferentially in mild cases, and normally resolution is obtained with longer treatments.

On the contrary, open surgery leads in the majority of cases to percentage of high recovery in a shorter time with really low or none rate of complications. In sight of this consideration, our conduct begins with correct information of the relatives on all the possibilities, and with suggestion of an initial period of night splinting and in cases of incomplete recovery the purpose of open surgical release.

Normally relatives accept willingly the period of orthesis to try to have a simple way towards resolution. Anyway usually, due to little compliance of the babies and to prospective of really long treatments, relatives usually switches happily to a surgical solution.

Surgery is quite simple, it could be performed under slight sedation and local anaesthesia. It provides a small transversal incision at the MPJ

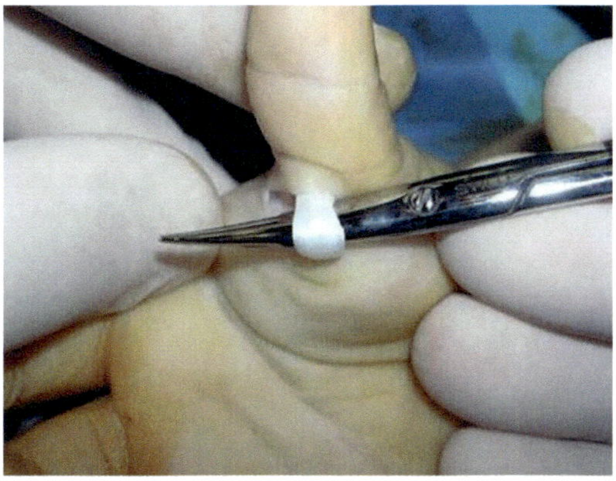

Fig. 4.3 Surgical procedure for thumb a1 pulley release

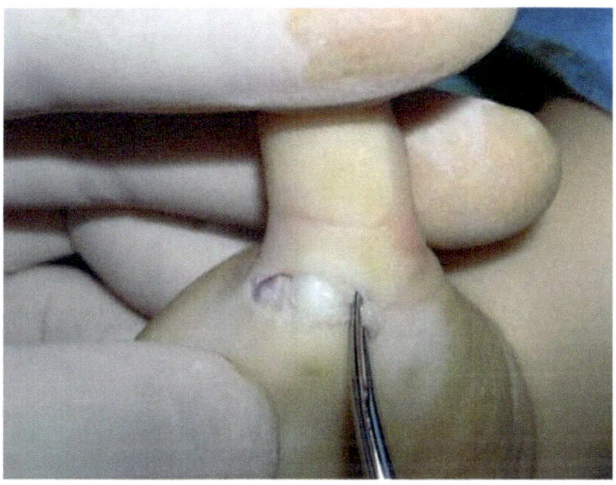

Fig. 4.2 Surgical procedure for thumb a1 pulley release

volar surface of the thumb, the identification of the tight A1 pulley and its surgical release (Figs. 4.2 and 4.3). Often it is possible to identify the Notta nodule, but once the pulley is open no procedures are required on the nodule. Immediately after the complete pulley releases, the finger shows complete extension of IPJ.

Regarding outcomes, a systematic review of outcomes reported on 17 retrospective studies and 1 prospective study of trigger thumb treatments. The authors found full IP joint motion reported in 95% of patients treated surgically, 67% treated with orthesis and 55% treated with exercise and concluded that open surgery yields the most reliable outcomes [6].

A recent large retrospective review of 173 consecutive patients treated with surgical release of trigger thumb demonstrated full extension in all thumbs with IP joint hyperextension in 6, no recurrences and no digital nerve injuries [7].

A total of 79 families returned questionnaires at an average of 4 years after their children's surgery. Ninety-nine percent of parents who responded to the survey would recommend the surgery for other children with trigger thumbs.

Recurrence of paediatric trigger thumb after open release is negligible provided that the release is complete at the time of surgery.

Moreover, surgical release can lead to good outcomes even several years after the presentation as literature reported [8].

A potential complication is injury to the radial digital nerve during surgical dissection. Careful placement of the incision and careful dissection render this evenience really minimal.

4.1 Trigger Finger

Paediatric, or congenital, trigger finger, presents as a digit, other than the thumb, that locks in flexion.

As paediatric trigger thumb, although described as congenital by some authors, there are no clear records of this condition being present at birth [9, 10]. It has been reported as presenting between the ages of 3 weeks and 11 yrs [11]. Many papers suggest the pathological cause is due to anatomic anomalies but this does make it hard to explain why the condition presents with a delay and not at birth.

The management of this condition has varied from conservative splinting [12, 13] to operative exploration and correction of the offending structures [11, 14, 15].

There is no really clear literature on outcomes of splinting in trigger finger due to the fact that literature compares often conservative treatment of series of trigger thumb and trigger finger together, rendering not pure the analisis [9, 12, 16].

What is clear from literature [14], is that aetiology of congenital trigger finger is different from congenital trigger thumb and adults' condition. It is reported that anatomic mechanical condition such as mutual relationships among flexor digitorum profundus (FDP) and flexor digitorum superficialis (FDS), or anatomical anomalies of pulleys causes and sustains the triggering. So that the application of the operative principles applied in paediatric trigger thumb and adult trigger finger consisting in releasing of the A1 pulley only could lead to insufficient results.

Children who present with trigger fingers could have an underlying condition responsible for the triggering. Triggering has been associated with mucopolysaccharidosis, juvenile rheumatoid arthritis, Ehlers–Danlos syndrome, down syndrome and central nervous system disorders such as delayed motor development [14, 17–19].

In addition to generalized syndromes, which should be checked in the diagnostic pathway, there are multiple anatomic anomalies that have been described as causes of the pathology. The predisposing anatomic problem can either be overcrowding of the contents of the sheath or a narrow pulley system. These anatomical conditions could be widely listed below:

- Tendon structural anomaly (Nodule on FDS/FDP; Widening of FDS/FDP).
- Abnormal relationship between FDS/FDP (Decussation of the FDS proximal to A1 pulley; Aberrant attachments between FDS/FDP; FDS ulnar or radial slip abnormality; aberrant lumbrical muscles such as insertion of the lumbrical into the FDS).
- Thickening or stenosis of the pulley system (A1; A2; A3).

In view of these findings, surgery is quite often indicated and a step-wise approach through a Bruner's incision is therefore necessary.

Surgery could be performed under a soft sedation and local anaesthesia. The surgical approach allows the possibility to have a complete view of the flexor apparatus; either tendon structures and pulley system must be carefully analized or triggering must be evocated during surgery in order to be sure that the procedure undertaken has eliminated each possible cause of tendon friction (Figs. 4.4, 4.5, and 4.6).

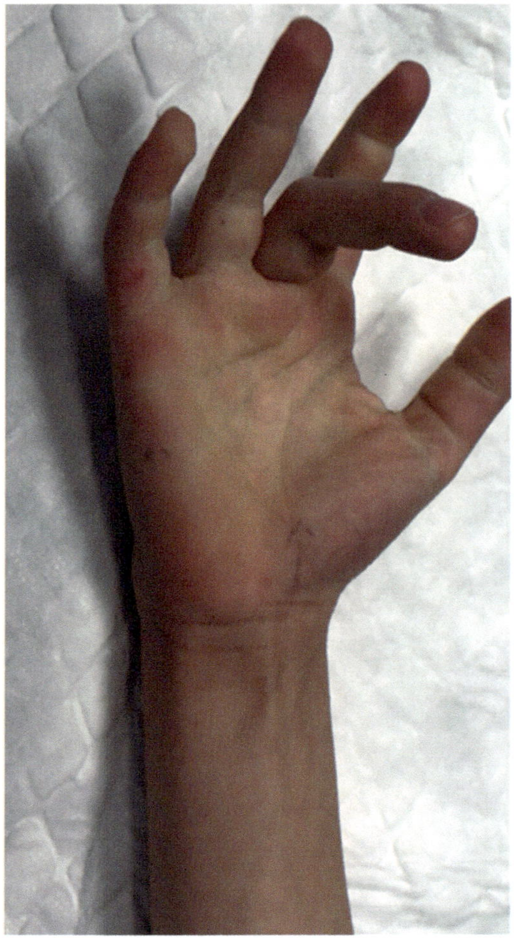

Fig. 4.4 Clinical condition of paediatric trigger digits

Some authors have suggested an algorithm that should be used during surgery in order to

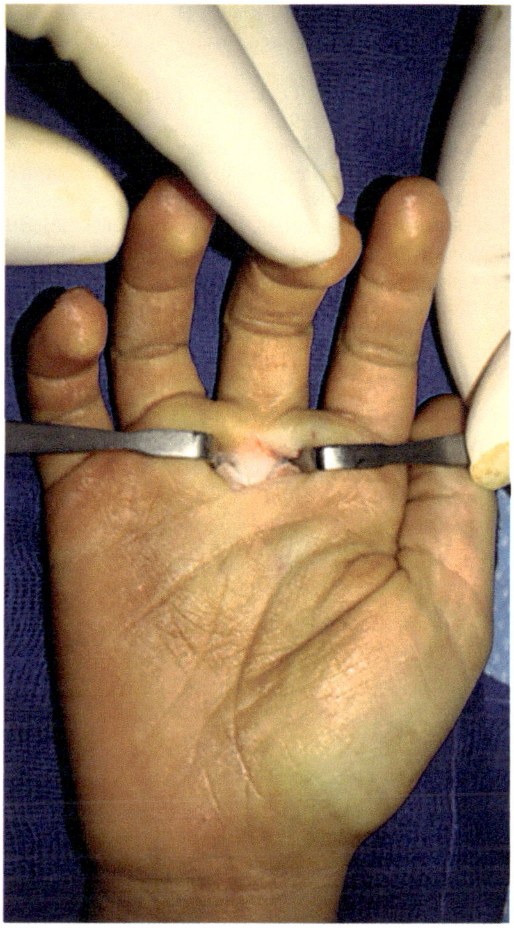

Fig. 4.5 Intraoperatory findings: surgical approcach

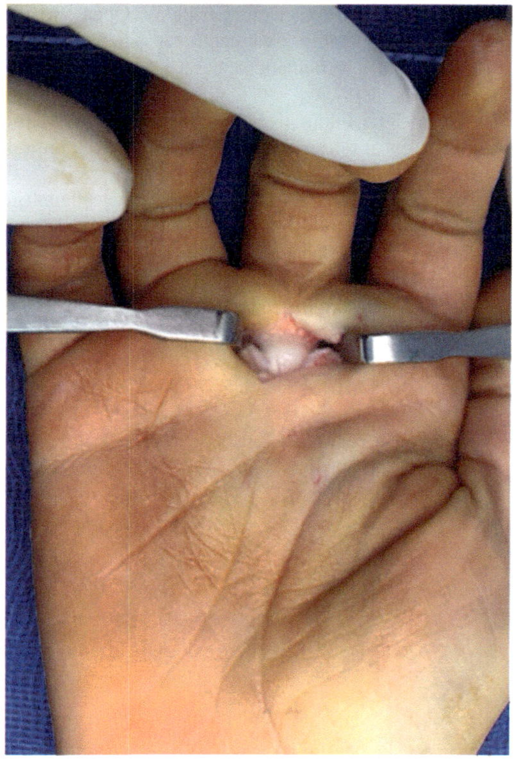

Fig. 4.6 Intraoperatory findings: FDS intratendinous cysts

explore and test all the possible conditions involved in triggering and to release them minimizing all the possibility of recurrences.

Literature focusing on the operative management of this condition, and focusing on paediatric trigger finger alone, [9–11, 14] has placed weight on three factors (1) conservative management is unlikely to work in the long-term as this is an anatomic problem; (2) unlike paediatric trigger thumb and trigger finger in the adult population, release of the A1 pulley alone may not relieve symptoms; and (3) a more extensive surgical exposure is required and failure to recognize this will lead to inadequate release with recurrence of the condition.

Intra-operative findings will dictate the extent of surgical exposure and which structures need release or correction.

References

1. Kikuchi N, Ogino T. Incidence and development of trigger thumb in children. J Hand Surg Am. 2006;31(4):541–3.
2. Slakey JB, Hennrikus WL. Acquired thumbflexion contracture in children: congenital trigger thumb. J Bone Joint Surg Br. 1996;78(3):481–3.
3. Shim VC, Admire AA, Heidenreich RA, Samimi KJ. Autosomal dominant inheritance pattern for trigger thumb. Plast Reconstr Surg. 2002;109(1):240–1.
4. Khoshhal KI, Jarvis JG, Uhthoff HK. Congenital trigger thumb in children: electron microscopy and immunohistochemical analysis of the first annular pulley. J Pediatr Orthop B. 2012;21(4):295–9.
5. Verma M, Craig CL, DiPietro MA, et al. Serial ultrasound evaluation of pediatric trigger thumb. J Pediatr Orthop. 2013;33(3):309–13.

6. Farr S, Grill F, Ganger R, Girsch W. Open surgery versus nonoperative treatments for paediatric trigger thumb: a systematic review. J Hand Surg Eur. 2014;39(7):719–26.
7. Marek DJ, Fitoussi F, Bohn DC, Van Heest AE. Surgical release of the pediatric trigger thumb. J Hand Surg Am. 2011;36(4):647–652.e2.
8. Han SH, Yoon HK, Shin DE, Song DG. Trigger thumb in children: results of surgical treatment in children above 5 years of age. J Pediatr Orthop. 2010;30(7):710–4.
9. Moon WN, Suh SW, Kim IC. Trigger digits in children. J Hand Surg Br. 2001;26:11–2.
10. Rodgers WB, Waters PM. Incidence of trigger digits in newborns. J Hand Surg Am. 1994;19:364–8.
11. Cardon LJ, Ezaki M, Carter PR. Trigger finger in children. J Hand Surg. 1999;24A:1156–61.
12. Nemoto K, Nemoto T, Terada N, et al. Splint therapy for trigger thumb and finger in children. J Hand Surg Br. 1996;21:416–8.
13. Tsuyuguchi Y, Tada K, Kawaii H. Splint therapy for trigger finger in children. Arch Phys Med Rehabil. 1983;64:75–6.
14. Tordai P, Engkvist O. Trigger fingers in children. J Hand Surg Am. 1999;24:1162–5.
15. Steenwerckx A, De Smet L, Fabry G. Congenital trigger digit. J Hand Surg Am. 1996;21:909–11.
16. Paaske BP, Søe-Nielsen NH, Noer HH. Release of trigger finger in children. Long term results. Scand J Plast Reconstr Surg Hand Surg. 1995;29:65–7.
17. Cardon LJ, Ezaki M, Carter PR. Trigger finger in children. J Hand Surg Am. 1999;24(6):1156–61.
18. Cheung JP, Fung BK, Mak KC, Leung KH. Multiple triggering in a girl with Ehlers-Danlos syndrome: case report. J Hand Surg Am. 2010;35(10):1675–7.
19. Van Heest AE, House J, Krivit W, Walker K. Surgical treatment of carpal tunnel syndrome and trigger digits in children with mucopolysaccharide storage disorders. J Hand Surg Am. 1998;23(2):236–43.

5 Camptodactyly

Chiara Parolo, Elisa Rosanda, and Giorgio Pajardi

Abstract

Camptodactyly is a relatively rare hand anomaly that involves varying degrees of congenital or acquired flexion contracture of the fingers at the proximal interphalangeal (PIP) joint, unilaterally or bilaterally. The cause of the deformity is obscure. Specific anatomic abnormalities have been implicated. Camptodactyly can also be divided into *simple* and *complex* types. Simple camptodactyly consists only of the flexion deformity of the PIP joint, whereas in complex camptodactyly, there are also other deformities such as syndactyly or combinations of clinodactyly and camptodactyly. Treatment can be either conservative, surgical or a combination regimen in which only certain patients undergo surgery, depending on its clinical severity. Nonoperative treatment is favoured in most cases whereby the PIP contracture is less than 40 degrees, and it includes passive stretching and splinting. Outcomes are variable but more favourable with early intervention.

Surgery should be reserved for patients with a preoperative PIP joint contracture of more than 60°.

Keywords

Camptodactyly · Flexion contracture · Stiffness · Flexion deformity · Hand anomaly

Camptodactyly was first described by Tamplin in 1846 in his 'Lectures on the Nature and Treatment of Deformities' at the Royal Orthopaedic Hospital, London. The term camptodactyly is of Greek origin means 'bent finger' and was used by Landouzy in 1906 to describe an irreducible flexion contracture affecting the proximal interphalangeal (PIP) joints in young girls.

Camptodactyly is a relatively rare hand anomaly that involves varying degrees of congenital or acquired flexion contracture of the fingers at the proximal interphalangeal (PIP) joint, unilaterally or bilaterally (Fig. 5.1). The metacarpophalangeal (MCP) and distal interphalangeal (DIP) joints are not affected, although compensatory deformities may develop. Involvement of either the distal interphalangeal joint or the metacarpophalangeal joint suggests a post-traumatic cause rather than camptodactyly. Likewise, camptodactyly should not be confused with Kirner's deformity or with clinodactyly. Contractures may be present at birth or develop in childhood or even adulthood; they may be stationary or progressive.

C. Parolo (✉) · E. Rosanda
Milan, Italy
e-mail: chiara.parolo@multimedica.it; elisa.rosanda@multimedica.it

G. Pajardi
Department of Hand Surgery and Rehabilitation, S. Giuseppe Hospital IRCCS MultiMedica, Milan University, Milan, Italy
e-mail: gpajardi@centrostudimano.it

G. Pajardi (ed.), *Pediatric Hand Surgery*, https://doi.org/10.1007/978-3-031-30984-7_5

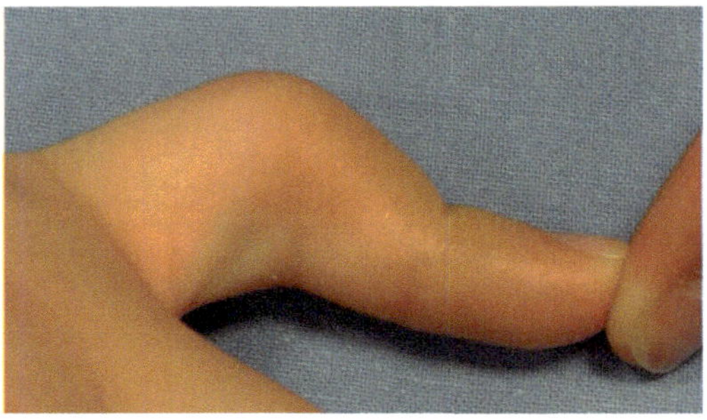

Fig. 5.1 Camptodactyly

The fifth finger is most commonly involved although the incidence decreases toward the radial side of the hand.

Camptodactyly can occur independently or have a syndromic association. Recently, several syndromes that include finger contractures along with many other features have been given a primary designation of camptodactyly, which may be confusing. These include Tel Hashomer camptodactyly syndrome (camptodactyly, distinctive facial features, dermatoglyphic changes and musculoskeletal anomalies), which is inherited in inbred Arab and Brazilian families in autosomal recessive manner; Guadalajara camptodactyly I (camptodactyly, intrauterine growth retardation, mental retardation, unusual facies and musculoskeletal anomalies), which is inherited as an autosomal recessive; and Guadalajara camptodactyly II (camptodactyly, intrauterine growth retardation, mental retardation, short second toe and musculoskeletal changes), which is inherited as an autosomal recessive disorder. In addition, camptodactyly has been reported as a recessive disorder with ichthyosis, and as a dominant with scoliosis, with symphalangism and with brachydactyly.

Camptodactyly is seen as a feature of more than 50 conditions and is frequently associated with chromosomal anomalies.

The prevalence is less than 1% although De Haas reported an incidence varying from 2 in 3000 to 58 in 239. The location is unilateral in 33% of cases or bilateral in 66%. Bilateral camptodactyly can be either symmetric or asymmetric. Camptodactyly can have an early or late onset, and it has been proven to show an autosomal dominant pattern of inheritance with variable expressivity and incomplete penetrance.

5.1 Pathogenesis

The cause of the deformity is obscure. Hereditary factors, tuberculosis, rheumatoid disease and ischemia have been cited in the literature. Specific anatomic abnormalities have been implicated including abnormal lumbricals; abnormal (adherent, hypoplastic) flexor digitorum superficialis (FDS) insertion, which is often accompanied by subsequent or associated skin shortening; tight fascial bands; a deficient dorsal central slip extensor mechanism; and changes in the distal interphalangeal joint or metacarpophalangeal joint. Todd stated that the stiffness of the joint seemed to be entirely due to changes in the soft tissue parts and that the principal contracture seemed to be in the capsule of the joint. Oldfield also blamed the soft tissue on the flexor surface of the affected fingers. The FDS has been implicated as a significant factor by Stoddard (abnormal shortness), Scott (tight flexor tendon under the skin), Herbert (slow retraction of the flexor tendon) and Smith and Kaplan (contracture of FDS). McFarlane et al. suggested that an abnormal lumbrical insertion is the major deforming force. Korean et al. believed that extensor mechanism anomalies are primary and the palmar manifestations of a tight FDS tendon and contractures of the palmar soft tissue are secondary. Millesi believed that abnormal development of the central slip and dorsal aponeurosis over the PIP joint was the cause of flexion contracture deformity. The theory of disturbed equilibrium between flexor and extensor forces has been accepted by Engber and Flatt, Koman et al. and Miura et al., although the primary cause is still unclear. McCash pointed out three main factors: skin shortage on the volar side, congenital fibrous substrate present beneath the skin and muscle imbalance.

5.2 Classification

Camptodactyly has been divided into three categories (Table 5.1). A type I deformity is the most common form and becomes apparent during infancy. The deformity is usually an isolated finding that is limited to the small finger. This 'congenital' form affects males and females equally. A type II deformity has similar clinical features, although they are not apparent until preadolescence. This 'acquired' form of camptodactyly develops between the ages of 7 and 11 years and affects females more than males. This type of camptodactyly usually does not improve spontaneously and may progress to a severe flexion deformity. A type III deformity is often a severe deformity that usually involves multiple digits of both extremities and is associated with a variety of syndromes. This 'syndromic camptodactyly' can occur in conjunction with craniofacial disorders, short stature, and chromosomal abnormalities.

Camptodactyly can also be divided into *simple* and *complex* types. Simple camptodactyly consists only of the flexion deformity of the PIP joint, whereas in complex camptodactyly, there are also other deformities such as syndactyly or combinations of clinodactyly and camptodactyly.

According to Foucher, camptodactyly can be classified as follows (Table 5.2).

TYPE IA early presentation and fix contracture.

Table 5.1 Benson classification of camptodactyly

Type	Manifestation	Description
I	Congenital	Apparent during infancy. Usually limited to the fifth finger.
II	Preadolescence	Develops between the ages of 7 and 11 years. Does not improve spontaneously and may progress to a severe flexion deformity of 90 degrees.
III	Syndromic	Multiple digits of both extremities are affected. Associated with a variety of syndromes, such as craniofacial disorders, short stature, and chromosomal abnormalities.

Table 5.2 Classification of Foucher

Classification	
TYPE IA	Early and stiff
TYPE IB	Early and correctable
TYPE IIA	Late and stiff
TYPE IIB	Late and correctable
TYPE III	First ray camptodactyly
TYPE IV	Camptodactyly in Syndromes

Goffin D, Lenoble E, Marin-Broun F, Foucher G. Camptodactylie: classification et résultats thérapeutiques d'une sérle de 50 cas. Ann. Chir. Main 20:13, 1994

TYPE IB early presentation and passively correctable flexion deformity.

TYPE IIA late presentation and fix contracture.

TYPE IIB late presentation and passively correctable flexion deformity.

TYPE III first ray camptodactyly.

TYPE IV camptodactyly in syndromes.

5.3 Clinical Exam

Symptoms often go unnoticed, as usually only the small finger is affected and is very rarely associated with any significant compromise in function.

Camptodactyly is typically painless and without motor/sensory deficits. This condition often does not cause functional impairment, meaning that patients seek medical attention for concerns relating to cosmesis.

The PIP joint is assessed for extension lag and flexion contracture with the wrist in neutral position. Extension lag is the maximum extension measurement when performing *active* motion testing. Flexion contracture is the maximum extension measurement when performing *passive* motion testing. A perfectly straight PIP joint is considered to have 0 degrees of lag or contracture. Extension lag and flexion contracture measurements are not mutually exclusive. A joint may have an extension lag of 60 degrees, but passive testing may reveal a joint correctable to a 30-degree flexion contracture.

Assessing the finger with the metacarpophalangeal (MCP) in flexion and extension is performed next. For patients with camptodactyly, when the MCP joint is in extension the finger assumes a flexed posture at the PIP. Passive extension of the PIP may produce blanching of the skin, which implies a skin deficiency. Additionally, if passive flexion of the MCP improves PIP extension, the aetiology of the contracture is outside the PIP joint. This can mean skin deficiency, subcutaneous fibrous bands, or tightness of the extrinsic finger flexors, principally the FDS. If passive extension is not improved with MCP flexion, there is some component of primary joint contracture that will need to be surgically addressed.

A compensatory hyperextension deformity of the MCP is frequently found with a PIP flexion deformity. With the Bouvier manoeuvre, the examiner corrects the hyperextension by passively placing the MCP in neutral or slight flexion. If this restores full PIP active extension, this implies the MCP hyperextension as the cause of the PIP flexion deformity and may be secondary to an intrinsic muscle abnormality. An FDS transfer to the lateral band is the procedure of choice. This increases MCP flexion and PIP extension forces.

For patients with passively correctable flexion deformities, the extensor tenodesis effect is checked to assess the extrinsic extensor integrity. The wrist is placed in full flexion along with full flexion of the MCP joints. In a normal finger, this manoeuvre should produce full PIP extension through passive stretch on extensor digitorum communis. If it does not, this implies a laxity or hypoplasia of the central slip.

The FDS of the little and ring finger may have a tendinous interconnection, which prohibits independent PIP joint flexion of the little finger. Classically, if a patient cannot flex the little finger while holding the ring finger in full extension, this is thought to mean an absence of an FDS to the little finger. The test should be repeated with the liberation of the ring finger and similar assessment of active PIP joint flexion. If the patient is able to isolate PIP flexion of the ring finger and the small finger simultaneously flexes at the PIP, this indicates an interconnected FDS. The small finger FDS must be separated from the ring finger at the time of surgery to be a suitable donor for transfer.

During the physical exam flexion deformity of small finger PIP joint with a flexible (correctable) or fixed (non-correctable) deformity that progressively worsens over time if untreated and may rapidly worsen during growth spurts.

Typically in camptodactyly, strength, sensation and perfusion are normal. DIP and MCP joint alignment are normal however compensatory contractures can develop. No swelling, erythema or warmth associated with inflammation are noticed.

Radiographs are often normal, especially in early stages. In later stages, a decrease in the proximal phalangeal head convexity can be noticed and a volar subluxation can occur (Fig. 5.2).

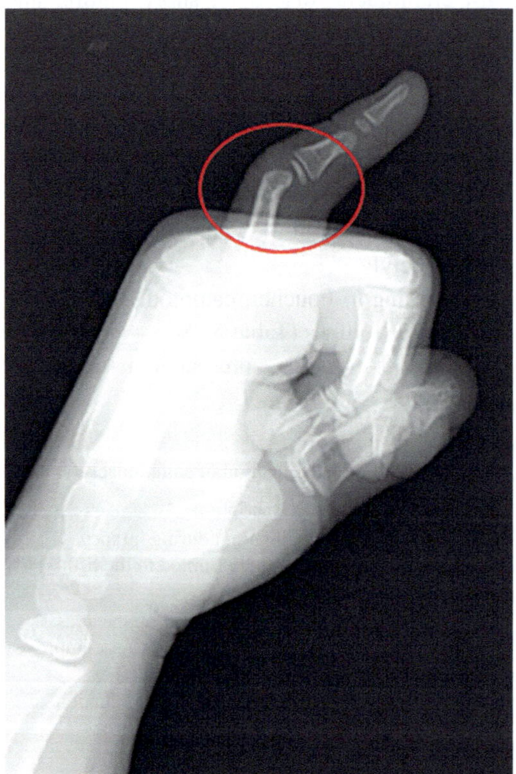

Fig. 5.2 Proximal phalangeal head convexity in Camptodactyly

5.4 Treatment

Treatment can be either conservative, surgical or a combination regimen in which only certain patients undergo surgery, depending on its clinical severity. These diverse techniques range from splinting or stretching exercises to release of tendons, fascial bands, muscle transfer and tenotomy.

Nonoperative treatment is favoured in most cases whereby the PIP contracture is less than 40 degrees, and it includes *passive stretching and splinting*. Outcomes are variable, but more favourable with early intervention.

Surgery should be reserved for patients with a preoperative PIP joint contracture of more than 60°. Operative treatment includes *FDS tenotomy ± FDS transfer*. It is indicated when the deformity is progressive and leading to functional impairment. FDS tenotomy or FDS transfer to radial lateral band is indicated if full active PIP extension can be achieved with MCP flexion.

Osteotomy or arthrodesis is indicated in severe fixed deformities.

Hori et al. advocated using a dynamic splint worn 24 h a day until full extension of the PIP joint was achieved, followed by a regimen in which the splint is worn 8 h a day. Contracture tended to recur when the dynamic splint was no longer used. This raises the question of when to tell the patient to stop wearing the splint. Siegert et al. performed release of the FDS according to Smith and Kaplan's recommendations, which was followed by a palmar capsulotomy and collateral ligament release if necessary (Figs. 5.3 and 5.4). Engber and Flatt advocated a combination of volar soft tissue releases: some combination of skin, subcutaneous tissue, flexor tendon sheath, FDS, PIP collateral ligament and volar plate release. Osteotomy was used occasionally.

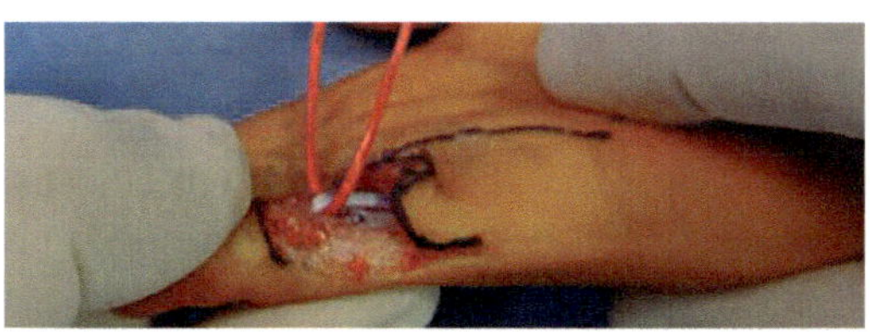

Fig. 5.3 Collateral band release

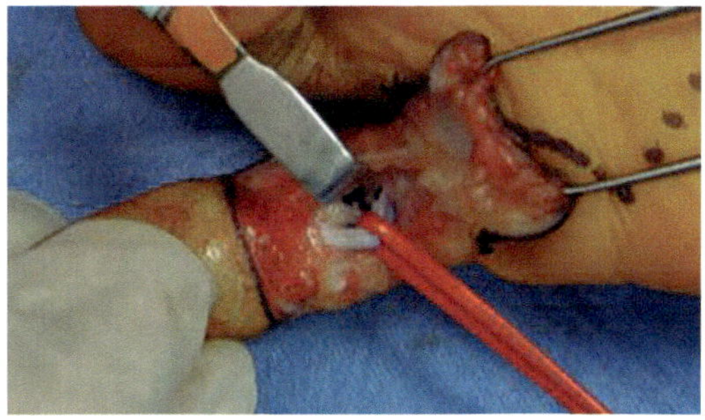

Fig. 5.4 Palmar capsulotomy

Various tendon transfers and lengthenings have been used. McFarlane et al. advocated FDS transfer of the fifth finger to the extensor mechanism after an anomalous insertion of the lumbrical muscle had been sought. Koman et al. lengthened or transferred the FDS tendon and reconstructed the extensor mechanism. Gupta and Burke recommended the extensor indicis proprius (EIP) transfer to the radial side of the extensor expansion in an attempt to strengthen the intrinsic action. Results of treatment are difficult to compare owing to lack of objective data in most studies. McFarlane et al. reported perfect results in 22% of cases after 1 year.

Preoperative joint contractures play an important role both in treatment indications and outcomes. We now reserve surgical intervention for cases with PIP joint contracture of more than 60°. Surgery on patients who have minor contractures is more likely to produce complications than to produce benefits. Postoperative rehabilitation is important, as loss of flexion is a disaster. It is also important to instil a sense of realism in patients at the onset of treatment by explaining that they will be fortunate to obtain a correction of the deformity and that if they do, they should regard it as an unexpected bonus. It should be explained that the real aim of surgery should be to prevent further progressive deterioration.

5.5 Conservative Treatment

In our department, different types of splints are used based on the classification of Foucher. For reducible contractures (type IA) a static night

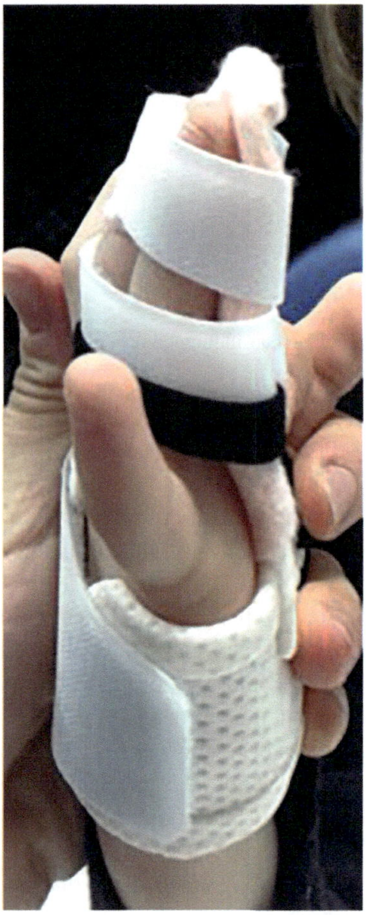

Fig. 5.5 Static splint

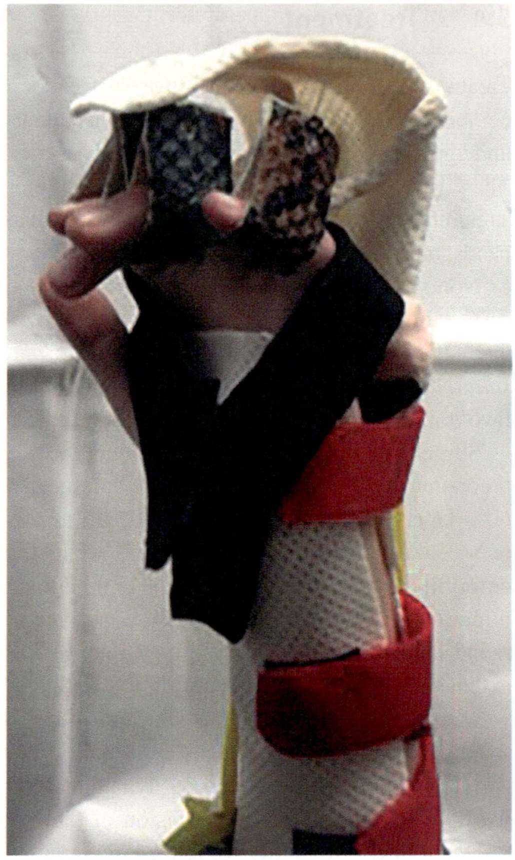

Fig. 5.6 Dynamic splint

splint is used (Fig. 5.5), while for irreducible ones (type IB) a dynamic splint in extension with circular base module, wrist included and Levame type bar as dynamic tractions is custom made (Fig. 5.6). It is very important that the splint is worn correctly. The splint in PIP extension must have dorsal closure stabilizing the V metacarpal very well and positioning the MPJ at about 50° of flexion. In fact, in addition to the bending stiffness of the PIPJ, there is often a compensatory attitude in hypertension of the MPJ Furthermore, the dynamic bar must pull the middle phalanx on the proximal phalanx by means of a velcro ring with a perfectly perpendicular force.

The difficulty of realization is linked to the complexity of the orthosis and the size of the fifth finger of a child (or a newborn). The splint is often worn from the early months of life and used during the night and during the afternoon nap.

The initial choice of the type of splint is therefore not a definitive choice. A type IB camptodactyly may become reducible after a few months of treatment with the use of a dynamic splint and therefore a static type will be chosen. During development stiffness may recurr and a dynamic splint should be applied again.

5.6 Surgical Technique

A volar linear incision is used and converted to multiple z-plasties, placing the central limbs over the flexion creases of the joints. On reflecting the skin, the shortened retinaculum is visualized; it is released, including the bony attachment of Grayson's ligaments. At this stage, the lateral bands of the intrinsic apparatus and interosseous muscles are freed from their abnormal and widespread attachment to the sides of the proximal phalanx. It is this attachment that prevents the extension of the PIP joint. On its release, proximal pull on the lateral bands will confirm that PIP extension can now occur. Some attenuation of the central slip may have occurred and is probably secondary, as in other forms of prolonged PIP joint contracture. Its presence can be confirmed by the central slip tenodesis test. It involves flexing the wrist and the MP joints. In the normal hand, the PIP joint will automatically fully extend, owing to tension on the central slip insertion. If the central slip is attenuated, there will be an extensor lag at the PIP joint. In such patients, the central slip can be treated by appropriate postoperative splinting. The lumbrical muscle is abnormally inserted and often adherent to the proximal phalanx. It may also have an abnormal origin and occasionally may be inserted into the FDS tendon proximal to the A1 pulley. The FDS tendon is tested by a tenodesis test to ascertain whether it is short. If the PIP joint cannot be fully extended when the wrist is in extension, the FDS is short and must be released. Two types of FDS abnormalities exist: (1) one in which the FDS is merely short, and (2) the other in which only the distal portion of the FDS is present, there is proximal aplasia, and the distal part of the FDS acts as a tenodesis, producing a flexion contracture of the PIP joint. In such cases, complete surgical release by division is undertaken. A small minority may require release of the flexor tendon sheath, volar plate or even the accessory collateral ligaments. The central slip attenuation responds to postoperative extension splinting.

From 2002 to 2018, we have treated 54 patients and 88 fingers affected by camptodactyly.

In total, 59 fingers were affected by the flexible form. Twentynine fingers were affected by the rigid form.

A total of 85 fingers underwent conservative treatment (59 flexible and 26 fixed).

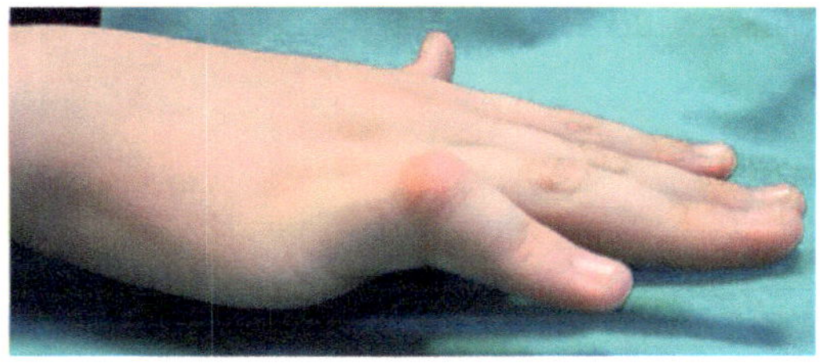

Fig. 5.7 Pre-op

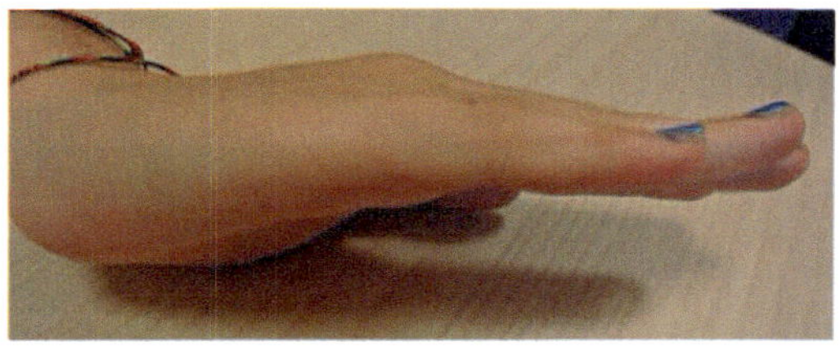

Fig. 5.8 Post-op

Among this series, 67 fingers concluded the conservative treatment with success (56 with no lack of extension—excellent result; 11 fingers with an extensor lag minor than 20°—good result) (Figs. 5.7 and 5.8). Conservative treatment failed in 18 fingers (lag of extension major than 20°). Ten fingers (seven from the conservative group plus three from the fixed group never treated with splinting) underwent surgery with a lag of extension of more than 40°.

Results were excellent in two digits (no lag of extension), good in three (lag of extension less than 20° and poor in five (lag of extension more than 20°) (Table 5.3).

In all of our series, there was an improvement after treatment and the quality of results depended upon the severity of the contracture and protocol compliance.

The conservative approach leads to gains in function. Hand therapy and custom-made splinting are essential to obtain and maintain improvement of passive extension and to regain active extension both in conservative and surgical treatment. Continuous monitoring, constant use of splints and manipulation are important to maintain the achieved results.

Table 5.3 Results of treatment

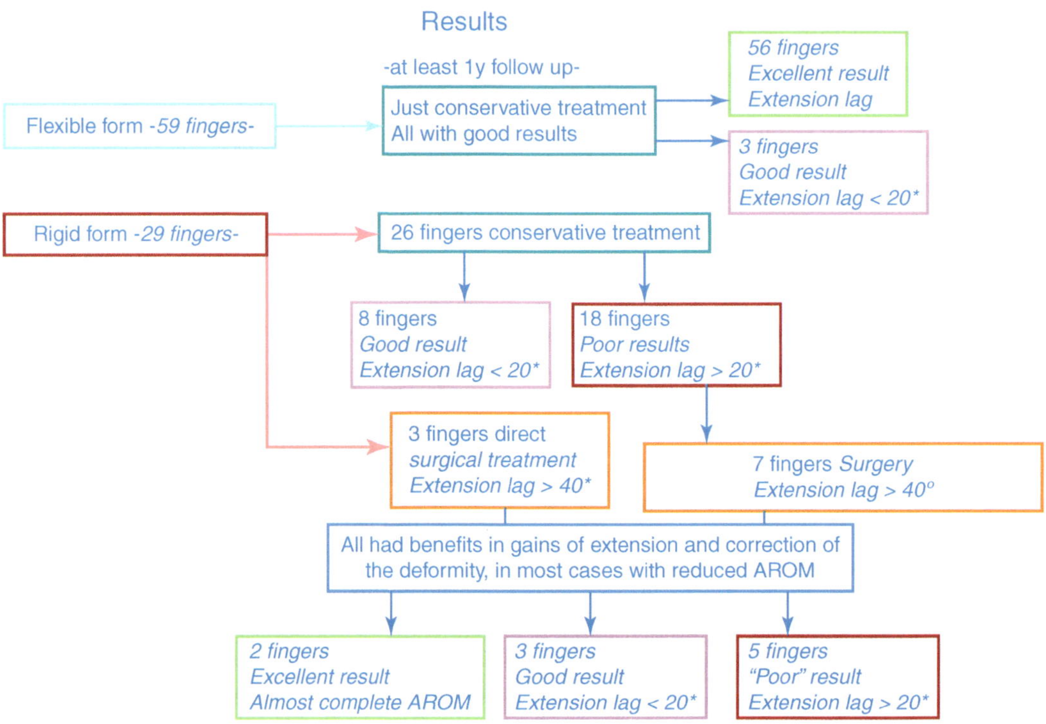

Further Reading

Courtemanche AD. Campylodactyly: etiology and management. Plast Reconstr Surg. 1969;44:451–4.

Dautel G. Camptodactylies. Chir Main. 2003;22:115–24.

De Haas WHD. Camptodactylie Nederlands tijdschr Geneesk. 1957;101:2121–4.

Doffin G, Lenoble E, Foucher G, et al. Camptodactylie: classification et résultats thérapeutiques. Ann Chir Main (Ann Hand Surg). 1994;13(1):20–5.

Engber WD, Flatt AE. Camptodactyly: an analysis of sixty-six patients and twenty-four operations. J Hand Surg. 1977;2:216–24.

Gupta A, Burke FD. Correction of camptodactyly. J. Hand Surg. 1990;15B:168–70.

Hori M, Nakamura R, Inoue G, et al. Nonoperative treatment of camptodactyly. J Hand Surg. 1987a;12A:1061–5.

Inoue G, Tamura Y. Camptodactyly resulting from paradoxical action of an anomalous lumbrical muscle. Scand J Plast Reconstr Hand Surg. 1994;28:309–12.

Koman LA, Toby EB, Poehling GG. Congenital flexion deformities of the proximal interphalangeal joint in children: a subgroup of camptodactyly. J Hand Surg. 1990;15A:582–6.

Maeda M, Matsui T. Camptodactyly caused by an abnormal lumbrical muscle. J Hand Surg. 1985;10B:95–6.

McCash C. Congenital contractures of the hand. In: Stack HG, Botton H, editors. The proceedings of the Second Hand Club, British Society for Surgery of the Hand. London; 1975. p. 399–401.

McFarlane RM, Curry GI. Evans HBAnomalies of the intrinsic muscles in camptodactyly. J Hand Surg. 1983;8:531–44.

McFarlane RM, Classen DA, Porte AM, Botz JS. The anatomy and treatment of camptodactyly of the small finger. J Hand Surg. 1992;17A:35–44.

Minami A, Sakai T. Camptodactyly caused by abnormal insetion and orgin of lumbrical muscle. J Hand Surg. 1993;18B:310–1.

Miura T. Nontraumatic flexion deformity of the proximal interphalangeal joint: its pathogenesis and treatment. Hand. 1983;15:25–34.

Miura T, Nakamura R, Tamura Y. Long-standing extended dynamic splintage and release of an abnormal restraining structure in camptodactyly. J Hand Surg. 1992;17B:665–72.

Miura T, Nackamura R, Tamura Y. Long standing Extended Dynamic splintage and release of an abnormal restraining structure in camptodactyly. J Hand Surg Br. 1992;17B:665–72.

Ogino T, Kato H. Operative findings in camptodactyly of the little finger. J Hand Surg. 1992;17B:661–4.

Oldfield MD. Camptodactyly: flexor contracture of the fingers in young girls. Br J Plast Surg. 1956;8:312–7.

Scott J. Hammer finger with notes of seven cases occuring in one family. Glasgow Med J. 1903;60:335–44.
Siegert JJ, Cooney WP, Dobyns JH. Management of simple camptodactyly. J Hand Surg. 1990;15B:181–9.
Siegert JJ, Cooney WP, Dobyns JH. Management of simple camptodactyly. J Hand Surg Br. 1990;15B:181–9.
Smith PJ. Ross DAThe central slip tenodesis test for early diagnosis of potential Boutonniere deformities. J Hand Surg. 1994;19B:88–90.
Smith RJ, Kaplan EB. Camptodactyly and similar atraumatic flexion deformities of the proximal interphalangeal joints of the fingers: a study of thirty-one cases. J Bone Joint Surg. 1968;50A:1187–203.
Stoddard EE. Nomenclature of hereditary crooked fingers: Streblomicrodatyly and camptodactyly—are they synonyms? J Hered. 1939;30:511–2.
Todd AH. Hereditary contracture of the little fingers (Kamptodactyly). Lancet. 1929;2:1088–9.

Syndactyly

6

Daniel M. Weber

Abstract

Syndactyly is a common hand anomaly that affects 1 in 2000–3000 live births. It has a spectrum from simple syndactylies with fusion of the skin and soft tissues only, complex syndactylies with fusion of bones and nails to complicated syndactylies which are often associated with syndromes.

This chapter covers the epidemiology, classification, and diagnostic workup of syndactylies. It presents treatment strategies for surgical corrections of syndactylies, including techniques with skin grafts, without skin grafts, and with skin substitutes.

Keywords

Syndactyly · Child · Hand · Surgery · Release

6.1 Introduction

Syndactyly is a congenital limb anomaly that is characterized by an incomplete separation of digits, caused by abnormal interdigital connections. The term is derived from the Greek words *syn*, meaning together and *dactylos*, meaning digit.

D. M. Weber (✉)
Division of Hand Surgery, Department of Pediatric Surgery, University Children's Hospital, Zurich, Switzerland
e-mail: Daniel.Weber@kispi.uzh.ch

6.2 Epidemiology

Syndactylies are among the most common hand anomalies, with an estimated incidence of 1 in 2000–3000 live births, affecting both hands in 50%. Ten to 40% have a positive family history with a clear male predominance.

The basic principles of segmentation of the hand are fairly well understood. The apical ectodermal ridge controls the proximodistal outgrowth of the limb, whereas the development and differentiation along the radio-ulnar axis are controlled by the zone of polarizing activity (ZPA). The ZPA and the AER work in a close feedback loop, resulting in a hand plate that becomes visible in the fifth week of development. During the elongation process, digits form through condensation, whereas tissues in between are removed by apoptosis in a distal to proximal orientation. Only a perfect equilibrium between the Bone Morphogenic Proteins (BMPs) that suppress fibroblast growth factors (FGFs), thereby inducing apoptosis, and the BMP inhibitors enable a normal development. Interference with or mutations of BMPs, FGFs, and BMP inhibitors suppress controlled apoptosis and can therefore induce syndactylies, sometimes associated with polydactylies or synostoses [1, 2].

There are over 300 known syndromic anomalies causing syndactylies with etiologies that remain poorly understood, mainly due to their phenotypic and genetic diversity. Within fami-

G. Pajardi (ed.), *Pediatric Hand Surgery*, https://doi.org/10.1007/978-3-031-30984-7_6

lies and even individuals, phenotypes may be severe or mild, unilateral or bilateral, and affect both or either hands and feet [1]. Geneticists classify syndactylies on Temtamy and McKusick's system which has been extended to nine non-syndromic forms of syndactylies, seven of them with autosomal dominant inheritance, variable expressivity and incomplete penetrance and two autosomal recessive forms. Syndactyly type I is the most common non-syndromic syndactyly, usually affecting the third web space on the hands and the second web space on the feet. The most common subtype 1 has been associated with the locus 3p21.31 but no disease-causing genes have been identified [1].

6.3 Classification

Simple clinical classifications help surgical planning. The differentiation into *complete syndactyly* includes the fingertips and *partial syndactyly* with a web space that can reach anywhere between a normal web space and the fingertips can describe all forms of syndactyly. Furthermore, syndactylies can be classified into simple syndactylies, complex syndactylies, and complex complicated syndactylies (Fig. 6.1). Simple syndactylies are characterized by only cutaneous and soft tissue fusions of the fingers and well-developed, separated fingernails. Usually, the segmentation of the digits, tendons, and pulleys is normal with occasional distalisation of the bifurcation of the neurovascular bundles. Complex syndactylies involve the nail and osseous phalanges and may be associated with segmentation anomalies of tendons and a distalisation of the bifurcation of the neurovascular bundles. Complex complicated syndactylies have a severely disturbed anatomy not only of the osseous elements but also of the neurovascular bundles and musculotendinous structures. They are often associated with syndromes, such as in Apert's syndrome.

As mentioned above, some geneticists and pediatricians adhere to the classification which is based on Temtamy and McKusick.

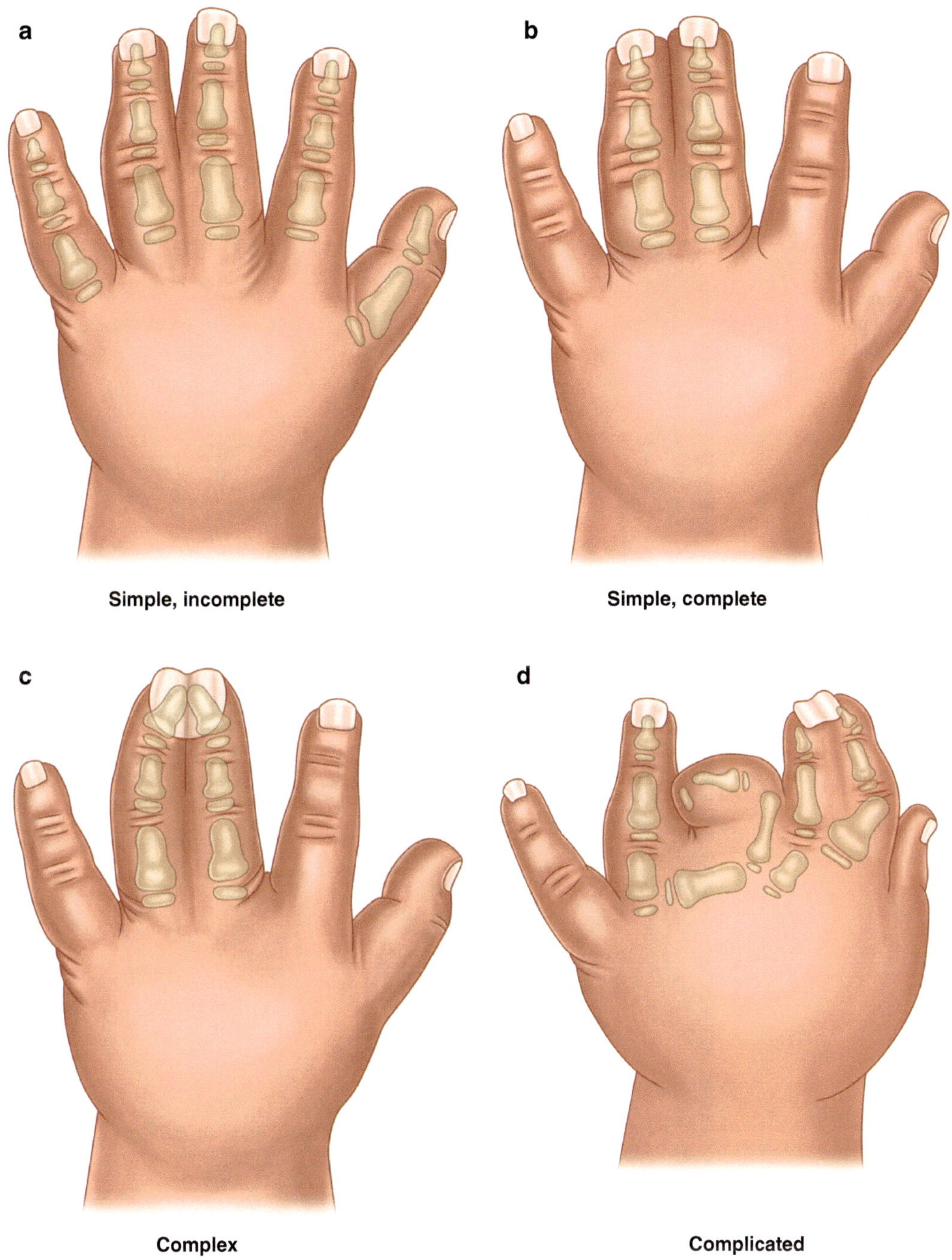

Fig. 6.1 Classification of syndactylies: (**a**) Simple, incomplete; (**b**) Simple, complete; (**c**) Complex; (**d**) Complicated. (From Upton J: Management of disorders of separation-syndactyly. In: Hentz VR, editor. The hand and upper lim (Part2) in: Mathes SJ, editor. Plastic surgery vol. 8. Philadelphia: Saunders Elsevier; 2006. P. 140)

6.4 Diagnostic Workup

Simple syndactylies of the fingers with a full mobility of the IP joints don't need a further workup, since a regular anatomy of tendons and neurovascular bundles can be anticipated. However, if in doubt, an X-ray is recommended, because the complexity can be underestimated as illustrated in Fig. 6.2 with a patient with a familial synpolydactyly. A pediatric or genetic workup is recommended for complicated syndactylies and can be considered in complex syndactylies.

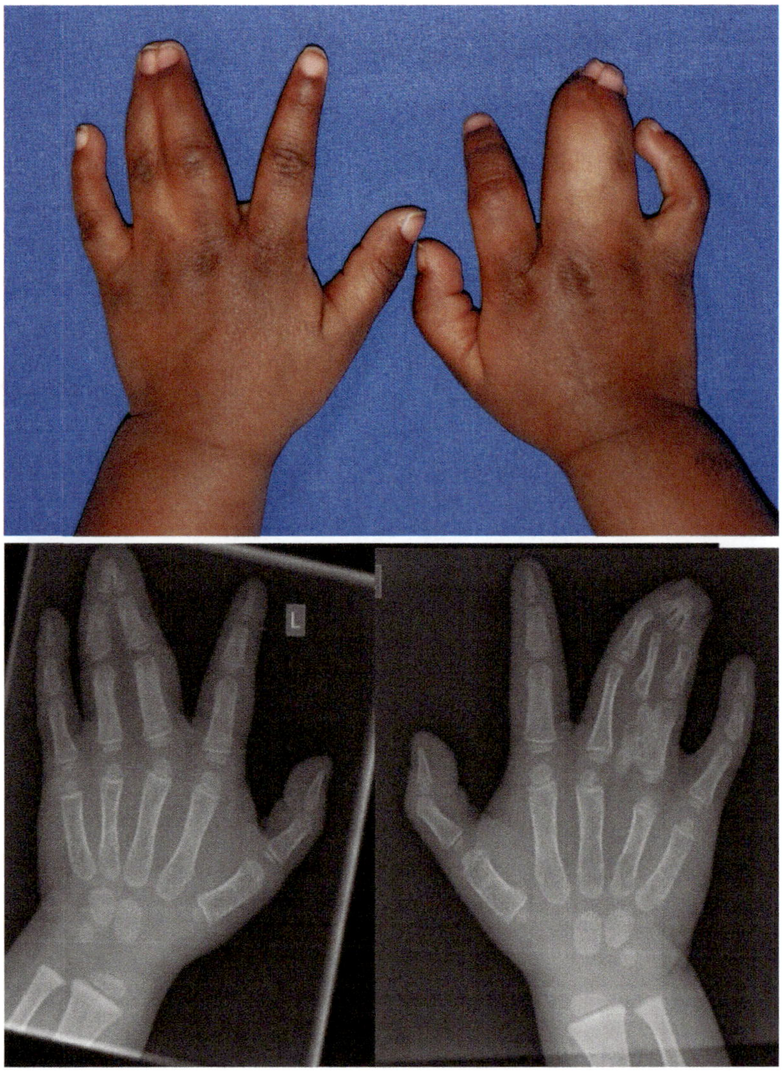

Fig. 6.2 The X-ray reveals the complexity of this complete, complex, complicated syndactyly in a child with a synpolydactyly

6.5 Treatment

The aim of surgical separation of web spaces is improving or maintaining function while optimizing the appearance of the hand by separating all digits.

6.5.1 General Principles

Irrespective of the localization and type of the syndactyly, some principles of reconstruction must be respected.

6.5.1.1 Flap Coverage of the Web

The proximal definition of the web should be covered with a wide, well-vascularized flap to avoid scar formation and "web creep", a secondary syndactyly that narrows or distalizes the new commissure. The width of the flap should ensure a round configuration and avoid a V-shaped web space. Dorsally based flaps can be mobilized easily since they have hardly any fascio-cutaneous adherence and have the advantage of bringing pigmented skin to the dorsal and well-visible aspect of the web space. Ideally, they mimic the natural proximal to distal and dorsal to palmar inclination of the web.

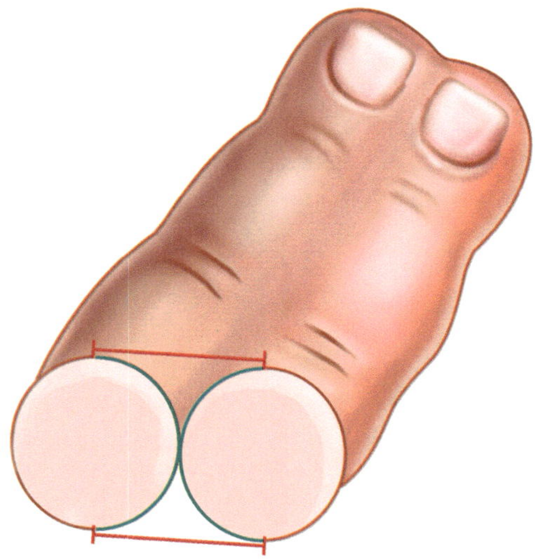

Fig. 6.3 A simple hand-drawn sketch illustrates to parents the shortage of skin

6.5.1.2 Skin Grafts and Substitutes

There is a shortage of interdigital skin when separating syndactylies. This becomes evident on a hand drawn sketch and can be explained and demonstrated to parents easily (Fig. 6.3). Various flap designs have been recommended to separate partial and complete syndactylies without skin grafts. Partial syndactylies up to the PIP joint can be separated reliably without using skin grafts or substitutes [3] (technique see below), whereas separation of complete syndactylies without skin grafts may be associated with higher risks of complications and a less favorable outcome.

Large skin defects on the hand result in scars that retract and may distort the neighboring skin flaps. Exceptionally, skin defects may be tolerated in stiff fingers, when contractures are not an issue, such as in Apert's hands with symphalangism. Traditionally, skin defects are covered with autologous skin grafts. Full-thickness skin grafts are preferred over split skin grafts, because they hardly shrink. The pigmentation, texture, and hair bearing of the donor skin must match the recipient site on the hand and the donor site must be inconspicuous. Traditionally, full-thickness skin grafts are taken from the ulnar volar aspect of the wrist, the cubital fossa, or the groin. It is important to remember that the skin from the groin may grow pubic hair after puberty, particularly when being taken medially.

An excellent donor site that is not used commonly is retroauricular skin (Fig. 6.4). It is hardly hair bearing and has a superior color match when compared with groin skin (Fig. 6.5) [4]. The ellipsoid incisions should be marked with a pen so that 1/3 of the skin is taken from the ear. Injection of a local anesthetic with a vasoconstrictor (such as bupivacaine + adrenaline) facilitates harvesting of the skin graft. After a two-layer wound closure with resorbable subcutaneous and intracutaneous sutures, a light dressing may be applied for a day or two. Experienced surgeons may harvest the retroauricular skin graft before operating on the hand to minimize tourniquet time and avoid leaving the draped hand to raise a skin graft.

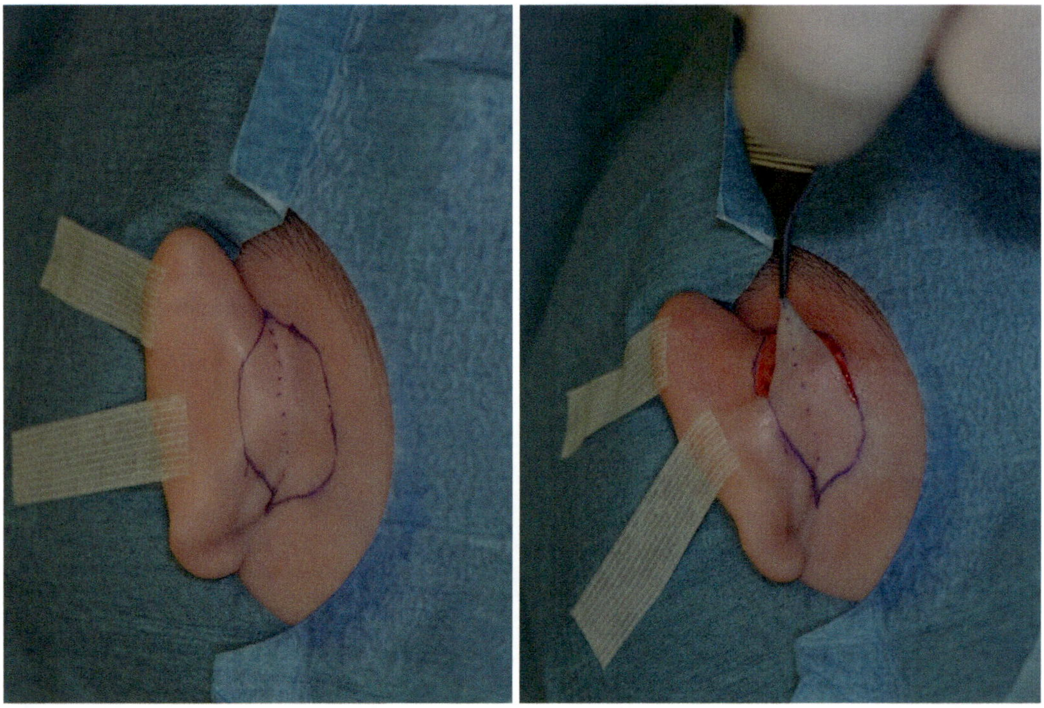

Fig. 6.4 Full-thickness retroauricular skin graft

Dermal substitutes or a hyaluronic scaffold can be used as an alternative to skin grafts. It shortens operating time and avoids donor site scars. Application by suture fixation is easy and spontaneous resorption of the hyaluronic acid is followed by spontaneous epithelialization with a good color match (Fig. 6.6). Good results were published [5]; however, no studies have compared the results of skin substitutes with skin grafts.

6.5.1.3 Fingertip and Nail Wall Reconstruction

Complete complex and complete complicated syndactylies often have fused nails and therefore lack a lateral nail fold. Spontaneous scarification of the nail fold or scarification after application of full-thickness skin grafts after separation of the nails results in nail growth disturbance. Flap coverage of the defect protects nail growth and creates a natural-looking nail fold. Buck-Gramcko published symmetrical flaps from the neighboring fingertips [6]. They provide excellent results in children with well-developed fingertips. However, quite often, there is not enough volume and the author prefers doing asymmetrical flaps with a transverse Buck-Gramcko flap from one fingertip, asymmetrical longitudinal incisions between the pulps and a simple translation of the pulp on the donor fingertip (Fig. 6.7). It is important not to mobilize the fasciocutaneous adherence extensively to avoid wobbly fingertips. Sutures on the nail fold should never be tight and small defects that heal secondarily are acceptable.

6.5.1.4 Exposure and Separation of Neurovascular Bundles

Dissection in a bloodless field with a tourniquet allows a good visualization of the neurovascular bundles. In simple syndactylies, the bifurcation of nerves and vessels is usually deep in the web space and does not limit the opening of the web space. In complex syndactylies, such as, for example, in Apert syndrome, one may find just one interdigital artery with a distal bifurcation that necessitates ligation of one digital artery. Before ligating one branch, one may apply a

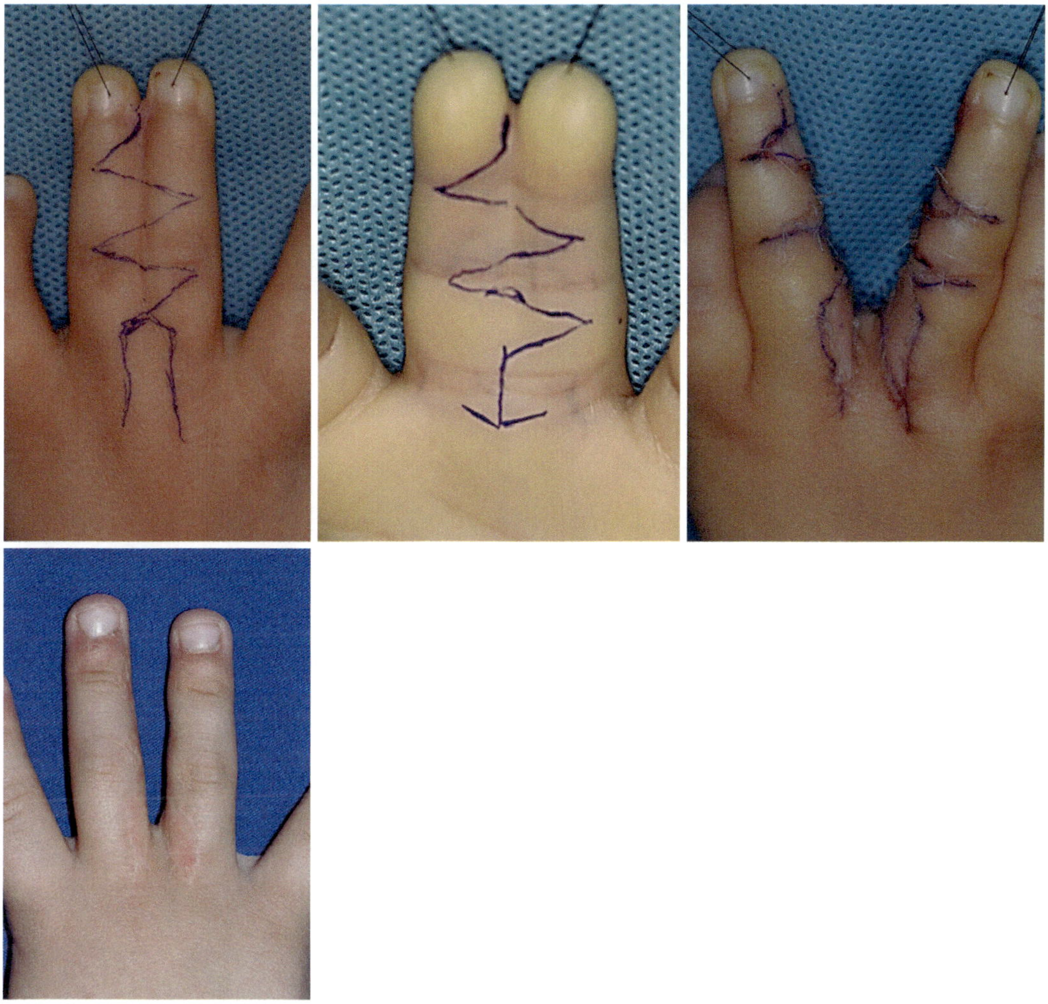

Fig. 6.5 Simple syndactyly can be separated with a dorsal Omega flap and triangular interdigital flaps. The skin defects can be covered with full-thickness skin grafts

microvascular clamp and open the tourniquet to reassure sufficient vascularization of both digits. Distal bifurcation of digital nerves can be treated by interfascicular longitudinal dissection and separation with a scalpel under loup (3.5×) or microscopic magnification.

6.5.1.5 Simultaneous Separation of Multiple Syndactylies

Traditionally, the separation of multiple adjacent syndactylies was avoided to prevent digital ischemia due to simultaneous dissection on the radial and ulnar neurovascular bundle. Nevertheless, simultaneous separation of adjacent syndactylies may be considered as long as there is a good visualization of the neurovascular bundles during dissection. If all fingers are syndactylized, simultaneous separation may not be optimal due to the limited skin and soft tissue coverage. A two-stage procedure, starting with the first and third and followed by the second and fourth web space in a second stage, should be considered in these hands.

6.5.1.6 Dressings and Dressing Changes

Dressings protect the wound and secure skin grafts. Application under tourniquet is acceptable

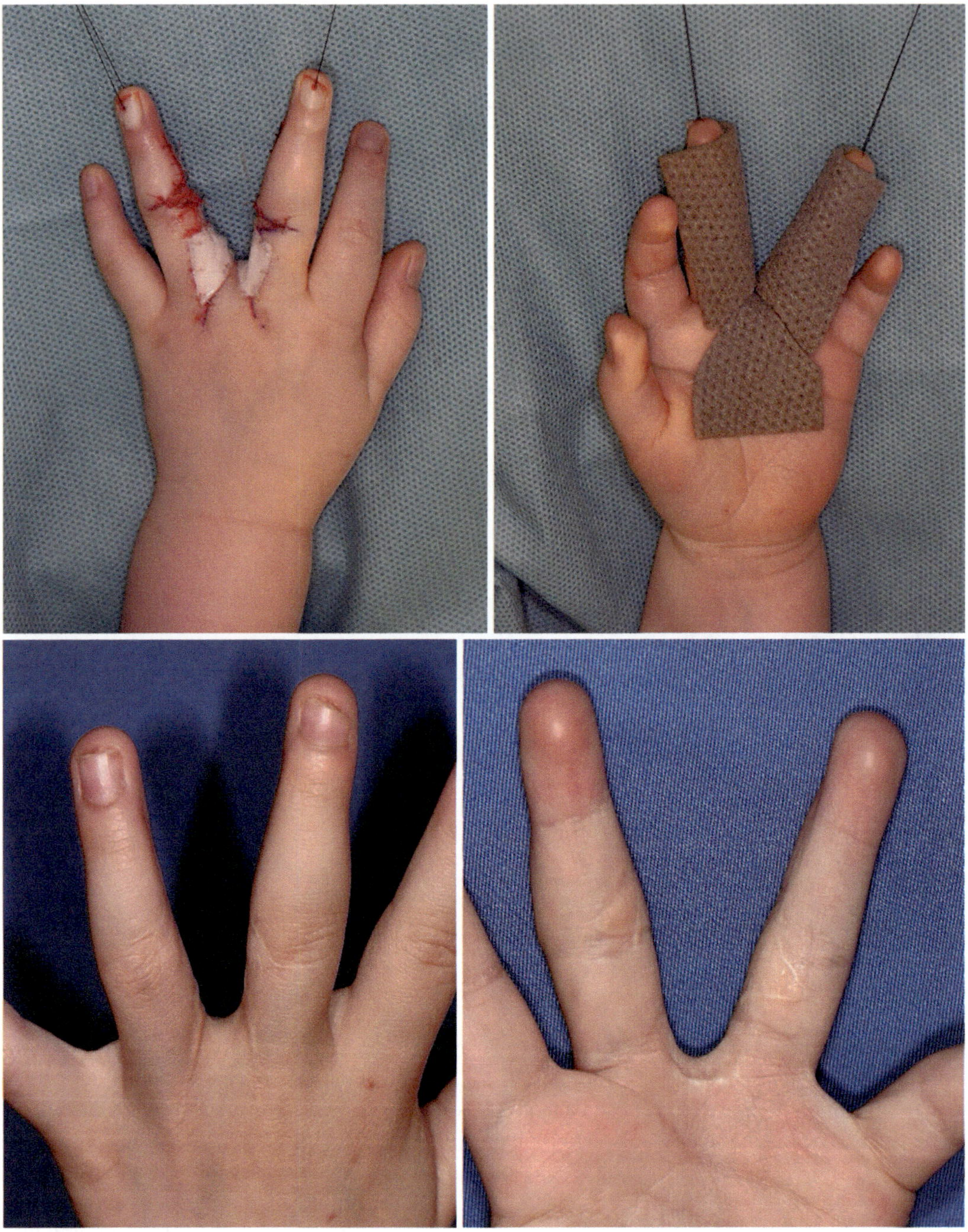

Fig. 6.6 Skin substitutes such as hyaluronic scaffolds can give similar results to full-thickness skin grafts, however, the time to primary wound healing may be prolongated

as long as the surgeon feels confident regarding flap vascularity and if recapillarization of the fingertips can be observed with the dressing. Both traditional wound dressings with fat gauze and cotton, as well as more elaborate wound dressings with synthetic dressings such as Mepilex Silver Transfer® (Fig. 6.6) give similar results in the author's hands. Tie-over dressings are not needed to secure digital skin grafts in hands. However, dressings must be well secured and may be stuck

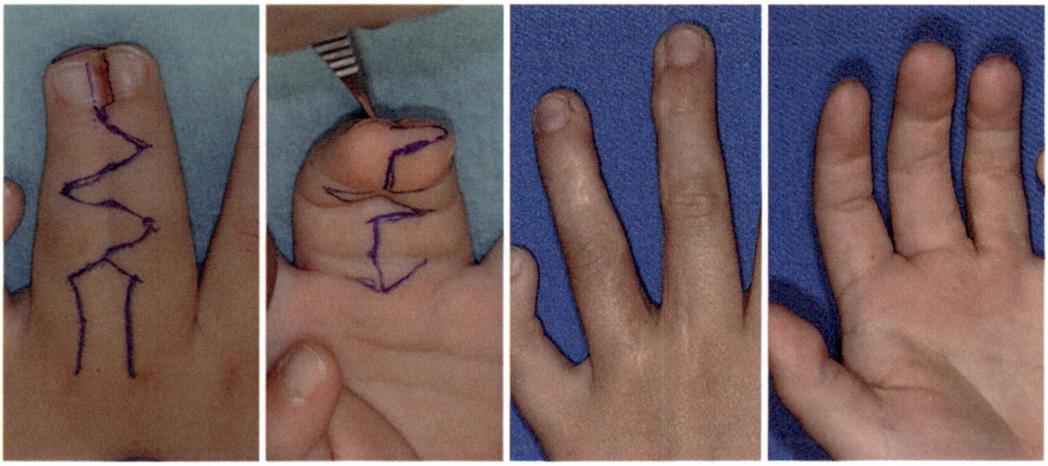

Fig. 6.7 Asymmetrical finger pulp flaps, modified after the Buck-Gramcko technique result in a good nail wall reconstruction and unimpaired nail growth

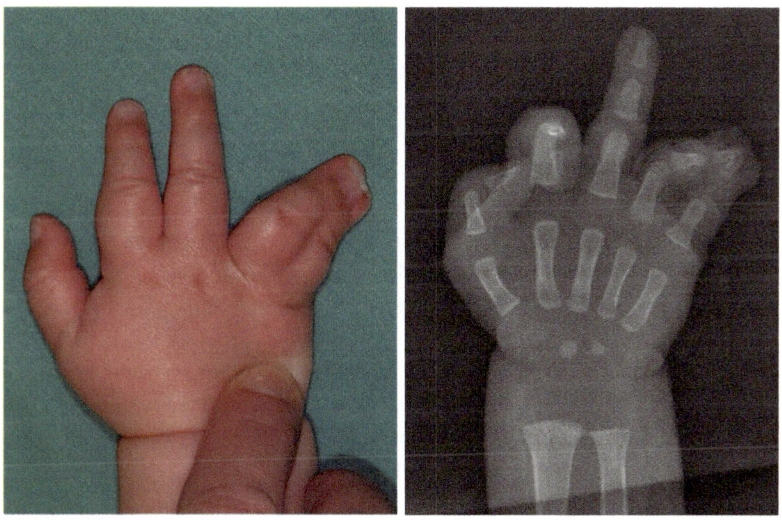

Fig. 6.8 Complete syndactylies of digits with unequal length should be separated early to avoid progression of clinodactyly

directly on the skin. An additional stocking on top of the first dressing can be changed by the parents. The thumb should be left under the stocking and the arm should be immobilized in a sling to prevent the use of the hand and inadvertent removal of the first dressing. Splint or cast immobilization is reserved for complex cases with osteotomies and K-wire insertion.

The first dressing change can be planned after 2 to 3 weeks. The author recommends the use of resorbable sutures such as, for example, Vicryl-Rapid 6–0®, so that no routine anesthesia is needed for the first dressing change and removal of the stitches [7]. At the first dressing change, a similar dressing as that during surgery can be applied together with some ointment, followed by further dressing changes as needed. Parents are encouraged to massage the scars with ointment or silicone gel. Prophylactic splinting with silicone application at night for up to 6 months may be considered if hypertrophic scars are anticipated.

6.5.1.7 Timing of Surgery

Syndactylized fingers of unequal length tend to get a progressive clinodactyly and should be separated early, preferentially around 6 months of age (Fig. 6.8). All other syndactylies can be operated ideally from about the first birthday until the age of 18 months. Anesthesia at an earlier age is more demanding and may bear higher risks [8]. The determined will of children between the ages of 18 months and 4 years and yet the limited understanding of the goal of surgery makes elective surgery and immobilization difficult in this age group and may pose a major burden to the children and their families.

6.5.2 Surgical Techniques

6.5.2.1 The First Web Space of the Hand

Syndactylies of the first web space are usually associated with syndromes, such as Apert's syndrome, or other anomalies, such as symbrachydactyly, thumb hypoplasia, or amniotic bands. Separation of the first web space must therefore always incorporate treatment of all aspects of the anomaly. The associated narrowing of the first web space is not only due to the cutaneous syndactyly but also due to contractures of the adductor pollicis and the first dorsal interosseous muscle. The fascia of these muscles must be incised during the exposure of the first web space and the insertion of the adductor on the third metacarpal may need to be released. Fibrous bands, resembling interglenoid ligaments between the thumb and index, can be found and must be released when present. An artery that runs in the first web space and bifurcates to the thumb and index far distally is a common finding. Before the ligature of one arterial branch, it may be clamped and the perfusion checked after release of the tourniquet.

In a relatively proximal partial syndactyly, local "Z-flaps" and a "VY-flap" in the first web space may be sufficient. More distal forms and narrow web spaces need large flaps such as the dorsal rotation-advancement flap (Fig. 6.9) and eventually a full-thickness skin graft. A microsurgical flap may be considered in very tight first web spaces with complete syndactyly.

6.5.2.2 The Second to Fourth Web Spaces of the Hand

Dozens of techniques and flap designs to separate syndactylies have been published [9]. The author recommends surgeons to limit themselves to a few techniques and to become familiar with them before eventually trying other flap designs. The standard armamentarium should comprise a technique for complete syndactylies with full-thickness skin grafting or skin substitutes (Figs. 6.5 and 6.6) [10] and graftless techniques for partial syndactylies until the PIP joint (Fig. 6.10) or slight distalization of the web space (Fig. 6.11) [3]. Irrespective of the flap design, it is important to make a deep, i.e., proximal web space since it always tends to migrate distally again. Short fingers, such as in symbrachydactyly, look longer if the web space is slightly too proximal.

6.5.2.3 Syndactyly of the Feet

The incidence of simple, partial syndactylies of the second web space of the feet is x per 10,000 live births. Most concerns consider appearance of the foot, since functional problems or pain is exceptional. Although surgical separation of syndactylies of the feet follows the same principles as that of the hands, indications should be kept restrictive: The complication rate after syndactyly repair, particularly for infections, is higher on the feet than on the hands. Scars can be very cumbersome at sports, particularly with athletic shoe wear. The authors therefore recommend the separation of syndactylies between the second and third toes only at the patient's wish at an older age and not upon parental desire only.

Surgical separation is recommended for the first web space, since syndactyly fuses the biphalangeal first toe the biphalangeal second toe and because web space is functional for wearing flip-flop sandals. Furthermore, the separation of toes of unequal length, mostly in the third web space, should be considered, because fusion of unequal toes results in progressive clinodactyly and may be associated with pain or clavus formation.

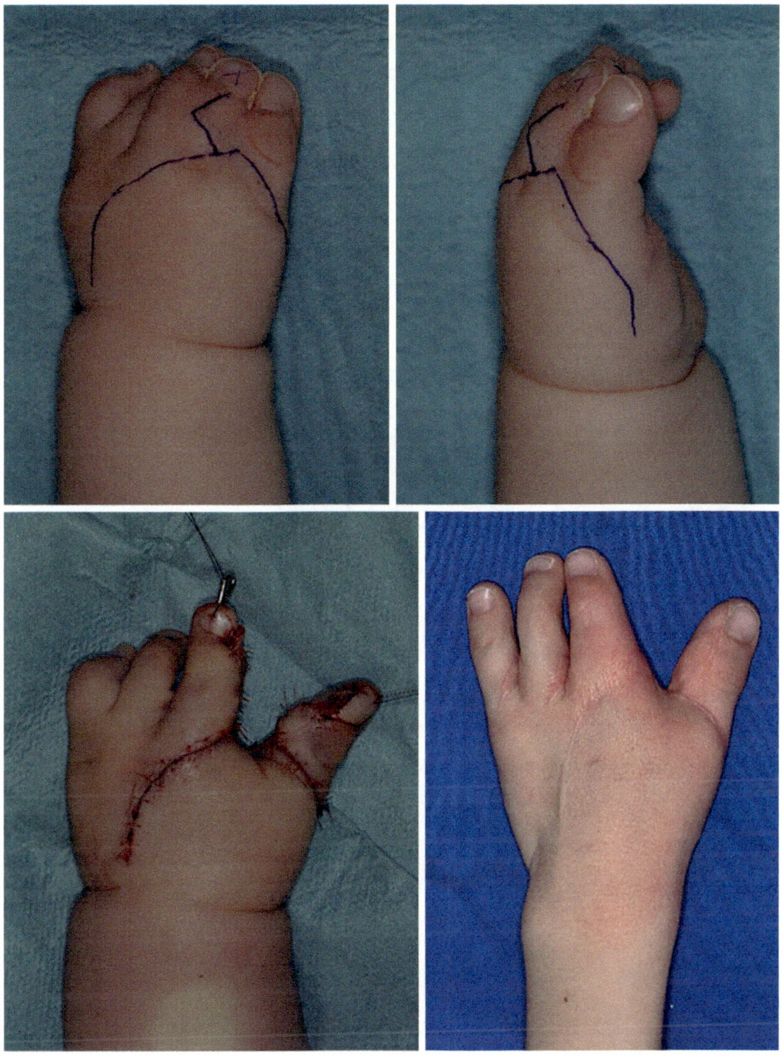

Fig. 6.9 Wide, dorsal rotational advancement flap to liberate the first web space in a patient with symbrachydactyly

Associated anomalies, such as postaxial polysyndactyly, should be excluded with an X-ray before surgery. Interdisciplinary evaluations together with a pediatric orthopedic surgeon should be considered in complex syndactylies of the feet, particularly in children with syndromes, such as, for example, Apert syndrome. We recommend early syndactyly repair at the age of 9 to 12 months, before children start walking, since this makes care much easier for the families. Surgical principals are the same as those for hands, with an emphasis of a good flap coverage in the web space. Small full-thickness skin grafts may be taken below the lateral malleolus, if needed (Fig. 6.12).

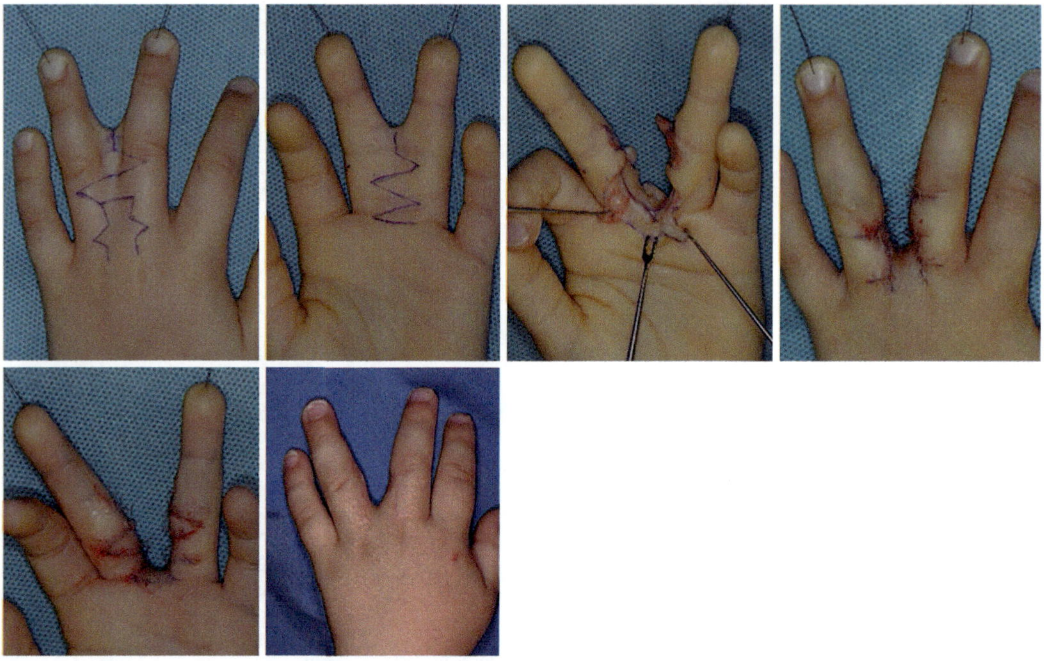

Fig. 6.10 Repair of partial syndactylies up to the PIP joint with primary skin closure without skin grafts

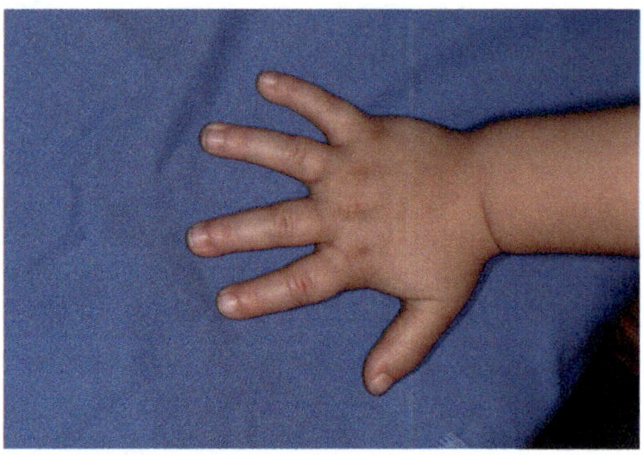

Fig. 6.11 Web deepening for proximal forms of partial syndactylies with multiple Z-plasties (trident flaps) without skin grafts

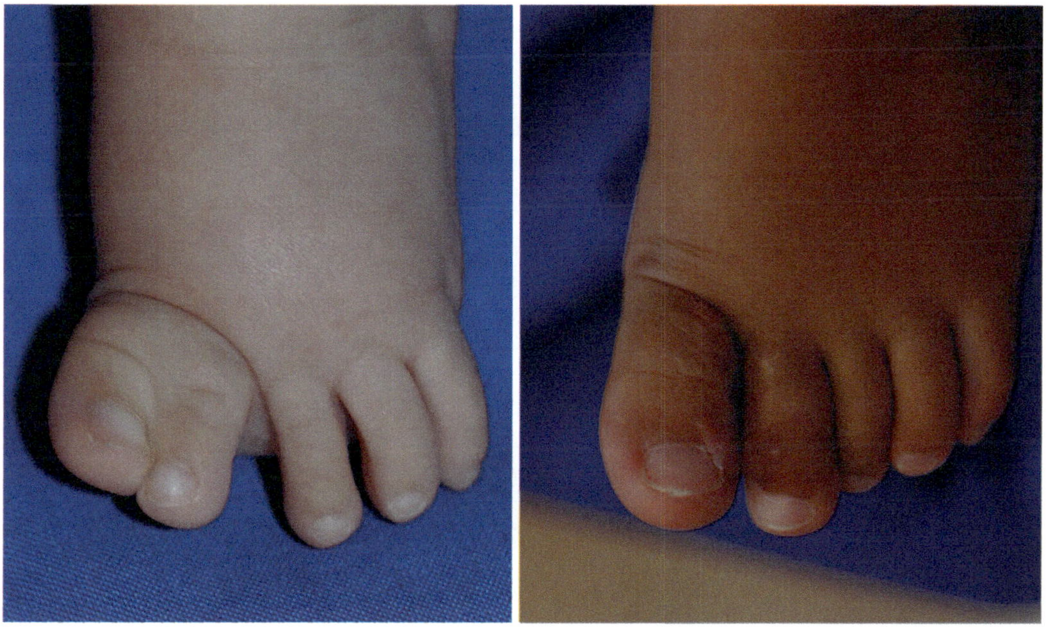

Fig. 6.12 Syndactyly repair of the feet is warranted for the first web space. It follows similar principles as that of the hands with wide commissural flaps and full-thickness skin transplants

6.6 Complications

Injury to digital arteries or tension of skin flaps may delay wound healing, promote infections, and result in the loss of skin grafts. Severe scarring and web creep can be the consequences and lead to functional as well as esthetic deficits that require reoperations [11]. Scars may not inhibit hand function initially. However, tight scars do not grow with the child and may result in contractures, clinodactyly, and even luxation of joints years after the initial surgery (Fig. 6.13) Therefore, splinting at night is recommended in children with difficult scars after syndactyly release. Keloid formation is an unusual complication after syndactyly release. A study by Muzaffar et al. demonstrated, that primary digital enlargement is a highly predictive risk factor for keloid formation and that standard treatment with pressure, topical or intralesional corticosteroids may not be sufficient to control keloids [12].

Reoperations for scar contractures or hypertrophic scars should be delayed until the maturation of the scars, which does not occur until 6 months postoperative.

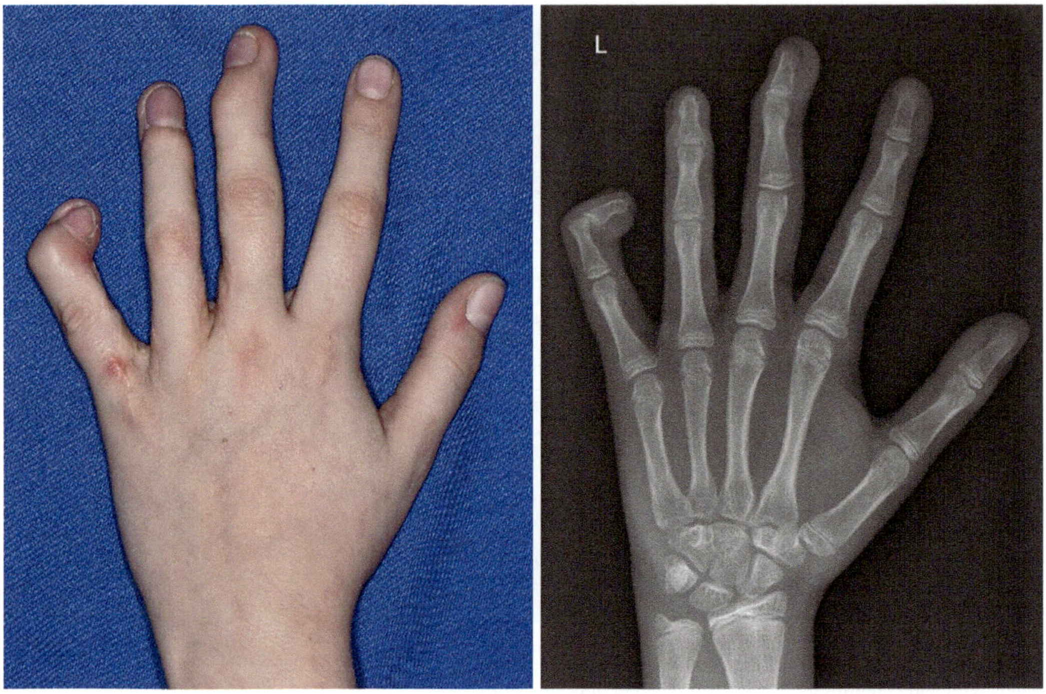

Fig. 6.13 Severe late complication with clinodactyly and subluxation of the DIP due to scar contractures

References

1. Ahmed H, et al. Genetic overview of syndactyly and polydactyly. Plast Reconstr Surg Glob Open. 2017;5(11):e1549.
2. Oberg KC, et al. Developmental biology and classification of congenital anomalies of the hand and upper extremity. J Hand Surg Am. 2010;35(12):2066–76.
3. Tonkin MA. Failure of differentiation part I: syndactyly. Hand Clin. 2009;25(2):171–93.
4. Sulser PS, Kalisch M, Weber DM. Retroauricular full-thickness skin grafts in syndactyly repair: outcome and comparison with inguinal full-thickness skin grafts: retrospective (cross-sectional) study. J Plast Surg Hand Surg. 2016;50(5):281–5.
5. Landi A, et al. Hyaluronic acid scaffold for skin defects in congenital syndactyly release surgery: a novel technique based on the regenerative model. J Hand Surg Europ. 2014;39(9):994–1000.
6. Errol G. Syndactyly. In: Dieter B-G, editor. Congenital malformations of the hand and forearm. London: Churchill Livingstone; 1998. p. 131–40.
7. Weber DM, Schiestl CM. Absorbable sutures help minimise patient discomfort and reduce cost in syndactyly release. Eur J Pediatr Surg. 2004;14(3):151–4.
8. Davidson A, Vutskits L. The new FDA drug safety communication on the use of general anesthetics in young children: what should we make of it? Paediatr Anaesth. 2017;27(4):336–7.
9. Samson P, Salazard B. Syndactyly. Chir Main. 2008;27(Suppl 1):S100–14.
10. D'Arcangelo M, Gilbert A, Pirrello R. Correction of syndactyly using a dorsal omega flap and two lateral and volar flaps. A long-term review. J Hand Surg Br. 1996;21(3):320–4.
11. Canizares MF, et al. Complications and cost of syndactyly reconstruction in the United States: analysis of the pediatric health information system. Hand (N Y). 2017;12(4):327–34.
12. Muzaffar AR, et al. Keloid formation after syndactyly reconstruction: associated conditions, prevalence, and preliminary report of a treatment method. J Hand Surg Am. 2004;29(2):201–8.

Symbrachydactyly

7

Elisa Rosanda, Chiara Parolo, and Giorgio Pajardi

Abstract

Symbrachydactyly is a congenital hand defect where there is both syndactyly and brachydactyly. The clinical manifestations have many variations, from a hand with hypoplastic fingers to a severe form of adactylous hand. Symbrachydactyly is typically unilateral, characterized by failure of the formation of fingers and presence of rudimentary nubbins that include elements of nail plate, bone, and cartilage.

The etiology is still unknown, but vascular dysgenesis during fetal development is a leading hypothesis.

The treatments vary based on the degree of malformation and family needs. When surgical treatment is needed, syndactyly release is the most frequent procedure. In monodactyly type or adactyly type pinch function can be created with non-vascularized free phalangeal transfer procedure or microsurgical toe-to-hand transfers.

E. Rosanda (✉) · C. Parolo
University Department of Hand Surgery and Rehabilitation, San Giuseppe Hospital MultiMedica IRCCS, Milan University, Milan, Italy
e-mail: elisa.rosanda@multimedica.it; chiara.parolo@multimedica.it

G. Pajardi
Milan, Italy
e-mail: gpajardi@centrostudimano.it

Keywords

Symbrachydactyly · Congenital hand · Poland syndrome · Toe-to-hand transfer · Non-vascularized free phalangeal transfer

7.1 Introduction

Symbrachydactyly is a congenital hand defect where in which there is both syndactyly and brachydactyly.

The clinical manifestations have many variations, from a hand with hypoplastic fingers to severe form of adactylous hand.

Symbrachydactyly is typically unilateral, characterized by failure of formation of fingers, and presence of rudimentary nubbins that include elements of nail plate, bone, and cartilage. In the past was called also atypical cleft hand for the absence of the central digits and presence of the digit of the border [1].

Symbrachydactyly was first described by Poland in 1841. He described a syndrome in which there was a combination of absence or hypoplasia of long finger, syndactyly, and hypoplasia of pectoralis major (Fig. 7.1) [2]. Pol in 1921 was the first who used the terms Symbrachydactyly and described two different forms: with or without the association of hypoplasia or aplasia of pectoralis major [3].

G. Pajardi (ed.), *Pediatric Hand Surgery*, https://doi.org/10.1007/978-3-031-30984-7_7

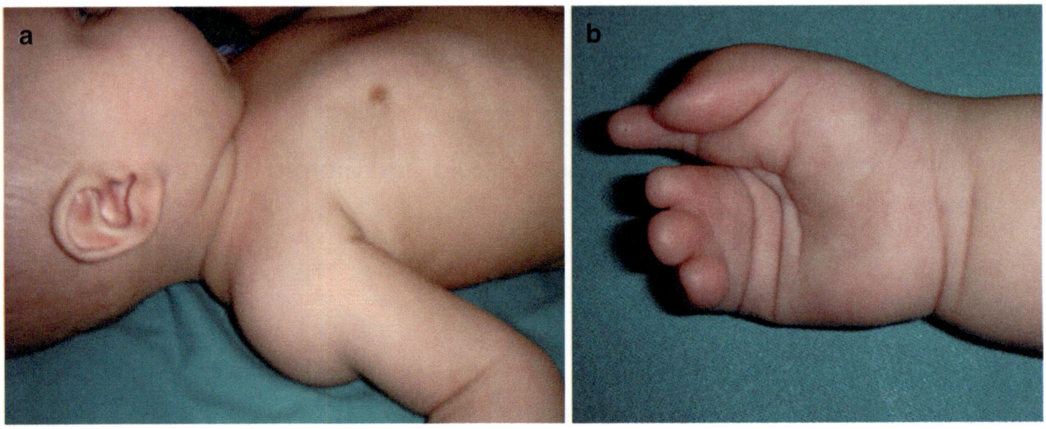

Fig. 7.1 Poland syndrome: (**a**) hypoplasia of pectoralis major and (**b**) symbrachydactyly

Today, the symbrachydactyly is classified in the Oberg, Manske, and Tonkin (OMT) classification as an undergrowth or failure of axis formation.

7.2 Epidemiology

The diverse morphologic characteristics of symbrachydactyly make accurate incidence difficult. A study from Brazil reported a 0.054% incidence of symbrachydactyly in Caucasians and 0.043% in African Americans [4]. Two studies from Japan reported an incidence of 1 in every 20,000 to 30,000 births [5] and 1 in 10,000 birth [6]. Other survey estimates an incidence of approximately 0.6 per 10,000 in live births. In total, 73% of cases are males. The condition is usually unilateral with the left upper limb alone involved in 67% of cases, the right in 27%, and 1% to 7% bilateral [7]. A total of 7% of cases have associated anomalies such as Poland syndrome, in which hypoplasia or absence of the pectoralis major occurs with additional variable abnormalities [2]. In 7% of cases, there is a positive family history of symbracydactyly [7–9].

Associated syndrome [71]
Poland syndrome
Moebius syndrome
Langer-Giedion syndrome
Trisomy 9p syndrome
Deletion 5p syndrome

Associated syndrome [71]
Cohen syndrome
Aglossia-adactyly syndrome
Coffin–Siris syndrome
Dyggve–Melchior–Clausen syndrome
Grebe syndrome
CHILD syndrome
Duplication 9p syndrome

7.3 Etiology

The etiology of symbrachydactyly is still unknown, but vascular dysgenesis during fetal development ("subclavian artery supply disruption sequence") is a leading hypothesis [10].

In support of this theory, a study of eight patients with Poland syndrome showed decreased blood flow velocity in affected limbs [11]. Other studies suggest different etiologies: one study showed that giving 5-fluorouracil early in pregnancy produced symbrachydactyly in rats [12]. Another study showed that injection of busulfan produced rats with central clefts, osseous syndactyly, and symbrachydactyly [13, 14].

Based on the current understanding of upper limb development, symbrachydactyly likely arises through disruption of the apical ectodermal ridge (AER) of the developing limb bud. The AER, a thickening of ectodermal cells at the distal end of the limb bud, directs proximal-distal limb development through a complex cascade of growth factors and genetic signaling, while controlling aspects of mesenchyme cell differentiation [15]. In animal models, disruption of the AER and its signaling pathways causes transverse deficiencies, including symbrachydactyly [16–18].

Although limb development occurs in a proximal-distal manner, there may be some regenerative capacity of distal limb elements after a partial or complete insult to the AER that may result in the characteristic "nubbins" or rudimentary digits seen in symbrachydactyly [18, 19].

7.4 Classification

The International Federation of Societies for Surgery of the Hand (IFSSH) has adopted the OMT classification system [20]. In the OMT system, symbrachydactyly is categorized as a failure of formation of the proximal-distal axis, which can involve the entire upper limb or the hand plate [21]. In the previous IFSSH system, symbrachydactyly was classified under I (failure of formation), II (failure of differentiation), and V (undergrowth) categories [22].

Over the years, several classifications of symbrachydactyly have been described: The first was Pol in 1921 who classified symbrachydactyly into two groups: those with and without a pectoral muscle defect [3]. Blauth and Gekeler [23] refined Müller's original concepts [24] into a classification system for symbrachydactyly that included 4 phenotypes, and is the most commonly used classification:

1. *Short finger type* (brachymesophalangia): presence of thumb and four short coalesced stiff digits that may have one or more missing phalanges, most often the middle.
2. *Oligodactylic type* (atipical cleft hand): the central part of the hand is aplastic with a relatively intact thumb and fifth digits.
3. *Monodactyly type*: the thumb is present; the fingers are absent or aplastic.
4. *Peromelic type*: adactyly with complete absence of all digits at the metacarpal level with rudimentary nubbins (Fig. 7.2).

Yamauchi and Tanabu [25] described a more elaborate classification of 7 types based on the morphological and radiographic bony deficiency but not providing guidance for treatment.

Foucher [26] modified the Blauth classification. He subdivides the four groups into subcate-

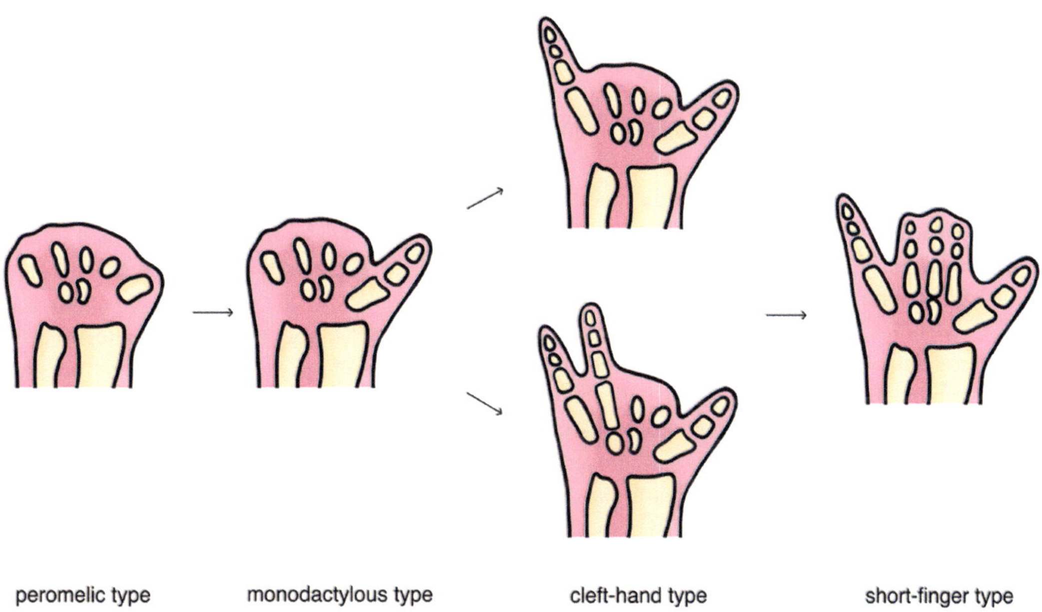

Fig. 7.2 Blauth and Gekeler classification

Table 7.1 Foucher's Classification

Type	Features	Thumb	Ulnar digit	Interventions
I	All bones and digits present, brachydactyly and syndactyly	Normal	Bones present, brachydactyly or syndactyly	Syndactyly release
II A	≥2 fingers. Normal thumb, hypoplastic fingers	Normal	Hypoplastic, syndactyly	Non-vascularized toe phalanx transfers, ablation, or stabilization
IIB	Functional border digits, variable central nubbins	Normal	Present, variable hypoplasia and stability	Surgery rarely indicated
IIC	"Spoon hand", thumb conjoined with hypoplastic ulnar digit	Present (±stability)	Hypoplastic, clinodactyly	Variable
IIIA	Monodactyly	Normal	Absent	Vascularized toe-to-hand transfer
IIIB	Monodactyly	Hypoplastic and/ or unstable	Absent	Variable, vascularized toe-to-hand transfer, thumb stabilization, thumb lengthening
IVA	Peromelic, wrist mobility	Absent	Absent	Surgery not indicated
IVB	Peromelic, no wrist mobility	Absent	Absent	Surgery not indicated

gories describing the functionality of thumb and ulnar digit and giving the indication for surgery (Table 7.1).

7.5 Differential Diagnosis

Symbrachydactyly can be confused with other different hand conditions. The most difficult differential diagnosis is with the constriction ring syndrome. There are some elements that differ within these two malformations.

In the constriction ring syndrome:

- fenestrated syndactyly (acrosindactily) may be present
- nails are absent in the amputated finger
- the upper limb isn't hypoplastic
- there are the signs of a constriction band
- more than one limb is typically involved

Central deficiency is another differential diagnosis: symbrachydactyly was previously called "atypical cleft hand" due to morphological similarities [27]. Central deficiency is an autosomal dominant condition in which the central rays are absent, it is usually bilateral and often associated with cleft feet. Other conditions in the differential diagnosis of symbrachydactyly include Apert Syndrome, ulnar longitudinal deficiency, and hypodactyly [28].

7.6 Treatment

The treatments of symbrachydactyly vary based on the degree of malformation and family needs. It is important at the beginning of the clinical relationship with the family to discuss all the possible surgical and nonsurgical treatments and the correct timing of these. It is known that a correction of the grip must be in the early childhood for maximizing function. Many manual skills are developed by the age of 3, including pinch [29, 30].

Finally because the malformation is usually unilateral sometimes families choose to simply await development and observe how their child progresses.

7.6.1 Nonoperative Treatment

In symbrachydactyly, nonoperative interventions are hand therapy, psychomotricity, and prostheses. An occupational and psychomotricity therapist can help children with unilateral malformations to increase their ability in the activities of daily life while increasing self-esteem and gaining independence.

In symbrachydactyly, the use of prostheses is limited, primarily because it is typically unilateral and the prostheses cannot provide sensation. In bimanual activity, children prefer to use the affected hand to assist the contralateral hand particularly if it has wrist motion and/or at least one sensate digit.

In adactylous hand with no wrist mobility, the prostheses may be helpful because they provide a surface to grip against. There are passive hand prostheses and myoelectric hand prostheses.

Without surgical intervention, these are the ability levels that children typically develop [31]:

- *Adactylous hand:* unable to perform single-hand prehension. Assist the contralateral extremity in performing tasks, stabilizing objects on a flat surface or against the body, and using the wrist to hook or hold objects.
- *Monodactylous hand:* usually has a thumb and may have a normal palm width with intact metacarpals. May have more stable bimanual hand tasks and may be able to hook and press with the finger. The child may be able to pinch between the thumb and palm.
- *Bidactylous hand:* usually has a thumb and a single ulnar digit. The ulnar digit, if long enough and stable, will provide a pinch against the thumb, and these children usually can hold objects in the hand and perform 2-finger or palm pinch. They cannot perform cylindrical pinch and grip strength is usually weak compared with the uninvolved side.
- *3-functioning-digit hand:* usually have tip, palm, and cylindrical grip with more strength compared with the 2-fingered hand, though power grip may be limited.
- *4- and 5-digit hands:* have greater power grip than other types. The fingers may have unstable interphalangeal joints but are capable of single-hand prehension.

7.6.2 Operative Treatment

The treatment of symbrachydactyly depends on the clinical appearance, function, radiological findings, and perceived patient needs. The specific aspect of symbrachydactyly that the treatment addresses can be used to help categorize the surgical treatments: nubbins, syndactyly and web contracture, brachydactyly, digit instability, thumb in the plane of the hand, and absence of fingers.

7.6.2.1 Nubbins

Symbrachydactyly can result in severely hypoplastic digits, referred to as nubbins. They consist of a small balloon-like digit with a hypoplastic nail and a small bit of cartilage or distal phalangeal bone connected to the hand by a relatively narrow skin sleeve.

The nubbins can cause difficulties with respect to nail care and may impede prehension if they are located in an area of palmar contact or web space. Some parents choose to remove the abnormal appearing digits some not, because they are considered as fingers by the child (Fig. 7.3).

7.6.2.2 Syndactyly

Syndactyly and web contractures are treated to improve independent digital function, grasp span, and appearance. Depending on the type of symbrachydactyly, the syndactyly could be complete and incomplete for example usually in the Type I (Blauth and Gekeler) is incomplete. The syndactyly release could be challenging because vessels are often hypoplastic or have an abnormal course. For incomplete simple syndactyly of the digits, twofold or fourfold Z-plasty is usually sufficient [32]. For complete syndactyly, the choice of flap depends on surgeon preferences. We prefer Flatt's technique [33] (Fig. 7.4).

In cases of tight syndactyly, to allow the skin release and limit the need for skin grafting, the authors use tissue distraction performed using an external distraction device (Cube-Fix distractor) developed for Apert Syndrome [34, 35]. The device is referred to as the "magic cube" since the distraction results in extra skin that makes subsequent separation easier (Fig. 7.5).

7.6.2.3 Web Contracture

Release of the web space in symbrachydactyly can be more challenging than similar releases performed for other congenital disorders due to a lack of local skin available. Usually, the web space may benefit from deepening and widening. Priority is given to the first web space to facilitate the thumb function. A 4-flap z-plasty is useful for

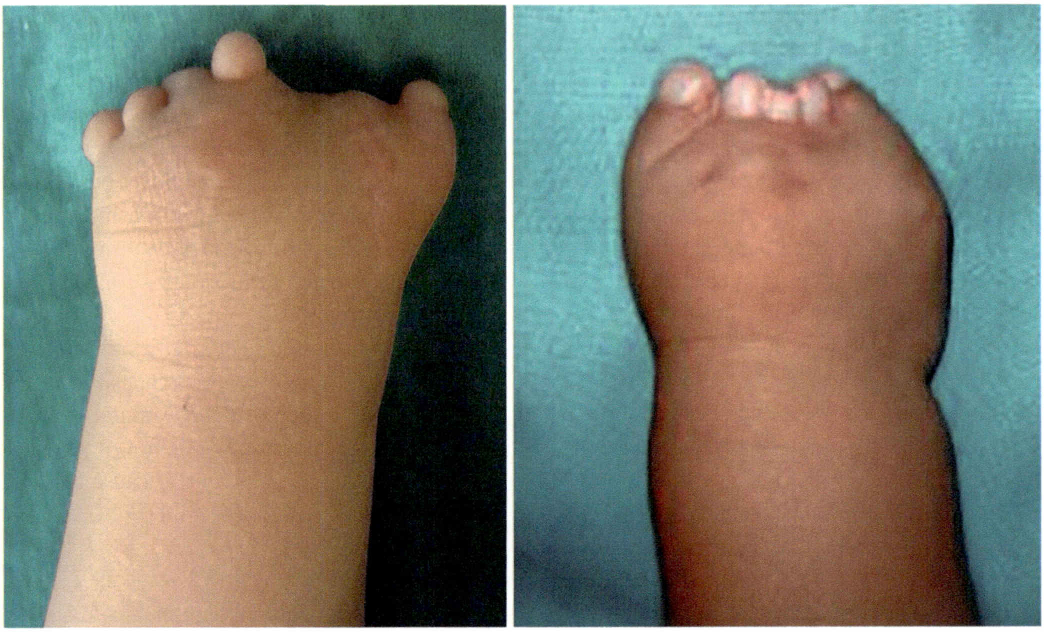

Fig. 7.3 symbrachydactyly: nubbins

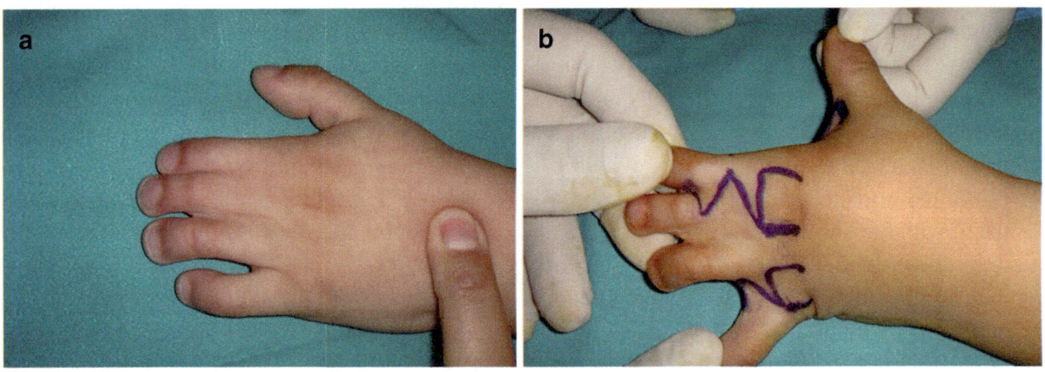

Fig. 7.4 Syndactyly release with Flatt's technique: (**a**) preoperative photograph of type I symbrachydactyly. (**b**) Preoperative planning of syndactyly release, Flatt's flap is used for 2° web space

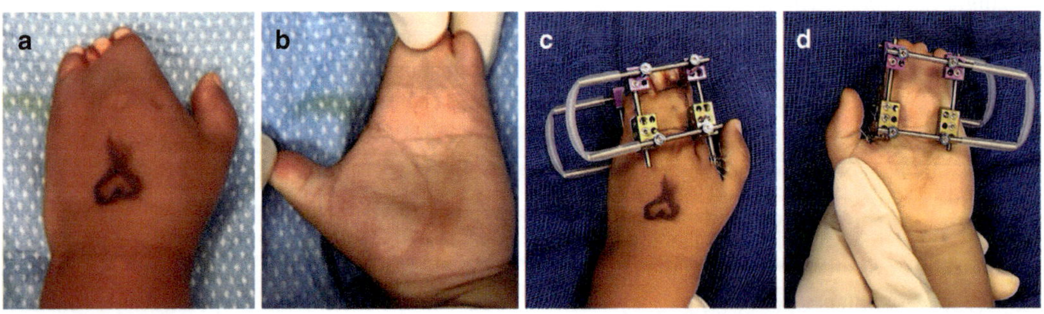

Fig. 7.5 Cube-Fix distractor as the first step of tight syndactyly release: (**a**) preoperative photograph of type I symbrachydactyly, dorsal view and (**b**) palmar view; (**c**) and (**d**) postoperative result of positioning of cube-fix

deepening the first web space; for widening the first web space the authors prefer jumping man flap (5-flap z-plasty). In more severe cases, a dorsal rotation flap will bring additional skin into the first web [36]. Finally, there are more complex advancement techniques [37–39]. After the skin incision is important to release the fascia and tight soft tissue. The other web spaces can be treated with multiple Z-plasties, jumping man flap (5-flap z-plasty), Ostrowsky flaps, and more complex advancement techniques [40–42]. Deepening web spaces greater than the normal level gain the illusion of a longer digit and aid function (Figs. 7.6 and 7.7).

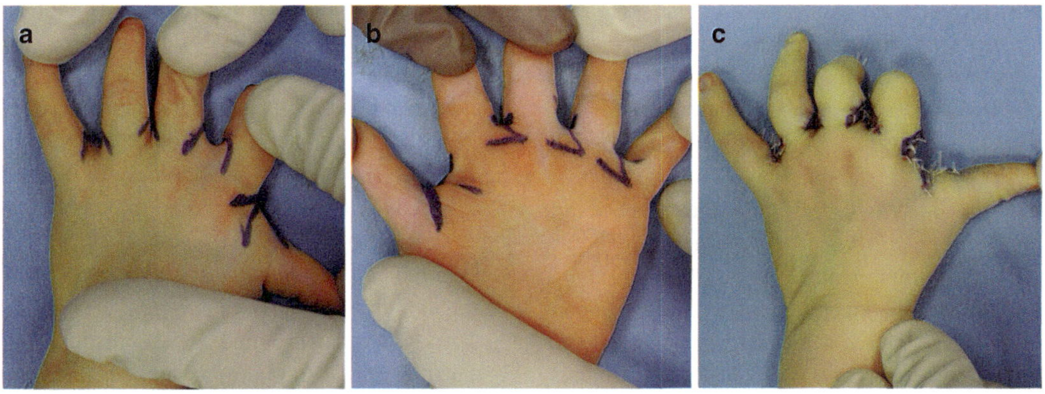

Fig. 7.6 Web spaces deepening using Ostrowsky flaps: (**a**) preoperative planning of the flaps dorsal view and (**b**) palmar view; (**c**) postoperative result

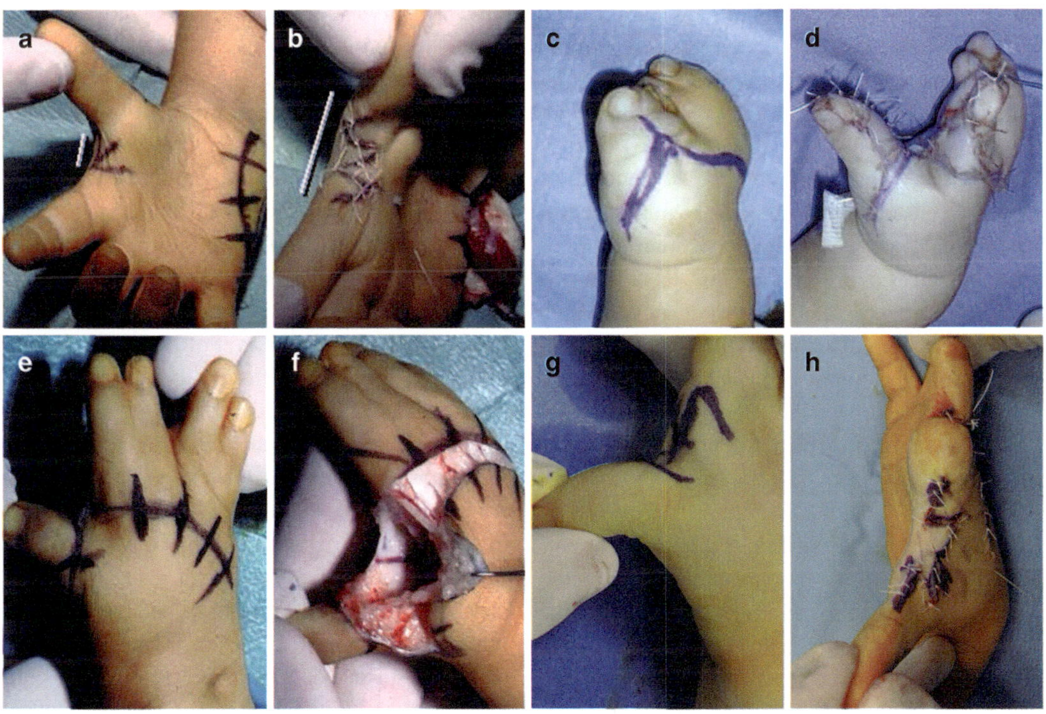

Fig. 7.7 First web release technique: (**a**) preoperative photograph of 4-flap z-plasty and (**b**) postoperative appearance. (**c**) Preoperative photograph of modified Buck Gramcko flap and (**d**) postoperative result. (**e**) Preoperative planning of Buck Gramcko flap and (**f**) intraoperative appearance. (**g**) Preoperative photograph of 5-flap z-plasty and (**h**) postoperative result

7.6.2.4 Thumb in the Plane of the Hand

In symbrachydactyly, thumb is usually hypoplastic and in the plane of the hand.

To improve the position and function of the adducted thumb, it is necessary to release soft tissue in the first web. When the thumb is also retropulsed, osteotomy may reposition the thumb in a more appropriate position for pinch. Langer et al. [43] reported the results of the first web space deepening combined with an abduction-rotational osteotomy of the thumb metacarpal in 5 of 14 children. The osteotomy repositioned the metacarpal in an average of 73° of palmar abduction and 60° to 90° of pronation to facilitate pulp-to-pulp pinch. In this series, all hands were able to perform key pinch and lateral pinch and showed subjective improvement in hand function and appearance. Iba et al. [44] also reported a small series of patients in whom improvement in pinch and thumb function was noted after web-plasty and rotation osteotomy of the first metacarpal.

When the thumb is ipoplastic, it is possible to combine first web deepening with Huber muscle transfer or other procedures to gain stability and force as thumb metacarpal lengthening, thumb interphalangeal joint arthrodesis, long finger metacarpal lengthening.

7.6.2.5 Digit Instability

Floppy or unstable digits occur in symbrachydactyly. Chondrodesis, or fusion of the two cartilaginous surfaces, may stabilize these digits. Arthrodesis can be performed in unstable, floppy skeletally fingers without disturbing physeal growth once the epiphysis has ossified.

7.6.2.6 Brachydactyly and Absence of Fingers

Non-Vascularized Free Toe Phalanx Transfers

The objective of this operation is to augment the length and stability of the fingers to improve prehension and appearance. Non-vascularized toe phalangeal bone grafts provide additional length for short hypoplastic digits in which the skin sleeve is longer than the skeletal elements. Such digits usually have ossification only in the distal phalanx. This operation may be useful in type IIA symbrachydactyly, when the base of the proximal phalanx is present along with a generous soft tissue envelope.

The procedure was first described in 1919 by Noesske and recently used by Goldberg and Watson [45]. The procedure must be performed in early childhood. Goldberg and Watson demonstrated that for patients between 6 and 18 months at the time of surgery, 91% of phalanges had radiographically radiolucent physes and these phalanges showed growth between 83% and 100% of the contralateral undisturbed phalanx. In children 18 months to 5 years old, only 67% of transferred bones had open physes, whereas children more than 5 years of age had only 50% radiographically open physes; however, the percentage of growth was the same [45].

Buck-Gramcko reported similar results with better outcomes in children younger than 12 months [46].

The procedure involves the entire proximal phalanx of the fourth or third toe being extraperiosteally harvested with its proximal collateral ligaments and plantar plate, and then positioned articulating against the metacarpal head. The plantar plate and collateral ligaments are secured to the host metacarpal. Primitive flexor and extensor tendons in the hypoplastic digit are sutured to the transferred phalanx [31]. Then all is secured with a Kirschner wire from proximal to distal.

To reduce shortening on the finger at the donor site, authors prefer to suture flexors and extensor tendons together at the level of bone draw. Other option is the interposition of bone graft in the phalangeal void within the toe.

The use of non-vascularized free toe phalanx in symbrachydactyly is debated; the literature reveals variable results, with longer-term follow-up showing more disappointing outcomes. The most frequent complications or issues are reabsorption of the transposed graft (more often observed if the graft does not include the distal articular surface), donor site morbidity, poor functional results, and instability of toe phalanx [47] (Fig. 7.8).

Garagnani et al. studied 40 children with a mean follow-up of 10 years, they noted consid-

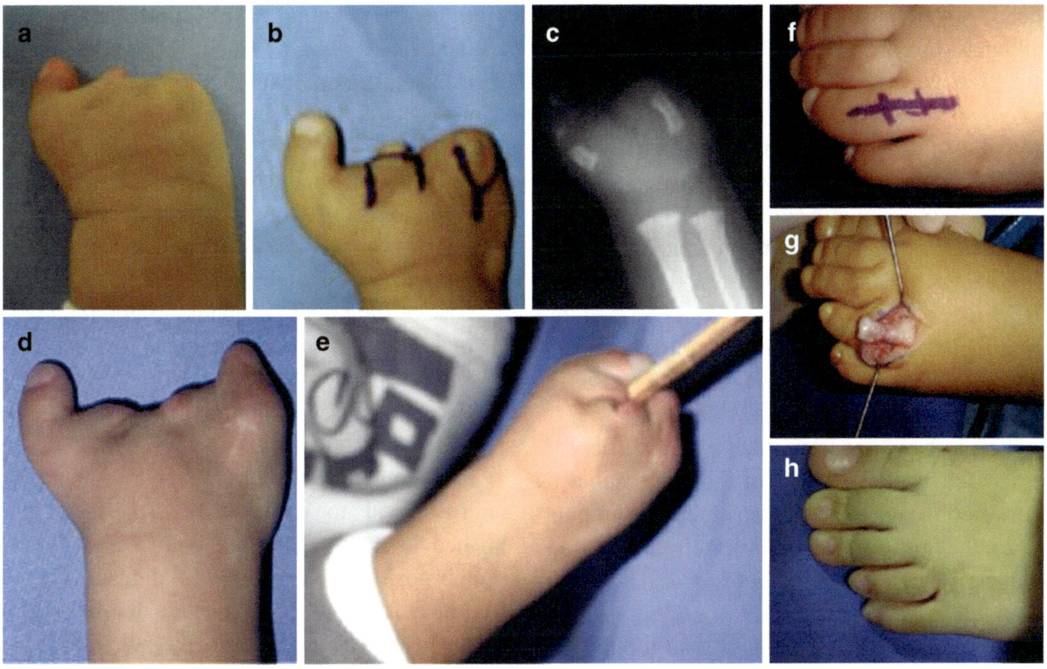

Fig. 7.8 Non-vascularized free-toe phalanx transfers technique: (**a**) A patient with a monodactylous hand with hypoplastic thumb; (**b**) preoperative planning of phalanx transfer on the ulnar ray (**c**) preoperative radiographs (**d**) postoperative results (**e**) thumb to ulnar digit pinch (**f**) preoperative planning of donor site (**g**) intraoperative photograph of phalanx drawing (**h**) long term follow-up of donor site appearance

erable long-term donor site morbidity after toe phalangeal harvest with many donors toes floppy, unstable, and short with deformities in adjacent toes [48]. Patients and families reported varying degrees of dissatisfaction with the appearance and durability of the foot as well as cosmetic and physical problems with regard to the toes [48].

Distraction Lengthening

Bone distraction is potentially useful for the treatment of short fingers in symbrachydactyly. However, the high rate of complications makes the indications debated [49]. This treatment rarely normalizes appearance and the literature shows mixed results with little information to indicate whether this procedure improves function and appearance.

Foucher [50] reviewed results of distraction lengthening in 41 patients, 22 cases with symbrachydactyly. He reported an average gain of 2.3 cm over 4 months. Complications observed were infection, nonunion, or fracture in 32%. Miyawaki [51] reported successful cases of metacarpal lengthening in patients with types IIA, IIB, and IIIA, noting improved pinch strength with no major complications; Heo [52] reported a series of 24 metacarpal and 27 phalangeal lengthening procedures with a 31% complication rate, including nonunion, fracture, premature consolidation, angulation, and hardware failure. Others authors have reported angulation of the lengthened bones, with unsatisfactory appearance [53].

Seitz [54] reported a large series reflecting his long-term experience with distraction lengthening in the arm, forearm, and hand for children with a wide range of conditions. He demonstrated that in most cases the procedure increase length; the family and child are satisfied despite of complex and arduous procedure and high rate of complication (50% minor, 9% major).

Given the high rates of complications reported for distraction lengthening and the paucity of evidence to support significant functional gains, authors rarely perform this procedure in symbrachydactyly.

Microsurgical Toe-to-Hand Transfers

Toe-to-hand transfer is well-accepted for the treatment of traumatic amputations in adults and children. The indication for congenital hand malformations remains more debated.

O'Brien and colleagues [55] described the first toe-to-hand transfer for a congenital hand anomaly in 1978, and several series have subsequently been reported [56, 57].

Toe-to-hand transfer could be more difficult in symbrachydactyly despite of other anomalies as constriction ring syndrome or traumatic amputations: the host nerves, blood vessels, and tendons may be hypoplastic, anomalous, or absent in children with symbrachydactyly.

In 1988, Lister [58] described 12 toe-to-hand transfers in children with various congenital hand differences, including three cases of symbrachydactyly, and noted unique neuro-vascular anatomic variations in each patient.

Others have reinforced that there is a wide variation in the neurovascular structures in symbrachydactyly [58–60].

The optimal age for toe transfers remains unknown, but most experienced surgeons believe toe transfers between 2 and 3 years of age have the best cortical integration [60], although transfers have been successfully reported in older children [61].

The indications for toe-to-hand transfers are still being established for unilateral symbrachydactyly. Jones and Kaplan [60] proposed a morphologic framework of indications for vascularized toe transfer in congenitals. There are three indications for considering microsurgical reconstruction of an absent thumb:

1. isolated absence of the thumb, distal to the metacarpal base with preservation of the carpometacarpal joint and thenar muscles and with four normal or relatively normal fingers
2. absence of the thumb as well as the index, middle, and ring fingers, but with one or two fingers remaining on the ulnar side of the hand
3. unilateral and extremely rarely bilateral absence of all five digits

There are two indications for considering toe transfers to reconstruct absent fingers:

1. Absence of all four fingers proximal to the base of the middle phalanges, but with a normal thumb (correspond to types IIIA and IVA symbrachydactyly)
2. Complete absence of all five digits

Providing pinch to the adactylous hand by microsurgical toe transfer is usually accomplished in two stages, first with a digit in the thumb position and then with a digit positioned for pinch using the second toe transfer most commonly [62]. Other authors have suggested that the simultaneous transfer of bilateral second toes has the advantage of not having to dissect the previously anastomosed vessels in a second procedure. Results show that toe to hand transfer is a safe procedure: reported survival rates are greater than 96% [63–66].

The range of motion of the transferred toes can be unpredictable and Is the most common indication for secondary revision. Passive range of motion exceeds the active range of motion. Despite this finding, tenolysis is rarely useful [65, 67]. The transferred toes usually have minimal active distal interphalangeal motion and an extension deficit at the proximal interphalangeal joint. A fixed flexion deformity of the toe transfer is a frequent outcome.

Vilkki [68] reported that 14 of 17 patients had the ability to pinch, whereas Van Holder et al. [69] documented a mean extension deficit of 20° in 28 transfers at the distal joint and active total flexion of proximal and distal joints of 80°. Foucher et al. [64] reported on 65 toe transfers with 25° of extensor lag and approximately 38° of active motion.

Growth and sensation are usually satisfactory. Kay et al. [67, 70] documented that transferred toes can reach up to 100% length of the

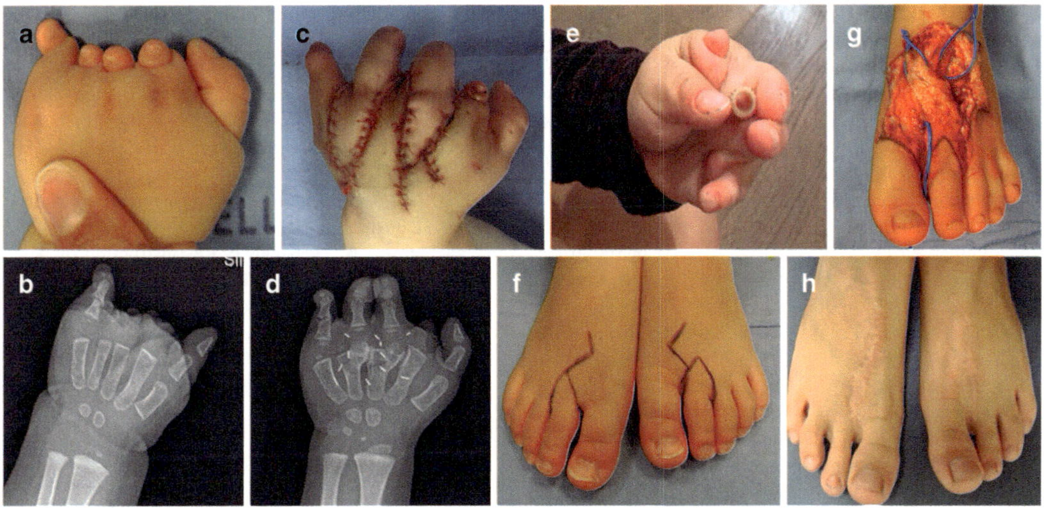

Fig. 7.9 Microsurgical toe-to-hand transfers: (**a**) A patient with a monodactylous hand with hypoplastic thumb; previous operation a non-vascularized free toe phalanx transfers to ulnar digit; (**b**) preoperative radiographs; (**c**) postoperative appearance after double toe to hand transfers; (**d**) postoperative radiographs (**e**) thumb to "new" fingers pinch (**f**) preoperative planning of donor sites (**g**) intraoperative photograph of toe harvest drawing (**h**) long term follow-up of donor sites appearance

contralateral toe with normal growth, whereas other authors reported the length range from 60% to 100% [65].

Foucher et al [64] reported mean two-point discrimination of 5 mm. Kay and Wiberg [67] found that all of the children recovered protective sensibility and the majority recovered good levels of two-point discrimination and light touch perception.

With regards to the psychological affects, Kay et al. demonstrated a high level of satisfaction for appearance, function, donor site, reaction of others, and psychological well-being in parents and children [67] (Fig. 7.9).

References

1. Gupta A, Kay SP, Scheker LR. The growing hand: diagnosis and management of the upper extremity in children. Maryland Heights, MO: Mosby; 2000.
2. Poland A. Deficiency of the pectoralis muscles. Guys Hosp Rep. 1841;6:191–3.
3. Pol R. "Brachydaktylie" – "Klinodaktylie" – Hyperphalangie und ihre Grundlagen: Form und Enstehung der meist unter dem Bild der Brachtdaktylie auftretenden Varietaten Anomalien und Mißbildungen der Hand und des Fußes. Virchows Arch Path Anat. 1921;229:388–530.
4. Fraser FC, Ronen GM, O'Leary E. Pectoralis major defect and Poland sequence in second cousins: extension of the Poland sequence spectrum. Am J Med Genet. 1989;33:468–70.
5. Al-Qattan MM. Classification of hand anomalies in Poland's syndrome. Br J Plast Surg. 2001;54:132–6.
6. Ireland D, Takayama N, et al. Poland's syndrome. A review of fortythree cases. J Bone Joint Surg. 1976;58A:52–8.
7. Ekblom AG, Laurell T, Arner M. Epidemiology of congenital upper limb anomalies in Stockholm, Sweden, 1997 to 2007: application of the Oberg, Manske, and Tonkin classification. J Hand Surg Am. 2014;39(2):237–48.
8. Cobben JM, Robinson PH, van Essen AJ, van der Wiel HL, ten Kate LP. Poland anomaly in mother and daughter. Am J Med Genet. 1989;33:519–21.
9. Darian VB, Argenta LC, Pasyk KA. Familial Poland's syndrome. Ann Plast Surg. 1989;23:531.
10. Bavinck JN, Weaver DD. Subclavian artery supply disruption sequence: hypothesis of a vascular etiology for Poland, Klippel-Feil, and Möbius anomalies. Am J Med Genet. 1986;23(4):903–18.
11. Bouvet JP, Leveque D, Bernetieres F, Gros JJ. Vascular origin of Poland syndrome? A comparative rheographic study of the vascularization of the arms in eight patients. Eur J Pediatr. 1978;128(1):17–26.
12. Iwagawa S. Symbrachydactyly: review of 50 cases and definition. Hiroshima J Med Sci. 1980;29:105–15.

13. Ogino T, Ischii S, Minami M, et al. Congenital anomalies of the hand. The Asian perspective. Clin Orthop. 1996;323:12–21.
14. Ogino T. Teratogenic mechanisms of longitudinal deficiency and cleft hand. Handchir Mikrochir Plast Chir. 2004;36:108–16.
15. Fernandez-Teran M, Ros MA. The apical ectodermal ridge: morphological aspects and signaling pathways. Int J Dev Biol. 2008;52(7):857–71.
16. Summerbell D. A quantitative analysis of the effect of excision of the AER from the chick limb-bud. J Embryol Exp Morphol. 1974;32(3):651–60.
17. Winkel A, Stricker S, Tylzanowski P, et al. Wnt-ligand- dependent interaction of TAK1 (TGF-beta-activated kinase-1) with the receptor tyrosine kinase Ror2 modulates canonical Wnt-signalling. Cell Signal. 2008;20(11):2134–44.
18. Goodell PB, Bauer AS, Sierra FJ, James MA. Symbrachydactyly. Hand (NY). 2016;11(3):262–70. Epub 2016 Sep 1. Review
19. Gardiner DM, Holmes LB. Hypothesis: terminal transverse limb defects with "nubbins" represent a regenerative process during limb development in human fetuses. Birth Defects Res A Clin Mol Teratol. 2012;94(3):129–33.
20. International Federation of Societies for Surgery of the Hand. IFSSH scientific committee on congenital conditions. J Hand Surg Eur Vol. 2014;39(6):676–8.
21. Tonkin MA, Tolerton SK, Quick TJ, et al. Classification of congenital anomalies of the hand and upper limb: development and assessment of a new system. J Hand Surg Am. 2013;38(9):1845–53.
22. Swanson AB. A classification for congenital limb malformations. J Hand Surg Am. 1976;1(1):8–22.
23. Blauth W, Gekeler J. Morphology and classification of symbrachydactylia. Handchirurgie. 1971;3(4):123–8.
24. Müller W. Die angeborenen Fehlbildungen der menschlichen Hand: Erb-und Konstitutionsbiologie der Hand. New York, NY: Thieme; 1937.
25. Yamauchi Y, Tanabu S. Symbrachydactyly. In: Buck-Gramcko D, editor. Congenital malformations of the hand and forearm. London: Churchill Livingstone; 1998. p. 149–58.
26. Foucher G, Medina J, Pajardi G, Navarro R. Classification and treatment of symbrachydactyly. A series of 117 cases. Chir Main. 2000;19(3):161–8.
27. Flatt AE. The care of congenital hand anomalies. St. Louis, MO: Quality Medical Publishing; 1994.
28. Knight JB, Pritsch T, Ezaki M, Oishi SN. Unilateral congenital terminal finger absences: a condition that differs from symbrachydactyly. J Hand Surg Br. 2012;37(1):124–9.
29. Case-Smith J. Clinical interpretation of "development of in-hand manipulation and relationship with activities". Am J Occup Ther. 1995;49(8):772–4.
30. Gordon A, Forssberg H. Development of neural mechanisms underlying grasping in children. In: Connolly K, Forssberg H, editors. Neurophysiology and neuropsychology of motor development. London: MacKeith Press; 1997. p. 214–31.
31. Woodside JC, Light TR. Symbrachydactyly - diagnosis, function, and treatment. J Hand Surg Am. 2016;41(1):135–43.
32. Gulgonen A, Gudemez E. Reconstruction of the first web space in symbrachydactyly using the reverse radial forearm flap. J Hand Surg Am. 2007;32(2):162–7.
33. Flatt AE. Treatment of syndactylism. Plast Reconstr Surg Transplant Bull. 1962;29:336–41.
34. Nachemson A, Hessman P. Reconstruction of Apert hands with Cube fix distractor. In: Proceedings 8th World Symposium on Congenital Malformations of the Hand Upper Limb, Hamburg. 2009.
35. Kvernmo HD, Haugstvedt JR. Treatment of congenital syndactyly of the fingers. Tidsskr Nor Laegeforen. 2013;133(15):1591–5.
36. Friedman R, Wood VE. The dorsal transposition flap for congenital contractures of the first web space: a 20-year experience. J Hand Surg Br. 1997;22(4):664–70.
37. Brown PW. Adduction—flexion contracture of the thumb: correction with dorsal rotation flap and release of contracture. Clin Orthop Relat Res. 1972;88:161–8.
38. Caroli A, Zanasi S. First web-space reconstruction by Caroli's technique in congenital hand deformities with severe thumb ray adduction. Br J Plast Surg. 1989;42(6):653–9.
39. Chang SM, Hou CL, Zhang F, Lineaweaver WC, Chen ZW, Gu YD. Distally based radial forearm flap with preservation of the radial artery: anatomic, experimental, and clinical stud- ies. Microsurgery. 2003;23(4):328–37.
40. Flatt AE, Wood VE. Multiple dorsal rotation flaps from the hand for thumb web contractures. Plast Reconstr Surg. 1970;45(3):258–62.
41. Waters PM, Bae DS. Pediatric hand and upper limb surgery: a practical guide. Philadelphia, PA: Wolters Kluwer Health/Lippincott Williams & Wilkins; 2012.
42. Ostrowski DM, Feagin CA, Gould JS. A three-flap web-plasty for release of short congenital syndactyly and dorsal adduction contracture. J Hand Surg Am. 1991;16(4):634–41.
43. Langer JS, Manske PR, Steffen JA, Hu C, Goldfarb C. Thumb in the plane of the hand: characterization and results of surgical treatment. J Hand Surg Am. 2009;34(10):1795–801.
44. Iba K, Wada T, Aoki M, Yamashita T. Improvement in pinch function after surgical treatment for thumb in the plane of the hand. J Hand Surg Eur Vol. 2012;37(2):145–8.
45. Goldberg NH, Watson HK. Composite toe (phalanx and epiphysis) transfers in the reconstruction of the aphalangic hand. J Hand Surg Br. 1982;7(5):454–9.
46. Buck-Gramcko D. The role of nonvascularized toe phalanx transplantation. Hand Clin. 1990;6(4):643–59.
47. Cavallo AV, Smith PJ, Morley S, Morsi AW. Non- vascularized free toe phalanx transfers in congenital hand

deformities—the Great Ormond Street experience. J Hand Surg Br. 2003;28(6):520–7.
48. Garagnani L, Gibson M, Smith PJ, Smith GD. Long-term donor site morbidity after free nonvascularized toe phalangeal transfer. J Hand Surg Br. 2012;37(4):764–74.
49. Matev IB. Thumb reconstruction in children through metacarpal lengthening. Plast Reconstr Surg. 1979;64(5):665–9.
50. Foucher G, Pajardi G, Lamas C, Medina J, Navarro R. Progressive bone lengthening of the hand in congenital malformations. 41 cases. Rev Chir Orthop Reparatrice Appar Mot. 2001;87(5):451–8.
51. Miyawaki T, Masuzawa G, Hirakawa M, Kurihara K. Bone-lengthening for symbrachydactyly of the hand with the technique of callus distraction. J Bone Joint Surg Am. 2002;84-A(6):986–91.
52. Heo CY, Kwon S, Back GH, Chung MS. Complications of distraction lengthening in the hand. J Hand Surg Eur. 2008;33(5):609–15.
53. Matsuno T, Ishida O, Sunagawa T, Ichikawa M, Ikuta Y, Ochi M. Bone lengthening for congenital differences of the hands and digits in children. J Hand Surg Br. 2004;29(4):712–9.
54. Seitz WH Jr, Shimko P, Patterson RW. Long-term results of callus distraction-lengthening in the hand and upper extremity for traumatic and congenital skeletal deficiencies. J Bone Joint Surg Am. 2010;92(Suppl 2):47–58.
55. O'Brien BM, Black MJ, Morrison WA, et al. Microvascular great toe transfer for congenital absence of the thumb. Hand. 1978;10:113–24.
56. Nyarady J, Szekeres P, Vilmos Z. Toe-to-thumb transfer in congenital grade III thumb hypoplasia. J Hand Surg [Am]. 1983;8:898–901.
57. Schenker M, Wiberg M, Kay SP, et al. Precision grip function after free toe transfer in children with hypoplastic digits. J Plast Reconstr Aesthet Surg. 2007;60:13–23.
58. Lister G. Microsurgical transfer of the second toe for congenital deficiency of the thumb. Plast Reconstr Surg. 1988;82:658–65.
59. Richardson PW, Johnstone BR, Coombs CJ. Toe-to-hand transfer in symbrachydactyly. Hand Surg. 2004;9:11–8.
60. Jones NF, Kaplan J. Indications for microsurgical reconstruction of congenital hand anomalies by toe-to-hand transfers. Hand. 2013;8(4):367–74.
61. Spokevicius S, Radzevicius D. Late toe-to-hand transfer for the reconstruction of congenital defects of the long fingers. Scand J Plast Reconstr Surg Hand Surg. 1997;31(4):345–50.
62. Jones NF, Hansen SL, Bates SJ. Toe-to-hand transfers for congenital anomalies of the hand. Hand Clin. 2007;23(1):129–36.
63. Gilbert A. Reconstruction of congenital hand defects with microvascular toe transfers. Hand Clin. 1985;1:351–60.
64. Foucher G, Medina J, Navarro R, et al. Toe transfer in congenital hand malformations. J Reconstr Microsurg. 2001;17:1–7.
65. Gilbert A. Toe transfers for congenital hand defects. J Hand Surg [Am]. 1982;7:118–24.
66. Chang J, Jones NF. Radiographic analysis of growth in pediatric microsurgical toe-to-hand transfers. Plast Reconstr Surg. 2002;109:576–82.
67. Kay SP, Wiberg M, Bellew M, Webb F. Toe to hand transfer in children. Part 2: functional and psychological aspects. J Hand Surg Br. 1996;21(6):735–45.
68. Vilkki S. Advances in microsurgical reconstruction of the congenitally adactylous hand. Clin Orthop Relat Res. 1995;314:45–8.
69. Van Holder C, Giele H, Gilbert A. Double second toe transfer in congenital hand anomalies. J Hand Surg (Br). 1999;24:471–5.
70. Kay SP, Wiberg M. Toe to hand transfer in children. Part 1. Technical aspects. J Hand Surg (Br). 1996;21:723–34.
71. Rayan GM, Upton III J. Congenital hand anomalies and associated syndromes. Berlin: Springer; 2014.

Central Synpolydactyly

8

Andrea Jester, Tatiana Y. Jacomel,
Michail Vourvachis, and Jeannette W. C. Ting

Abstract

Central synpolydactyly (CSPD) is a rare and heterogeneous, autosomal dominant congenital hand condition thought to be attributed to the Homeobox-D13 (HOXD13) gene. There are multiple clinical and radiological classification systems for syndactyly and CSPD although none of these comprehensively describe the complexity of the condition. The degree of flexion, deviation and rotation at birth has a significant influence on the eventual form and function of the affected digits. Unlike syndactyly or polydactyly alone, CSPD patients often also have stiffness and flexion contractures of their interphalangeal joints, complicating their surgery and outcome. We describe our two preferred surgical approaches to CSPD depending on the patient's skin type.

Keywords

Central synpolydactyly · SPD 1 · SPD 2
SPD 3 · Syndactyly

A. Jester (✉) · T. Y. Jacomel · M. Vourvachis
J. W. C. Ting
Hands and Upper Limb Service, Birmingham Women's and Children's Hospital, Birmingham, UK
e-mail: andrea.jester@nhs.net

8.1 Introduction

Central synpolydactyly (CSPD) is a non-syndromic, complex and heterogeneous malformation of the hand that is rare and can be challenging to manage. CSPD involves fusion (syn) of the central axis digits (third and fourth rays only) with excess digits or parts of digits (poly). The accessory digit may arise from either the middle or ring finger. The terminology is often confusing in the literature as classically, CSPD is a type of synpolydactyly (SPD). SPD, in turn, is a subtype (II) of syndactyly [1–3].

As separate entities, both polydactyly and syndactyly are common, with an incidence of 5–17 [4] and 3–40 per 10,000 births [5], respectively. The true incidence of CSPD is unknown, but thought to be significantly rarer than polydactyly or syndactyly alone. CSPD is also associated with various forms of synpolydactyly of the toes and rarely, hypospadias, which is beyond the scope of this chapter and therefore will not be discussed [1, 6].

8.2 Genetics

CSPD is an autosomal dominant condition [1, 5, 6] which shows incomplete penetrance, variable expressivity and intra- and inter-familial variability [5, 7–9] (Fig. 8.1). Much of our understanding of the genetics behind CSPD has arisen from

G. Pajardi (ed.), *Pediatric Hand Surgery*, https://doi.org/10.1007/978-3-031-30984-7_8

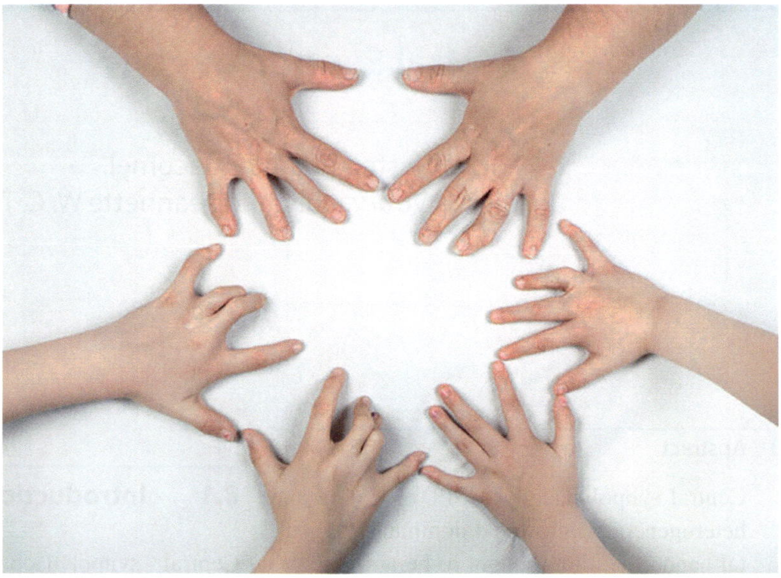

Fig. 8.1 A family of two sisters and mother all with CSPD. Note the intra-family variability commonly seen in CSPD

investigations of large affected Turkish and Chinese families as it is such a rare condition and therefore difficult to study in large populations [2, 6, 10]. The Homeobox (HOX) family of genes is the main family of genes affecting limb patterning that has been implicated in CSPD [1, 6, 11, 12]. It encodes for a family of transcription factors that affect downstream pathways, which in turn control axis formation during embryonic development [12, 13]. In humans, there are a total of 39 HOX genes. These are grouped into four clusters based on their location on four different chromosomes and named HOXA, B, C and D clusters [6]. The HOXD cluster, and more specifically, the HOXD13 gene at chromosome 2q31, is believed to be responsible for CSPD [6, 14]. The HOXD13 gene is also involved with other congenital hand conditions including certain subtypes of brachydactyly, brachysyndactyly syndrome, VACTERL and other forms of syndactyly [2, 3, 6, 12].

The phenotype of CSPD seen is dependent on whether the genetic abnormality of the HOXD13 genes is a result of polyalanine expansion, intragenic deletion, missense mutations or frameshift deletions [6]. Polyalanine expansion is when stretches of alanine (amino acid) increase in length beyond a threshold, resulting in mutant proteins that cannot fold and therefore bind normally [6, 10, 15–17]. In the HOXD13 gene, a minimum of seven alanine expansions will produce SPD [6, 11, 13] with the greater expansion leading to greater penetrance of phenotypic mutation and more limbs involved [1, 6, 11, 18]. Deletions, frameshifting and missense mutations are also attributed to atypical or milder forms of SPD and other congenital hand conditions by producing proteins that are unable to function normally [6, 19, 20].

Very few syndromic conditions are associated with CSPD. One of these is Pallister–Hall syndrome, a very rare autosomal dominant disorder with unknown prevalence that can present with postaxial SPD or CSPD [21, 22]. It is caused by mutations in the GLI3 gene, responsible for the shaping of many organs during the prenatal period [22, 23]. These patients universally present with hypothalamic hamartoma [24].

8.2.1 Classification

Several classification systems have been used over the years for SPD that are also applicable to CSPD.

The first classification system used for SPD, described by Stelling and Turek in 1963, classifies SPD according to the morphological skeletal abnormalities of the polydactylous component of SPD [25–27]. Type I is associated with no skeletal syndactylous attachment. Type II is characterised by a duplication of the common metacarpal or phalanx associated with (Subtype A) or without skeletal syndactyly (Subtype B). Type III refers to polydactyly associated with a complete duplication of the finger including the metacarpal [25–27].

Over two decades later, in 1989, Buck-Gramcko and Behrens [28] published a different classification of SPD based on radiological features rather than morphological features. Their aim was to be able to classify all polydactylies, including pre, central and postaxial variations. However, it does not include complex fusions, hypoplastic or incomplete digits [28].

In 2014, Zhou et al. [13] developed a classification with no genetic or precise radiological features. The types are classified according to predicted surgical difficulty. The mild form clinically presents with supplementary fingers, with normal outline of fingers and joints and no bony abnormalities or dysfunctions. The moderate form is associated with supplementary fingers, with a normal bony shape and webbed fingers or finger adhesions affecting joint movement. In severe forms, the extra digits are associated with bony deformity, resulting in compromised grip and function.

In 2016, Wall et al. [25] published a radiological classification for CSPD only, identifying types based on the bony level of the polydactylous digit and its associated characteristic skeletal deformities (Fig. 8.2 and Table 8.1). They do not, however, include additional clinical features such as flexion deformity, hypoplastic bones or soft tissue anomalies. They argue that their classification system not only facilitates the communication between the surgeons, but more importantly, it would allow for a more systematic approach towards CSPD than previous classification systems. Type I is characterised by the involvement of the metacarpals. It is divided into two subtypes: A (division of the metacarpal bone, affecting the ring and middle fingers) and B (extra digit between third and fourth fingers). In Type II, the affected level is the proximal phalanx. It is also divided into two subtypes: Type 2A involves duplication of the ring finger with a syndactyly with the middle finger. The proximal phalanx of the fourth digit is a "delta" phalanx. Type 2B, however, does not show a delta phalanx. Type III refers to the involvement of the middle or distal phalanx of the middle and ring fingers.

The main criticism of this classification system is that it does not take non-bony issues such as flexion deformity and soft tissue contractures into consideration. This is particularly relevant in CSPD where the severity of soft tissue features significantly affects the functional and cosmetic outcome of the fingers more so than syndactyly and polydactyly alone. A more ideal classification system would combine both Zhou's and Wall's principles to allow surgeons to compare conditions and outcomes meaningfully. This has yet to be described.

8.2.2 Surgical Considerations

CSPD patients present even within the same family with very a wide-ranging phenotypic expression. Various factors can have a significant impact on the final form and function of the hand. The outcome is significantly affected by the degree of flexion contracture as well as deviation or rotational deformity. Proximal and distal interphalangeal joints are not rarely partially or completely stiff. Even with meticulous separation of fingers, removal of accessory digits and intensive postoperative hand therapy, stiffness often remains.

Discussions with parents with regards to the surgery and outcome need to be individualised to the patient and conducted comprehensively and openly by a surgeon who understands these complexities. Parents should also be aware that although the aim of surgery is to maximise the outcome with a minimal number of operations, as the child grows, additional surgery may be required to accommodate for these changes.

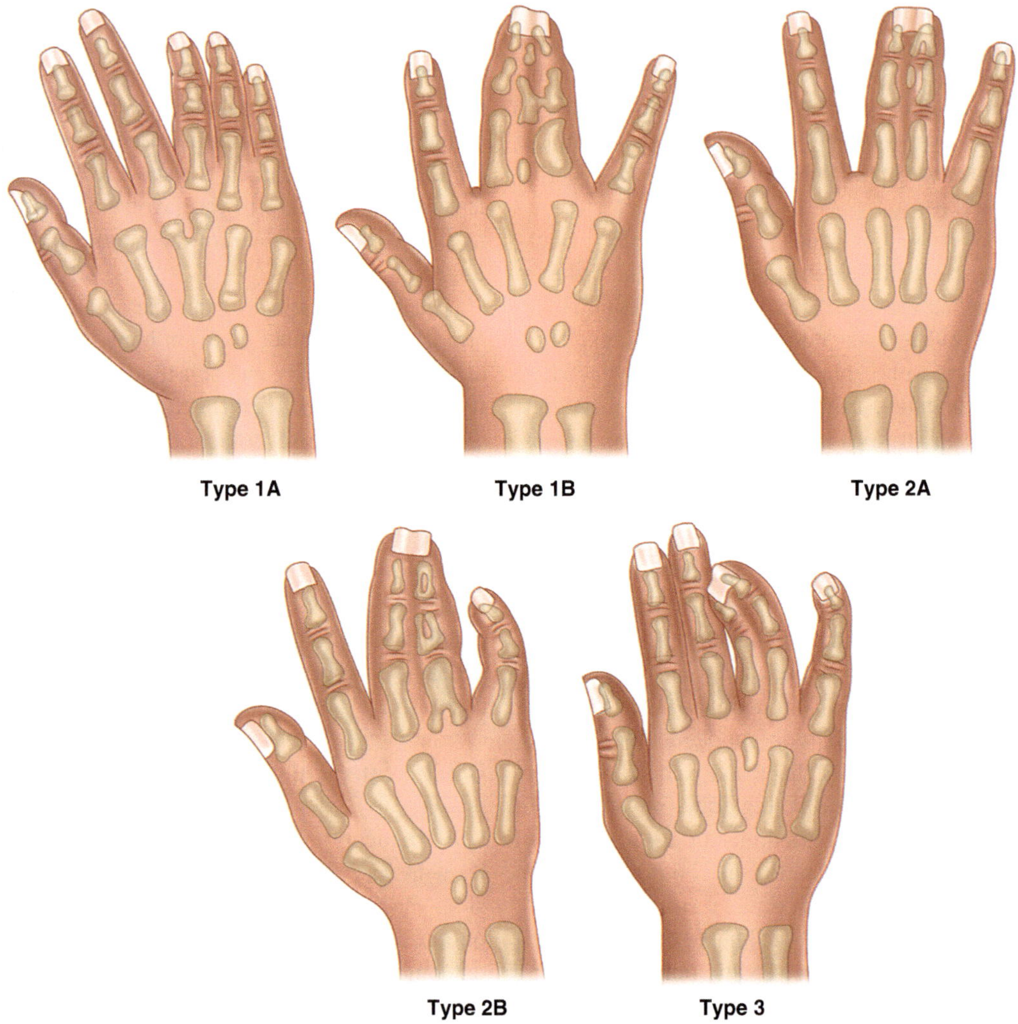

Fig. 8.2 Classification of Polysyndactyly. (From Wall et al., synpolydactyly of the hand: a radiographic classification. J Hand Surg Eur Vol 2016 Mar 41(3):301–307 [25])

Table 8.1 Classification of polysyndactyly. (From Wall et al., Synpolydactyly of the hand: a radiographic classification. J Hand Surg Eur Vol 2016 Mar 41(3):301–307 [25])

Classification type		Level of duplication	Description
1	A	Metacarpal	3rd metacarpal bifurcates Affects long and ring fingers
	B	Metacarpal	3-or 4-boned digits between long and ring fingers Syndactylised to ring or both ring and long fingers
2	A	Proximal phalanx	Duplication of ring finger Syndactyly may involve long finger Delta phalanx of ring P1
	B	Proximal phalanx	Duplication of ring or long fingers Parallel of divergent orientation
3		Middle or distal phalanx	Duplication at P2 or P3 level between long and ring fingers

8.3 Authors Preferred Method

The aim of CSPD surgery consists of the separation of the syndactylous middle finger from the ring finger as well as the removal of the duplicated finger. The duplication may be of either the middle or ring finger. The principles are to achieve an excellent cosmetic result and the best possible functional outcome, without compromising either. Scars should be hidden in the inter-digital space; grafts should be of similar colour as the recipient side. Palmar scars should furthermore not lead to an increase in flexion contractures. I tend to use two main techniques to separate the fingers, with the choice being dependent on the patient's skin colour. These techniques are also used in conventional syndactyly releases.

In fair-skinned patients, a palmar flap combined with inter-digitating zig-zag flaps is used to minimise visible dorsal scarring that is evident when the patient looks that their outstretched hand. The palmar flap is designed with the base of the flap just proximal to an imaginary arch connecting the palmar digital crease of the index and the little finger. The centre of the palmar flap is in the middle of the fused finger mass. The flap is slightly narrowed at the waist with the distal tip of the flap shaped like the gothic arch reaching up to the proximal inter-phalangeal (PIP) crease [29]. When raising the central palmar flap careful blunt dissection with the tip of the scissors aimed between the bones guarantees preservation of the perforators and the vascular bundle. The palmar incisions are matched by a dorsal straight-line incision, which begins proximally at a point halfway between the PIP joint and the metacarpal phalangeal (MCP) joint and ends distally at the PIPJ (Fig. 8.3a).

Narrow thin-tipped triangular flaps are designed distal to this, running up the centre of the syndactyly on the dorsal and corresponding volar surface. They extend to the middle of the finger. These zigzag incisions are made with acute angles deliberately, as they result in horizontal scars that eventually "vanish" in dorsal skin creases and therefore become very well hidden. More obtuse-angled flaps result in obvious oblique scars, especially on the dorsal surface. In the author's experience, there are no issues with flap viability and therefore can be used safely. Over the pulp, a straight-line incision continues into reciprocal triangular flaps. This is a variation of the technique first described by Lundkvist [30] and adapted by (and popularly known as flaps by) Buck-Gramcko (Fig. 8.3b) [31]. These flaps are used to recreate the nail folds.

Full-thickness grafts from the elbow crease are used to resurface only the wounds adjacent to the web space. All other raw areas are left to heal spontaneously. Post-operative management of these patients usually involves a dressing change 14–21 days after the surgery.

For dark-skinned patients, other than minimising dorsal scars, the additional complication to avoid is a colour mismatch. Dark-skinned patients have very light-coloured palmar skin compared to their darker dorsal skin. A palmar flap as described above would result in a lighter-coloured palmar skin being evident in the darker dorsal skin in the depth of the web space. A combination of both dorsal and palmar rectangular flaps is therefore used to avoid this and has been described by Flatt in 1974 [32]. Another advantage of this technique is that only one full-thickness graft is required compared to the two needed in the palmar flap. One of the disadvantages are more visible scars on the dorsum of the hand compared to the palmar only flap.

The removal of the polydactylous bone requires careful dissection and removal of all rudimentary part of the accessory digit, also known as the "Anlage". Incomplete removal of the cartilaginous Anlage, especially between the metacarpal bones may lead to regrowth and a mechanical block that prevents patients from being able to adduct their fingers. This unfortunately leads to visible extension of the scar on the dorsum.

The neurovascular bundles are not skeletonised and fully dissected to prevent inadvertent damage to these fine structures. Instead, a technique of gentle spreading with scissors is used to allow the vascular bundles to be guided into their respective fingers.

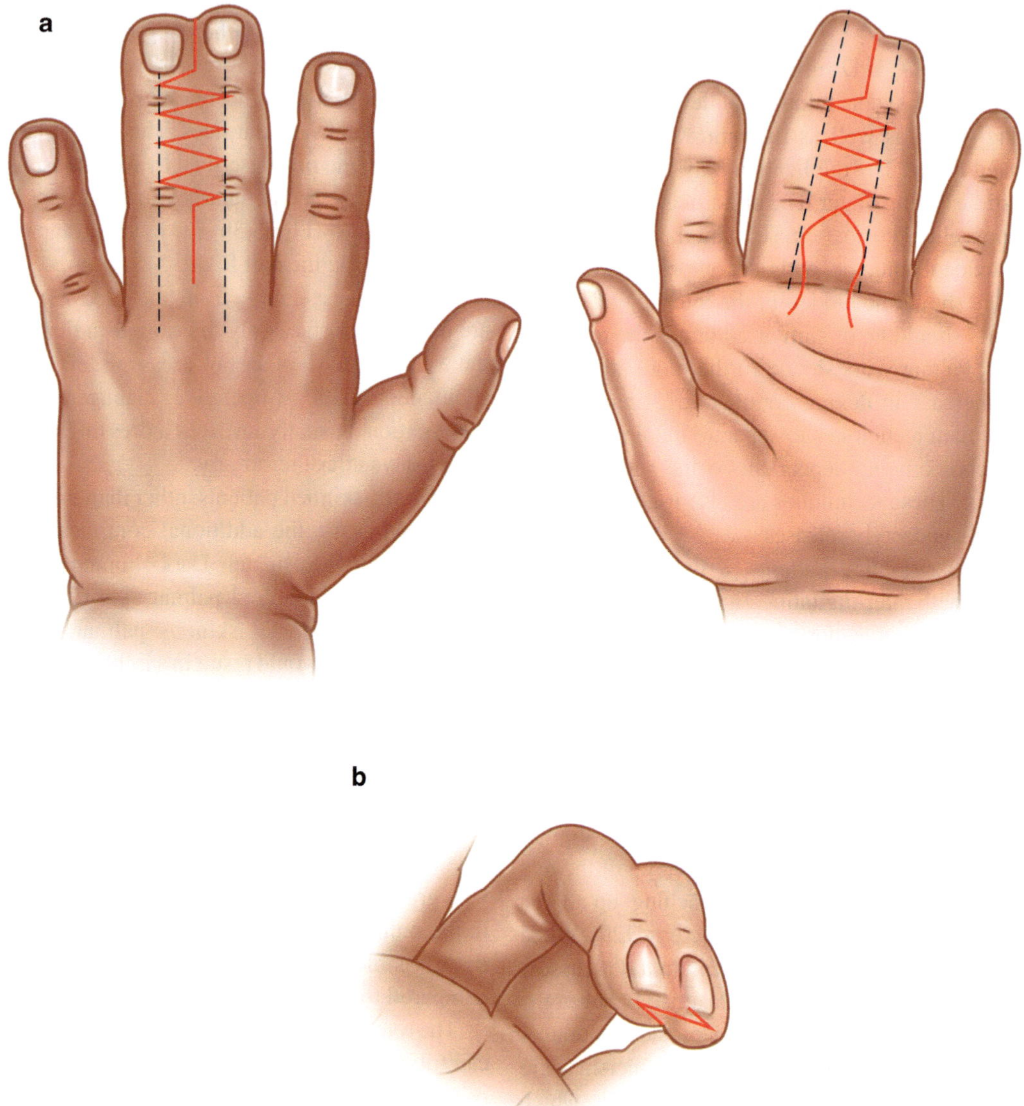

Fig. 8.3 (**a**) Planning of the incision and flaps for primary operation dorsal and palmar. (**b**) Planning of the fingertip incisions

For patients with obviously deviated fingers caused by an aberrant epiphysis (Fig. 8.3a) a decision needs be made as to be whether this can be corrected at the same time as the separation. We do recommend this despite the frequent need for further osteotomies at a later date. (Fig. 8.3c) The foot surgery is also usually done at the same time as primary hand surgery.

8.3.1 Secondary Surgery

As mentioned above, unlike patients with syndactyl or polydactyly alone, patients with CSPD often need secondary surgery. In the author's experience, children that are more likely to require this are those who presented initially with flexed and/or deviated synpolydactyly (Fig. 8.4). Cosmetically and functionally, centrally posi-

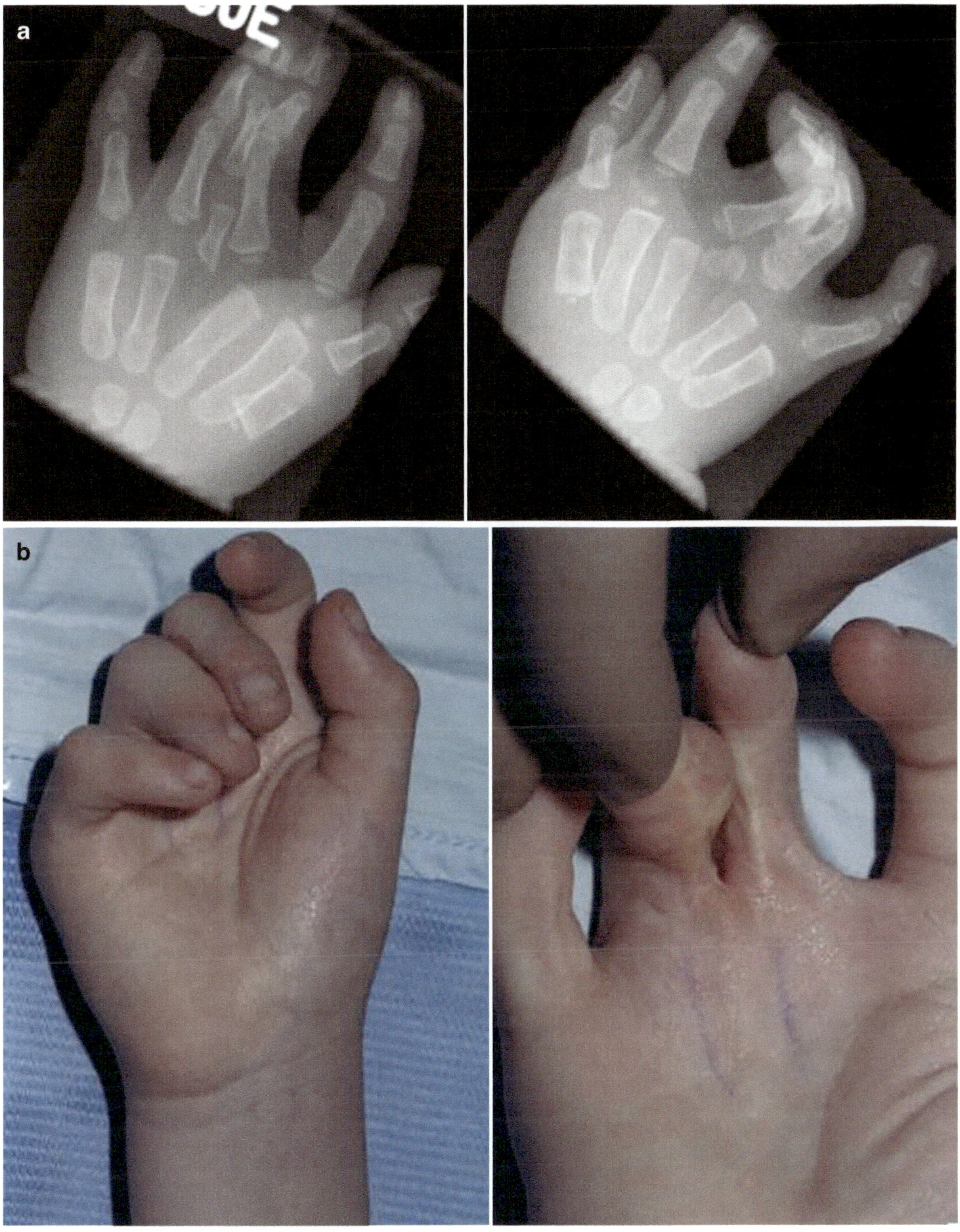

Fig. 8.4 Case 2: female, CSPD, Wall and Goldberg Type 1B. Initial radiographies (**a**). 2017: Pre-operative pictures (**b**) and intra-operative images (**c**). Actual clinical and radiological findings (**d**)

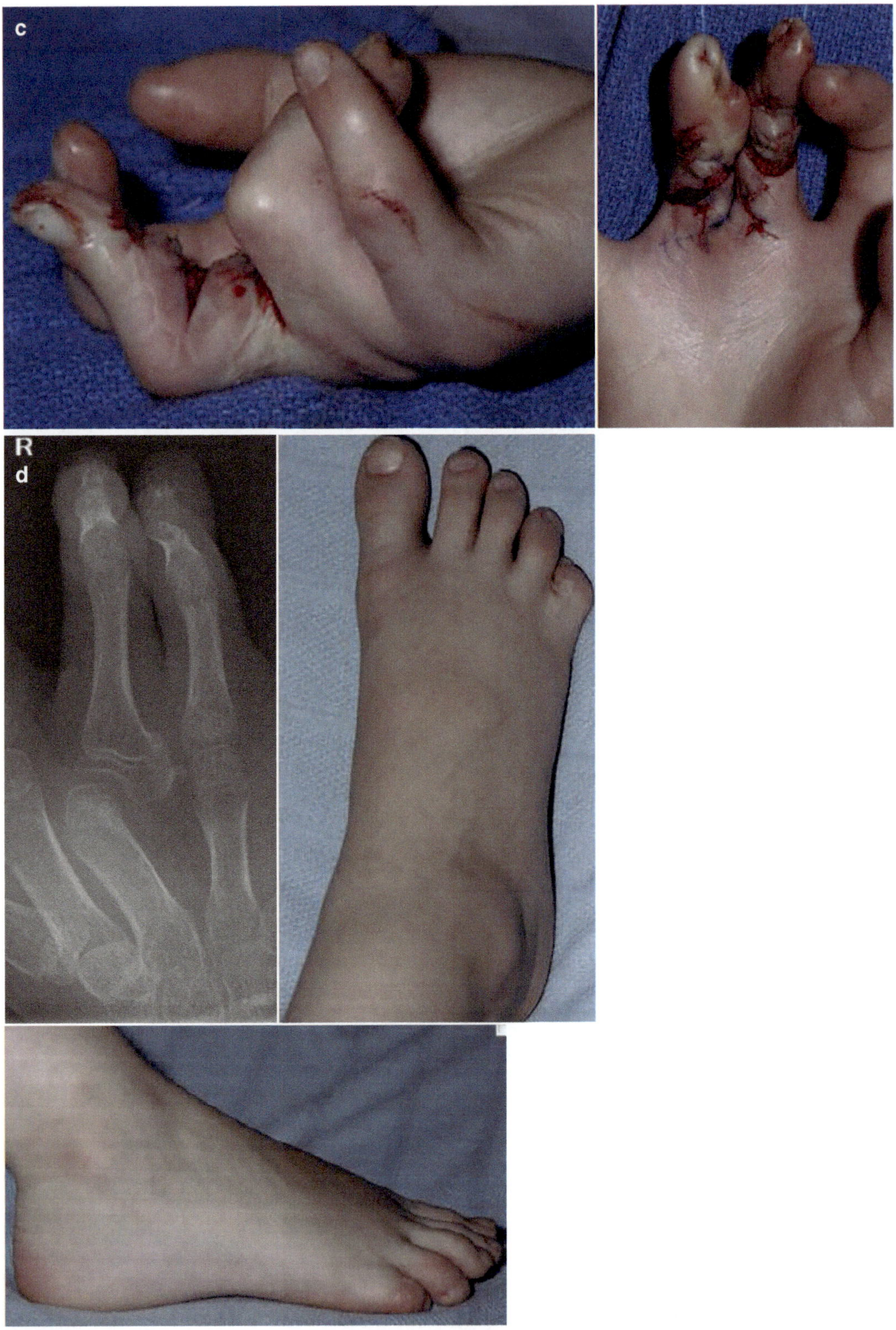

Fig. 8.4 (continued)

tioned flexed fingers are more bothersome to patients and parents than extended fingers. These patients also seem to have an increasing tendency to present with unfavourable palmar scar contractures and webbing that need revision surgery. A large generous full thickness grafting is usually required to prevent its recurrence as the patient continues to grow. Other more invasive procedures are also available to the patients, including straightening osteotomies. However, these procedures sacrifice grip in return for straighter digits and therefore, are not offered to children until they are fully grown and are able of making informed and considered decisions themselves. Deviated fingers may also need osteotomies at a later stage depending on whether the patients present with a cosmetic or functional issue (Figs. 8.5 and 8.6).

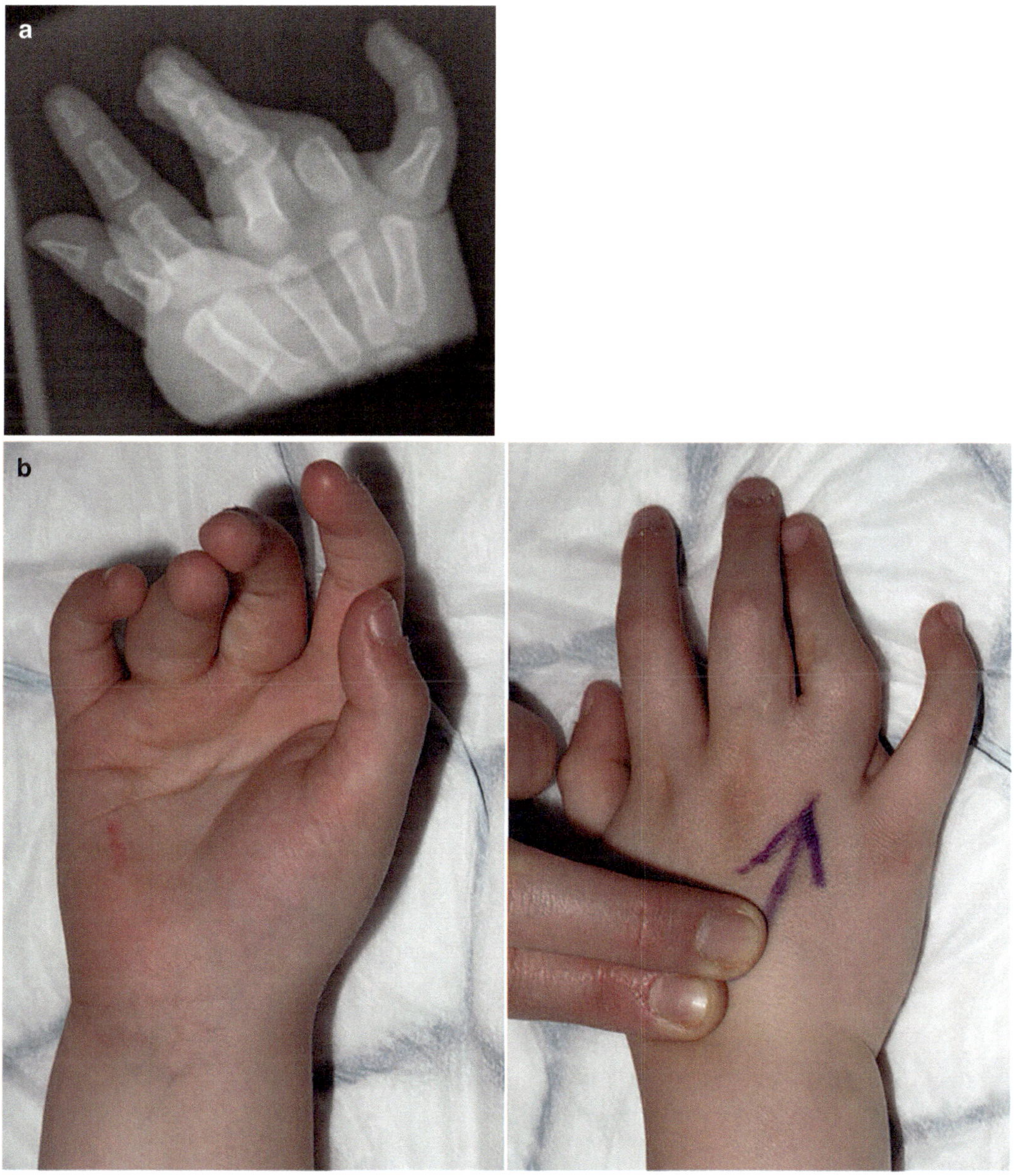

Fig. 8.5 Case 3: female, CSPD, Wall and Goldberg Type. Initial radiography (**a**) and clinical presentation (**b**). Intra-operative photos of second surgery (**c**). Post-operative images (**d**)

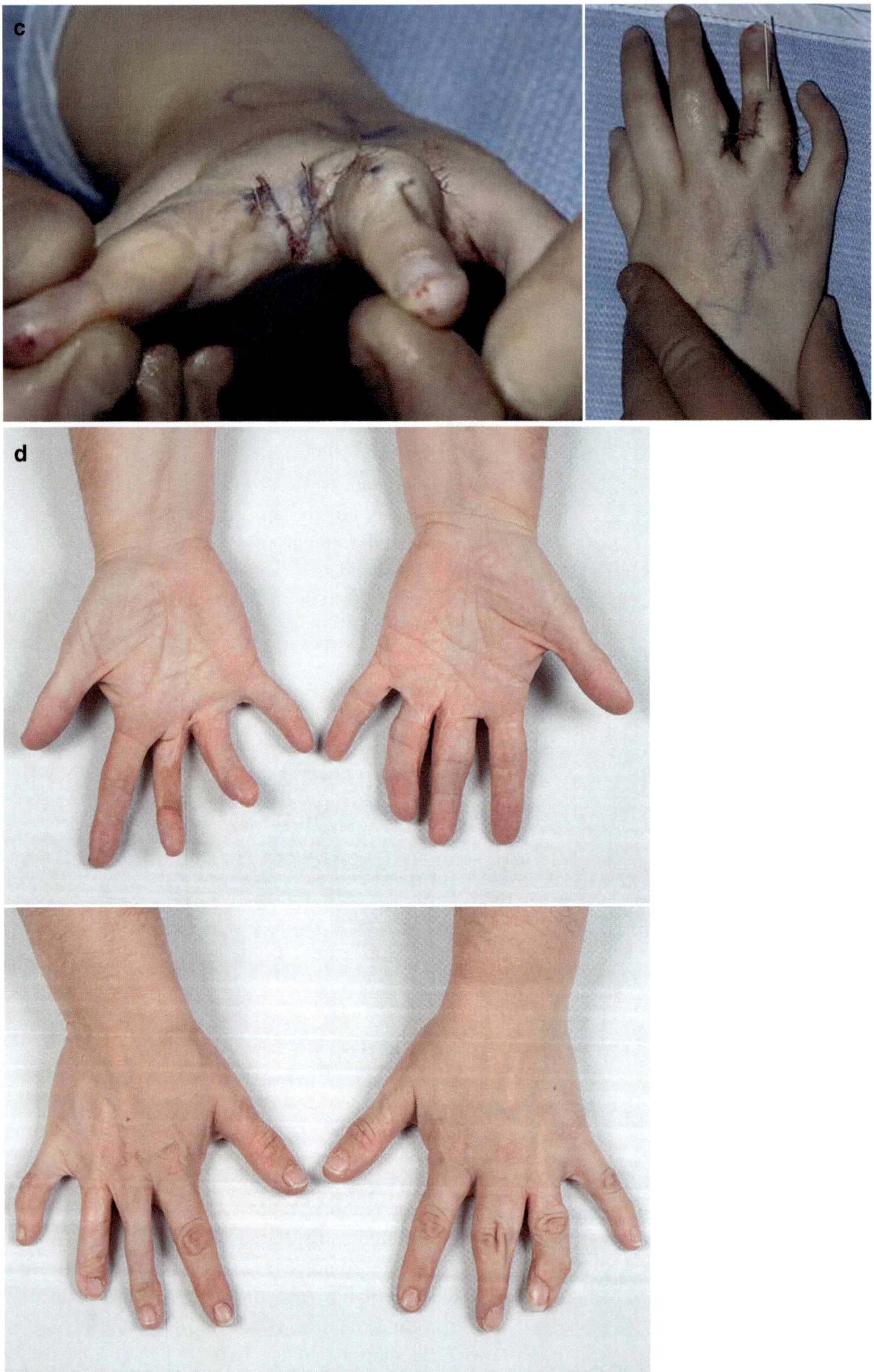

Fig. 8.5 (continued)

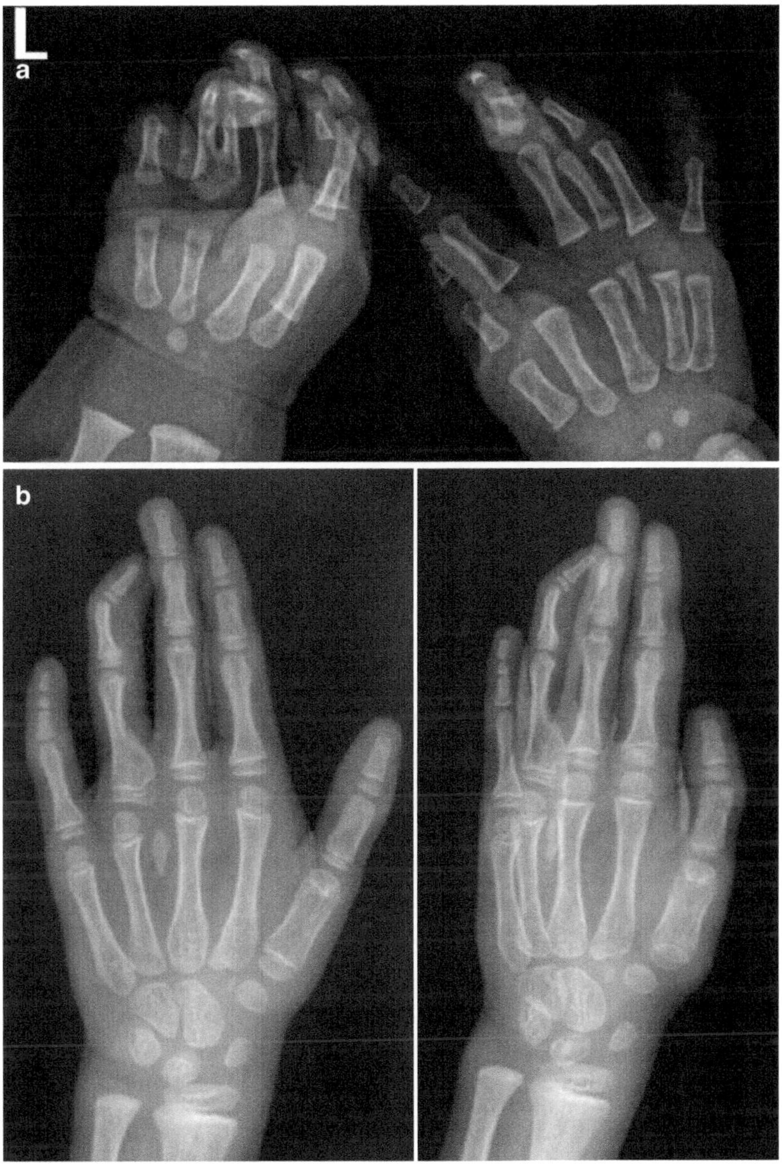

Fig. 8.6 Case 4: female, CSPD, Wall and Goldberg Type 2A. Initial radiographies (**a**). Actual radiographies left side (**b**) and clinical presentation (**c**)

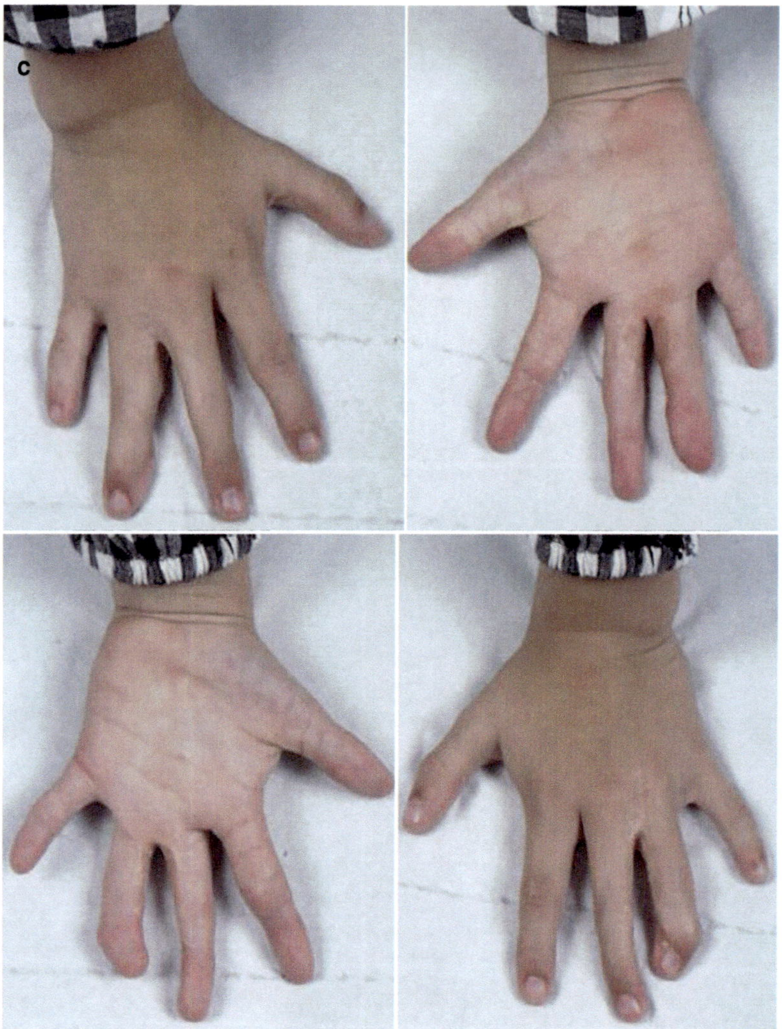

Fig. 8.6 (continued)

References

1. Jordan D, Hindocha S, Dhital M, Saleh M, Khan W. The epidemiology, genetics and future management of syndactyly. Open Orthop J. 2012;6:14–27.
2. Zhao X, Sun M, Zhao J, Leyva JA, Zhu H, Yang W, et al. Mutations in HOXD13 underlie syndactyly type V and a novel brachydactyly-syndactyly syndrome. Am J Hum Genet. 2007;80:361–71.
3. Ghoumid J, Andrieux J, Sablonniere B, Odent S, Philippe N, Zanlonghi X, et al. Duplication of chromosome 2q31.1-q31.2 in a family presenting syndactyly and nystagmus. Eur J Hum Genet. 2011;19:1198–201.
4. Zguricas J, Bakker WF, Heus H, Lindhout D, Heutink P, Hovius SE. Genetics of limb development and congenital hand malformations. Plast Reconstr Surg. 1998;101:1126–35.
5. Mali KS. Syndactyly: phenotypes, genetics and current classification. Eur J Hum Genet. 2012;20:817–24.
6. Quinonez SC, Innis JW. Human HOX genes disorders. Mol Genet Metab. 2014;111:4–15.
7. Sayli BS, Akarsu AN, Sayli U, Akhan O, Ceylaner S, Sarfarazi M. A large Turkish kindred with syndactyly type II (synpolydactyly). 1. Field investigation, clinical and pedigree data. J Med Genet. 1995;32:421–34.
8. Merlob P, Grunebaum M. Type II syndactyly or polysyndactyly. J Med Genet. 1986;23:237–41.

9. Yucel A, Kuru I, Bozan ME, Acar M, Solak M. Radiographic evaluation and unusual bone formations in different genetic patterns in synpolydactyly. Skelet Radiol. 2005;34:468–76.
10. Dai L, Heng ZC, Zhu J, Cai R, Mao M, Wang H, et al. Mutation analysis of HOXD13 gene in a Chinese pedigree with synpolydactyly. Zhonghua Yi Xue Yi Chuan Xue Za Zhi. 2005;22:277–80.
11. Mundlos S, Horn D. Synpolydactyly. In: Mundlos S, Horn D, editors. Limb malformations. An atlas of genetic disorders of limb development. Berlin: Springer; 2014. p. 38–40.
12. Barham G, Clarke NM. Genetic regulation of embryological limb development with relation to congenital limb deformity in humans. J Child Orthop. 2008;2:1–9.
13. Zhou J, Chen Y, Cao K, Zou Y, Zhou H, Hu F, et al. Functional classification and mutation analysis of a synpolydactyly kindred. Exp Ther Med. 2014;8:1569–74.
14. Sarfarazi M, Akarsu AN, Sayli BS. Localization of the syndactyly type II [synpolydactyly] locus to 2q31 region and identification of tight linkage to HOXD8 intragenic marker. Hum Mol Genet. 1995;4:1453–8.
15. Amiel J, Trochet D, Clement-Ziz M, Munnich A, Lyonnet S. Polyalanine expansions in human. Hum Mol Genet. 2004;13(Suppl 2):235–43.
16. Wajid M, Ishi Y, Kurban M, Dua-Awereh MB, Shimomura Y, Christiano AM. Polyalanine repeat expansion mutations in the HOXD13 gene in Pakistani families with synpolydactyly. Clin Genet. 2009;76:300–2.
17. Akarsu AN, Stoilov I, Yilmaz E, Sayli BS, Sarfarazi M. Genomic structure of HOXD13 gene: a nine polyalanine duplication causes synpolydactyly in two unrelated families. Hum Mol Genet. 1996;5:945–52.
18. Goodman FR, Mundlos S, Muragaki Y, Donnai D, Giovannucci-Uzielli ML, Lapi E, et al. Synpolydactyly phenotypes correlate with size of expansions in HOXD13 polyalanine tract. Proc Natl Acad Sci. 1997;94:7458–63.
19. Goodman F, Giovannucci-Uzielli ML, Hall C, Reardon W, Winter R, Scambler P. Deletions in HOXD13 segregate with an identical, novel foot malformation in two unrelated families. Am J Hum Genet. 1998;63:992–1000.
20. Debeer P, Bachelli C, Scambler PJ, De Smet L, Fryns JP, Goodman FR. Severe digital abnormalities in a patient heterozygous for both a novel missense mutation in HOXD13 and a polyalanine tract expansion in HOXA13. J Med Genet. 2002;39:852–6.
21. Hall JG, Pallister PD, Clarren SK, Beckwith JB, Wiglesworth FW, Fraser FC, et al. Congenital hypothalamic hamartoblastoma, hypopituitarism, imperforate anus and postaxial polydactyly—a new syndrome? Part I: clinical, causal and pathogenetic considerations. Am J Med Genet. 1980;7:47–74.
22. Chandra SR, Daryappa MM, Mukheem Mudabbir MA, Pooja M, Arivazhagan A. Pallister-Hall syndrome. J Paediatr Neurosci. 2017;12:276–9.
23. Kang S, Graham JM Jr, Olney AH, Biesecker LG. GLI3 frameshift mutations cause autosomal dominant Pallister-Hall syndrome. Nat Genet. 1997;15:266–8.
24. Hall JG. Pallister-Hall syndrome has gone the way of modern medical genetics. Am J Genet C Semin Med Genet. 2014;166:414–8.
25. Wall LB, Bae DS, Oishi SN, Calfee RP, Goldfarb CA. Synpolydactyly of the hand: a radiographic classification. J Hand Surg Eur. 2016;41:301–7.
26. Stelling F. The upper extremity. In: Furgusion A, editor. Orthopedic surgery in infancy and childhood. Baltimore: Williams & Wilkins; 1963. p. 304–8.
27. Turek S. Orthopedic principles and their application. Philadelphia: Lippincott; 1967.
28. Buck-Gramcko D, Behrens P. Classification of polydactyly of the hand and foot. Handchir Mikrochir Plast Chir. 1989;21:195–204.
29. Jose RM, Timoney N, Vidyadharan R, Lester R. Syndactyly correction: an aesthetic reconstruction. J Hand Surg Eur. 2010;35:446–50.
30. Lundkvist L, Barfred T. A double pulp flap technique for creating nail-folds in syndactyly release. J Hand Surg Br. 1991;16:32–4.
31. Buck-Gramcko D. Pollicization of the index finger. Method and results in aplasia and hypoplasia of the thumb. J Bone Joint Surg Am. 1971;53:1605–17.
32. Flatt A. Practical factors in the treatment of syndactyly. In: Symposium on reconstructive hand surgery, vol. 9. St Louis: Mosby; 1974. p. 144–56.

9 Thumb Polydactyly

Christianne van Nieuwenhoven
and Steven Hovius

Abstract

Thumb polydactyly or radial polydactyly is a congenital hand difference in which the patient presents with an extra digit at one or two thumbs. Together with syndactyly, clinodactyly and camptodactyly, thumb polydactyly is one of the most common congenital upper extremity differences.

To structure the variable phenotypic presentations of thumb polydactyly, several classification systems can be used. The most widely used is the Wassel classification, followed by the Rotterdam classification including different triphalangeal thumb phenotypes as well. Later evaluation of postoperative results of the different types of thumb polydactyly will be influenced by the choice in classification made.

In this chapter, the examination at first consultation is described since it is important to perform this systematically, not missing out on less conspicuous differences or even differences on the contralateral hand.

However seen as a relatively simple difference, its treatment can be very complex. The goal is to obtain a functional thumb, without instability and deviation, and is aesthetically close to normal. Except for the abnormal osseous structures, flexor and extensor tendons can have aberrant insertions and connections. The primary operation is the major one, addressing to all differences and avoiding corrective operations later in life.

Keywords

Radial polydactyly · Thumb · Congenital
Surgical treatment

9.1 Introduction

Thumb polydactyly, also radial polydactyly, refers to the disorder in which patients have an extra digit at the thumb aspect of the hand on at least one extremity. Polydactylous hands and footprints have been found when studying rock art and petroglyphs, some dated 1000AD. The first time that polydactyly was referred to in literature was in the Old Testament, where in a battle in Gath, a giant had six fingers on each hand, and six toes on each foot. A Dutch anatomist and alchemist, Theodor Kerckring, first described the difference in the seventeenth century. Since then, many reports have been made on polydactyly. The preaxial polydactyly can be separated into five types according genetic literature: thumb polydactyly; polydactyly of a triphalangeal thumb; polydactyly of an index finger; polysyndactyly and hallux polydactyly [1]. For this chapter, the focus will be directed toward the

C. van Nieuwenhoven (✉) · S. Hovius
Erasmus Medical Center Rotterdam,
Rotterdam, The Netherlands
e-mail: c.vannieuwenhoven@erasmusmc.nl

G. Pajardi (ed.), *Pediatric Hand Surgery*, https://doi.org/10.1007/978-3-031-30984-7_9

thumb polydactyly. Polydactyly with a triphalangeal thumb will be described in the chapter on the triphalangeal thumb.

According to the OMT classification, polydactyly of the hand is a Malformation with an Abnormal axis formation/difference of the Handplate, Radioulnar axis (2iii) [2]. Previously, polydactyly was categorized as radial, central and ulnar polydactyly in the modified Swanson classification in group III, Duplications as Radial polydactyly including triphalangeal thumb [2]. In the OMT classification, ulnar polydactyly has been categorized in the same group as the radial polydactyly, whereas the central polydactyly was proposed to be part of the unspecified axis iii. complex recently by Baas et al. [3].

Together with syndactyly, clinodactyly and camptodactyly, thumb polydactyly is one of the most common congenital upper extremity differences seen by dedicated congenital hand specialists.

The incidence of polydactyly depends on the population studied and the definition used. Region, ethnicity and combined numbers of all polydactylies, or only radial or ulnar-sided polydactyly, provide very different incidences in published series. The incidence is estimated to be 0.3–3.6 per 1000 live births and 1.6–10.7 per 1000 in the general population [4, 5], with males twice as often affected as females. Variability in incidence is based on the population studied and the definition used for thumb polydactyly. It is believed that the incidence of thumb polydactyly with or without a triphalangeal component is highest in people of Asian descent. Thumb polydactyly represents up to 90% of all polydactyly cases in the Chinese population [6].

In a recent Swedish population study, the thumb polydactyly is mentioned to have a relative incidence of 2.3 per 10,000 live births. The thumb polydactyly without a triphalangeal component was predominantly present in the male population (58%) with 56% on the left side and 15% bilaterally in this study [4]. In approximately 24% of cases, thumb polydactyly has an inherited pattern. Associated anomalies were seen in 22% of cases [4]. In our patient population, preaxial polydactyly characterized according to the OMT classification [2] was seen in 124 out of the 954 diagnoses with 29% bilaterally affected patients and 39% only right side affected and 32% only left side affected hands.

Thumb polydactyly mostly occurs as an isolated and sporadic anomaly, however, in the Online Mendelian Inheritance in Man ('OMIM') database, it is mentioned as part of over 125 distinct syndromes and phenotypical associations, including Holt–Oram syndrome, Townes–Brocks syndrome and Fanconi's anaemia. In our population, cases were additionally associated with craniofacialsyndromes, Greigcephalosynpolydacyly, Nager, Klippel–Feil and VACTERL. In the Human Phenotype Ontology (HPO) database, preaxial hand polydactyly as a patient's feature is related to 59 different diagnoses. Therefore, multidisciplinary knowledge on the phenotypes and syndromes is in our opinion mandatory to treat these patients with a high quality of care.

9.2 Embryology and Genetics

CULAs arise during upper limb development, which takes place between the fourth and eighth weeks of gestation. During these 4 weeks, a fully functional hand is formed along three axes of development: The proximal–distal axis, the dorsal–ventral axis and the anterior–posterior (or 'radial–ulnar') axis. Growth and differentiation of tissue along the axes are orchestrated through genetic and molecular signalling pathways, which arise from areas of specialized cells in the limb bud called 'signalling centres' [7–9].

In the development of polydactyly, the radial–ulnar axis is the most important. This axis is formed along the Zone of Polarizing Activity ('ZPA'), where Sonic Hedgehog ('SHH') proteins regulate ulnarization and widening of the limb (Fig. 9.1) [10]. Disruption of SSH signalling pathways may result in radial polydactyly. Moreover, mutations of SHH and GLI3 are associated with various phenotypes of radial polydactyly [11–13] and triphalangeal thumb [14–18]. The complex genetic and molecular interactions

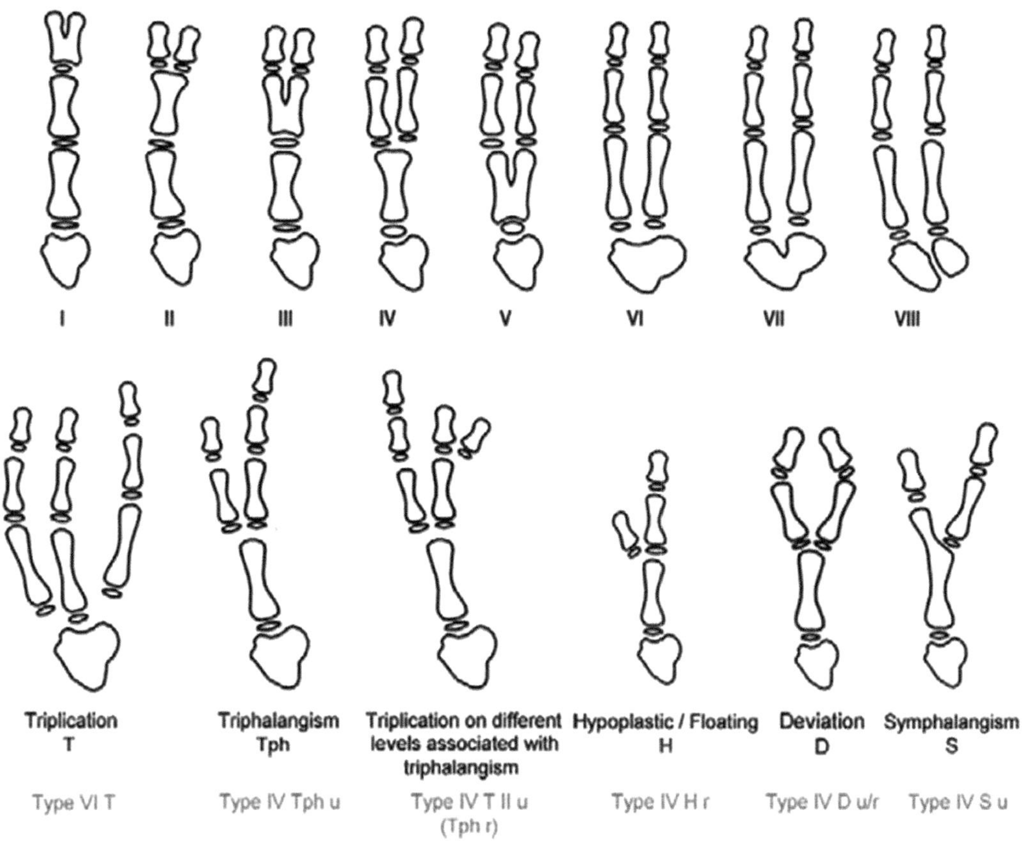

Fig. 9.1 Rotterdam classification for polydactyly

result in a highly variable clinical presentation of radial polydactyly, ranging from a rudimental skin tag to very complex triplications of the thumb.

9.3 Patient Presentation

The disorder is easily detected after birth leading to a cosmetic and functional concern with the parents and if not treated, to cosmetic concern of the affected child. Additionally, depending on the level of the duplication, it can cause functional impairment. Most parents or patients will pursue surgery for restoring functional anatomy, however, affected by abnormal embryological development of osseous structures and soft tissues, normal aesthetic and functional results are not to be expected. Results on functionality and aesthetics with regard to manual ability, participation and quality of life in patients with thumb polydactyly are scarce.

Nowadays, a growing number of polydactylies are seen with increasing ultrasound techniques and experience of examiners. Therefore, more parents might be referred to a congenital hand team to have more information on the difference and possible associated syndromes.

9.4 Classification

As mentioned before, polydactyly can be arranged according to a genetic classification into five types or classified as a part of the congenital hand differences in the OMT. These classifications might give information on the genetic and/or embryologic nature of the difference, but it doesn't give information on the phenotype and possible related surgical treatment options.

In order to structure the variable phenotypic presentation, thumb polydactyly cases can be categorized using different types of phenotypic-based classification systems. In choosing such a classification system, later evaluation of the results of the different types of thumb polydactyly is influenced by this choice.

Since soft tissue anomalies are harder to visualize, most classification systems are based on osseous configuration, which can be shown using X-rays. These classification systems play an important role in communication between specialists, in the evaluation of treatment outcomes, and in supporting clinical decision-making. However, in using the osseous-based classification systems, one should not overlook the additional soft tissue differences.

The most widely used system for thumb polydactyly is the Wassel classification [19]. Seven types of osseous configurations are described: types I–VI represent distal-to-proximal levels of thumb polydactyly, while type VII represents thumb polydactyly with a triphalangeal component. The three most common types of radial polydactyly are type IV (30–46%), type II (9–25%) and type VII (7–32%), with varying occurrence across different case series, e.g. areas in the world.

This classification is easy to apply, but the clinical relevance is limited by the inability to classify surgically important features of radial polydactyly (e.g. diverging components or hypoplasia), features that influence outcome. This has led to the introduction of many alternative classification systems [20, 21], such as the Rotterdam classification for radial polydactyly [20], integrating elements of the Wassel [19], Buck-Gramcko [22], and Upton [23] classification, into an all-embracing classification system for thumb polydactyly including triphalangeal components and triplications (Fig. 9.1) [24].

In a study, incorporating patients from two large European congenital hand units (Hamburg and Rotterdam), the occurrence of the different types of thumb polydactyly was investigated, evaluating a total of 520 available X-rays from both units from the period 1980 to 2012. Both the Wassel and Rotterdam classifications were applied. A comparative historical cohort was extracted from the literature, pooling 1723 eligible cases of thumb polydactyly to describe the frequency of the different types reported in the literature. A large part (40%) of the studied population could not be classified using the Wassel classification, compared to 6% studied in the literature. However, all study cases could be classified using the Rotterdam classification. All the unclassifiable cases had aberrant components: triphalangeal, deviating and hypoplastic. This implies that the Rotterdam classification is more suited for describing the entire spectrum of thumb polydactyly and guidance in surgical treatment. Both classifications show a good overall intra-observer and fair inter-observer reliability regardless of the experience of the person using the classification system.

According to these results, the Rotterdam classification is best suited for research purposes, even if an inexperienced observer performs analysis. However, for daily practice in non-research environment, the use might be too time-consuming.

9.5 Physical Examination

At first consultation, following medical history and general physical examination, both upper limbs are examined, and if indicated or a syndrome is expected, the lower limbs as well. If the fingers are normal, with normal hand and finger creases, and a normal hypothenar region, the examination can focus on the radial side of the hand. In our experience, it is worthwhile to perform this systematically, as quite often more anomalies are present. Don't be distracted by the major difference, overlooking the less major differences.

The examination is performed systematically. The *thenar* musculature varies widely from normal to severely hypoplastic. In Wassel I and II, the thenar musculature is mostly normal, in contrast to Wassel V, VI and VII.

Hypermobile joints should always be related to the other joints in the hands. It is important to look for creases on both the dorsal and palmar sides. If creases are present, then an active movement in that particular joint can be expected.

The *CMCJ* in polydactyly can be normal, stiff or hypermobile. If abnormalities in the CMCJ are present, they are mostly encountered in the more proximal polydactylies. If polydactyly is situated at the CMCJ, the MCPJ in the best thumb can be near normal. In these cases, the movement is dependent on the presence of a syndactyly between the duplication.

Depending on the location of the polydactyly, the *MCPJ* can be stiff, normal moving or hypermobile and hypoplastic. For instance, in a polydactyly involving the MCPJ, both thumbs move as a block. In most of these cases, the radial-sided thumb is hypoplastic and stiff, and the ulnar thumb is the better one.

Finally, the *IPJ* can present with normal movement, stiffness or hypermobility. If the duplication is at the IPJ, both parts can move as a block. The range of motion in those cases is typically less than in a normal IPJ. In an asymmetric duplication at the IPJ, the best-developed part usually moves better.

Normal examination includes extrinsic and intrinsic movement, but difficult to perform in a newborn. However, flexion and extension can be evaluated, as well as the presence of palmar abduction. In radial polydactyly, the flexor pollicis longus is Y-shaped in the majority of cases, with a less developed tendon to the most hypoplastic thumb. Therefore, flexion can be seen simultaneously in both thumbs. Moreover, the flexor tendon can have its insertion on the radial side for the ulnar thumb, and ulnar side of the radial extra thumb, causing a more deviating flexion in the IPJ. This is especially true for the type 4 and more proximal polydactylies.

The extensor apparatus is usually less developed or absent in the more hypoplastic thumb. It can be Y-shaped as in the flexor and asymmetrically attached, therefore, deviating the distal part. The fingertips can be either normal or asymmetric. The asymmetric side is typically found on the opposing sides of the two thumbs. The nails are smaller and asymmetrical in most cases. The first web is nearly always normal in the distal duplications. In more proximal polydactylies, the first web can be narrower than the normal contralateral side.

9.5.1 Patient Selection

Polydactylies are usually treated surgically. Functional impairment can vary from slight to severe, depending on the extent of the deformity. Polydactylies can be a nuisance in, for example, shaking hands, putting hands in pockets or narrow spaces and in wearing gloves. However, most parents visit the outpatient clinic with their child for aesthetic and social reasons. In patients with a syndrome with serious concomitant disease, surgery can be delayed or even be avoided.

9.5.2 Treatment/Surgical Technique

Thumb polydactyly is seen as a relatively simple difference; however, its treatment can be very complex. The aim of surgical intervention in thumb polydactyly is to obtain a functional thumb, without instability and deviation, and is aesthetically pleasing or acceptable. Except for the abnormal osseous structure with joint incongruence, the flexor and extensor tendons can have aberrant insertions, influencing the line of pull with regard to future deviations. In addition, aberrant and intricate connections may exist between flexors and extensors, affecting thumb movement. In the more proximal polydactyly types, intrinsic muscles might be hypoplastic or absent. In most cases, the thumb is inadequate in size, width and nail development compared to the non-involved opposite side in unilateral cases. However, it is difficult to address these latter hypoplastic features when reconstructing a thumb polydactyly.

Taking into account all the features of reconstruction in thumb polydactyly surgical approaches have been refined over the years. Different techniques to treat thumb polydactyly can be identified.

The timing of surgery is not fixed at a certain age. Surgery is recommended at the end of the first year of life by many authors, as it is important to be able to identify the structures properly and to minimize the anaesthetic risks. In a recent study, patients operated at an age older than 2 years had significantly better results than children before the age of 1 year regarding patient-reported scores. No such difference was found for patients operated between ages 1 and 2 years [25]. This suggests that timing might be best after the age of 1 year only taking the results into account, and even later if anesthesiologic and psychological risks are taken into account.

In the end, most essential for good long-term good results is the knowledge of patho-embryology and patho-anatomy [26, 27]. Try to visualize aberrant anatomy without too much dissection! In general, in evaluating results, experienced surgeons are reported to have better results in outcomes [25].

9.6 Operative Treatment

A number of principles in the treatment of thumb polydactyly can be listed in Table 9.1. The most versatile and widely applied surgical treatment for thumb polydactyly is the resection and reconstruction technique. The majority of cases can be treated using this technique, indicated whenever one of the extra thumbs is better developed than the other (floating-type thumb polydactyly excepted). In most cases, the ulnar thumb is better developed and the radial thumb is resected. Resection of the radial thumb has the added benefit of preserving the ulnar collateral ligament, playing a key role in stabilizing the MCPJ during pinch grip and prehension. Furthermore, the scar will be situated dorsally or on the radial side of the remaining thumb, not impeding with sensation of the ulnar-sided pulp of the thumb. Several techniques have been described to improve appearance and function, as well as attention to pulp size and girth [28], separate techniques for type III reconstruction [29], support of collateral ligaments in type IV [30] and rebalancing of tendons [31].

Table 9.1 Principles in treating thumb polydactyly

- "Make one thumb out of two. It is not a simple excision of one"
- Decide which thumb to be kept
- Preserve tendons, ligaments and skin of the discarded thumb to align, balance and augment the residual thumb
- Perform as much correction as possible and necessary during the first operation on both soft tissues and bones
- Be aware of and search for less obvious anatomical anomalies
- Align articular surfaces as axial and as congruent as possible by transverse and longitudinal osteotomies
- Perform ligament reconstructions or releases
- Balance tendon insertions
- Adjust skin cover as accurately as possible. Excess of skin will not disappear in time
- Postoperative dressings should be meticulously applied, protect the reconstruction and resistant to removal by the child

When analyzing literature on the long-term outcome of thumb polydactyly treatment, only few reports are found with overall outcome [32–34] and one only on thumb size and appearance [35]. In a recently published thesis, an extensive analysis was performed on the outcome of surgically treated thumb polydactyly [36]. Most important lessons were: reporting outcome starts with the implementation of a reliable and all comprising classification for thumb polydactyly regarding the pre-operative situation; and the use of a reliable and clinically weighted outcome assessment system [37–39]. If analyzed according to these conditions, type IV had worse functional outcomes than type II and IV-Tph if the thumb was operated only once. However, if multiple surgeries were needed, an overall worse outcome is to be expected. Furthermore, overall outcome significantly improves when the first operation is performed by an experienced surgeon, specialized in congenital upper limb anomalies [25]. Regarding the Bilhaut–Cloquet procedure, this technique is not worthwhile in cases where a reconstruction is a viable option. The Bilhaut–Cloquet does not give the beneficial strength as believed because of the MCP joint stability is improved. Furthermore, the overall appearance is scored less, with nail appearance being the most consistent factor [40].

The surgical techniques of Wassel type II and type IV are discussed extensively in several textbooks. For this chapter, we would like to discuss the treatment of different type IV thumb polydactylies. It is the most frequent type but does not have a single approach since it appears in different forms. For the principles of treatment, see Table 9.1.

9.6.1 Radial Polydactyly at the MCPJ (Type IV)

Type IV thumbs often demonstrate a hypoplastic or smaller extra thumb on the radial side. However, the degree of development and involvement of the extra thumbs varies widely, with an extra thumb only attached with a skin pedicle, to similar develop thumbs with deviation in the MCPJ and IPJ.

The operative technique is based on the previously mentioned principles, with as a goal to provide in one thumb, in alignment with the first metacarpal, with a stable MCPJ and IPJ and with movement along those joints in a normal fashion. However, in the depicted end result, one should take into account the initial situation, that is for instance, an ulnar thumb with deviation in the MCPJ and IPJ, deviant insertions of the tendons, with no flexion crease at the IPJ.

In Fig. 9.2, the radiographic appearance of four type IV polydactylies is depicted.

Type IV as shown in Fig. 9.2a is a type IV H r, implying a polydactyly at the level of the MCPJ with a hypoplastic thumb at the radial side. Surgical correction consists of simple ablation with inspection of the radial collateral band with respect to stability. In these cases, reefing of this collateral band is sometimes needed.

The thumb polydactyly shown in Fig. 9.2b seems to be equal (type IV H r) to the extra thumb in Fig. 9.2a, however, the proximal osseous structure is more related to the first MC, whereas this part was not ossified at the same age in case Fig. 9.2a. During the surgical correction, attention should be paid to the different soft tissue connections and bony structures at the MCPJ level. In this case, the insertion of the thenar muscles (outlined in Fig. 9.3a) at the base of the radial thumb is a giveaway for the need for more structural corrections than the first case. The thenar muscle attachment is dissected from the base of the radial thumb and released more proximal to evaluate the radial collateral band and joint sur-

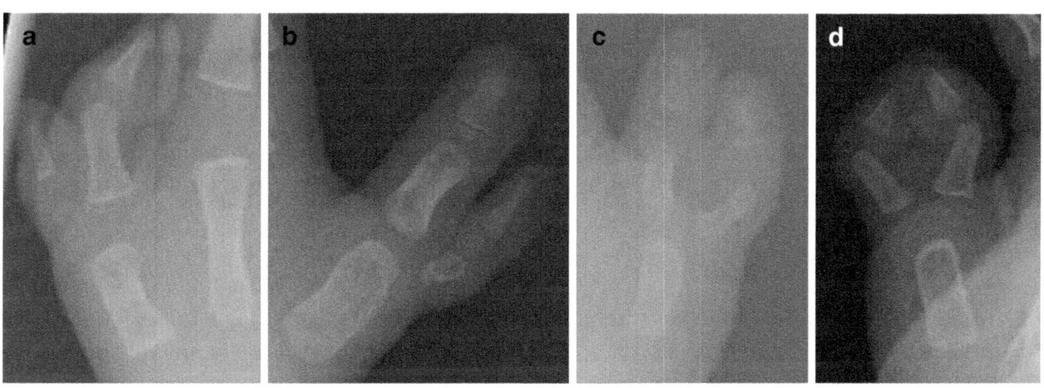

Fig. 9.2 (**a**–**d**) Four examples of type IV radial polydactylies with a different aspect and therefore different surgical approaches. (**a**) Type IV H r, implying a polydactyly at the level of the MCPJ with a hypoplastic thumb at the radial side. (**b**) Type IV H r, similar to the extra thumb in (**a**), however, the proximal osseous structure is more related to the first MC, implicating an additional procedure (see text). (**c**) Type IV D r, deviation of the radial thumb. (**d**) Type IV D r u, deviation of the radial and ulnar thumb

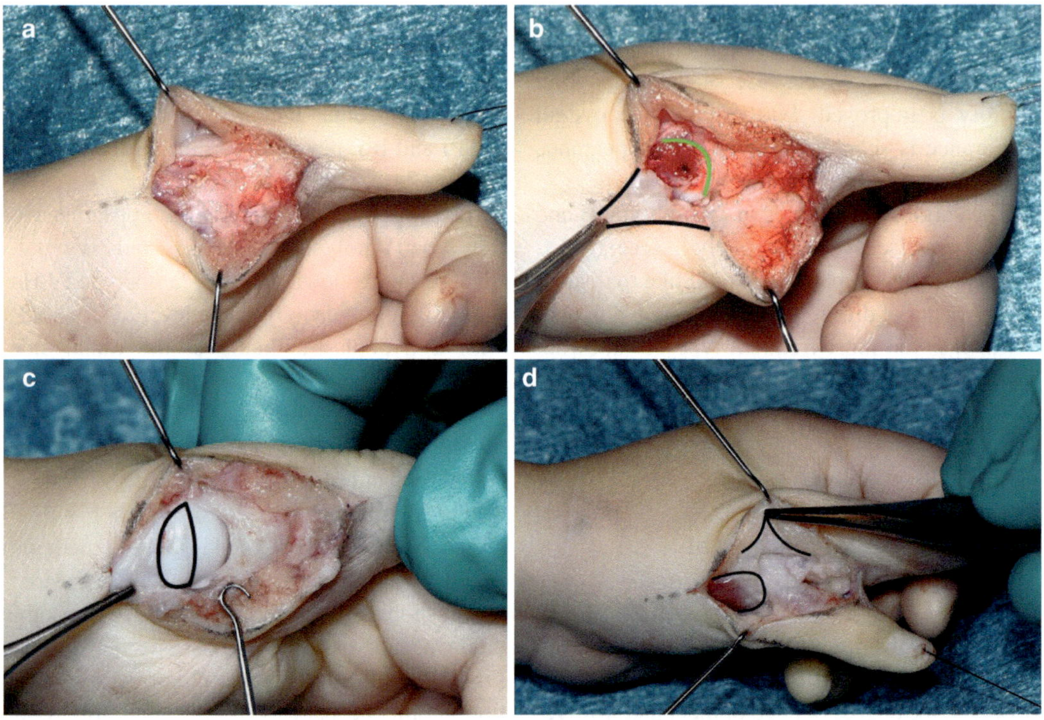

Fig. 9.3 (**a**–**d**) Surgical correction of a type IV D r polydactyly. (**a**) The insertion of the thenar muscles attached at the base of the radial thumb, and dorsal joint capsule (lifted in pincers). (**b**) Metacarpal head of the radial thumb with an insufficient radial collateral band. (**c**) After longitudinal osteotomy of the metacarpal head of the radial thumb to adjust the with and prevent future osseous bulging (green). The thenar muscle and collateral band previously attached to the proximal phalanx of the radial thumb (black). (**d**) After reconstruction of the collateral band and thenar muscle to the radial base of the proximal phalanx of the ulnar thumb

face. In this case, the radial collateral band was insufficient and a joint surface for the radial thumb was present (see Fig. 9.3b). Neglecting this presence will result in an instable thumb with an osseous prominence on the radial side at the distal first metacarpal level. Therefore, a longitudinal osteotomy needs to be performed (see Fig. 9.3c) in line with the joint surface of the ulnar thumb. The joint is stabilized by reinsertion of the collateral band to the base of the radial side of the ulnar thumb (see Fig. 9.3d). Whereas the previous example doesn't need postoperative immobilization, this case will need immobilization and protection up till 3 months after the intervention for high-impact activities. Postoperative protocols differ in congenital hand centres regarding the time needed for immobilization before a period of protection with a splint is introduced. However, it will take approximately 3 months until the radial collateral band has reached its maximal stability, and full exertion on the reconstructed ligament is allowed. Therefore, we recommend a gradual increase in load to this joint reconstruction, with a normal load allowed, 3 months after the operation.

The case in Fig. 9.2c, type IV D r, is approached in the same fashion as above. However, the osseous alignment of the ulnar thumb should be inspected, as well as the insertions of the flexor and extensor tendon of the ulnar thumb. Especially in the presence of a more distal syndactyly between the ulnar and radial thumb. In the case of a type IV D r u, as depicted in Fig. 9.2d, a correction osteotomy of the first MC and basal phalanx is necessary, together with reconstruction of the joint surface of the MCPJ, radial collateral band of the MCPJ and IPJ, as well as reattachment of the flexor and extensor tendons. This technique is described in detail by the authors in different textbook chapters [41].

9.6.2 Postoperative Care

The reconstructed thumb is immobilized for 4–6 weeks, allowing finger movement in the bandage. Following the initial 4–6 weeks and depending on the level and complexity of the reconstruction, further treatment consists of uninhibited full motion to a removable splint for several weeks. The child will exercise in play, and therefore hand therapy under supervision is not necessary. In a simple, 'floating type' hypoplastic thumb polydactyly, with no reconstruction of tendons or ligaments needed, a bandage is given for 2 days, as in regular wound care.

9.6.3 Outcomes, Prognosis and Complications

When reconstruction in a congenital hand is performed, definitive outcome can only be assessed after growth has been completed. Therefore, it is advisable to check children several times during growth, preferably after growth spurts. At our outpatient clinic, examination is performed thoroughly, in such a way that the modified JSSH classification for postoperative results in thumb polydactyly can be filled out [37]. Specific attention is paid to nail deformities, movement and stability of joints, active range of motion, appearance, broadness and malalignment of the skin. Older children and parents hardly complain of lack of function even though joints can be stiff [36]. Painful thumbs are very rare, although we did see occasionally problems with sustained writing. However, they do complain more about appearance, after they present with an insignificant functional complaint. Especially teenagers visit the outpatient clinic wishing for an esthetic improvement.

Outcome can be divided into unavoidable and avoidable results. In the unavoidable outcome in type II, the distal part of the thumb can be from nearly normal to hypoplastic, depending on the initial presentation. Insufficient pulp, smaller nails and less developed IPJs are inevitable. In nail bed reconstructions, the nail will never be completely normal.

Avoidable outcomes in type II relate to inappropriate alignment, resulting in nail deformities, scarring at the nail wall, and residual nail development. If the collateral ligament is constructed with cartilage or a small piece of bone from the excised phalanx, new formation of bone can be the result. At the IPJ, incongruent alignment causes deviation, instability or stiffness. Too much resection at the base of the distal phalanx damages growth of the remaining distal phalanx.

In the unavoidable outcome in type IV, the residual thumb is always lesser developed than the normal contralateral thumb. The pulp is often less developed, the nail is usually smaller, and motion can vary from nearly normal to stiff, especially at the IPJ. Goldfarb found only a difference in nail width; however, motion was not taken into account in this study. But even though the thumb appears smaller, patients are satisfied as long as it is well-shaped.

Avoidable outcomes in type IV also relate to inappropriate alignment. IPJ and MCPJ angulation decreases the aesthetic outcome. Deviations at either the IP or MP joint can mostly be prevented at initial operation by aligning the articular surfaces and balancing the thumb properly. Too much resection at the MP joint results in growth disturbances at the proximal phalanx of the remaining thumb. In late S- and zig-zag deformities, proper initial alignment has not been accomplished. Residual unstable IP- or MCPJs can develop following improper ligamentous reconstruction and tendon alignment at the initial stage.

Evaluating the reported outcome in thumb polydactyly according to the current standard is a challenge due to the different tools used. In classifying thumb polydactyly, most will choose the Wassel classification. But since not all thumb polydactylies can be classified according to this osseous anatomy-based classification, authors choose to modify it, all in a different manner. As a result, the base for being able to compare results of different types of thumb polydactyly is undefined, leading to incomparable evaluations of patient groups. The second step in evaluating outcome is choosing the right outcome assessment system, since reported results in the treatment of thumb polydactyly are dependent on the available tools used [39]. To be able to report valid and generalizable outcomes, the importance of the different items in assessment schemes should be weighted carefully, defined by careful statistical analysis as is performed for the modified JSSH outcome measure [37].

In an era of value-based health care, evaluating surgical result is the first step, followed by patient-related outcome measures such as manual ability, participation and quality of life. The reduced strength in thumb polydactyly patients does not influence their manual ability. However, the current questionnaires available for thumb polydactyly or hand differences as a whole are not specific and sensitive for the detection of activities that patients won't be able to perform. Are we asking the right questions? And do we need these results in shared-decision-making? Therefore, a group of congenital hand surgeons worked on an ICHOM evaluation set for congenital hand differences. This will give caregivers the opportunity to collect data on patient-reported outcomes based on the same questionnaires, generating outcomes that will be comparable worldwide and giving direction in how to treat these patients.

Most importantly, the primary operation for children with thumb polydactyly is the major one, not performing surgery before 1 year of age, correcting all differences and avoiding revision surgery, by experienced congenital hand surgeons.

References

1. Orioli IM, Castilla EE. Thumb/hallux duplication and preaxial polydactyly type I. Am J Med Genet. 1999;82(3):219–24.
2. Tonkin MA, Oberg KC. The OMT classification of congenital anomalies of the hand and upper limb. Hand Surg. 2015;20(3):336–42.
3. Baas M, Stubbs AP, van Zessen DB, Galjaard RH, van der Spek PJ, Hovius SER, et al. Identification of associated genes and diseases in patients with congenital upper-limb anomalies: a novel application of the OMT classification. J Hand Surg Am. 2017;42(7):533–45 e4.
4. Ekblom AG, Laurell T, Arner M. Epidemiology of congenital upper limb anomalies in 562 children born in 1997 to 2007: a total population study from Stockholm, Sweden. J Hand Surg Am. 2010;35(11):1742–54.
5. Goldfarb CA, Wall LB, Bohn DC, Moen P, Van Heest AE. Epidemiology of congenital upper limb anomalies in a Midwest United States population: an assessment using the Oberg, Manske, and Tonkin classification. J Hand Surg Am. 2015;40(1):127-32.e1-2.
6. Leung PC, Chan KM, Cheng JC. Congenital anomalies of the upper limb among the Chinese population in Hong Kong. J Hand Surg Am. 1982;7(6):563–5.
7. Bamshad M, Watkins WS, Dixon ME, Le T, Roeder AD, Kramer BE, et al. Reconstructing the history of human limb development: lessons from birth defects. Pediatr Res. 1999;45(3):291–9.
8. Riddle RD, Tabin C. How limbs develop. Sci Am. 1999;280(2):74–9.
9. Riddle RD, Ensini M, Nelson C, Tsuchida T, Jessell TM, Tabin C. Induction of the LIM homeobox gene Lmx1 by WNT7a establishes dorsoventral pattern in the vertebrate limb. Cell. 1995;83(4):631–40.
10. Riddle RD, Johnson RL, Laufer E, Tabin C. Sonic hedgehog mediates the polarizing activity of the ZPA. Cell. 1993;75(7):1401–16.
11. Radhakrishna U, Bornholdt D, Scott HS, Patel UC, Rossier C, Engel H, et al. The phenotypic spectrum of GLI3 morphopathies includes autosomal dominant preaxial polydactyly type-IV and postaxial polydactyly type-A/B: no phenotype prediction from the position of GLI3 mutations. Am J Hum Genet. 1999;65(3):645–55.
12. Debeer P, Peeters H, Driess S, De Smet L, Freese K, Matthijs G, et al. Variable phenotype in Greig cephalopolysyndactyly syndrome: clinical and radiological findings in 4 independent families and 3 sporadic cases with identified GLI3 mutations. Am J Med Genet. 2003;120A(1):49–58.
13. Lettice LA, Hill RE. Preaxial polydactyly: a model for defective long-range regulation in congenital abnormalities. Curr Opin Genet Dev. 2005;15(3):294–300.
14. Swanson AB, Brown KS. Hereditary triphalangeal thumb. J Hered. 1962;53:259–65.
15. Farooq M, Troelsen JT, Boyd M, Eiberg H, Hansen L, Hussain MS, et al. Preaxial polydactyly/triphalangeal thumb is associated with changed transcription factor-binding affinity in a family with a novel point mutation in the long-range cis-regulatory element ZRS. Eur J Hum Genet. 2010;18(6):733–6.
16. Wieczorek D, Pawlik B, Li Y, Akarsu NA, Caliebe A, May KJ, et al. A specific mutation in the distant sonic hedgehog (SHH) cis-regulator (ZRS) causes Werner mesomelic syndrome (WMS) while complete ZRS duplications underlie Haas type polysyndactyly and preaxial polydactyly (PPD) with or without triphalangeal thumb. Hum Mutat. 2010;31(1):81–9.

17. Klopocki E, Ott CE, Benatar N, Ullmann R, Mundlos S, Lehmann K. A microduplication of the long range SHH limb regulator (ZRS) is associated with triphalangeal thumb-polysyndactyly syndrome. J Med Genet. 2008;45(6):370–5.
18. Sun M, Ma F, Zeng X, Liu Q, Zhao XL, Wu FX, et al. Triphalangeal thumb-polysyndactyly syndrome and syndactyly type IV are caused by genomic duplications involving the long range, limb-specific SHH enhancer. J Med Genet. 2008;45(9):589–95.
19. Wassel HD. The results of surgery for polydactyly of the thumb. A review. Clin Orthop Relat Res. 1969;64:175–93.
20. Zuidam JM, Selles RW, Ananta M, Runia J, Hovius SE. A classification system of radial polydactyly: inclusion of triphalangeal thumb and triplication. J Hand Surg Am. 2008;33(3):373–7.
21. Kim JK, Al-Dhafer BAA, Shin YH, Joo HS. Polydactyly of the thumb: a modification of the Wassel-Flatt classification. J Hand Surg Eur. 2021;46(4):346–51.
22. Buck-Gramcko D. Congenital malformations of the hand and forearm. Chir Main. 2002;21(2):70–101.
23. Upton J, Shoen S. Triphalangeal thumb. In: Gupta A, Kay SP, Scheker LR, editors. The growing hand, diagnosis and management of the upper extremity in children. 1st ed. London: Mosby; 2000. p. 255–68.
24. Hu CH, Thompson ER, Agel J, Bauer AS, Moeller AT, Novotny SA, et al. A comparative analysis of 150 thumb polydactyly cases from the CoULD registry using the Wassel-Flatt, Rotterdam, and Chung classifications. J Hand Surg Am. 2021;46(1):17–26.
25. Dijkman RR, van Nieuwenhoven CA, Hovius SE, Hulsemann W. Clinical presentation, surgical treatment, and outcome in radial polydactyly. Handchir Mikrochir Plast Chir. 2016;48(1):10–7.
26. Saito S, Tsuge I, Yamanaka H, Morimoto N. Soft tissue abnormalities in Wassel type VI radial polydactyly: a detailed anatomical study. J Hand Surg Eur. 2021;46(4):352–9.
27. Crowley B, Stevenson S, Diogo R. Radial polydactyly: putting together evolution, development and clinical anatomy. J Hand Surg Eur. 2019;44(1):51–8.
28. Dautel G, Perrin P. Use of an axial flap to increase the girth of Wassel IV thumb reconstructions. J Hand Surg Am. 2015;40(7):1327–32.
29. Horii E, Hattori T, Koh S, Majima M. Reconstruction for Wassel type III radial polydactyly with two digits equal in size. J Hand Surg Am. 2009;34(10):1802–7.
30. Engelhardt TO, Baur EM, Pedross F, Piza-Katzer H. Supporting the collateral ligament complex in radial polydactyly type Wassel IV. J Plast Reconstr Aesthet Surg. 2013;66(1):104–12.
31. Xu YL, Shen KY, Chen J, Wang ZG. Flexor pollicis longus rebalancing: a modified technique for Wassel IV-D thumb duplication. J Hand Surg Am. 2014;39(1):75–82 e1.
32. Stutz C, Mills J, Wheeler L, Ezaki M, Oishi S. Long-term outcomes following radial polydactyly reconstruction. J Hand Surg Am. 2014;39(8):1549–52.
33. Patel AU, Tonkin MA, Smith BJ, Alshehri AH, Lawson RD. Factors affecting surgical results of Wassel type IV thumb duplications. J Hand Surg Eur. 2014;39(9):934–43.
34. Ogino O, Tsuchida H, Kashiwa H, Ishigaku D, Takahara M. Thumb polydactyly. Tech Hand Up Extrem Surg. 1999;3(4):278–85.
35. Goldfarb CA, Patterson JM, Maender A, Manske PR. Thumb size and appearance following reconstruction of radial polydactyly. J Hand Surg Am. 2008;33(8):1348–53.
36. Dijkman R. Radial polydactyly: double or nothing? Rotterdam: Erasmus University; 2016.
37. Dijkman R, Selles R, van Rosmalen J, Hulsemann W, Mann M, Habenicht R, et al. A clinically weighted approach to outcome assessment in radial polydactyly. J Hand Surg Eur. 2016;41(3):265–74.
38. Dijkman RR, van Nieuwenhoven CA, Selles RW, Habenicht R, Hovius SE. A multicenter comparative study of two classification systems for radial polydactyly. Plast Reconstr Surg. 2014;134(5):991–1001.
39. Dijkman RR, van Nieuwenhoven CA, Selles RW, Hovius SE. Comparison of functional outcome scores in radial polydactyly. J Bone Joint Surg Am. 2014;96(6):463–70.
40. Dijkman RR, Selles RW, Hulsemann W, Mann M, Habenicht R, Hovius SE, et al. A matched comparative study of the Bilhaut procedure versus resection and reconstruction for treatment of radial polydactyly Types II and IV. J Hand Surg Am. 2016;41(5):e73–83.
41. Hovius S, van Nieuwenhoven CA. Congenital hand IV: syndactyly, synostosis, polydactyly, camptodactyly, and clinodactyly. In: Chang J, Neligan PC, editors. Plastic surgery. 4th ed. Elsevier; 2018.

Ulnar Polydactyly

10

Scott N. Oishi and Terri Beckwith

Abstract

Ulnar polydactyly is the most common form of polydactyly among the pediatric population. The polydactylous digits are developmentally classified as Type A or Type B, with Type B more prevalent. Type A is more rare and is occasionally associated with syndromic conditions, thus a thorough initial evaluation is mandatory to assess for the possible associated findings. For those patients requiring general anesthesia (Type A and wide-based Type B), delay until at least 1 year of age is recommended to decrease potential anesthesia risk. Many Type B ulnar polydactylies can be treated in the clinic without the use of general anesthesia and can be performed within days of birth. The appropriate evaluation of these patients is mandatory in order to provide the best reconstructive option for them.

Keywords

Ulnar polydactyly · Postaxial · Pediatric hand Congenital hand · Type A · Type B

10.1 Introduction

Ulnar polydactyly is a congenital hand difference frequently encountered in a pediatric hand surgery practice. The incidence is estimated at about 1 in 1300 live births [1].

The general classification system currently used was developed by Temtamy and McKusick [2]. They categorized them into Type A and Type B based on the development of the polydactylous digit. Type B refers to a supernumerary digit that is rudimentary and loosely attached. Type A refers to a polydactylous digit that is well-developed and connects to the bony elements of the hand. Type B ulnar polydactyly is much more common than Type A and occurs ten times as frequent in individuals of African descent in which the incidence is 1 in 100 to 300 live births compared to 1 in 1500 to 3000 in white children [3]. The incidence of Type A is equal between individuals of African descent and Caucasians [4].

In general, Type B ulnar polydactyly is an isolated finding which can have a strong autosomal dominant inheritance pattern, affecting the feet as well as the hands. In contrast, Type A ulnar polydactyly has been associated with syndromes such as Greig's, Bardet–Biedl, Ellis–van Creveld,

S. N. Oishi (✉)
Texas Scottish Rite Hospital for Children, Dallas, TX, USA
e-mail: Scott.Oishi@tsrh.org

T. Beckwith (✉)
Center for Excellence in Hand, Upper Extremity and Microvascular Surgery, Texas Scottish Rite Hospital, Dallas, TX, USA
e-mail: Terri.Beckwith@tsrh.org

G. Pajardi (ed.), *Pediatric Hand Surgery*, https://doi.org/10.1007/978-3-031-30984-7_10

Table 10.1 Subtypes of Type A ulnar polydactyly of the hand [6]

Type A Ulnar Polydactyly Subgroup	Metacarpal type (Type I)	Metacarpophalangeal type (Type II)	Phalangeal type (Type III)	Intercalated type (Type IV)	Fully developed type (Type V)	Unclassified	Total
Number of patients	19	20	4	5	4	2	49[a]
Patients with bilateral Type A ulnar polydactyly	12 (63%)	4 (20%)	1 (25%)	2 (40%)	3 (75%)	1	18[a]
Patients with same subgroup type bilaterally	7	0	1	1	3	1	13
Patients with contralateral Type B ulnar polydactyly	7	8	0	0	1	0	16
Patients with combined hand and foot postaxial polydactyly of the feet	19	10	1	3	2	1	31[a]

[a]Because of bilateral Type A cases with two different subtypes, the total number of patients does not match the summation of the different subtypes

Smith–Lemhi-Optic, McKusick–Kaufmann, and others [5].

Pritsch et al. reviewed the phenotypic presentation of patients with Type A ulnar polydactyly and classified them based on bony anatomy (Table 10.1) [6]. Interestingly, they also found that in patients with bilateral involvement the type of ulnar polydactyly was not necessarily symmetric.

10.2 Evaluation

Hand surgeons are often the first practitioners to see these patients after birth. Although in many instances the ulnar polydactyly is an isolated finding, it is imperative to perform a thorough history and physical examination on these patients at initial evaluation. In African American children, a strong family history of ulnar polydactyly is frequently encountered. Lower extremity evaluation will also frequently reveal postaxial polydactyly.

As stated above, in patients with Type A ulnar polydactyly, a thorough examination must be performed as craniofacial, musculoskeletal, cardiac, renal, reproductive, and visual anomalies may be present warranting further investigation. In patients with any of these associated findings, a referral to a geneticist would be appropriate.

An example of this is Ellis Van Creveld syndrome (chondroectodermal dysplasia) where patients have characteristic nail, hair, and teeth anomalies in addition to the ulnar polydactyly (Fig. 10.1).

More importantly greater than 50% of these patients have a congenital heart defect and can also have cryptorchidism (males), chest, and spine anomalies.

In patients with straightforward narrow-based Type B ulnar polydactyly, radiographs are not necessary and treatment can easily be performed in the clinic setting. In patients that require surgical reconstruction, radiographs taken just prior to surgery are mandatory, especially in patients with Type A that will require more than just excision.

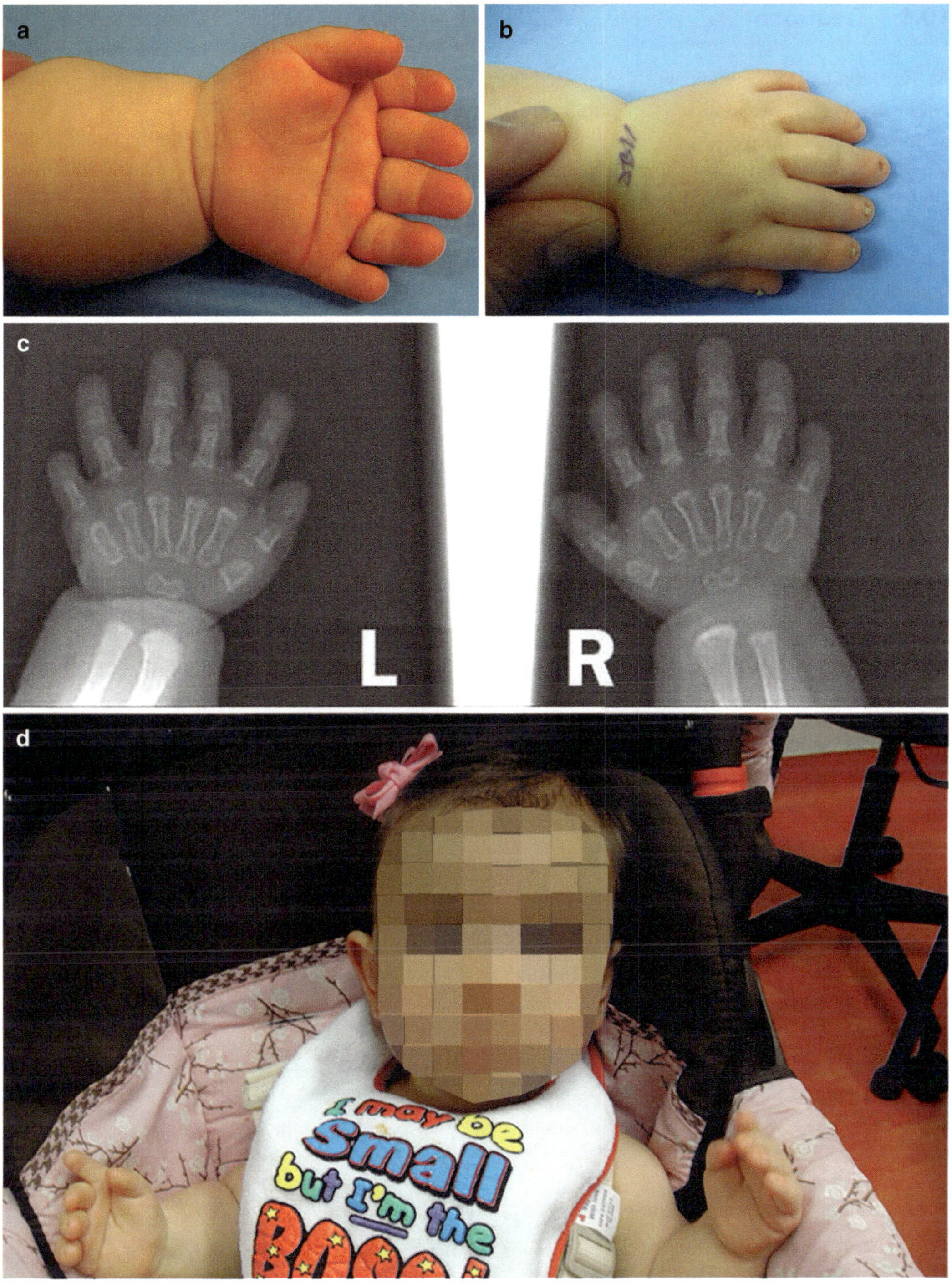

Fig. 10.1 Chondroectodermal Dysplasia (**a**, **b**), clinical appearance of a patient with chondroectodermal dysplasia. Note the brachydactyly and small nails. (**c**) Radiographs showing the short, broad middle phalanges and hypoplastic distal phalanges. (**d**) Clinical appearance of sparse, fine-textured hair and short upper lip

10.3 Treatment

At first evaluation patients with Type B, ulnar polydactyly must be assessed for suitability of treatment at that setting. Broad-based polydactylous digits are best left until after a year of age when the anesthetic risks related to safety issues sufficiently decrease (Fig. 10.2).

In patients with narrow-based polydactyly, several options exist. Suture ligature has been used with reliable results as far as the removal of the digit. However, significant scarring and neuroma formation has been reported in up to 23.5% of cases (Fig. 10.3).

Our preferred method is shown in Fig. 10.4. The base is injected with 1% lidocaine then 2–3 appropriately size ligaclips are applied as shown.

A gauze bandage is then wrapped around the area and the patient is seen back in 2 weeks. When the bandage is removed, usually the digit has already auto-amputated. If there is still some adherence of the digit, an 18-gauge needle bevel can be used for final removal. This procedure can be easily performed in the clinic and offers large cost savings when compared to an outpatient surgical procedure.

In our review of patients treated at our institution with ligaclip, application the incidence of neuroma formation was 7%, which is significantly less than that reported with the suture ligation technique [7]. No matter which technique is utilized near-normal function of the little finger is to be expected.

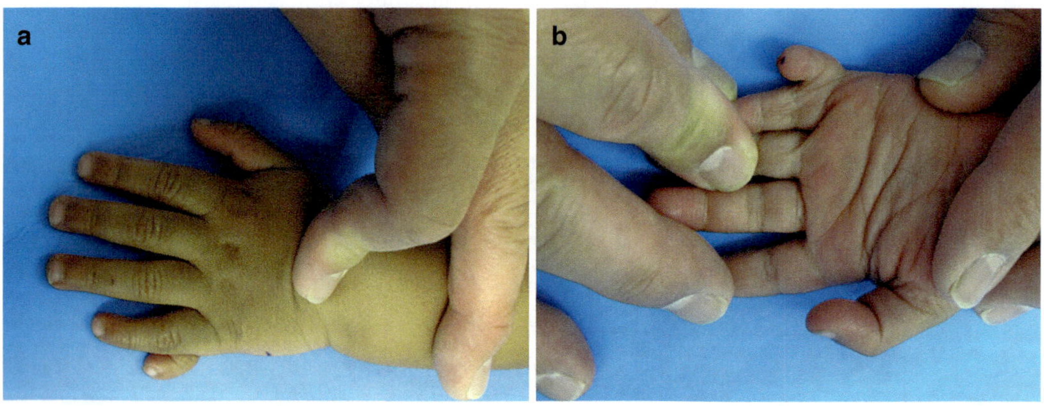

Fig. 10.2 Type B post-axial polydactyly. (**a**, **b**) Example of broad-based polydactyly not amenable to removal with suture ligature or ligaclip application

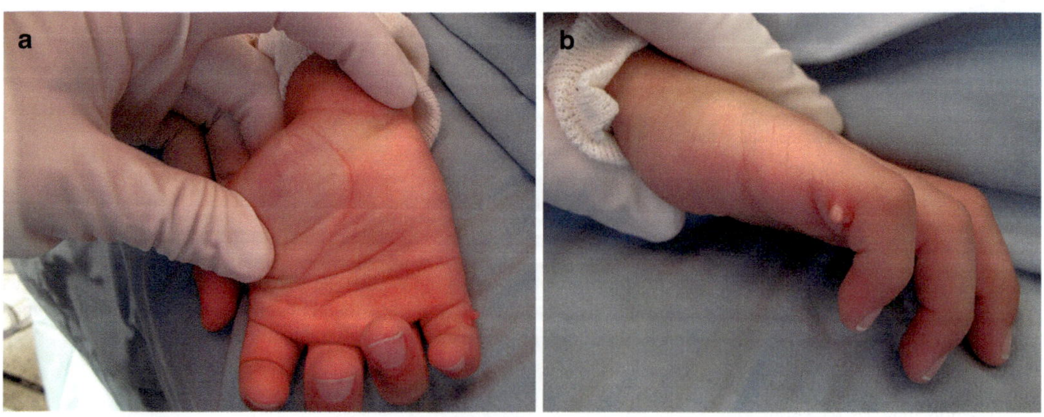

Fig. 10.3 (**a**, **b**) Neuroma formation after suture ligation

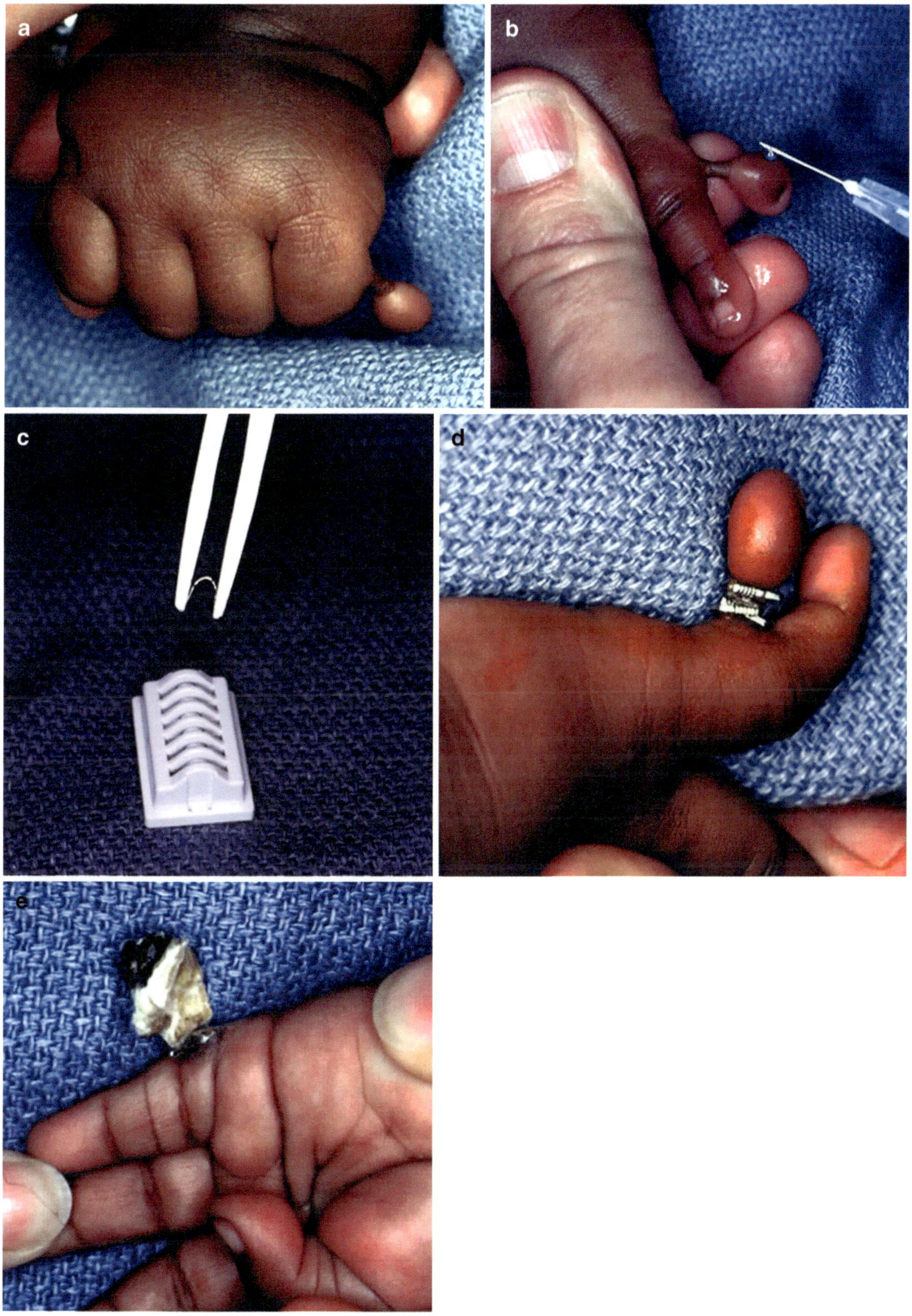

Fig. 10.4 Technique of ligaclip application. (**a**) Narrow-based Type B postaxial polydactyly. (**b**) Injection of the base with 1% lidocaine. (**c, b**) Application of ligaclips to base of digit. (**e**) Two weeks after ligaclip application

As discussed above, Type A ulnar polydactyly can present as many as different phenotypes and each patient must be individually assessed for reconstruction. In particular, symmetry may not exist between hands and/or between hands and feet. A single patient may have a combination of Types A and B polydactylous digits or different types of Type A. It is important for the parents to understand the difference between Types A and B, as many times decreased motion and stability will exist in the little finger after the reconstruction of Type A variants. In addition, many times this digit is also hypoplastic when compared to a normal little finger. Except in rare instances, surgery should be performed after a year of age because of the potential anesthesia consequences that can occur as well as size of structures.

Reconstruction can be very complex in these patients and can include osteotomy, ligament reconstruction, and tendon realignment. Pin fixation is often required as well as cast immobilization for a much longer time as compared to Type B reconstruction (Figs. 10.5 and 10.6).

In conclusion, ulnar polydactyly is frequently encountered in a pediatric hand surgery practice. Appropriate assessment is key to optimal reconstruction in these patients. In patients with Type A ulnar polydactyly, a high degree of suspicion for associated anomalies (syndromes) is mandatory with appropriate further testing and referrals as indicated. After reconstruction Type B ulnar polydactyly patients will have near-normal function, whereas Type A ulnar polydactyly patients may not. Proper counseling of parents is mandatory to assure realistic goals and expectations are agreed upon.

Fig. 10.5 Example of Type A (Type 4) postaxial polydactyly. (**a–c**) Preoperative clinical photographs and radiographs. Note the well-developed digit with shared metacarpal. Reconstruction of this digit involves reconstruction of the collateral ligament and hypothenar muscle insertion as well as metacarpal head chondroplasty for optimum outcome. In addition, flexor and extensor tendon anatomy must be assessed. (**d, e**) After reconstruction is performed. Note the pin to stabilize the ligamentous reconstruction

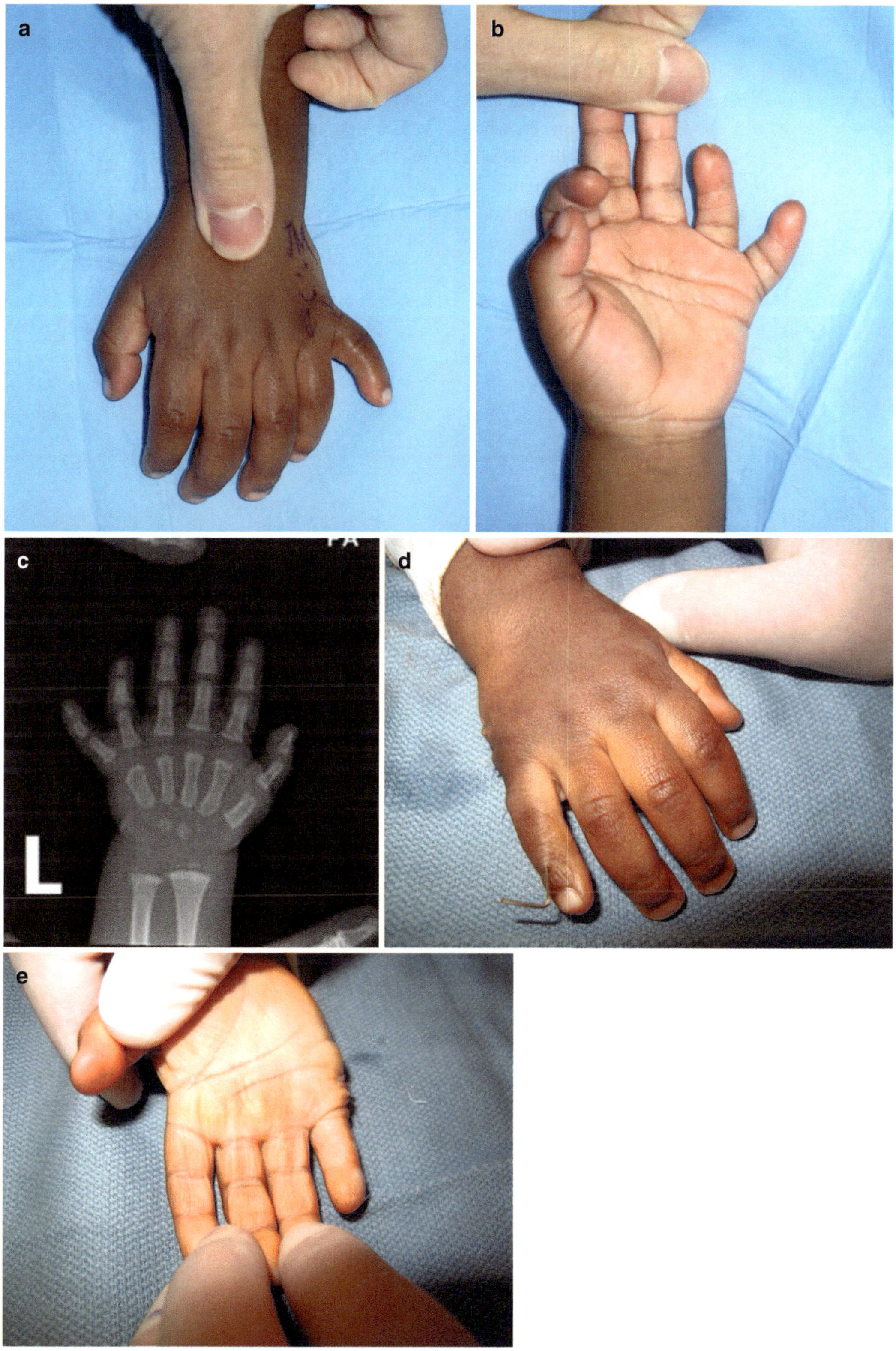
a
b
c
L
d
e

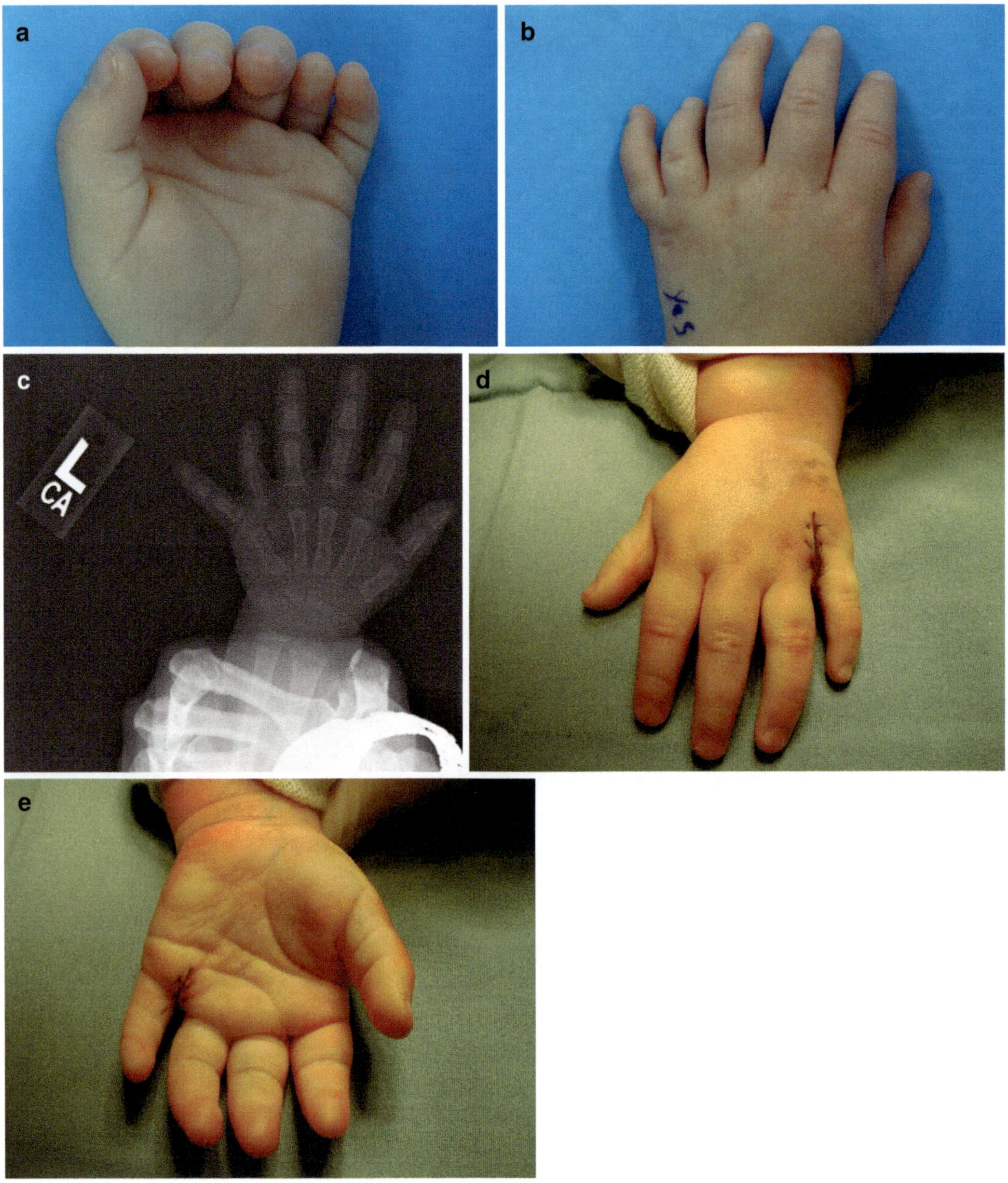

Fig. 10.6 Example of Type A postaxial (Type 2) polydactyly. (**a**–**e**) Preoperative clinical photographs and radiographs. Successful reconstruction requires extensor and flexor tendon assessment, collateral ligament reconstruction and intermetacarpal ligament reconstruction. Note that the reconstructed little finger is hypoplastic

References

1. Staff TSRH. Disorders of the upper extremity: ulnar polydactyly. In: Herring J, editor. Tachdjians pediatric orthopedics: from the Texas Scottish rite hospital for children. 4th ed. Philadelphia, PA: Elsevier Saunders; 2008. p. 556–8.
2. Temtamy SA, McKusick VA. The genetics of hand malformations. Birth Defects Orig Artic Ser. 1978;14(3):i–xviii, 1–619. Epub 1978/01/01.
3. Watson BT, Hennrikus WL. Postaxial type-B polydactyly. Prevalence and treatment. J Bone Joint Surg Am. 1997;79(1):65–8. Epub 1997/01/01
4. Woolf CM, Myrianthopoulos NC. Polydactyly in American negroes and whites. Am J Hum Genet. 1973;25(4):397–404. Epub 1973/07/01
5. Umm-e-Kalsoom, Basit S, Kamran-ul-Hassan Naqvi S, Ansar M, Ahmad W. Genetic mapping of an autosomal recessive postaxial polydactyly type A to chromosome 13q13.3-q21.2 and screening of the candidate genes. Human genetics. 2012;131(3):415–22. Epub 2011/08/31
6. Pritsch T, Ezaki M, Mills J, Oishi SN. Type A ulnar polydactyly of the hand: a classification system and clinical series. J Hand Surg Am. 2013;38(3):453–8. Epub 2013/02/23
7. Mills JK, Ezaki M, Oishi SN. Ulnar polydactyly: long-term outcomes and cost-effectiveness of surgical clip application in the newborn. Clin Pediatr. 2014;53(5):470–3. Epub 2013/12/19

11 Cleft Hand or Split Hand Foot Malformation

Stéfane Guéro

Abstract

Cleft Hand or Split Hand Foot Malformation (SHFM) is a sequence of phenotypes, from a minor shortening of the central digit to a complete absence of the third ray and, in the most severe cases, absence of two, three or four rays. It is a rare but spectacular presentation usually involving both hands and feet. Inheritance is primarily autosomal dominant but sporadic cases are also reported, resulting from a de novo mutation/deletion/duplication. Intra-familial clinical variability is the rule, with incomplete penetrance. X-linked or autosomal recessive inheritance has also been described. To date, seven subgroups of SHFM have been identified and seven loci are currently known. Anatomical records have enhanced our knowledge of this group of disorders of the hands and feet and allowed us to improve surgical procedures and long-term outcomes.

Keywords

Hand · Cleft hand · SHFM · Classification Congenital

S. Guéro (✉)
Institut de la Main, Paris, France

Paediatric Orthopaedic Unit, Hôpital Necker Enfants Malades, Université Paris Sorbonne-centre, Paris, France

11.1 Definition

Split hand foot malformations (SHFM) are complex congenital malformations, fortunately rare, most often of familial origin and of autosomal dominant inheritance. This spectacular presentation usually involves both hands and feet. SHFM is a sequence of phenotypes, from a minor shortening of the central digit to a complete absence of the third ray and, in the most severe cases, absence of two, three or four rays. The condition was first described by Isidore Geoffroy Saint-Hilaire (1832) [1] who gave the name ectrodactyly which is still used today. Many authors have described this malformation using terminology such as 'claw hand', 'lobster hand' or even 'lobster-claw hand' [2]; these may be descriptive terms but they are insulting to the children and should not be used anymore. Cleft hand is acceptable but we definitely prefer split hand foot malformation as it is shared with the Geneticists.

11.2 Incidence

The incidence has been reported by Adrian Flatt (1994) as 3.9% in his series of congenital hand anomalies [3]. However, the reported incidence varies greatly since confusion with symbrachydactyly remains. In the most recent publications, the incidence of SHFM varies from 1/8500 to 1/90000 living births, accounting for up to 15%

G. Pajardi (ed.), *Pediatric Hand Surgery*, https://doi.org/10.1007/978-3-031-30984-7_11

of all limb defects, depending on the terminology and whether the patients were seen by surgeons or clinical geneticists [4].

11.3 Clinical Presentation

The typical presentation of split hand is a bilateral deep, central cleft of the hands (Fig. 11.1a, b), but often with asymmetrical malformations. Adjacent fingers are usually abnormal, broad, deviated or rotated toward the cleft. Split hand cannot be summarized as a simple cleft as additional embryological disorders such as syndactyly, camptodactyly, clinodactyly with or without delta phalanges can be encountered [5]. Fusion and duplication of rays and some transverse bones, so-called 'cross bones' are also very specific to SHFM [6]. Feet are also often involved, without any correlation with the hand presentation (Fig. 11.2).

Typically, the deformity involves the four extremities but, on average, malformations of the hands are asymmetrical. Affections of the upper limb are sometimes very different from those of the lower limb, which is explained embryologically by the time lag between the appearance of the buds of the upper limb and inferior. It is thus possible to observe on the hands a median cleft and on the lower limb a central polydactyly. We

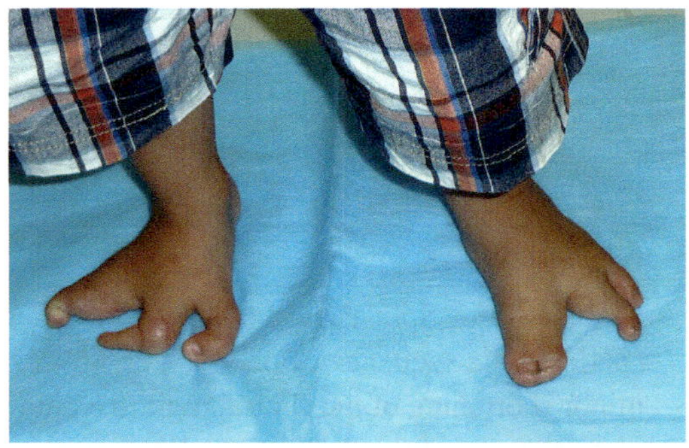

Fig. 11.2 Foot anomalies. Divergence of the first and fifth toe is the rule. Impairment of the shoe bearing comes very early, requiring the closure of the cleft with multiple metatarsal or phalanges osteotomies

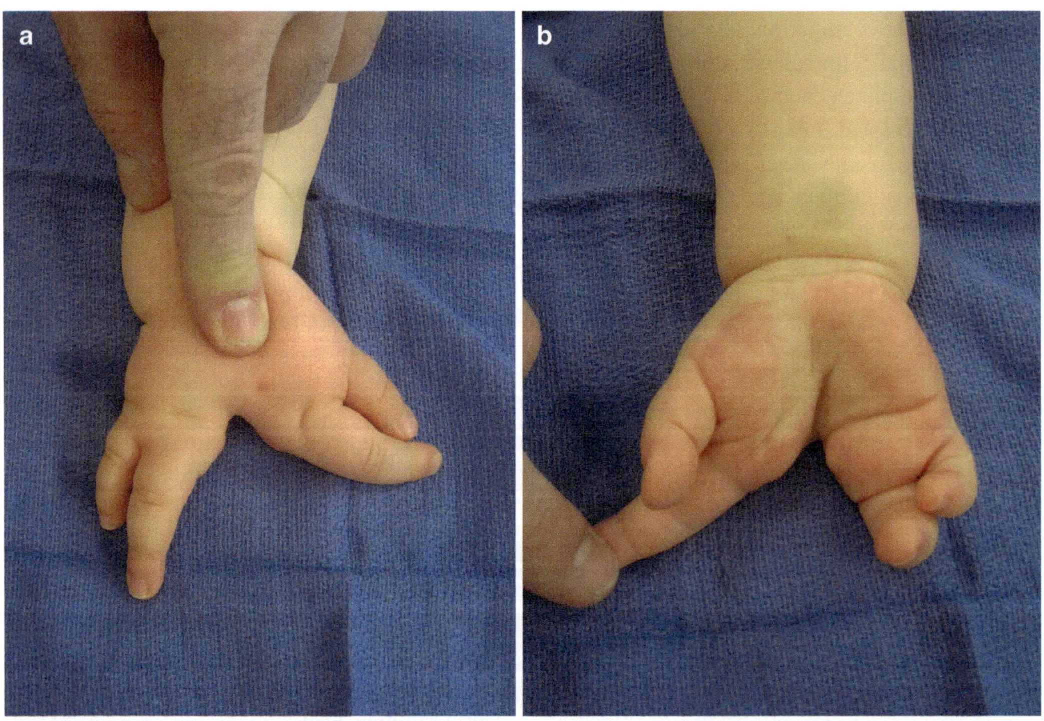

Fig. 11.1 SHFM, right hand. (**a**) Dorsal view of a SHFM with a moderate syndactyly of the first web. (**b**) palmar view

will come back to this notion in the classification chapter.

Sometimes there is cleft located on the fourth space; these cases are even more exceptional, but we will treat them in this chapter because they show similar problems, and their treatment follows the same principle.

It is true that the extremely 'bizarre' aspect of the hands or feet has a considerable psychological impact, and one of the first goals of the treatment should be to 'normalize' the overall appearance of the hand and feet. But in some severe and complex forms it is not even possible to plan a surgical correction. In congenital hand specialist meetings, most of the cases requiring discussion are SHFM.

11.3.1 Distinction Between True and False Median Clefts

The first classification proposed by Barsky (1964) [7] was an attempt to clarify the differences between 'typical' cleft hand and symbrachydactyly (atypical cleft hands). He described typical cleft hand as usually involving the third ray, bilateral and following an autosomal dominant inheritance pattern. There are also unilateral forms where the cleft is shown only on one hand, and these cases produce confusion with symbrachydactyly type 2 or 3 of Blauth's classification [8] modified by Foucher [9]. Anyway, the morphological differences between the typical cleft hand (SHFM) and the atypical cleft hand – which are symbrachydactylies [10]—have now been clearly established: (1) In the symbrachydactyly, the 'cleft' is U-shaped, whereas in the typical cleft, it is V-shaped. (2) If the malformation is unilateral and therefore does not involve the other limbs, it cannot be assessed as cleft. (3) In the monodactylous type of symbrachydactyly, the thumb is absent, and the fifth ray is present. All these characteristics are therefore opposed to the typical cleft hands (see Table 11.1). Diagnosis between typical and atypical types is usually straightforward for a hand surgeon trained in congenital anomalies [10]. This has not a simple connotation of classification interest, but the identity gives us indication to direct parents to genetic counselling. Indeed, a child with typical familial cleft hand or a cleft by de novo mutation has a high possibility to transmit this condition to the 50% of his descents, on the contrary symbrachydactylies are nonhereditary, probably teratological (viral?), and the approach for the relatives is completely different and more reassuring.

Table 11.1 Differences between typical cleft hand and symbrachydactyly (atypical cleft hand) according to Barsky. (Republished from J Hand Surg Eur Vol, 2019)

	Cleft hand	Symbrachydactyly
Rays involve	3rd ray	Three central digits
Monodactylous hand	5th	Thumb
Upper limb	Bilateral	Unilateral
Transmission	Dominant inheritance	No inheritance
Central defect	V shape	U shape
Feet involvement	Yes	No
Syndactylies	Frequent	Less frequent
Associated anomalies	Yes	No

11.4 Inheritance

SHFM can be inherited or sporadic. Inheritance is mostly autosomal dominant with intra-familial clinical variability but X-linked and autosomal recessive forms have been reported. Sporadic cases can be caused by de novo mutation/chromosome imbalances.

SHFM can be isolated and associated with some malformations or part of a syndrome. The most frequent syndromes are EEC (Ectrodactyly-Ectodermal dysplasia-Cleft lip and palate), LADD (Lacrimo-Auriculo-Dento-Digital), ADULT (Acro-Dermato-Ungual-Lacrimal-Tooth), CHARGE (Coloboma-Heart defect, Atresia choanae, Retarded growth and development-Genital hypoplasia-Ear), VACTERL (Vertebral-Anal-Cardiac-Tracheal-Esophageal-Renal-Limb defects), Cornelia de Lange [11, 12] and Smith–Lemli–Opitz [13]. Some rare cases of SHFM have been ascribed to teratogens, particularly after exposure to retinoic acid.

11.5 Genetic Classification

More recently, different aetiologies and subgroups of SHFM have been highlighted [14], based on genetic data. Sowinska-Seidler et al. [15] summarized the underlying genetics mechanisms. Indeed, seven subgroups have been identified as follows: SHFM1 at 7q21.2q22.1 (*DLX5* gene), SHFM2 at Xq26, SHFM3 at 10q24q25, SHFM4 at 3q27 (*TP63* gene), SHFM5 at 2q31 and SHFM6 as a result of variants in *WNT10B* (chromosome 12q13). Duplications at 17p13.3 are seen in SHFM7 when isolated or associated with long bone deficiency. As previously stated above, most cases of SHFM are following an autosomal dominant pattern of inheritance (types 1, 3, 4, 5 and 7), but autosomal recessive (type 1 and 6) and X-linked inheritance (type 2) have also been reported. SHFM can be identified as an isolated finding but can also be associated with other malformations or be part of a syndromic association. Genetic heterogeneity and clinical variability, even between individuals from the same family, is the rule. Incomplete penetrance is also quite common, which leads to difficult genetic counselling. We have summarized the different types in Table 11.2 [16], according to Sowinska-Seidler et al. SHFM1 can appear as isolated, associated with other malformations or syndromic. It is most commonly autosomal dominant and associated with deafness (35%) or ectodermal dysplasia. Autosomal recessive SHFM1 has also been reported in association with homozygous mutations within the *DLX5* gene. SHFM2 is the only X-linked form of SHFM and to date the underlying molecular mechanism is unknown, although there are two potential candidate genes (*FGF13* and *TONDU*). SHFM3 is the most frequent form of SHFM (with SHFM7). It is autosomal dominant and non-syndromic but can be associated with preaxial ray anomalies such as polydactyly or triphalangeal thumbs. SHFM4 is also autosomal dominant and linked with variants within the *TP63* gene (Fig. 11.3a–d). It can be isolated or part of EEC syndrome. SHFM5 is due to deletions encompassing the entire *HOXD* gene cluster. However, the phenotype is unclear (synpolydactyly/Split foot) as well as the pathogenesis. SHFM6 is following an autosomal reces-

Table 11.2 Different SHFM subgroups with their molecular and clinical characteristics

Sub-type	Chromosome	Inheritance	Gene	Frequency	Clinical presentation	Syndromic association
SHFM1	7q21.3-q22.1	AD/AR	*DLX5*	ND	SHFM	EEC, deafness, MR
SHFM2	Xq26	XR		One family	SHFM, syndactyly, metacarpal and phalangeal hypoplasia	
SHFM3	10q24	AD		20% of SHFM	SHFM, preaxial anomalies (triphalangeal thumb, duplicated thumb)	
SHFM4	3q27	AD	*TP63*	10–16% of isolated SHFM (93% of EEC with limb malformation)	SHFM, cleft lip and palate	EEC, ADULT, MR
SHFM5	2q31	AD		ND	SHFM	MR
SHFM6	12q13	AR	*WNT10B*	Three families and one sporadic case	SHFM	
SHFM7	17p13.3	AD	*BHLHA9*	12% of isolated SHFM (90% SHFLD)	SHFM/tibial aplasia or hypoplasia	SHFLD

AD autosomal dominant, *ADULT* acro-dermato-ungual-lacrymal-tooth syndrome, *AR* autosomal recessive, *EEC* ectrodactyly-ecto-dermal dysplasis-cleft lip/plate, *MR* mental retardation, *ND* no data, *SHFLD* split hand foot and long bone deficience, *SHFM* split hand foot malformation, *DR* X-linked recessive

Guero, S. and M. Holder-Espinasse, *Insights into the pathogenesis and treatment of split/hand foot malformation (cleft hand/foot).* J Hand Surg Eur Vol, 2019. 44(1): p. 80–87 sive mode of inheritance linked with homozygous mutations in the *WNT10B* gene. It is very rare and apparently isolated. SHFM7 is either isolated or associated with long bone deficiency. It is due to chromosome 17p13.3 duplication comprising the *BHLHA9* gene. Incomplete penetrance and sex bias have been commonly reported in this particular group. When a patient is seen in a Clinical Genetics setting, array CGH should be offered as a baseline test. This would very likely identify a chromosome 10q24 or 17p13 duplication is around 50% of cases (SHFM types 3 and 7). If negative, we would recommend *TP63* gene molecular testing, as this will identify SHFM type 4 in 10% of cases. If no underlying explanation is found at this stage, a karyotype should be offered to test for deletion/translocation involving chromosome 7 (SHFM type 1). Then, if inheritance appears to be autosomal recessive, molecular testing of *WNT10* and/or *DLX5* genes is relevant (SHFM types 1 and 6). An underlying explanation is currently identified in approximately 50–60% of cases therefore more loci are likely to be identified in the future. Whole-exome sequencing and whole genome sequencing on a research basis are obviously relevant, but since

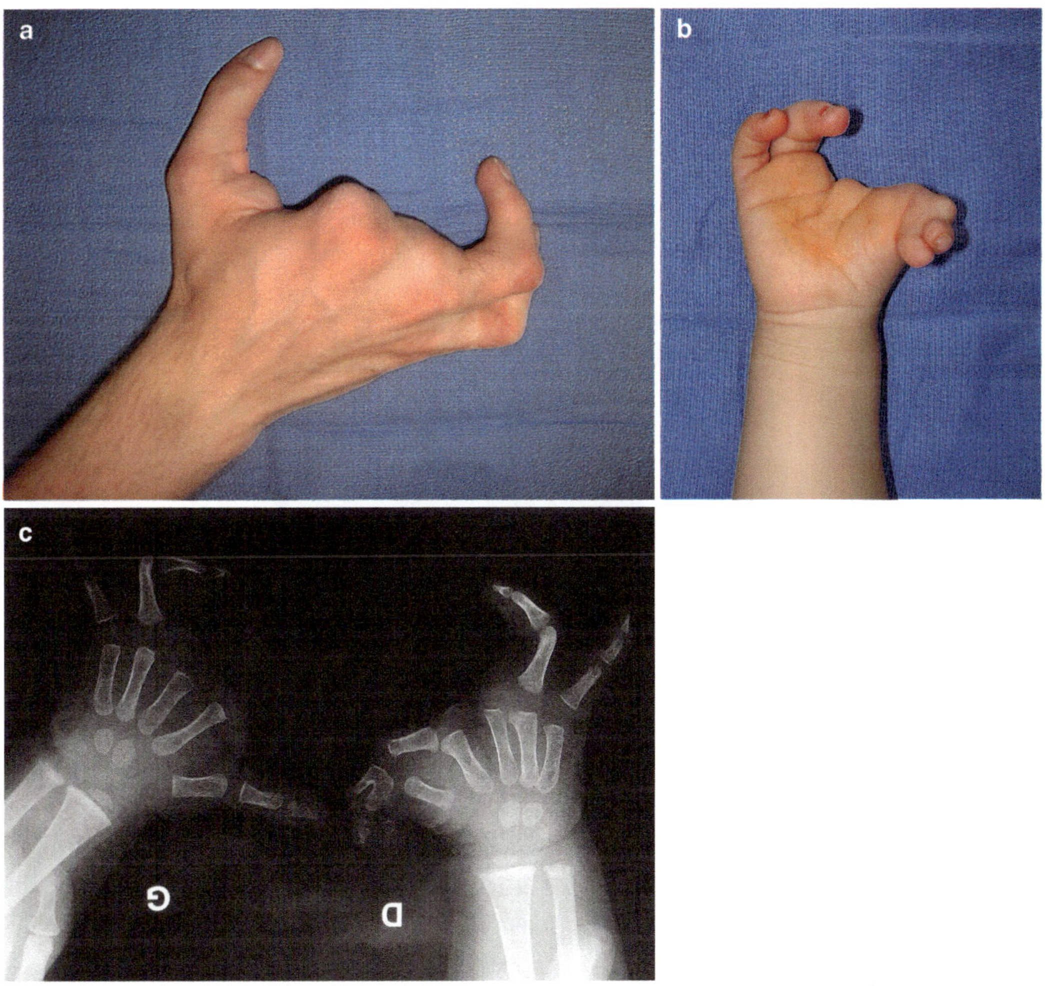

Fig. 11.3 Three members of a family with a SHFM type 4, with mutation on *TP63*, severe cleft hand and cleft foot, cleft palate and lip. (**a**) Right hand of the father. (**b**) Right hand of the son with a complete and complex syndactyly of the thumb and index. (**c**) X-ray of the son's right hand showing the bony fusions. (**d**) X-ray of the daughter's right hand. Tridactylous hand with absence of the index finger and superdigit on the 'fourth finger'

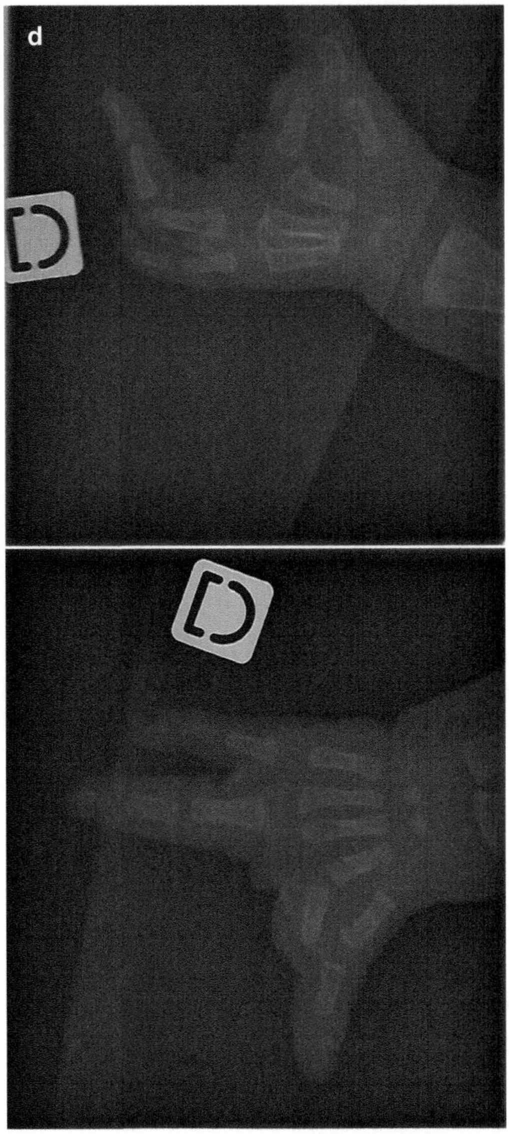

Fig. 11.3 (continued)

complex non-coding regulatory elements are involved in such malformations, other pathways need to be explored as well. The Department of Genetic Research of the Necker-Enfant Malades Hospital in Paris has recently reviewed the data of 22 patients with SHFM. A mutation was identified in only 50% of the children. The most frequent ($n = 4$), was on *TP63* (type 4), one patient had a deletion on *HOXD13* (type 5), another deletion was found in 7q21 (type1) one on *BHLHA9* (type 7). In five patients, a chromosomal rearrangement was found on chromosome 10 (type 3) but the gene involved has not been identified to date.

11.5.1 Embryological Hypothesis

Whatever the genetic mutation, the precise pathogenetic processes leading to phenotypic disruptions of the normal pattern of hands and feet remain unclear. Among morphogens involved in the formation of the autopod, DLX5 and DLX6 seem to be crucial for the persistence of the apical ectodermal ridge (AER) and are upregulated by TP63. In mice *Tp63* Null, the AER fails to stratify and the expression of the *Dlx* genes is strongly reduced [17]. Disorders in the pathways explain some similarities in the SHFM1 and SHFM4 phenotypes (EEC and developmental delay). Duijf et al. [18] have postulated that cleft hand is primarily due to a defect in the central part of the apical ectodermal ridge (AER) on the autopod; this was also suggested by Naruse et al. [19]. If the disruption of the central AER occurs precisely on the top of the median ray, one can observe a central polydactyly. When the disruption to the central portion of the AER becomes irregular and wider, the consequence is a failure of induction of finger rays and disorganization of the formation of the precartilaginous anlagen of the future central digits. The third or median anlage can fuse with the fourth or the second anlage or with both of them. In severe cases, some rays can be missing.

Another consistent finding in SHFM is the presence of extrinsic tendons and intrinsic muscles in the hand despite the absence of the bones, which raises questions about the close relationship of bones and tendons during development.

11.6 The Cleft Hand in the Classifications of the Congenital Hand Anomalies

The quarrels regarding classification and treatment of cleft hand since Swanson's classification (1968) [20] are in part due to the incredibly low incidence of this disorder. In this system previously adopted by the International Federation for Surgery of the Hand (IFSSH), cleft hands were classified as 'failure of formation of parts, longitudinal arrest, central ray'. This remained largely unchanged until Ogino (1990) [21] published the results of his experiment. In his work, Ogino exposed pregnant rats to an antimitotic agent (Busulfan) at different stages and observed central polydactyly or central clefts of various severity. His conclusion was that cleft hand and central polydactyly are derived from the same embryological mechanism, and that the aetiology is primarily not a failure of formation but a failure of differentiation of parts. Twice we observed, in child a medial cleft on one hand, bidactylous form, and an authentic central polydactyly on the other hand. Flatt [1] in his book shows an example of monozygotic twins with one twin presenting a central polydactyly, and the other twin a complete absence of the third ray. Indeed, the radiological analysis of some SHFM distinctly shows a separation in two of the third ray which migrates on the second and/or fourth finger, which evokes more a lack of separation than a real lack of formation of a ray (Fig. 11.4).

Ogino's publication sparked off controversial discussions between specialists; some decided to stay with the former classification whilst others decided to modify the position of cleft hand within Swanson's classification. More recently, and in light of recent knowledge gained from developmental biology, a new classification has been adopted by the IFSSH, namely, the Oberg–Manske–Tonkin or OMT classification [22]. Based on the three axes of development of the hand and upper limb, cleft hand is now classified within the category of 'Malformation, which is a failure of formation/differentiation, of unspecified axis and complex' [23]. With many colleagues, we have proposed to move SHFM to malformation; handplate; and proximal-distal axis (IB1iv).

11.7 Classification of Clinical Forms of SHFM

Concomitantly, many attempts had been made to classify the different types of 'typical' cleft hand. The most relevant have been those providing guidelines for surgical treatment, such as the classification by Glicenstein et al. [24] where it is divided into three groups: simple, complex and

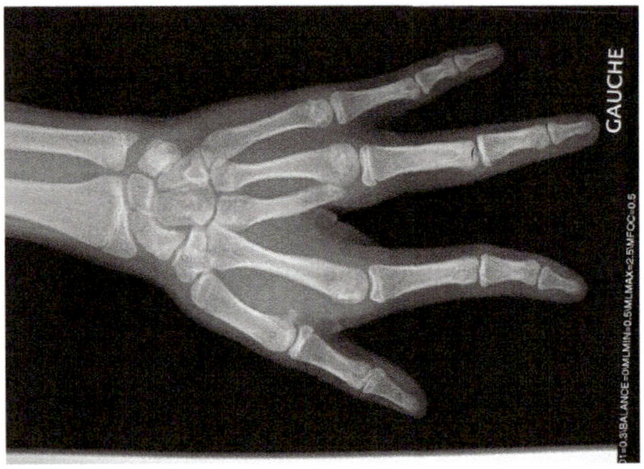

Fig. 11.4 SHFM with fusion of the third and fourth metacarpal, moderate central cleft and fist web syndactyly

severe. The simple type has a more or less marked cleft on the third ray, usually with the presence of the third metacarpal. Complex types are associated with membranous or complex syndactylies and/or with bone anomalies: transverse phalanges (cross-bones) [6], delta phalanges and bone fusions (Fig. 11.5). The severe types are the three-fingered or bidactylous or monodactylous forms (Fig. 11.6).

Another way of choosing a surgical treatment is to consider the state of the first web, as suggested by Manske and Halikis [25]. In type 1 (normal first web) or 2 (first narrow first web), a simple treatment of the cleft and/or syndactyly of

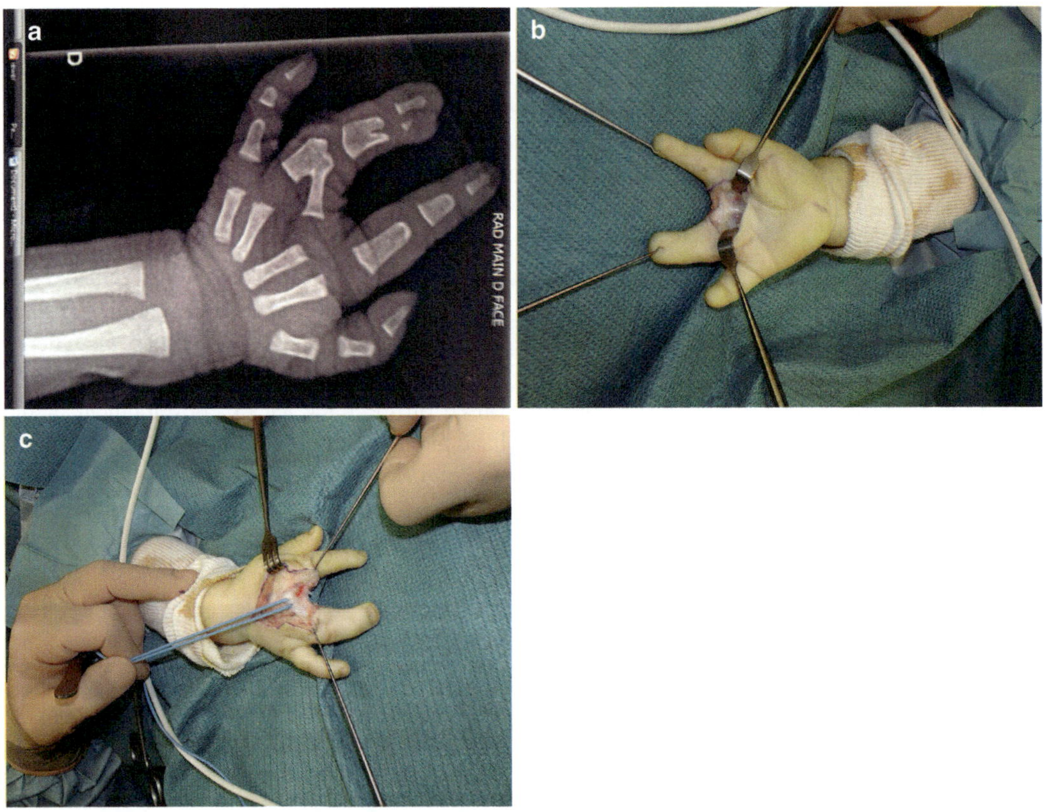

Fig. 11.5 'Simple closure' of a moderate SHFM. . (**a**) Pre-operative X-rays showing the migration of the third ray onto the fourth. (**b**) Per operative palmar view. Note the abnormal fibrous anlagen in the cleft and the remnant of the flexor tendon of the third digit running on the radial side of the fourth. This extra tendon limits the extension of the PIP joint. (**c**) Dorsal view demonstrating a central tendinous loop (blue silicone loop) and a supernumerary extensor tendon

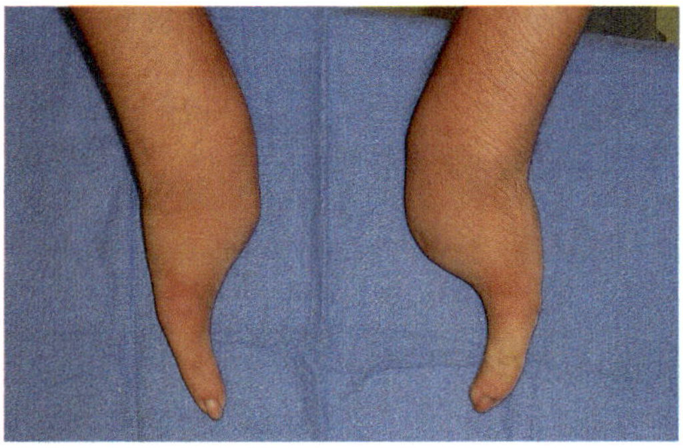

Fig. 11.6 Bilateral monodactylous hand. Feet have the same feature. No surgical solution. The child can write very nicely with a bimanual grasp

the first commissure is performed. In some more severe cases of type 2, a translocation of the second ray on the third metacarpal will be proposed, or we will simplify the hand resecting the second ray to achieve a three-fingered hand.

11.8 Principle of Treatment

As Adrian Flatt [3] said: 'cleft hand is a functional triumph but a social disaster'. The first surgical goal is to improve the disturbing appearance to an almost normal hand. After surgery, one ray might still be missing but with good closure of the cleft with a minimal amount of scar and by achieving parallelism of the long fingers, the hand anomaly will be barely noticeable. The second principle is to preserve the function by treating the thumb web or associated camptodactyly, but we should never compromise the child's former function. The third principle is to combine the two, cosmesis and function or a 'cosmetic function' by avoiding rotation of the fingers during flexion and preserving the normal skeletal structures (bones, joints, tendons) from the deleterious effects of the additional elements (bone fusions and supernumerary tendons).

11.8.1 Tendon Anomalies

Before considering the surgical treatment of such complex hands, it is necessary first to comprehend and understand anatomical abnormalities. As a rule, we must consider that growth can alter a result that was previously thought to be good. We must not dissociate aesthetics and function. The surgeon can make a hand that is aesthetically pleasing at rest but, looks abnormal during use, such as the rotation of the fingers during flexion. These are important notions that the surgeon must keep in mind before proposing a therapeutic schedule to families.

If bone abnormalities are visible on radiographs or CT scan with 3D reconstructions, tendon abnormalities are often neglected. It is imperative to explore the cleft and the adjacent fingers to make the distinction between the normal elements of each ray and the supernumerary elements which will have to be largely resected.

We previously had the opportunity to perform a dissection of a human specimen with SHFM [26]. The patient presented with bilateral SHFM, and bidactylous hands; little other information was available. The thumbs were slightly hypoplastic whereas the ulnar digit was broad, probably resulting from the fusion of two rays (superdigit) [27]. Before dissection, skeletal radiographs of the upper limbs and computer-tomographic scans with three-dimensional reconstruction of the images were performed. The wrist and forearm bones were normal, but arthrosis on the proximal-inter-phalangeal joint of the most ulnar digit was noted. During the dissection, we were able to identify all muscles and tendons in the forearm, even flexor and extensor tendons for the missing fingers. These tendons were present in the forearm and travelled to the hand but ended in the cleft, forming a few loops in the middle of the cleft or tendon plexuses onto the lateral side of the two digits.

This observation was of major interest for our current practice in reconstructive surgery, as we noted that extrinsic flexor and extensor tendons could be formed even in the absence of some rays in the hand. During surgery, additional tendons could join together in the centre of the cleft and migrate on the lateral side of the adjacent fingers in the presence or absence of cross-bones. These extra tendons could be partially responsible for camptodactyly and rotation of the adjacent fingers during flexion. Careful division of the cleft and of the lateral side of the fingers with removal of additional tendons greatly improved the cosmetic and functional outcomes of patients with split hands.

Bone anomalies: it is necessary to remove the abnormal elements which are more or less fused with the adjacent fingers, especially the transverse phalanges or cross-bones which have a physeal plate often very active and whose growth can cause a divergence of neighbouring metacarpals, further aggravating the deformity. These transverse phalanges must be removed carefully, they often share joints with neighbouring metacarpophalangeal joints (MP joints). It is advisable to keep a limited portion of these phalanges to avoid an instability of the MP joints. Delta phalanges can be treated either by osteotomy or Vicker's procedure.

If a divergence of the metacarpal remains, the surgeon should not hesitate to perform a closing wedge osteotomy at the base to achieve a complete parallelism, which will grant a harmonious growth. On the contrary, in the first commissure, it will sometimes be necessary to release the intrinsic muscles to increase the divergence between the first and second metacarpals, or perform a metacarpal osteotomy or, in some cases, remove the second metacarpal and perform an index translocation on to the third ray.

Interventions should be started early in infancy. Whenever possible, the first web must be corrected between 12 and 18 months. For complex translocations, it is not illogical to wait until 2 to 3 years old. Usually, we operate only on one hand to leave the child using the contralateral hand. Commonly we perform surgery on one hand and on the ipsilateral foot in the same stage.

11.9 Surgical Procedures

11.9.1 Simple Forms

In the simple type of Glicenstein or the type 1 of Manske, we perform a simple closure of the cleft. We have seen that this 'simple closure' is in appearance: it will require a parallelism of the second and fourth metacarpal, resect the third metacarpal if present, and rebuild an intermetacarpal ligament. This is facilitated by a complete exploration of the fingers to identify the flexor tendon sheeths. Their fascial expansions at the neck of the metacarpals must be preserved to be sutured at the end of the procedure.

We try to preserve the periosteum around the third metacarpal, even if there is a risk of reossification in the following years, this ossification never deforms the hand. The periosteum is a very resistant fabric for a 'paletot' suture, from the base of the metacarpals to the neck [28].

The procedure begins with a dorsal approach. The skin incision itself does not require any sophisticated flap for closure. Our drawing tends to leave only enough skin taken from the lateral side of the adjacent fingers to achieve a longitudinal scar. The final level of the web will be decided following comparisons with the other webs. We found that attempts of local flaps ended with contractures, imposing a revision surgery to 'redig the cleft'!

Neurovascular pedicles are identified, and careful division of the cleft is a very important step for the identification of any additional tendons. A central loop between flexor and extensor tendons might be found and should be fully removed. We examine the normal tendons of digits 2 and 4 and then resect any abnormal additional tendons. In some cases, we would observe an improvement of the flexion and rotation of the PIP joints. If there remains any abnormal flexion or rotation, we would completely remove the third metacarpal bone. Our goal is to achieve a good parallelism of the metacarpal bones (Fig. 11.7a–d). If digits 2 and 4 remain divergent, we would consider performing a closing wedge osteotomy of the base of one of the metacarpal bones. We carefully divide the flexor tendon sheets at the pulley A1 level to reconstruct the deep transverse metacarpal ligament by using two ligamentous flaps made out of the flexor tendon sheaths of the index and ring fingers to prevent future migration of the fingers. Although the flexor sheaths are strong structures, they are insufficient for a stable clo-

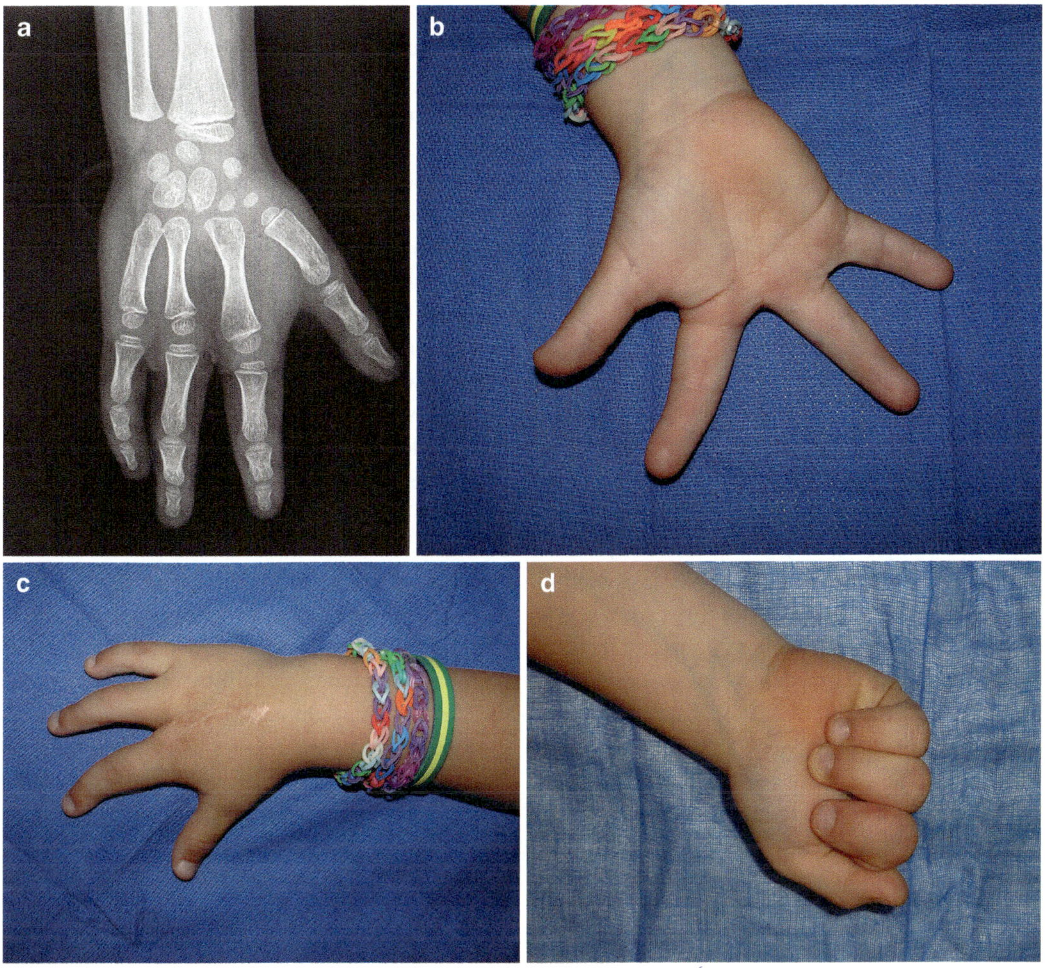

Fig. 11.7 Two years follow up after closure of a 'simple cleft'. (**a**) Plain radiograph showing the good parallelism of the second and fourth metatarsal. (**b**) Hand in full abduction. Good level of the central web. No flap has been performed but a straight longitudinal line of suture. (**c**) Dorsal view. Scar on the social face of the hand. (**d**) Fingers in flexion. No rotation thanks to the removal of abnormal fibrous anlagen and tendons

sure of the inter-metacarpal space. We used to partially preserve the periosteum of the former third metacarpal bone to reconstruct two periosteal flaps [28]. The dorsal aspect is closed with 'paletot' sutures, using an absorbable suture such as Monocryl® or PDS®, Ethicon, Cincinnati, USA. After which a passive flexion force is applied to check if the suture limits the range of motion of the MP joints. Fatty pads in the palm of the hand are removed to avoid any unaesthetic folds. The skin incisions are then sutured with absorbable stitches. At the end of the procedure, passive flexion of fingers is used to verify that there is no more rotation and that all fingertips converge in flexion towards the tubercle of the scaphoid (Fig. 11.7d). An occlusive bandage is left for 2 or 3 weeks in cases in which we have done an osteotomy. K-wires on the base of the metacarpal bones can be removed if radiographs confirm bone healing. After release of the first bandage, we leave the fingers free to move but strongly recommend a transverse bandage, with an elastic tape or a self-cohesive bandage, at the metacarpal heads level for another 3 weeks to protect the closure of the intermetacarpal space. For most cases, physiotherapy is not necessary as we have allowed motion from the second or third week onwards.

When all these steps are fulfilled, it is advisable that the result remains stable during growth. This harmonious four-fingered hand is hardly noticed by relatives and friends. This agreeable reconstruction significantly reduces the psychological impact of the congenital morphological condition on the child in the difficult time of childhood and adolescence.

11.9.2 Complex Forms

For complex cases with syndactyly of the first web, there are two options according to the severity of the narrowing of the web. If the syndactyly is proximal and loose, it can be released with any appropriate flap (Z plasty or combined Z plasties or a rotation-transposition flap) in association with closure of the cleft, as described above. For severe narrowing, the rule is to transpose the second ray onto the third metacarpal bone (if present). It is necessary to resect the distal two-thirds of the third metacarpal and to transfer the second metacarpal and the index on the base of the third metacarpal (as an on-top plasty) after performing a microsurgical dissection of the pedicles of the index. Osteosynthesis is usually performed with two oblique K-wires at the base and sometimes by transverse pins joining the second and fourth metacarpals. We no longer use a Snow-Littler procedure [29] owing to the poor viability of the palmar flap [30]. We have routinely performed the Miura and Komada technique [31], with satisfactory results (Fig. 11.8a, b), and our preference is now for the technique as described by Upton [32], through a distal approach to allow a limited dorsal scar. We usually try to avoid any dorsal incision since the dorsum of the hand is the part of the hand most often seen by others and by the patient himself (Fig. 11.9).

With this technique, we obtain both functional and natural hands and results which are stable with growth.

The exploration of the cleft is the same as in the simple closure and, before the translocation, it is necessary to remove all the supernumerary elements to keep only the normal elements and ensure a natural function to the future hand. In the case of a transverse bone, we would remove it partially, leaving parts of it in continuity with the metacarpal joints, in order to avoid damage to the collateral ligaments, instability or stiffness.

It is necessary, in certain cases, to correct the clinodactylies of the fingers and in particular to identify ‘delta’ phalanges which are frequent in the SHFM. This is often difficult on X-rays of very young children. If the delta phalanx is confirmed radiologically or, better, by ultrasound, we can propose, before the age of 7 years, Vickers procedure. This procedure consists in removing part of the C-shaped bracketed epiphysis, after resecting an epiphyseal triangle and lateral

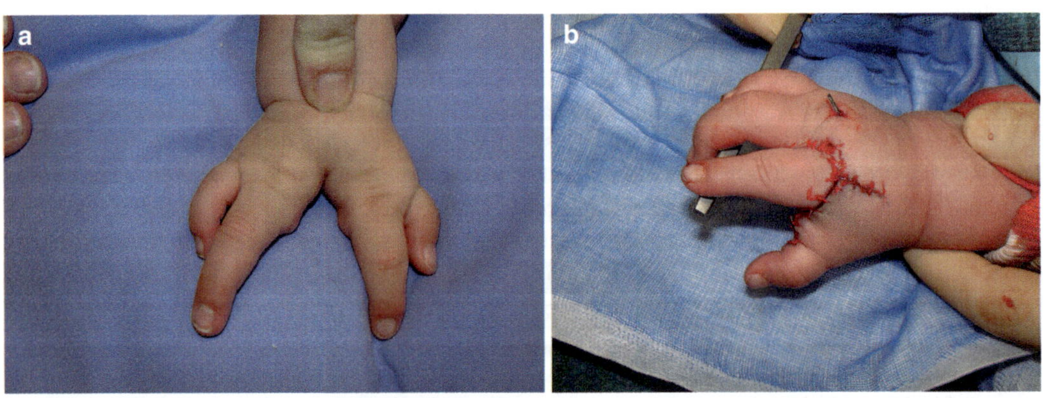

Fig. 11.8 Complex SHFM type 7. Miura’s procedure. (**a**) Pre-operative view. Deep central cleft and syndactyly of the first web. (**b**) Per-operative view after index transposition. Good opening of the first web and well-balanced cosmetic appearance of the hand

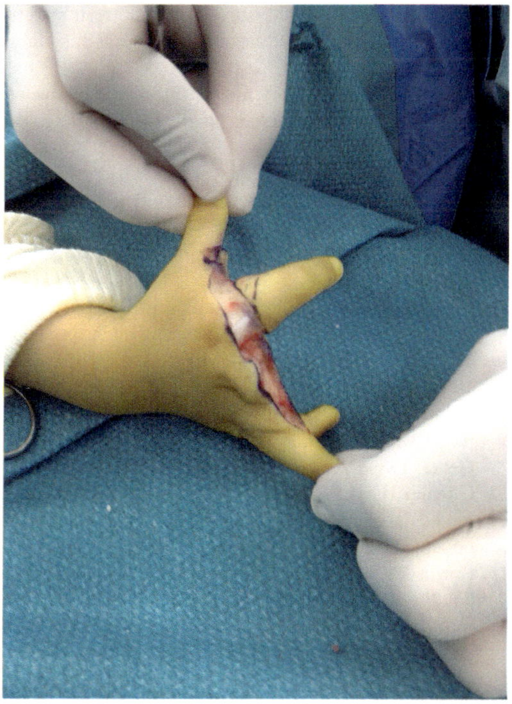

Fig. 11.9 Upton's approach for index transposition and closure of the web. This distal incision gives an excellent view on the cleft, the first web and avoid the dorsal scar

growth cartilage to the diaphyseal cancellous bone, a small amount of fatty tissue is interposed. This pearl prevents a re-ossification of the bracketed epiphysis. The locker is then released on the proximal and distal physeal plate. A spontaneous correction of the deviation is observed after a few years [33]. If the child is too old, a reverse osteotomy can be proposed by taking a bone triangle on the base of the triangular phalanx. The graft is returned and placed in the apex of the phalanx delta. This technique avoids the shortening created by a closing wedge osteotomy.

11.9.3 Severe Types

For severe forms with three, two or a finger, surgical indications are discussed with the parents and, if possible, with the child. It is sometimes useful to do nothing to avoid compromising the function. In particular, closing cleft at all costs could, on the contrary, limit the possibilities of grip. Sometimes we just 'simplify' some rays to reduce the monstrous nature of the hand and possibly facilitate prosthetic equipment for social life. A toe transfer would be a good option, but feet are usually abnormal. We used this procedure in two children with a monodactylous hand and bidactylous feet. Harvesting the hallux was much more difficult than in normal feet. The vascular network was difficult to divide despite the pre-operative angio-CT scan. One child is still painful on the donor site. It is wise to discuss complex malformations on a case-by-case basis with other specialists in congenital hand surgery. For some patients, the best option might be to accept the situation.

11.9.4 Central Clefts of the Feet

Foot treatment deserves attention as well, and much earlier correction than it was traditionally thought. Children are very quickly hampered by the width of the forefoot and painful calluses on the lateral faces of the toes which are found in the plantar position. It is therefore necessary, in the first years, to close the cleft by using staged osteotomies on the metatarsals and phalanges. The principle of closing the cleft is the same as at the level of the hand.

11.10 Conclusions

Median cleft hand is a complex but rare malformation requiring a multidisciplinary management. Genetics input has recently allowed to identify seven SHFM subgroups and provide better insight about associated malformations and inheritance for each type. If an infant is primarily referred to a hand surgeon, a thorough clinical examination should be carried out in order to identify additional malformations and/or a syndromic association. Referrals for genetic counselling and to various specialists might be necessary, such as paediatricians, ophthalmologists, ENT, dermatologists, plastic and orthopaedic surgeons. Function in the cleft hand is impaired because of the anatomical changes but not necessarily compromised, as children adapt very well to most congenital malformations. However, the unusual cosmetic appearance can have a marked psychological impact on patients. Surgical techniques have now allowed to improve the hand aspects and to become 'socially' acceptable. It is also now possible to correct any remaining stiffness by removing additional skeletal structures and to avoid rotation when digits are flexed by modifying the abnormal tendon anatomy. Indeed, even when rays are missing, it is important to bear in mind that the tendons are still formed and present in the cleft as a loop or on the adjacent digits and would need to be addressed for a good functional result. It is therefore important to have a good knowledge of the anatomical particularities for optimal treatment and growth stability.

The very severe malformations will be the subject of discussions between the specialized surgeons and in certain cases the therapeutic abstention will be the most reasonable option.

References

1. Geoffroy Saint Hilaire I. In: Histoire générale et particulière des anomalies de l'organisation chez l'homme et les animaux, J.B. Baillière, editor. Paris; 1832.
2. Maisels DO. Lobster-claw deformities of the hands and feet. Br J Plast Surg. 1970;23(3):269–82.
3. Flatt AE. The care of congenital hand anomalies. 2nd ed. St. Louis: Quality Medical Publishing, Inc; 1994. p. 466.
4. Ekblom AG, Laurell T, Arner M. Epidemiology of congenital upper limb anomalies in Stockholm, Sweden, 1997 to 2007: application of the Oberg, Manske, and Tonkin classification. J Hand Surg Am. 2014;39(2):237–48.
5. Wood VE, Flatt AE. Congenital triangular bones in the hand. J Hand Surg Am. 1977;2(3):179–93.
6. Wood VE. The treatment of crossbones of the hand. Handchir Mikrochir Plast Chir. 2004;36(2–3):161–5.
7. Barsky AJ. Cleft hand: classification, incidence, and treatment. Review of the literature and report of nineteen cases. J Bone Joint Surg Am. 1964;46:1707–20.
8. Blauth W, Gekeler J. Morphology and classification of symbrachydactylia. Handchirurgie. 1971;3(4):123–8.
9. Foucher G, et al. Classification and treatment of symbrachydactyly. A series of 117 cases. Chir Main. 2000;19(3):161–8.
10. Miura T, Suzuki M. Clinical differences between typical and atypical cleft hand. J Hand Surg Br. 1984;9(3):311–5.
11. Maruiwa M, et al. Cornelia de Lange syndrome associated with Wilms' tumour and infantile haemangioendothelioma of the liver: report of two autopsy cases. Virchows Arch A Pathol Anat Histopathol. 1988;413(5):463–8.
12. Pfeiffer RA, Correll J. Hemimelia in Brachmann-de Lange syndrome (BDLS): a patient with severe deficiency of the upper and lower limbs. Am J Med Genet. 1993;47(7):1014–7.
13. Singer LP, Marion RW, Li JK. Limb deficiency in an infant with smith-Lemli-Opitz syndrome. Am J Med Genet. 1989;32(3):380–3.
14. Gurrieri F, Everman DB. Clinical, genetic, and molecular aspects of split-hand/foot malformation: an update. Am J Med Genet A. 2013;161A(11):2860–72.
15. Sowinska-Seidler A, Socha M, Jamsheer A. Split-hand/foot malformation - molecular cause and implications in genetic counseling. J Appl Genet. 2014;55(1):105–15.
16. Guero S, Holder-Espinasse M. Insights into the pathogenesis and treatment of split/hand foot malformation (cleft hand/foot). J Hand Surg Eur. 2019;44(1):80–7.
17. Lo Iacono N, et al. Regulation of Dlx5 and Dlx6 gene expression by p63 is involved in EEC and SHFM congenital limb defects. Development. 2008;135(7):1377–88.
18. Duijf PH, van Bokhoven H, Brunner HG. Pathogenesis of split-hand/split-foot malformation. Hum Mol Genet. 2003;12:R51–60.
19. Naruse T, et al. Early morphological changes leading to central polydactyly, syndactyly, and central deficiencies: an experimental study in rats. J Hand Surg Am. 2007;32(9):1413–7.
20. Swanson AB, Barsky AJ, Entin MA. Classification of limb malformations on the basis of embryological failures. Surg Clin North Am. 1968;48(5):1169–79.
21. Ogino T. Teratogenic relationship between polydactyly, syndactyly and cleft hand. J Hand Surg Br. 1990;15(2):201–9.
22. Oberg KC, et al. Developmental biology and classification of congenital anomalies of the hand and upper extremity. J Hand Surg Am. 2010;35(12):2066–76.
23. Tonkin MA, et al. Classification of congenital anomalies of the hand and upper limb: development and assessment of a new system. J Hand Surg Am. 2013;38(9):1845–53.
24. Glicenstein J, Guero S, Haddad R. Median clefts of the hand. Classification and therapeutic indications apropos of 29 cases. Ann Chir Main Memb Super. 1995;14(6):253.

25. Manske PR, Halikis MN. Surgical classification of central deficiency according to the thumb web. J Hand Surg Am. 1995;20(4):687–97.
26. Durand S, et al. Anatomic variations in a cleft hand of an elder cadaveric specimen. Surg Radiol Anat. 2009;31(2):145–8.
27. Wood VE. Super digit. Hand Clin. 1990;6(4):673–84.
28. Dowd CN, IX. Cleft hand: a report of a case successfully treated by the use of periosteal flaps. Ann Surg. 1896;24(2):210.2–216.
29. Rider MA, et al. An experience of the Snow-Littler procedure. J Hand Surg Br. 2000;25(4):376–81.
30. Oberlin C, et al. Digitalization of the second finger in type 2 central longitudinal deficiencies (clefting) of the hand. Tech Hand Up Extrem Surg. 2009;13(2):110–2.
31. Miura T, Komada T. Simple method for reconstruction of the cleft hand with an adducted thumb. Plast Reconstr Surg. 1979;64(1):65–7.
32. Upton J. Simplicity and treatment of the typical cleft hand. Handchir Mikrochir Plast Chir. 2004;36(2–3):152–60.
33. El Sayed L, et al. Physiolysis for correction of clinodactyly with delta phalanx: early improvement. Hand Surg Rehabil. 2019;38(2):125–8.

12 Brachydactyly Types D and E

Zavarukhin V. Ivanovich

Abstract

The J. Bell's classification describes two types of hand ray shortening, namely, brachydactyly types D and E, which have a lot in common. When a child suffers either of these diseases, he/she is born with a hand that appears to be absolutely healthy, but when he/she is between four and 7 years of age, his/her parents notice the first signs of progressive shortening of one or several fingers. Although these pathologies are differentiated as two brachydactyly types, they are just different manifestations of the same disease with common etiology and pathogenesis, with similar complaints, and with similar surgical-treatment approaches.

Brachydactyly type E is shortening of one or several metacarpals and is also known as brachymetacarpia.

Brachydactyly type D is shortening of distal phalanx in the thumb where the nail plate looks extremely short but wide.

Indications for surgical treatment are mainly cosmetic for brachydactyly type E and are only cosmetic for brachydactyly type D.

The preferred treatment for both types of brachydactyly is distraction lengthening.

Keywords

Brachydactyly · Brachymetacarpia
Lengthening · Distraction · Shortening · Stub thumb

12.1 Introduction

The J. Bell's classification [1, 2] describes two types of hand ray shortening, namely, brachydactyly types D and E, which have a lot in common. When a child suffers either of these diseases, he/she is born with a hand that appears to be absolutely healthy, but when he/she is between 4 and 7 years of age [3–6], his/her parents notice the first signs of progressive shortening of one or several fingers. Although these pathologies are differentiated as two brachydactyly types, they are just different manifestations of the same disease with common etiology and pathogenesis, with similar complaints, and with similar surgical-treatment approaches.

Brachydactyly type E is shortening of one or several metacarpals and is also known as brachymetacarpia.

Brachydactyly type D is shortening of distal phalanx in the thumb where the nail plate looks extremely short but wide [7].

Z. V. Ivanovich (✉)
Candidate of Medical Sciences, Head of the Department of Traumatology N3, St. Petersburg State University Hospital, St Petersburg, Russia

G. Pajardi (ed.), *Pediatric Hand Surgery*, https://doi.org/10.1007/978-3-031-30984-7_12

12.2 Background

Brachydactyly type E (also known as *Brachymetacarpia*) was first described in 1908 when P. Mathew reported a clinical case of "hereditary brachydactyly" for a 31-year-old female patient who experienced shortening of the third, fourth, and fifth metacarpals on both hands [8]. C.P. Gillette was the first who reported in his article in 1931 that a child with brachymetacarpia was born with normal hands, and no progressive ray shortening was observed until adolescence. He has described a clinical case of inherited third-metacarpal shortening on both hands. All family members affected had no signs of such deformation until the age of seven [9]. Only in 1969 surgeons paid closer attention to this disease, and the first publication appeared regarding metacarpal lengthening based on osteotomy and bone grafting [10].

The first reports on *brachydactyly type D* appeared back in the 1920s [11, 12]. However, we have not found any description for surgical treatment of this pathology.

12.3 Epidemiology and Classification

When describing *brachydactyly type E*, almost all authors point out that this pathology is very rare [4, 6] with an occurrence rate under 1 out of 1000 [5, 13] which can probably explain why there are so few publications about brachymetacarpia and even less about its surgical treatment. According to many authors [3, 14, 15], metacarpal shortening is more common among girls, and, according to different data, the ratio between male and female patients varies between 1:5 [5, 13] and 1:25 [16]. Most authors emphasize that the fourth metacarpal is the most prone to this disorder [3–5, 13]. Moreover, some authors report that shortening can affect phalanxes of any fingers at random and in any combination in addition to metacarpals [17]. However, the distal phalanx of the thumb (brachydactyly type D) is the most common target for shortening.

Similar changes can occur on feet and are known as brachymetatarsia or metatarsal shortening [3, 18, 19]. The combined brachymetacarpia and brachymetatarsia occurrence rate is at least 1:1000 [5].

As to the isolated occurrence rate, *brachydactyly type D* is a rather common disease with an occurrence rate between 0.41 and 4% in the population [2].

The J. Bell's classification differentiates brachydactyly type E from type D; in addition to it, we have found only a brachydactyly type E classification suggested by Hertzog [20]. He differentiates three kinds of brachydactyly type E [20]. However, such classification does not account for all possible forms of this pathology. We have examined 53 patients and suggested a classification for brachydactyly type E (brachymetacarpia) which also includes related damages to hand ray phalanxes [21].

Brachymetacarpia classification:

1. Isolated forms:
   (a) Mono-osseous forms
   (b) Polyosseous forms
2. Combined forms accompanied by brachydactyly:
   (a) With distal-phalanx shortening of the thumb (type D).
   (b) With phalanx shortening of three-phalanx fingers.

Examination of patients has allowed us to determine the occurrence rate for various anatomy-based brachymetacarpia forms (Table 12.1).

We have established that the most common form of metacarpal brachymetacarpia is the mono-osseous one (72% of all cases). Its most common manifestations are shortening of the fourth metacarpal (50%), fifth metacarpal (18.3%), and combined shortening of the fourth and fifth metacarpals (12.2%). When examining the occurrence rate for individual metacarpals, we have found that the fourth metacarpal is affected more frequently (56.8%).

Among combined brachydactyly forms, the highest occurrence rate was associated with distal-phalanx shortening of the thumb (brachydactyly type D) which is 28.3%. The isolated

Table 12.1 Occurrence rate for various brachymetacarpia forms

Brachymetacarpia forms	Occurrence rate	
	Cases	%
Mono-osseous forms		
Isolated shortening of the third metacarpal	3	3.7
Isolated shortening of the fourth metacarpal	41	50.0
Isolated shortening of the fifth metacarpal	15	18.3
Total	59	72
Polyosseous forms		
Combined shortening of the first and fourth metacarpals	2	2.4
Combined shortening of third and fourth metacarpals	4	4.9
Combined shortening of the third and fifth metacarpals	1	1.2
Combined shortening of the fourth and fifth metacarpals	10	12.2
Combined shortening of the third, fourth, and fifth metacarpals	6	7.3
Total	23	28
Combined forms accompanied by brachydactyly		
With distal-phalanx shortening of the thumb	22	26.8
With phalanx shortening of three-phalanx fingers	12	14.6
Total number of hands affected by brachymetacarpia:	82	100.0

form of this disorder occurred on the contralateral hand (2.4% of all cases) and was not accompanied by metacarpal shortening. Combined forms (brachymetacarpia accompanied by some type of brachydactyly) were more common for polyosseous forms (56.5%).

12.4 Etiology

A number of hypotheses have been proposed to explain why one or several fingers become shorter in several years even if the child was born with absolutely healthy hands; their authors agree that the metacarpal or phalanxes affected have a progressive-shortening mechanism which is connected with early epiphyseal growth-plate closure [3–6]. Medical observations were made for children with a family history of this disease; their results have shown that the first pathology signs can be seen on X-ray films as early as at the age of two while closed growth areas can be observed by the age of four, which indicates that the bones affected keep growing after the birth, and the growth area becomes closed just in several years after birth [22]. At the moment, most authors tend to believe that early closure of the growth area is caused by an impaired mechanism of interaction between the parathyroid hormone and its receptor [23].

12.5 Clinical Presentation and Indications

Brachydactyly type E results in changes that make the patient come to the doctor; most of them can be seen with the naked eye. At that time, patients notice an abnormal shape of their straight hand when looking at the line formed by its finger tips (Fig. 12.1). Metacarpal shortening is the most obvious when the head of the metacarpal bone is pulled in (it is supposed to protrude when metacarpal joints are bent) (Fig. 12.2).

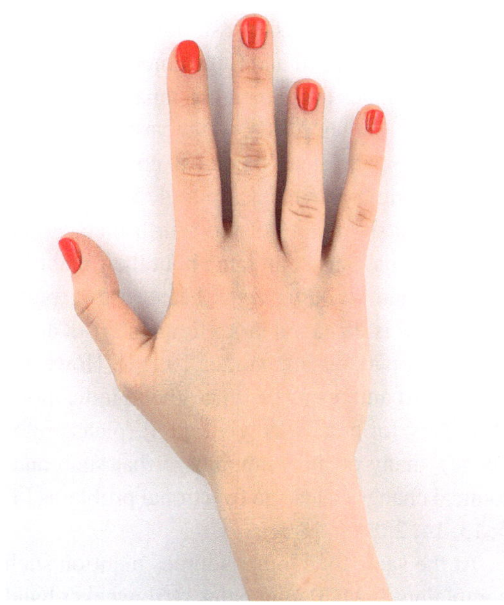

Fig. 12.1 Brachydactyly type E with shortening of the fourth metacarpal

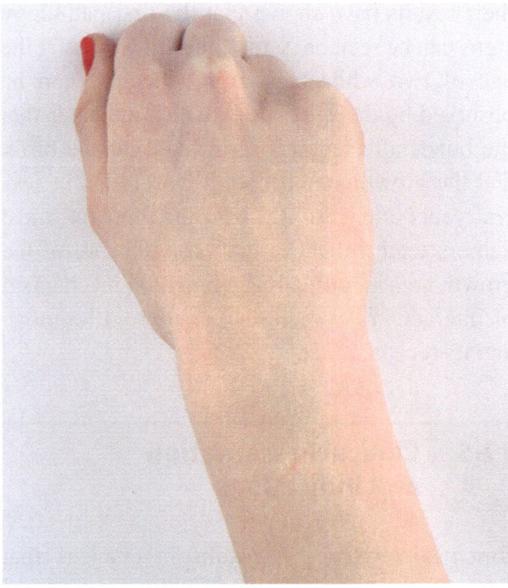

Fig. 12.2 Brachydactyly type E, the head of the fourth metacarpal bone is pulled in

S. Temptamy and M. Aglan describe the following clinical test for shortening of the fourth metacarpal: When the hand forms a fist, and a pencil touches the protruding areas of the third and fourth metacarpals, it does not touch the head of the fourth, shortened metacarpal (Fig. 12.3). It is also a sign which the authors suggest to look for on X-ray films by drawing a straight line between the heads of the third and fourth metacarpals [2].

Such changes make patients unhappy with the appearance of their hands, so the vast majority of authors describe it as the most common complaint during brachymetacarpia [4, 5, 13–15, 24, 25]. If it is shortening of the fourth metacarpal, then many patients complain about their inability to wear their wedding rings because the fourth metacarpal is damaged more frequently; in addition, most patients are women [6, 13]. However, while most authors agree on aesthetic indications to surgery for brachydactyly type E (please refer above), many of them emphasize that such anatomical changes cause no functional problems [4, 5, 13, 14, 25].

At the same time, other sources mention such complaints as MCP joint pains [15], weaker hand grip [4], or limited flexion in MCP joints [3, 6, 24, 26].

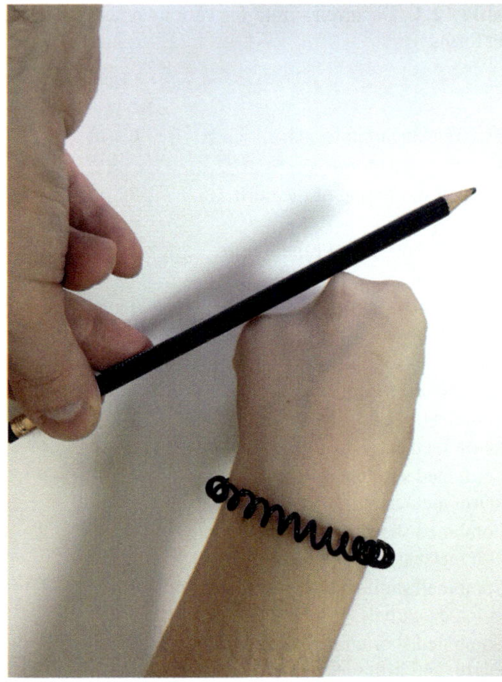

Fig. 12.3 Brachydactyly type E, "pencil test" demonstrating shortening of the fourth metacarpal

For our group of 53 patients, we found that all of them were unhappy with the appearance of their hand; it was also the most common complaint. When such complaints were analyzed according to the Visual Analog Scale, it was found that the patients were unhappy with their hand appearance the most when it was caused by shortening of the third, fourth, or both third and fifth metacarpals. We have found that mono-osseous forms are the ones which result in the bitterest complaints about the hand appearance.

In 28% of all cases, there were complaints when certain types of load were applied. It was the most common complaint among patients with shortening of the fourth metacarpal (62.8%); this symptom was also frequently observed for shortening of the fifth metacarpal (33.3%). In addition, it was found that this symptom is more common for mono-osseous forms of this disease.

Rapid fatigue was observed for polyosseous forms more often than for mono-osseous ones (57.1 vs. 18.0%).

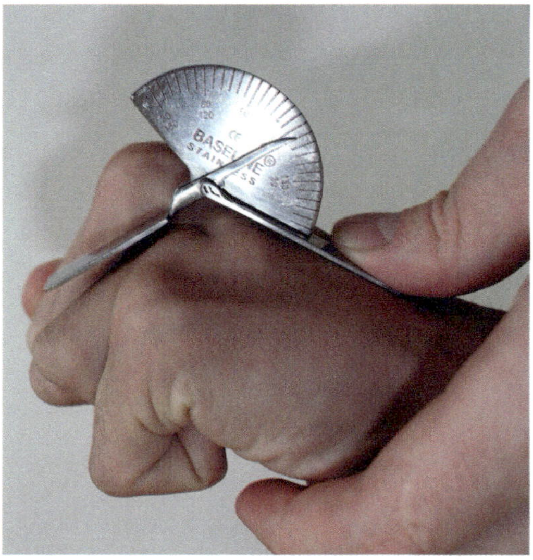

Fig. 12.4 Brachydactyly type E, limitation of fourth MCP flexion

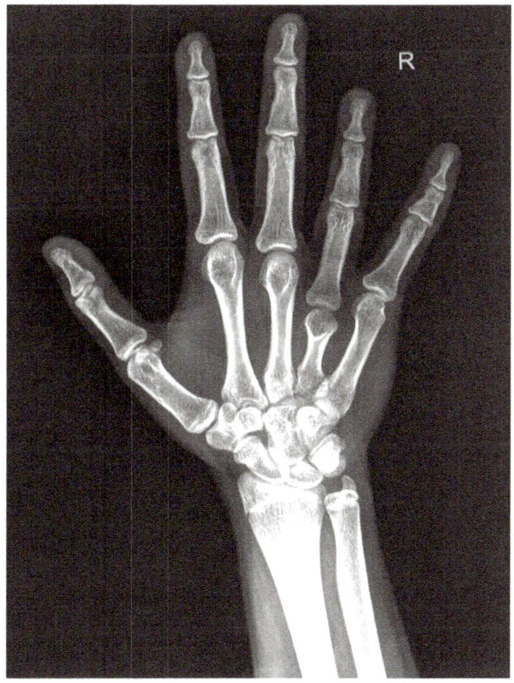

Fig. 12.5 Brachydactyly type E, X-ray of the hand with shortening of the fourth metacarpal

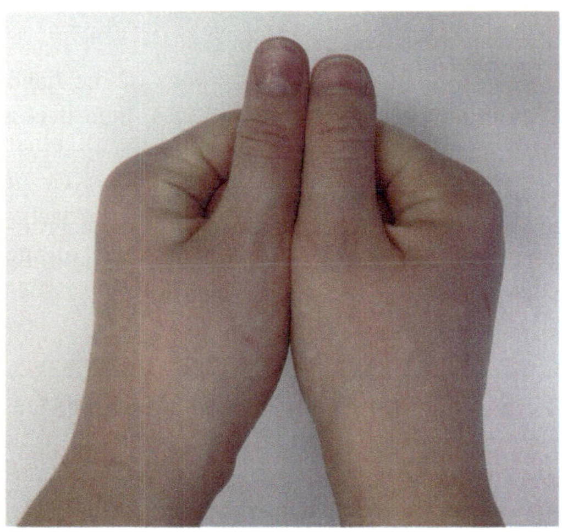

Fig. 12.6 Brachydactyly type D with shortening of the distal phalanx of the right thumb. The nail plate looks wider and shorter than on the left side

In addition, 12.9% all patients had special complaints related to problems with special types of motor activities such as playing musical instruments.

All patients exhibited a limited motion range for the MCP joints in the ray affected (Fig. 12.4); it was caused by flexion limitations which, on an average, were about 120° (it is a 30-degree limitation as compared to the physiological standard).

Hand-grip measurements have shown that 57.1% of all patients with brachymetacarpia have lower results for affected hands. It has been also noticed that the hand grip tends to be significantly weaker among patients with polyosseous forms of brachymetacarpia.

The X-ray analysis has shown that the average shortening was 15.3 mm for patients older than 10 years; it is more than 25% (or 10 mm) of the estimated metacarpal length (Fig. 12.5).

For *brachydactyly type D*, shorter and wider distal phalanxes of the thumbs result in complaints about the thumb appearance only, which is coined in such unpleasant slang expressions as stub thumb, shovel thumb, Dutch thumb, hammer thumb, potter's thumb, and even murderer's thumb (Fig. 12.6). Sometimes, nail plates look like a ski jump due to distal-phalanx deformation; therefore, it was first described as "standing nail deformity" [7]. The distal-phalanx shortening is between 6 mm and 10 mm for brachydactyly type D or between 30 and 50% of the normal phalanx length (Fig. 12.7).

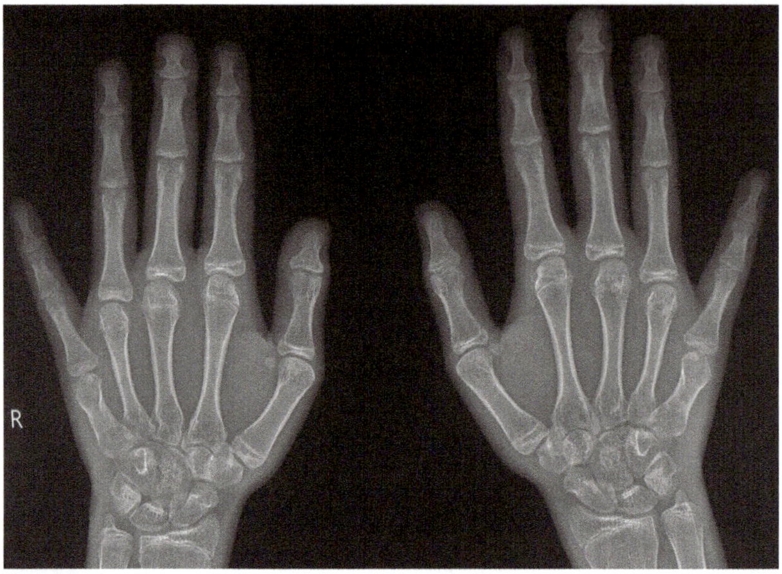

Fig. 12.7 Brachydactyly type D and E on the X-ray with shortening of the distal phalanxes of the right thumb and both middle fingers, shortening of the fifth metacarpals

We believe that any brachydactyly type E is an absolute indication to surgical treatment if there are function-related complaints.

Relative (aesthetic) indications to surgical treatment are either any form of brachydactyly type E when there are no function-related complaints or brachydactyly type D.

We decided that if other bones of the hand contain any unclosed growth plates, then it is a contraindication to treatment (except general surgical ones) because the continuing growth of unaffected bones does not allow us to predict reliably how much the bone affected should be lengthened.

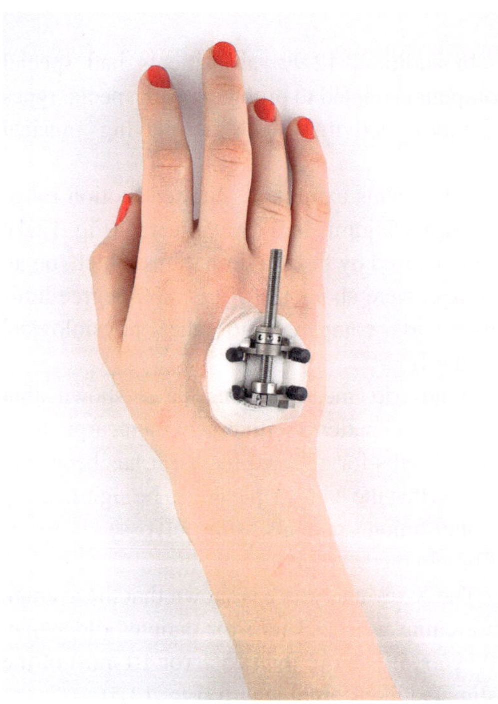

Fig. 12.8 Brachydactyly type E with shortening of the fourth metacarpal during the lengthening with external distractor placed on the dorsal side of the hand

12.6 Surgery Technique (Author's Preferred Method)

12.6.1 Brachydactyly Type E

We employ the Ilizarov method and use our patented distractor (Russian patent No. 2508063 of October 31, 2011) to restore the metacarpal length during brachymetacarpia. The distractor should be placed on the dorsal side of the hand (Fig. 12.8); no pins may run through the palmar surface of the hand or through the finger extensor mechanism. It is better to do osteotomy in the proximal part of the metacarpal. We perform osteotomy in a closed manner under C-Arm control (Fig. 12.9). There is no need to use a wire to immobilize finger joints or fix the joints in the distractor during distraction or to immobilize it otherwise (Fig. 12.10). On the contrary, when active or passive exercises are made in joints of the ray extended, it prevents lengthen-

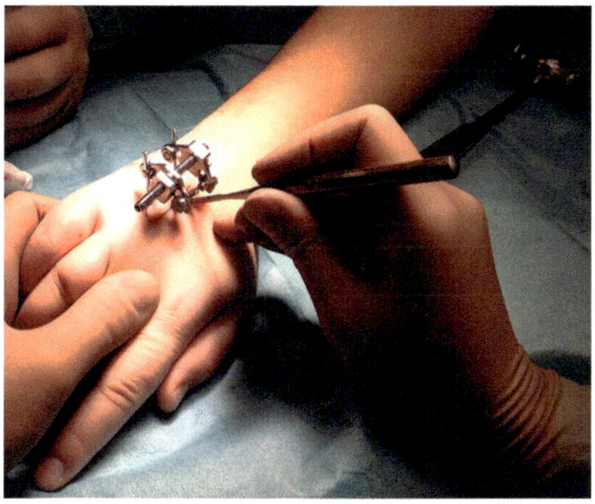

Fig. 12.9 Brachydactyly type E with shortening of the fourth metacarpal. "Close" osteotomy with 2 mm osteotome

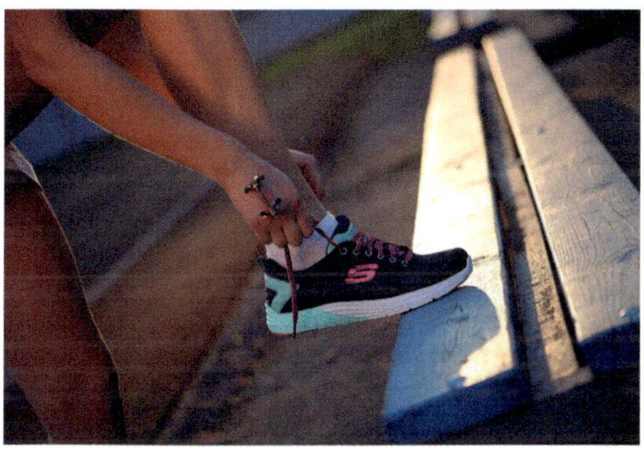

Fig. 12.10 Brachydactyly type E with shortening of the fourth metacarpal during the lengthening with external distractor without any immobilization

ing-induced stiffness. The distraction starts in 7 up to 10 days with an initial rate between 0.75 mm and 1 mm per day and is divided into three or four phases; later on, the distraction rate can be adjusted according to the X-ray results. The osteosynthesis index was 91.1 ± 10.6 day/cm in our group. The average fixation index was 64.0 ± 10.2 day/cm.

12.6.2 Brachydactyly Type D

We have not found any description of surgical treatments for brachydactyly type D in the available literature. So, for brachydactyly type D, we also apply the distraction-lengthening technique to restore an aesthetic appearance of the finger. A tiny distractor is used for these purposes (Fig. 12.11); one of its benefits is that there is no need to run pins by segments because a short distal phalanx does not allow to use monolateral distractors. The pins start on the palmar surface, and special care should be taken to prevent the nail bed from damaging when running the pins through the dorsal cortical plate. It is a closed osteotomy procedure, and it is critical not to damage the nail matrix (Fig. 12.12). Our distraction rate is 0.5 mm per day. The total lengthening value depends on changes in the finger appearance and is, on an average, between 8 mm and 10 mm.

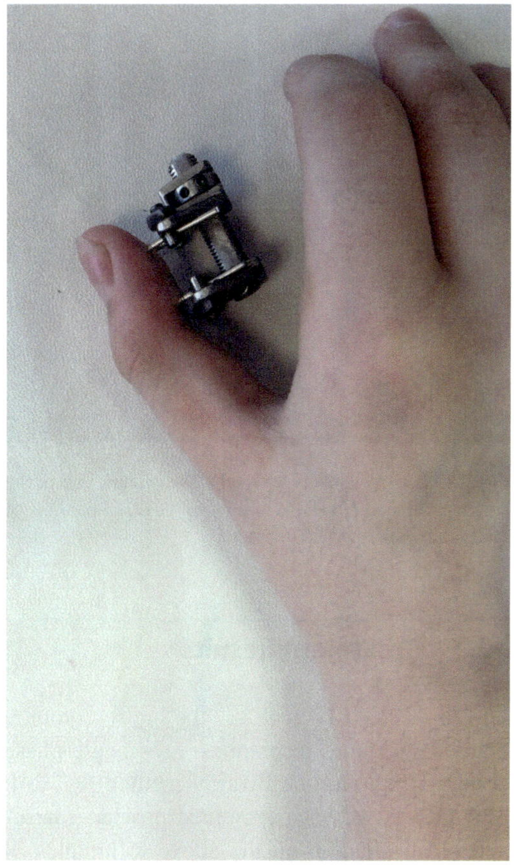

Fig. 12.11 Brachydactyly type D with shortening of the distal phalanx of the thumb during the lengthening with external distractor

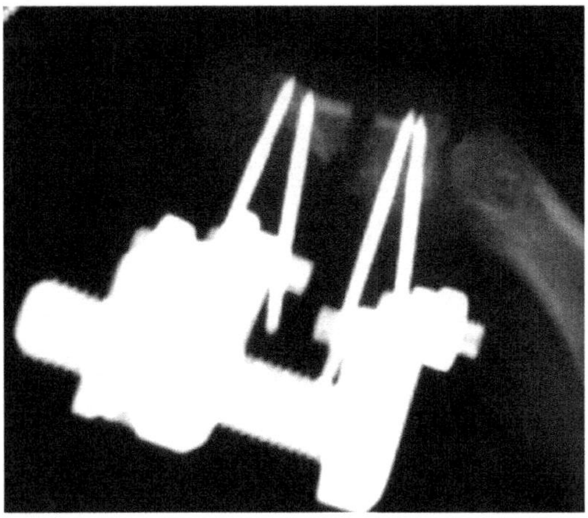

Fig. 12.12 Brachydactyly type D. X-ray at the end of the surgery with completed osteotomy of the distal phalanx of the thumb with external distractor

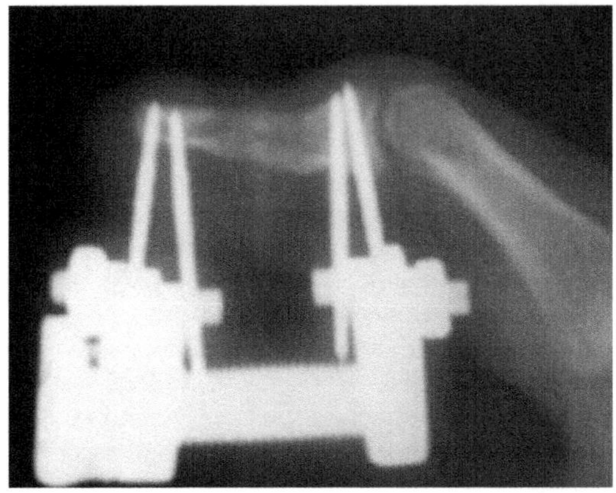

Fig. 12.13 Brachydactyly type D with callus formation after distraction lengthening

12.7 Treatment Results

For *brachydactyly type E*, the most common bone-lengthening techniques are single-phase bone grafting and the Ilizarov method [17, 26]. The sources we have examined provide controversial information on the above techniques as method of choice for surgical treatment of brachymetacarpia.

Therefore, we have conducted a prospective cohort study for 12 patients treated by applying the Ilizarov method and a retrospective cohort study for 13 patients treated by employing the bone-grafting method to compare treatment results.

In case of brachymetacarpia, the direct objective of surgical treatment is to restore the length of the metacarpal shortened. The Ilizarov's distraction osteosynthesis method was applied in the main experimental group and allowed to completely restore shortened metacarpal bones to an anatomic length in 100% of cases due to controllability during the entire treatment period; the anatomic length was calculated according to A. Aydinlioglu et al. [27] with an accuracy of 1 mm (Fig. 12.13). When X-ray film archives were examined for patients who had undergone surgery according to the single-phase bone-grafting method, it was found that there was no single case where anatomic metacarpal length was restored completely and that, on an average, the third, fourth, and fifth metacarpals were 4.66 mm up to 5.56 mm shorter (between 8.37 and 11.68%) than the estimated anatomical length after the surgery (Fig. 12.14). It correlates

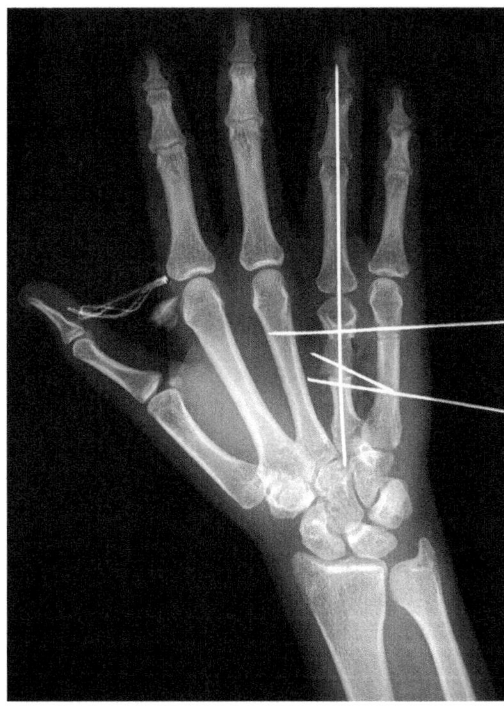

Fig. 12.14 Brachydactyly type E with shortening of the fourth metacarpal. X-ray after treatment by single-phase bone grafting. The shortening of the fourth metacarpal is preserved

with data reported by other authors and indicates that the metacarpal lengthening cannot exceed 10 mm in a single-phase process, which is insufficient in case of brachymetacarpia where the average shortening value varies between 15 mm and 18 mm [3, 4, 14, 17, 26].

When a long-term treatment outcome was evaluated for patients with brachymetacarpia treated by applying the distraction lengthening and single-phase bone-grafting methods, significant differences between study groups were found for most parameters.

For instance, although both techniques have improved the hand appearance according to patients' reports, the complaint analysis has proven that the distraction osteosynthesis technique allowed the surgical treatment to achieve better aesthetic, statistically significant results (Fig. 12.15).

When function-related complaints were analyzed, even a bigger difference was found between the study groups. When the distraction osteosynthesis method was applied during the surgical treatment, statistically significant improvements were observed: a lower occurrence rate and intensity of load-induced pain, longer periods without fatigue or some other specific complaints. On the contrary, when the single-phase bone-grafting method was employed, patients made more such function-related complaints as smaller hand force and rapid fatigue in the hand operated. In the control group, 76.7% patients complained about limited movements in joints operated and, sometimes, in adjacent rays although no patient had brought such complaints before the treatment.

Objective long-term studies have been conducted for patients after distraction lengthening; they have shown statistically significant increase in active-movement range for the MCP rays operated which has resulted from the flexion increase (Fig. 12.16). On the contrary, a double decrease in the movement range was observed in the group of patients after bone grafting both due to decrease in the active-flexion angle and due to extension (Fig. 12.17).

Hand-grip measurements have also shown a statistically significant reduction in the number of patients whose hand-grip force has become smaller after the surgery; their percentage has decreased from 75% down to 15.8% of the total number of patients in the group. In the control group, 78.9% of patients had a hand grip below the developmental norm for their age after the bone-grafting surgery.

Long-term X-ray studies have found no secondary changes in the osteoarticular structure of the hands after distraction lengthening. In the control group, 10% of patients had secondary deformations of the metacarpal lengthened, and 40% had a shorter length as compared to the one on the X-ray films made right after the surgery; it means that there are changes in the autogenous bone during its rearrangement and that it is hard to predict the surgical-treatment results when a single-phase bone-grafting method is employed.

After surgical treatment of *brachydactyly type D*, all patients have reported about improvements in the appearance of the finger operated and in its nail shape and length (Fig. 12.18). Although nail-plate deformation was observed in four out of ten cases upon the distraction-phase completion, it has disappeared in three cases within 2 or 3 months. In addition, one female patient had a moderate distal-phalanx angulation.

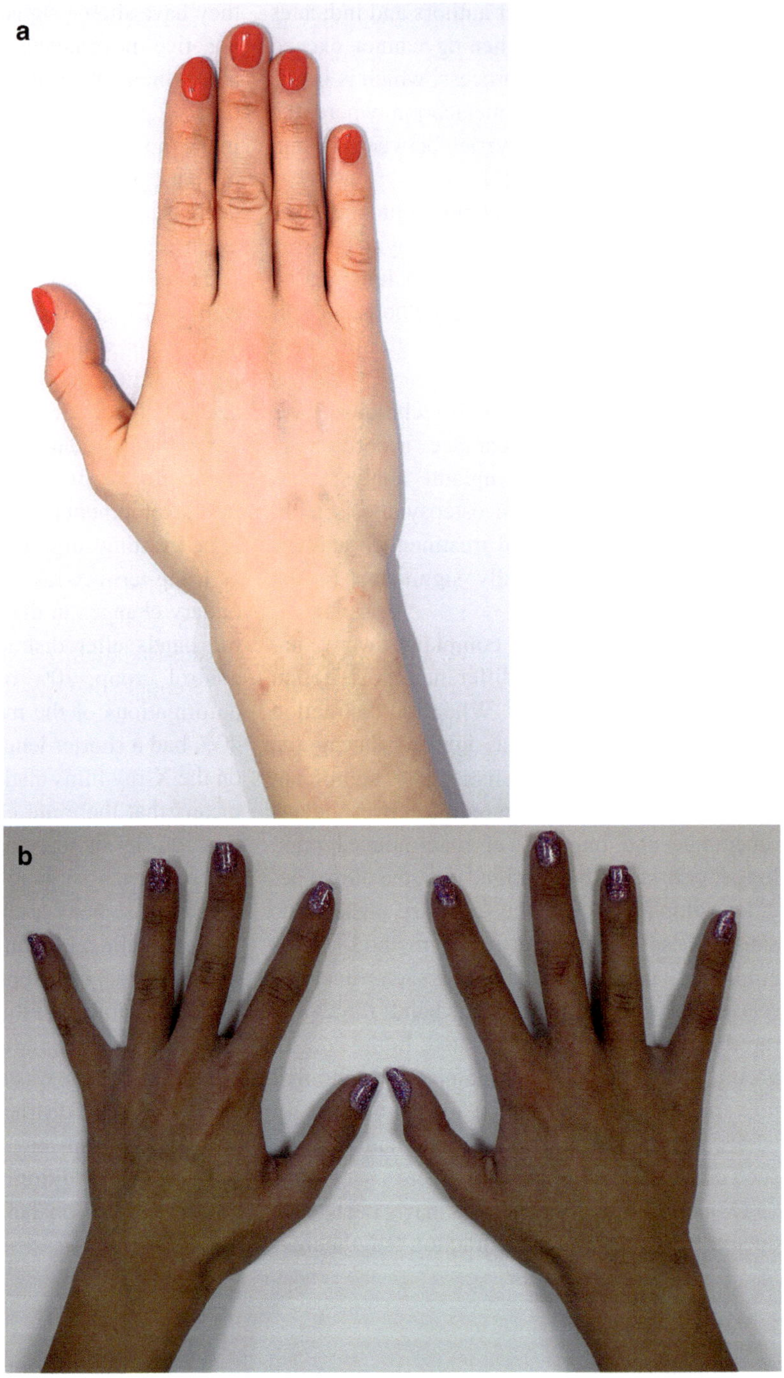

Fig. 12.15 Brachydactyly type E with shortening of the fourth metacarpal after treatment: (**a**) by distraction lengthening. The shortening of the fourth metacarpal is completely reduced, (**b**) by single-phase bone grafting. The shortening of the fourth metacarpal is preserved

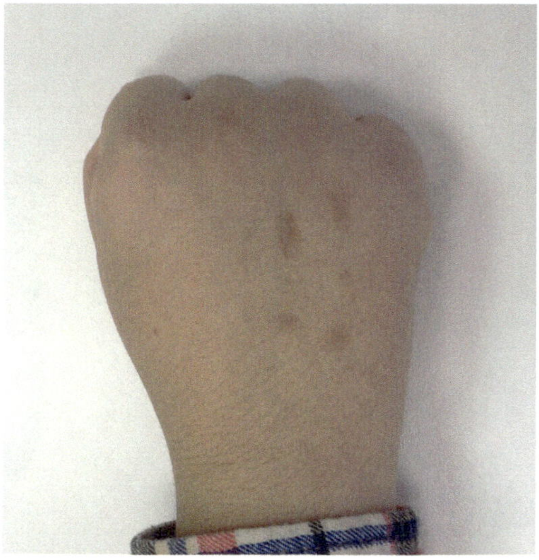

Fig. 12.16 Brachydactyly type E with shortening of the fourth metacarpal after treatment by distraction lengthening. Full flexion in MCP

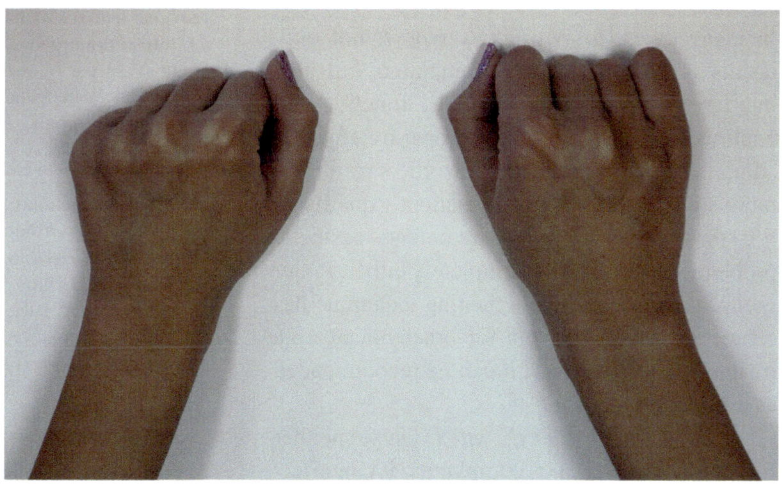

Fig. 12.17 Brachydactyly type E with shortening of the fourth metacarpal after treatment by single-phase bone grafting. The limitation of flexion in the fourth and allied MCP has been observed

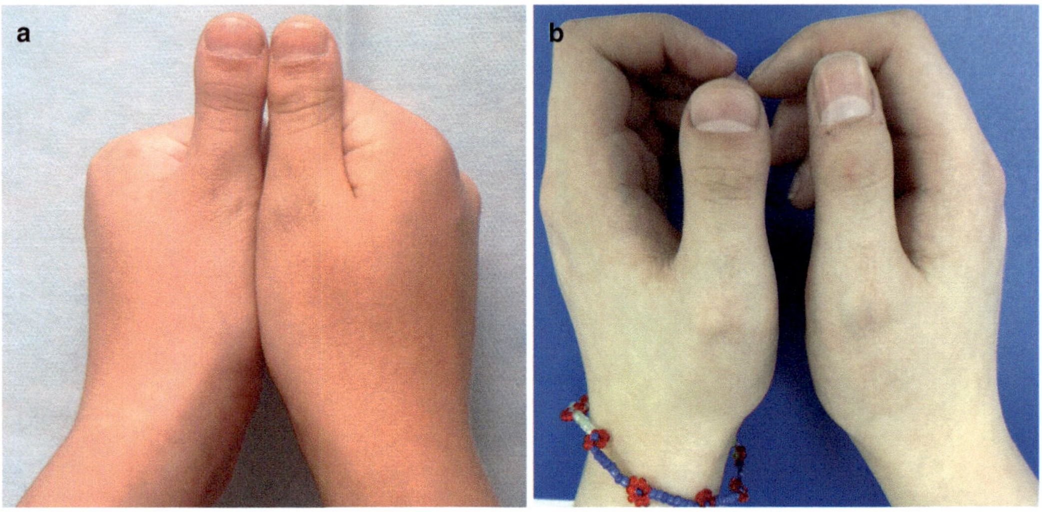

Fig. 12.18 Brachydactyly type D: (**a**) with shortening of the distal phalanxes of the thumb on both hands, (**b**) after distraction lengthening of the distal phalanx of the right thumb

12.8 Conclusion

In many cases, *brachydactyly type E* not only results in aesthetic-related complaints but also interferes with the patients' hand function and quality of life. However, if improper treatment is administered, then functional disorders result in a more significant reduction of patient's qualify of life than before surgical treatment; aesthetic problems are not solved completely either. In our group, the distraction-lengthening technique has clearly shown its benefits for brachymetacarpia treatment and, therefore, it can be recommended as a method of choice.

Although *brachydactyly type D* causes neither functional disorders nor complaints, it can affect patients' quality of life if there are high requirements for hand appearance. This deformation can be also treated successfully by employing the technique described herein.

References

1. Bell J. On brachydactyly and symphalangism. In: Pensore LS, editor. Treasury of human inheritance, vol. 5. London: Cambridge University Press; 1951. p. 1–31.
2. Temtamy S, Aglan M. Brachydactyly, Orphan J Rare Dis. 2008;3(15):1–16. https://doi.org/10.1186/1750-1172-3-15.
3. Bozan M, Altinel L, Kuru I, et al. Factors that affect the healing index of metacarpal lengthening: a retrospective study. J Orthop Surg. 2006;14(2):167–71. https://doi.org/10.1177/230949900601400212.
4. Bulut M, Ucar Y, Azboy I, et al. Lengthening by distraction osteogenesis in congenital shortening of metacarpals. Acta Orthop Traumatol Turc. 2013;47(2):79–85.
5. Erdem M, Sen C, Eralp L, et al. Lengthening of short bones by distraction osteogenesis – results and complications. Int Orthop. 2009;33(3):807–13. https://doi.org/10.1007/s00264-007-0491-x.
6. Southgate G, Holms W. Metacarpal lengthening. J Hand Surg. 1985;10B:391–2.
7. Okazaki M, Shiokawa I, Sasaki K et all. Standing nail deformity of the great toes with multiple brachymetacarpia and brachyphalangia of the hand. J Plast Surg Hand Surg 2010; 44: 4–5: 260–264. doi:https://doi.org/10.3109/02844311003679646.
8. Mathew PW. A case of hereditary brachydactyly. Br Med J. 1908;2:969.
9. Gillette CP. An inheritable defect of the human hand. J Hered. 1931;22:189–90.
10. Mansoor IA. Metacarpal lengthening: a case report. J Bone Joint Surg. 1947;51(8):1630–40.
11. Breitenbecher JK. Hereditary shortness of thumbs. J Hered. 1923;14:15–21.
12. Thomsen O. Hereditary growth anomaly of the thumb. Hereditas. 1928;10:261–73.
13. Volpi A, Fragomen A. Percutaneous distraction lengthening in brachymetacarpia. Orthopedics. 2001;34(8):424–7. https://doi.org/10.3928/01477447-20110627-29.
14. Arslan H. Metacarpal lengthening by distraction osteogenesis in childhood brachydactyly. Acta Orthop Belg. 2001;67(3):242–7.

15. Kawoosa AA, Nasir A, Dhar SA, et al. Metacarpal lengthening by distraction osteogenesis. JK-Practitioner. 2004;11(1):32–4.
16. Davidson RS. Metatarsal lengthening. Foot Ankle Clin. 2001;6:499–518.
17. Ogino T. Brachydactyly. In: Buck-Gramcko D, editor. Congenital malformation of the hand and forearm. London: Churchill Livingstone; 1998. p. 331–4.
18. Ridgeway S, Tai C, Singh D. A case report of brachydactyly types D and E: a new variation of brachydactyly. Foot Ankle Int. 2004;25(6):419–22. https://doi.org/10.1177/107110070402500610.
19. Shim J, Park S. Treatment of brachymetatarsia by distraction osteogenesis. J Pediatr Orthop. 2006;26(2):250–4. https://doi.org/10.1097/01.bpo.0000214922.18186.06.
20. Hertzog KP. Brachydactyly and pseudopseudohypoparathyroidism. Acta Genet Med Gemellol. 1968;17:428–38.
21. Zavarukhin VI. Korrektsiya dliny lucha kisti u detey pri brakhimetakarpii. Kand, Diss. [Correction of the length of finger rays in case of brachymethacarpia in children. Cand. Diss.]. Saint-Petersburg. 2017; 203.
22. Nagasaki K, Asami T, Kikuchi T, et al. Longitudinal growth of the short bones of the hand in a girl with pseudohypoparathyroidism type Ia. Clin Pediatr Endocrinol. 2007;16(1):23–9. https://doi.org/10.1297/cpe.16.23.
23. Mundlos S, Horn D, Limb malformation. An atlas of genetic disorders of Limb development. Berlin, Heidelberg: Springer; 2014. https://doi.org/10.1007/978-3-540-95928-1.
24. Saito H, Koizumi M, Takahashi Y, et al. One-stage elongation of the third or fourth brachymetacarpia through the palmar approach. J Hand Surg. 2001;26:518–24. https://doi.org/10.1053/jhsu.2001.22527.
25. Suresh S, Abraham R, Ravi P. Isolated symmetrical brachymetacarpia of the thumb – case report. Hand. 2009;4:424–6. https://doi.org/10.1007/s11552-009-9185-8.
26. Kato H, Minami A, Suenaga N. Callotasis lengthening in patients with brachymetacarpia. J Pediatr Orthop. 2002;22(4):497–500.
27. Aydinlioglu A, Akpinar F, Tosun N. Mathematical relations between the lengths of the metacarpal bones and phalanges: surgical significance. Tohoku J Exp Med. 1998;185(3):209–16.

13 Surgical Management of the Blauth 1 to 3A Thumb Hypoplasia

Stéphane Guéro

Abstract

Thumb Hypoplasia is a sequence of congenital abnormalities, from minor hypoplastic thumb with a preserved function to complete thumb aplasia. We only discuss in this chapter the management of the Thumb Hypoplasia type 1 to 3A according to the modified Blauth's classification. Their common feature is the conservative treatment, in opposition with severe hypoplastic thumbs usually treated by index pollicization. Whatever is the degree of hypoplasia, patients should be carefully examined for bilaterality, other anomalies and syndrome. Surgical treatment, when indicated, requires systematically widening of the first web space, stabilization of the metacarpophalangeal joint and restoration of opposition and extension. Reconstruction of the infant thumb should be started in the first year of life. Functional result depends on the degree of hypoplasia and differs dramatically whether if the thumb hypoplasia is isolated or associated with a radial club hand.

S. Guéro (✉)
Institut de la Main, Paris, France

Paediatric Orthopaedic Unit, Hôpital Necker Enfants Malades, Université Paris V René Descartes, Paris, France
e-mail: sguero@me.com

Keywords

Thumb · Child · Hypoplasia · Congenital abnormality · Tendon transfer

13.1 Introduction

Thumb hypoplasia is relatively frequent congenital malformations that associate various degrees of cutaneous, bone, tendon, joint and ligament abnormalities. They can be isolated or associated with regional malformations such as longitudinal radial aplasia or radial club hands (RCH). They can be part of many syndromes of which they sometimes represent the only visible part. We will therefore immediately state the following dogma: discovery of a thumb hypoplasia requires a radiological, biological and, above all, cardiac evaluation, which can lead to genetic counselling and multidisciplinary management.

We will only treat moderate hypoplasia here, excluding the forms that belong to a pollicization of the index. The preservation of the thumb will be the rule but depending on the degree of hypoplasia, it will often be difficult to obtain a strictly normal thumb [1].

G. Pajardi (ed.), *Pediatric Hand Surgery*, https://doi.org/10.1007/978-3-031-30984-7_13

13.2 Definitions

It is necessary to distinguish between flexus adductus thumb and true hypoplasia because confusion is frequent. These are distinct entities with different prognoses and treatments.

13.3 Flexus Adductus Thumb

The flexus adductus thumb or clasped thumb of the Anglo-Saxon is actually a vicious attitude on an anatomically normal thumb. The diagnosis is clinical and radiological. Clinically, the child presents with one or two thumbs in the palm (Fig. 13.1). The parents usually consult after 3 months, when they notice the deformation. Recall that the thumb in the palm is physiological in the infant up to 2 months. This archaic attitude disappears spontaneously from the development of prehension, in variable time, because the child begins to catch with a cubital grip and then with long fingers. The release of the thumb of the palm is therefore between 3 and 6 months, ending when the child begins to pinch between thumb and index finger.

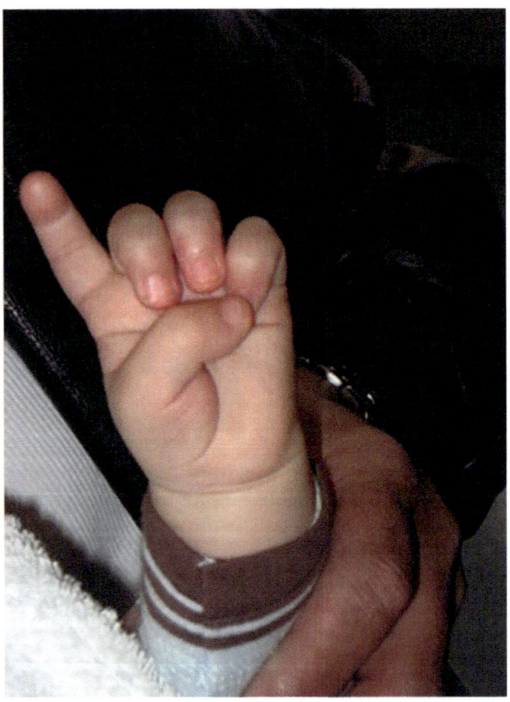

Fig. 13.1 Flexus adductus thumb. It is a lack of active extension and abduction but it is a transitory condition within the first 12 months. The thumb is normal both clinically and radiologically. Prognostic is excellent if hand therapy and manipulations by parents are started early

The clinical examination requires a lot of patience because it must be verified that the thumb can be gently brought into extension and abduction and that there is therefore neither first web contracture, articular stiffness nor pathological laxity. It is then necessary to stimulate the child and try to observe an active extension of the thumb. Usually, the child extends willingly its interphalangeal joint (IP) but it is an extension of the metacarpophalangeal (MP joint), even fugacious, which signs the presence of the extensor pollicis brevis (EPB). Plain radiography will confirm the diagnosis of thumb flexus adductus if no skeletal abnormalities are found, especially at the level of the first metacarpal. The radiological analysis is more difficult if the child is very young or if the deformity is bilateral. It is therefore necessary to remain cautious with the parents, because the only really positive argument for the diagnosis is evolutionary: it is the complete recovery of the function of the thumb, spontaneously or after physiotherapy. Given this, our management of flexus adductus thumb depends on evolution:

- Before 6 months we just observe the child by advising the parents some manipulations and stimulating the use of the thumb.
- Between 6 months and 1 year of age, it is advisable to have the thumb manipulated by a physiotherapist once a week while the parents will have daily to reproduce the manipulations taught by the physiotherapist.
- After 1 year, which is in practice quite rare, we perform a splint in abduction. We do not practice splints before 1 year for two reasons: (1) because they are very delicate on a small child and (2) because many children will be cured through manipulation. Even for apparently severe forms, correction of the flexus adductus thumb by splinting is usually

achieved in 2 months if observance is good. The child starts using his EPB and can grab large objects.

The thumb flexus adductus is therefore a transitory deformity due probably to a delay of the voluntary command of the extensor pollicis brevis and abductor pollicis longus, on a normal skeleton and whose prognosis is excellent, thanks to a simple conservative treatment.

13.4 Thumb Hypoplasia

Classification and anatomical abnormalities.

Blauth's classification (1967) [2] in five types is the reference in the literature. It is inspired by Müller's classification in four stages published in 1937 (quoted by Dautel [3]). Blauth's classification is based on clinical and radiological aspects, but his division in sub-types is still controversial and leads to many arguments in the literature [4–7]. We will describe only the first three types that concern the subject of our article.

Type 1: the thumb is a little bit shorter and slimmer than normal but harmonious. The tip of the thumb reaches half of the proximal phalanx of the index finger. There is no retraction of the first web, the joints are stable, and the extrinsic muscles are normal. The thenar muscles are slightly hypoplastic but present. The function is normal.

X-rays show a slight shortening of the first metacarpal bone and phalanges, which is more evident if the contralateral thumb is normal.

Type 2: the thumb is looking small; the shortening is clear. The first commissure is narrow, and the possibilities of passive abduction are limited. The absence of external thenar leads to a visible amyotrophy of the thenar eminence (Figs. 13.2a, b). There is more or less marked laxity of the ulnar collateral ligament of the metacarpophalangeal joint (MP joint). Abduction at the level of the MP joint or pollex adductus is frequent. It was emphasized by Lister [8], making suspect with an abnormal path of the flexor pollicis longus (FPL) on the radial edge of the thumb and adhesions with the extensor apparatus. Abnormalities of the extrinsic muscles are observed: the tendon of the FPL can be present and well centred but without synovial sheath, it can be interrupted on the retinaculum of the flexor tendons and, as we have seen, have a lateralized path on the radial edge, adhering to the extensor tendons.

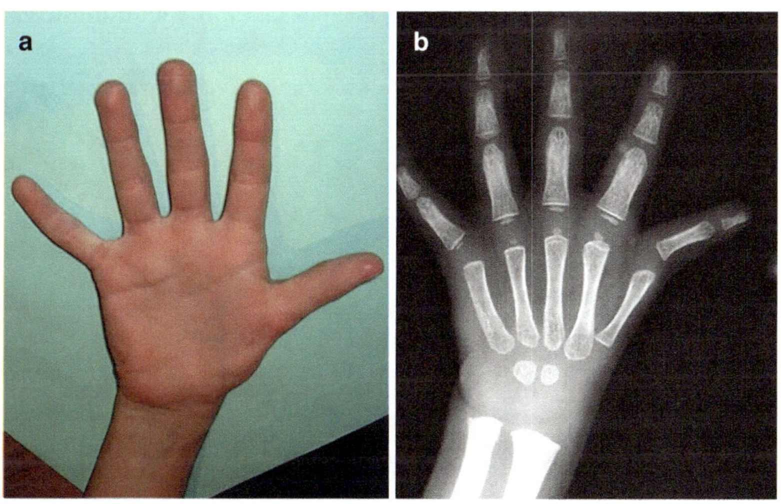

Fig. 13.2 Blauth type 2 hypoplasia. (**a**) Note the thenar eminence hypoplasia. Mild first web narrowing and thumb shortening. Extrinsic muscles are weak but active. (**b**) Plain X-ray showing the closure of the angle between the first and second metacarpal. Note the shortening of the distal radius (radial club hand type 1) and the abductus thumb with a severe instability of the ulnar collateral ligament of the MP joint

The EPB tendon may be loose or absent and the MP joint is in flexion. Active extension is possible only partially, thanks to the extensor pollicis longus (EPL). Lister also reports the inconsistent presence of a supernumerary muscle on the index. This muscle is derived from the tendon of the FPL and runs transversely in the first commissure to join the dossiere of the extensor of the index. Vascular and nerve abnormalities are reported: absence of motor branch of the median nerve [9], single proper palmar digital artery [10]. Despite these numerous muscular anomalies, the adults say they are not functionally very much bothered because they are adapted to their malformation.

Radiologically, the first metacarpal is stocky, phalanges are moderately short. There are no carpal anomalies.

Type 3: Since thumb hypoplasia is a spectrum of highly polymorphic abnormalities, some authors have proposed to add subclassifications in type 3 to better specify surgical indications. In 1995, Manske and McCarrol [11] divided this type into two subgroups according to the stability of the carpometacarpal joint (CMC) [6]. In group 3A, the CMC is stable and there are major abnormalities of the extrinsic muscles. In group 3B, the CMC is unstable because the base of the first metacarpal bone is absent. Buck-Gramcko has added a 3C subgroup where only the head of the first metacarpal is present. This group 3A created a storm in a cup since many authors pointed the abnormal radiological feature of the base of the first metacarpal and deducted that it was systematically associated with an instability of the CMC [5, 7, 12–14].

In all types 3, the muscular abnormalities are major: the intrinsic muscles are absent and the extrinsic are slender or absent. The thumb is almost parallel to the index as the first commissure is brief (Figs. 13.3a, b). The function is very reduced, or even nil depending on the subtypes. In type 3A, the conservation and motorization of the thumb are theoretically possible but for types 3B and 3C all authors agree to advocate a thumb removal and practice pollicization of the index.

If the interest of a classification is to be a guideline for the surgical treatment, one can wonder why the border between conservative thumb reconstruction and pollicization sits within type 3. It would seem more logical to include type 3A in type 2. The latter could be characterized as a short thumb with muscles anomalies but without bone anomalies (excerpt the hypoplasia and the joint instability). Type 2 would be divided into two sub-types: 2A without extrinsic abnormalities and 2 B with extrinsic abnormalities. I

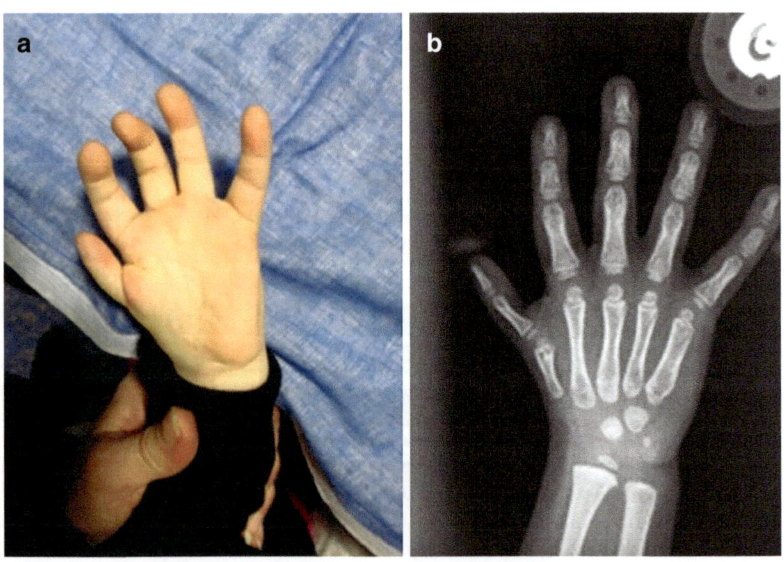

Fig. 13.3 Blauth type 3 hypoplasia. (**a**) Narrow first web, very short thumb. Absence of intrinsic and extrinsic muscles. Multiplanar MP joint instability. (**b**) Since the CMC is stable, it should be classified as a 3A in Blauth's modified classification but would be type 2B in our personal classification

agree that type 2C could be added for the thumb with a demonstrated CMC instability. Type 3 would be characterized radiologically by the presence of bone abnormalities in the base of the first metacarpal and therefore instability of TM. This is just a personal suggestion [15] that only entails the responsibility of the author but which has the merit of clarifying the surgical indications: types 1 and 2 (without or with anomalies of the extrinsic muscles) would be preserved and types 3, 4 and 5 would be resected with pollicization of the index. Readers will judge the merits of this simplification.

13.5 Incidence

For Lister, it would be 4.5% of congenital malformations of the hand. The incidence of thumb hypoplasia is actually underestimated. Indeed, type 1 often goes unnoticed and does not require any treatment. They are ignored in the therapeutic coding. It is not uncommon when examining parents of a child with hypoplasia to find that they have type 1, while they consider the size of their thumb to be normal. Even more, it has often happened to us to note an amyotrophy of the thenar eminence signing type 2 but held negligible by one of the parents.

There is a predominance of boys and the right side is a little more affected than the left.

13.6 The First Consultation

The first consultation of a child with a congenital malformation is important and takes time because many answers must be provided, according to the following plan in four steps:

1. What is the congenital malformation?
2. Is this hereditary?
3. Will my child be 'handicapped'?
4. What treatment can we offer and at what age?

The diagnosis of thumb hypoplasia is usually easy, based in most cases on clinical examination and, for minor forms, on plain radiographs. The parents do not usually consult for a hypoplasia but for a small unstable thumb or for another pathology (radial deviation of the wrist ...). It is important to distinguish with a thumb flexus adductus as previously described and then to specify the type of hypoplasia.

13.7 Physical Examination

Inspection: Sufficient for the diagnosis of hypoplasia by examining:

1. Size: The diagnosis is easy in severe hypoplasia, or in case of unilateral involvement, compared to the contralateral thumb. For minor bilateral forms, the thumb size is estimated relative to the IPP joint and the proximal phalanx of the index finger.
2. The volume of the thumb: lower than the neighbouring fingers giving a slender appearance.
3. The axes of the thumb: the thumb may be too parallel to the index and abnormally derotated.
4. The decrease or absence of inter-phalangeal folds is indicative of tendon abnormalities.
5. The thenar eminence may be the seat of obvious amyotrophy.

13.8 Palpation

This is a crucial step since it specifies the severity of hypoplasia. The palpation of the thumb should be gentle taking advantage of the 'interval of patience' of the infant.

1. First web: we appreciate the cutaneous brevity and we record the angle of passive abduction.
2. Stability of MP JOINT. Lateral and antero-posterior stability are tested. The existence of instability of the ulnar collateral ligament conditions the function of the thumb and the choice of palliative transplant. The instability of the radial slope must not be neglected. A stiff thumb can be helpful. An unstable thumb

is excluded. The child prefers the pinch between the index finger and the middle finger or sometimes another pinch and excludes his thumb.
3. Passive mobility of MP JOINT and IP joints: Parents must be aware of pre-operative joint stiffness and thus be informed that the thumb will never become normal after surgery. Some unrealistic hopes should be avoided.

Active Mobility: record of active range of motion is very difficult in infants. Children must be stimulated and observed for a long time while manipulating objects, toys and cakes to assess functional deficits: lack of extension, flexion, abduction or complete immobility.

Wrist and forearm: for any hypoplasia of the thumb, one must have the reflex to examine the wrist and the forearm. In a series of 160 patients, James, McCarrol and Manske [16] have reported 59% of radial dysplasia. It is compulsory to look for a radial deviation, a flessum of the wrist and to systematically test the passive pro-supination.

13.9 General Examination

The frequency of syndromic forms is high. The child should be fully examined for vertebral, genital, facial dysmorphia, cardiac auscultation and lower extremity malformations. Two syndromes are common: Holt Oram syndrome with RCH, thumb hypoplasia and atrial septal defect or ventricular septal defect and a classic association, the VATER syndrome (vertebral, anal, tracheoesophageal fistula, oesophageal atresia, renal and radial limb abnormalities) or VACTERL (vertebral, anal, cardiac, tracheoesophageal fistula, oesophageal atresia, renal and limb).

The contralateral upper limb is frequently affected [16]. Bilateral hypoplasia is found in 2/3 of the cases, in association with a thumb duplication, a triphalangeal thumb or a RCH.

Parental examination: as mentioned before, it is important to seek any even discreet and neglected malformation on parents. If this research is positive, the family must be offered genetic counselling, especially in the case of visceral associations.

13.10 Imaging and Para-Clinical Explorations

13.10.1 X-Rays of the Hand

Plain X-rays of the hand (antero-posterior and three-quarter views) confirm the diagnosis in the minor forms and allow the classification of hypoplasia among the different types and subtypes of the Blauth's classification.

In type 1, the diagnosis is based on comparative pictures. In bilateral cases, with a little habit, we find a broad and concave appearance of the first metacarpal that confirms the clinical impression.

With look for synostosis of the fourth and fifth metacarpal, a contralateral triphalangeal or duplicated thumb or some wrist anomalies [17].

X-rays of the forearm: radiological examination should be systematically supplemented with forearm radiographs to detect hypoplasia of the radius at a subclinical stage, or to confirm and classify a proven RCH. Indeed, the rehabilitation of RCH is an emergency and the treatment of the wrist takes priority over that of the thumb [18].

13.10.2 Other Imaging

In case of RCH, it is mandatory to look for a hemi vertebra on the cervical spine. Thus, a congenital scoliosis can be detected and treated earlier.

13.10.3 Essential Para-Clinical Explorations

Whether hypoplasia of the thumb is isolated or is part of an external longitudinal aplasia, one always asks:

- a blood test,
- a renal and cardiac ultrasound.

Other more specialized examinations are required depending on the clinical context: bronchial fibrescopy, digestive and urological explorations.

13.10.4 Genetic Counselling

At the end of this check-up, if we find any visceral involvement, facial dysmorphism and family history, parents should be referred to genetic counselling in order to assess the risk for future pregnancies and for the offspring of the child. It is also the geneticists who will strive to the slightest doubt in front of a longitudinal radial aplasia, to eliminate a Fanconi syndrome with a life-threatening prognosis (pancytopenia).

13.11 Treatment

13.11.1 Conservative Treatment

13.11.1.1 Manipulations

Although less essential than for the flexus adductus thumb, it seems important to minimize retraction of the first web and joint stiffness, particularly the interphalangeal (IP), by performing daily manipulations.

Occupational therapy is not mandatory but recommended, at first, to educate the parents. These are encouraged to manipulate their child daily, sometimes during the nap. Stimulate the extrinsic muscles will be recommended so that they develop the maximum activity. One should soften the first web but without worsening an instability of the MP joint, if present. Therefore, it is necessary to hold the thumb at the head of the first metacarpal and to exert traction outside.

13.11.1.2 Splints

Splints have little indication preoperatively because they are very difficult to perform in children under 1 year of age and they could aggravate an instability of the MP joint. On the other hand, they have an important place post-operatively in type 2 because, after release of the first web, secondary retractions may cause a partial recurrence in adduction of the thumb. Trained orthotists are required to ensure that splints do not result in exaggerated retraction of the thumb or compromise the instability of the MP joint. For this reason, we only use static splints molded into the first commissure as soon as skin healing is obtained. These splints are often maintained 4–6 weeks day and night and then night for at least 2 months.

13.11.2 Surgical Treatment

13.11.2.1 Techniques

Release of the First Web

Depending on the degree of retraction, either Z-plasty or its derivates (four-flap Z-plasty or Trident plasty [19]) or 'pseudo-kite' plasty [20] will be used.

For severe retractions, we recommend the use of Buck-Gramcko's dorsal flap, which is distally extended on the proximal third of the dorsal and radial aspect of the index finger. This flap is of excellent reliability, with a technical pearl: during the dorsal dissection, do not undermine until the base of the flap but only on its distal half to preserve the dorsal proximal perforating vessels which ensure a perfect blood supply to the flap. Thanks to this precaution, we have never had to deplore in our experience the slightest distal necrosis of the flap.

All these techniques of the first web release usually give a sufficient view on the aponeurotic and muscular elements of the first commissure as well as on the ulnar side of the MP joint. To obtain a complete opening of the commissure, the muscles must be carefully divided. If a supernumerary transverse muscle is found, he must be largely resected. The fibrous and aponeurotic formations which tend to limit the commissural opening, in particular the fascia of the first dorsal interosseous, are longitudinally divided, and the insertion of the adductor of the thumb into the third metacarpal may sometimes be disinserted, taking care not to injure the motor branch of the ulnar nerve. We can also partially disinsert the insertion of the first dorsal interosseous on the first metacarpal bone.

Exploration and Rerouting of Extrinsic Tendons

If there is no active flexion of the IP, an abnormal fusion of the flexor and extensor on the radial face of the thumb should be strongly suspected. A lateral incision on the first metacarpal and the first phalanx allows us to explore the FPL and the EPL (Figs. 13.4a, b). If they are fused, they are detached and recentralized. One can attempt to reconstruct a T1 pulley on the FPL although the results of the reconstruction of the flexor tendon apparatus are often disappointing [8]. FPL dissection will continue proximally if there are adhesions that prevent normal tendon sliding. We have sometimes had to release this tendon to the wrist before obtaining the natural elasticity caused by the muscular body. In some cases, the so-called FPL tendon takes an aberrant course [21] and moves towards the dorsal side of the wrist and forearm and its release never resulted in a restoration of the flexion of the thumb.

Opposition Transfers

Transfer of the abductor digiti minimi muscle (ADM) was described by Huber in 1921 [22].

This muscle and tendon transfer has the advantage of being both functional and aesthetic. Indeed, the muscular body partially restores the relief of the thenar eminence. On the other hand, it has the disadvantage of being a little short imposing a technical pearl: by a zigzag incision on the ulnar edge of the hand then of the first phalanx, one disinserts the terminal tendon on the first phalanx the most distally possible, possibly taking a periosteal slip to lengthen it as much as possible (Figs. 13.5a–e). The dissection is then easy, from distal to proximal, taking care not to injure the neurovascular bundle which enter the muscle by its deep face. The pedicle is divided and the dissection continues proximally to disinsert the muscle from the pisiform while keeping continuity with the flexor carpi ulnaris (FCU) fibres. A subcutaneous tunnel is then realized, and the transfer is recovered by a counter incision on the lateral face of the MP joint of the thumb. It is reinserted, depending on the case and according to the length, on the distal strip of the abductor pollicis brevis (APB) or on the articular capsule on the lateral face of the base of the proximal phalanx. Takayama sometimes used it both as a plasty of opposition and of stabilization of the ulnar collateral ligament of the MP joint [23]. To be able to transplant the ADM more distally, this author transposes the muscular body very radially and reattach it to the retinaculum of the flexor tendons. The tendon is then passed under the EPL and reinserted on the fascia of the adductor pollicis on the ulnar slope of the MP JOINT.

Transfer of the flexor communis superficialis (FCS) tendon of the fourth finger. As described

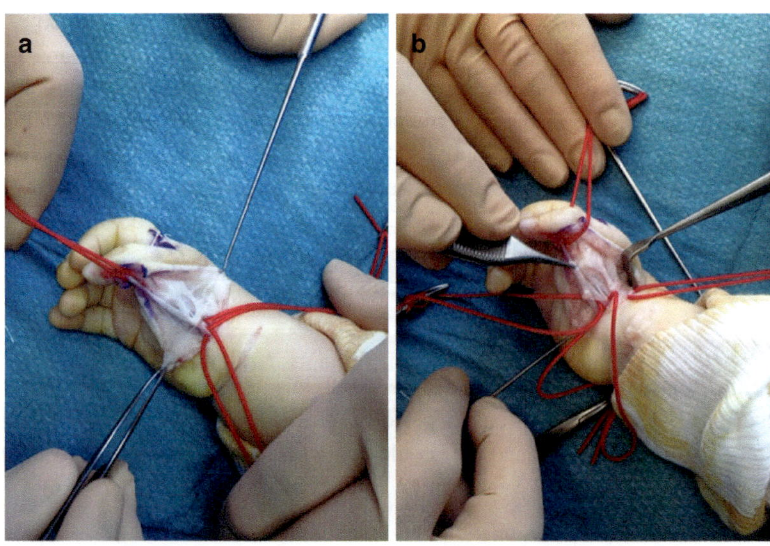

Fig. 13.4 Abductus thumb. (**a**) Multiple adherences between the flexor and extensor apparatus, realizing a radial plexus tendinosum. Absence of flexor tendon sheet and pulley. (**b**) Separation of the flexor and extensor tendons. Note the abnormal path of the FPL, heading to the radial edge of the wrist

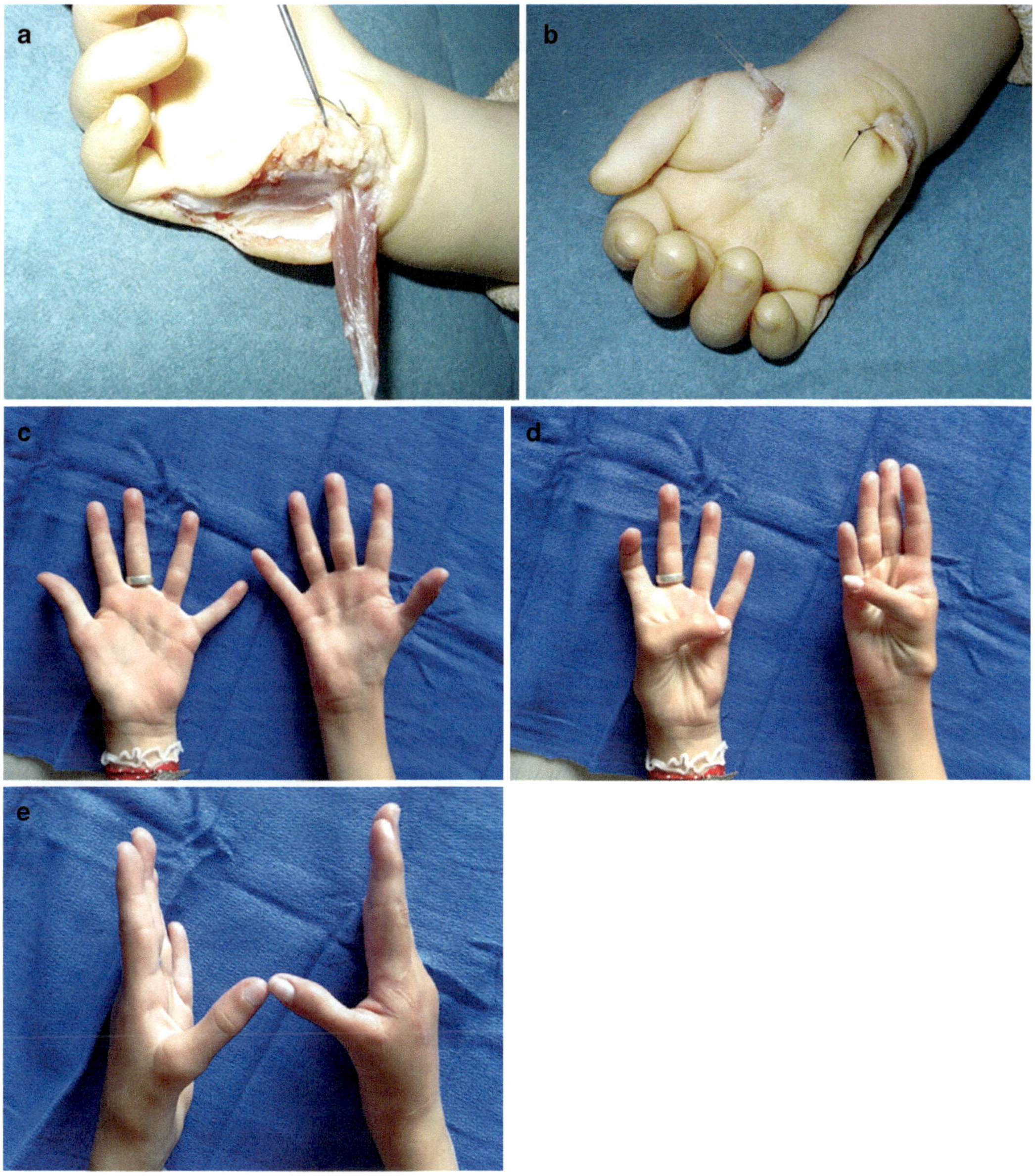

Fig. 13.5 Huber transfer; *abductor digiti minimi* (ADM). (**a**) division of the ADM from distal to proximal. One can lengthen the transplant by harvesting a periosteal slip of the ulnar base of the proximal phalanx. (**b**) the transfer is dragged subcutaneously to the radial side of the MP joint of the thumb. (**c**) Same girl right hand; result after 10 years. (**d**) Kapandji's score is 8. (**e**) True active antepulsion up to 40°

by Royle [24], it is a pure tendon transfer, which gives a longer transplant and is frequently used to restore opposition and stabilize the ulnar collateral ligament (UCL) [25]. The two lateral strips of the FCS can be disinserted distally at the intermediate phalanx but now we prefer avoiding an incision on the finger. We perform a transverse incision on the distal fold of the palm, proximal to the A1 pulley, we isolate the FCS tendon and by pulling strongly with a silicone loop, with the fourth finger in flexion, it is possible to bring the chiasma into the palm and cut it. It is then easy to harvest the tendon. Another transverse proximal incision is realized to identify the transplant at the exit of the carpal tunnel (Figs. 13.6a–i) and a buttonhole is made in the middle of the retinacu-

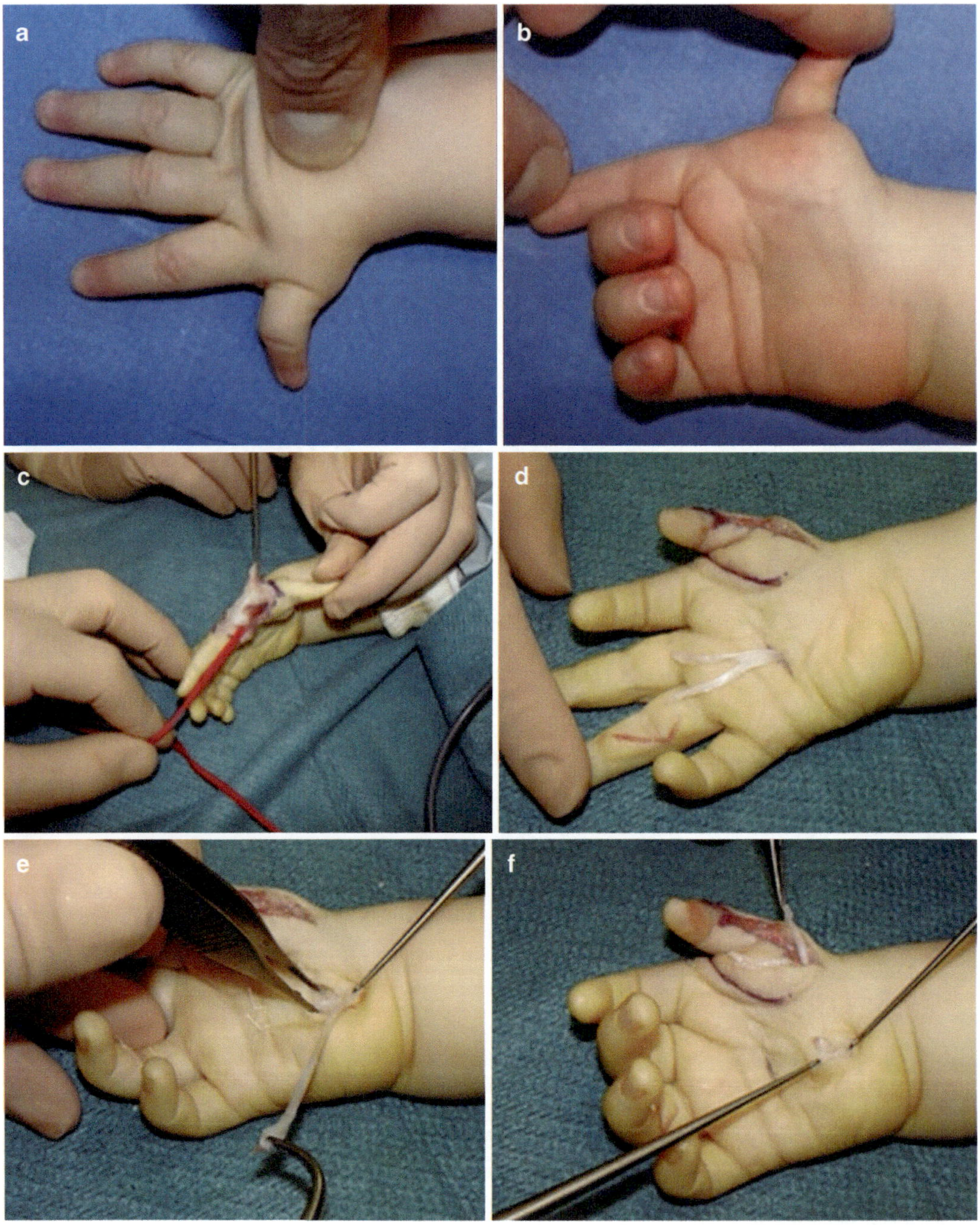

Fig. 13.6 Flexus adductus thumb on type 3A. Transfer of the sublimis of the fourth finger (Royle transfer). (**a**) Dorsal view. (**b**) palmar view showing the lateral passive hyper-laxity. (**c**) opening of the first web with resection of a supernumerary transverse muscle. (**d**) Harvesting of the two slips of the FCS of the fourth finger. We no longer open the fourth finger since we are able to harvest the FCS by pulling strongly the tendon in the palm and cutting the chiasma. (**e**) Making a pulley by opening a buttonhole in the flexor tendon retinaculum. (**f**) the transfer is dragged to the radial edge of the MP joint. One slip is sutured very proximal to the base of the proximal phalanx, while the other is dragged through a hole in the metacarpal head, from radial to ulnar, to reconstruct the UCL. (**g–i**) Same child; 2 years follow up with a true active antepulsion and opposition

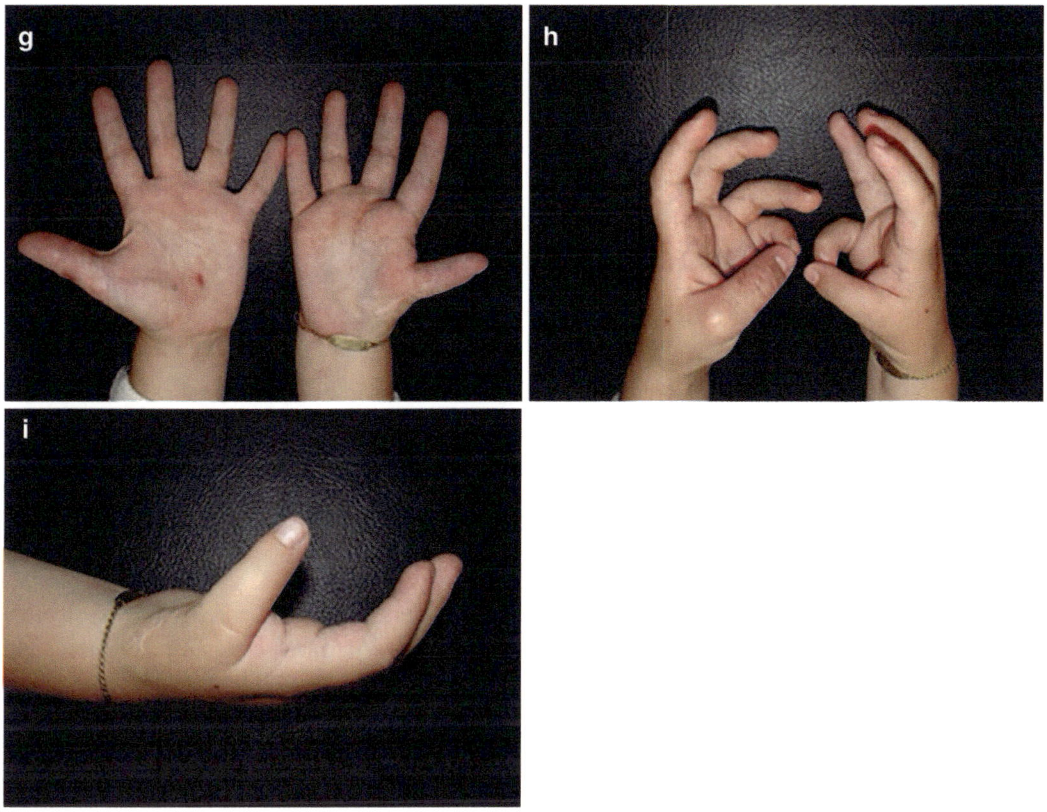

Fig. 13.6 (continued)

lum which will serve as reflection pulley. The tendon is then dragged to the lateral face of the MP joint and of the proximal phalanx of the thumb to be reinserted on the supposed distal insertion of the APB.

To stabilize the MP joint, many authors perform a transosseous tunnel in the head of the first metacarpal bone and use one of the strips to reconstruct the ulnar collateral ligament.

The removal of FCS tendon does not compromise the flexion of the fourth finger, nor create any instability of the PIP joint.

Extension Transfer

This transfer is largely underestimated in the literature. In case of EPB aplasia, if children have the extension through the EPL, it is often inadequate to cause a correct opening of the first web. In this case, we can use the extensor indicis proprius (EIP) after checking preoperatively that the child has an independent extension of the index. As reported in the Japanese publications, the interest of this transfer is to improve the thumb extension and to stabilize the ulnar side of the MP joint.

Harvesting the EIP is easy. We start distally by separating the distal insertion of the EIP on the MP joint of the index. The tendon is then dragged by a small incision on the dorsal surface of the wrist or taken directly when opening of the first web. It is then slipped on the dorsal and ulnar side of the first metacarpal and then inserted on the base of the proximal phalanx by making numerous mooring points on the ulnar part of the capsule of the MP joint becoming both an active transfer of extension and of joint stabilization.

Stabilization of the MP Joint

It should be checked pre-operatively if it is a simple ulnar or multi-directional instability. In this latter case, it is illusory to attempt to reconstruct the ligaments. It is better to perform a chondrodesis between the head of M1 and the base of P1, but this 'arthrodesis at pediatric age' must be carried out with care so as not to damage the growth cartilage at the base of P1.

If it is stability only on the ulnar side, the two techniques mentioned above will be carried out: stabilization transfer of the EIP, transfer of the FCS and for some Huber transfer (ADM).

Cosmetic improvement: thenar eminence augmentation. As mentioned before, the Huber transfer can correct the thenar muscle amyotrophy but very partially, to be honest. In order to restore the thenar relief, I have performed some fat grafts according to Coleman with satisfactory results. This should be proposed only at the end of growth. Upton [26] has published an adipofascial island flap in pollicization but it could be performed in type 2 or 3A as well.

13.11.2.2 Indications

Whatever the type of hypoplasia, treatment should be early, started in the first year and ideally completed before 2 years of age [27].

Type 1

For type 1, as we have seen, the function is normal. There is therefore no surgical indication.

Type 2

For type 2, the treatment systematically comprises three components:

- Opening of the first commissure with skin flaps and musculo-aponeurotic release.
- Thumb opposition transfer and possibly palliative extension.
- Stabilization of the MCP.

The reconstruction of the first web space is not the subject of any controversy. The choice of the type of opposition and the stabilization of the MCP depend on the habits of the authors. Paul Smith [28] proposed an algorithm of therapeutic decisions according to the type of instability of the MP joint. In case of uni-axial instability, he proposes the transfer of the FCS of the fourth finger with a transosseous passage of one of the strips to reconstruct the ulnar collateral ligament. It is also our method of choice. If the instability is multi-axial, he recommends a chondrodesis of the MCP and a Huber-type opposition transfer.

In our experience, the use of chondrodesis is rarely necessary in type 2, because we have the habit, in case of multi-axial instability with deficit extension of the MCP to practice at first the transfer of the 'EIP to restore the extension [29] and perform a transfer of the FCS of the fourth finger while the FPL of the thumb actively stabilize the MCP.

Type 3

We only mention the type 3 A case since the 3 B and 3 C are treated by index pollicization for the vast majority of authors.

For type 3A, multi-axis instability of the MP joint is the rule and chondrodesis is most often required. The intrinsic tendons are all absent and the extrinsic tendons are very slender. It is therefore imperative to restore the opposition and the extension of the thumb as previously described.

The opening of the first commissure most often requires a 'generous' flap-type Buck Gramcko.

The closure of the angle between the first and second metacarpal bone (M1 and M2) is so important that we could be tempted to perform M1-M2 arthrodesis by bicortical trapezoidal bone graft. However, this technique can only be performed at adolescence because it would block the physeal plate and thus the growth of the base of M1.

Key Points

- Do not confuse a flexus adductus thumb whose orthopaedic treatment with manipulations and splinting is always favourable with a true thumb hypoplasia that requires release of the first web, stabilization of the MP joint and restoration of the opposition and extension of the thumb.
- Take time to check if instability of the MP joint is only passive or both passive and active. If the child can stabilize actively his joint with

a proper contraction of his intrinsic or extrinsic muscles, there is no need for a ligament reconstruction.

- Regardless of the type of hypoplasia, even in type 1, keep in mind that the malformation of the thumb is rarely isolated, requiring a complete examination of the child, of his ipsi- and contra-lateral upper limb, and of the parents.
- The choice of the tendon transfer is made according to the stability of the MCP.
- Any kind of procedure requires a postoperative immobilization by splinting for several months to avoid a secondary retraction of the first web.
- It should not be forgotten that the functional result depends on the severity of the hypoplasia and especially if associated with a RCH.

References

1. Light TR, Gaffey JL. Reconstruction of the hypoplastic thumb. J Hand Surg Am. 2010;35(3):474–9.
2. Blauth W. The hypoplastic thumb. Arch Orthop Unfallchir. 1967;62(3):225–46.
3. Dautel G. Thumb hypoplasia. Chir Main. 2006;25(1):1–15.
4. Buck-Gramcko D. State of the art: congenital malformation of the hand and forearm. Part III. Eur Med Hand Surg. 1993;3:7–31.
5. Smith P. Lister's the hand. Diagnosis and indications. London: Churchill Livingstone; 2002. p. 505–12.
6. Soldado F, Zlotolow DA, Kozin SH. Thumb hypoplasia. J Hand Surg Am. 2013;38(7):1435–44.
7. Tonkin MA. On the classification of congenital thumb hypoplasia. J Hand Surg Eur Vol. 2014;39(9):948–55.
8. Lister G. Pollex abductus in hypoplasia and duplication of the thumb. J Hand Surg Am. 1991;16(4):626–33.
9. Dellon AL, Rayan G. Congenital absence of the thenar muscles. Report of two cases. J Bone Joint Surg Am. 1981;63(6):1014–5.
10. Rayan GM. Congenital thumb hypoplasia. J Okla State Med Assoc. 1994;87(12):546–50.
11. Manske PR, McCarroll HR Jr, James M. Type III-A hypoplastic thumb. J Hand Surg [Am]. 1995;20(2):246–53.
12. Hovius SE, van Nieuwenhoven C. Commentary on Tonkin. On the classification of congenital thumb hypoplasia. J Hand Surg Eur Vol. 2014;39(9):956–7.
13. Smith P. Re: Tonkin, M. A. On the classification of congenital thumb hypoplasia. J Hand Surg Eur. 2014, 39: 948–55. J Hand Surg Eur Vol. 2015;40(4):427.
14. Tonkin MA. Re: Tonkin, M. A. On the classification of congenital thumb hypoplasia. J Hand Surg Eur. 2014, 39: 948-55. Reply. J Hand Surg Eur Vol. 2015;40(4):427–8.
15. Guero S. Conduite à tenir devant Une hypoplasie du pouce de type 1 à 3A [surgical management of the Blauth 1 to 3A thumb hypoplasia]. Chir Main. 2008;27(Suppl 1):S62–70.
16. James MA, McCarroll HR Jr, Manske PR. Characteristics of patients with hypoplastic thumbs. J Hand Surg [Am]. 1996;21(1):104–13.
17. Hall RF Jr, Keuhn D Jr, Prieto J. Congenital hypoplasia of the thumb ray with absent carpal navicular and hypertrophic styloid process of the radius: a case report. J Hand Surg Am. 1986;11(1):32–5.
18. James MA, et al. The association of radial deficiency with thumb hypoplasia. J Bone Joint Surg Am. 2004;86(10):2196–205.
19. Glicenstein J, Bonnefous G. La plastie en trident. Ann Chir Plast. 1975;20:257–60.
20. Foucher G, Gazarian A, Pajardi G. Reconstructive surgery of Blauth type III hypoplasia of the thumb. Chir Main. 1999;18(3):191–6.
21. Graham TJ, Louis DS. A comprehensive approach to surgical management of the type IIIA hypoplastic thumb. J Hand Surg Am. 1998;23(1):3–13.
22. Gupta A, et al. Treatment of the severely injured upper extremity. Instr Course Lect. 2000;49:377–96.
23. Takayama S, et al. Modified abductor digiti minimi opponensplasty in congenital hypoplastic thumb with laxity of metacarpophalangeal joint. Tech Hand Up Extrem Surg. 2002;6(4):166–70.
24. Royle ND. The functions of human voluntary muscles. Sydney: Angus & Robertson limited; 1938. p. 42.
25. Kozin SH, Ezaki M. Flexor digitorum superficialis opponensplasty with ulnar collateral ligament reconstruction for thumb deficiency. Tech Hand Up Extrem Surg. 2010;14(1):46–50.
26. Upton J, Sharma S, Taghinia AH. Vascularized adipofascial Island flap for thenar augmentation in pollicization. Plast Reconstr Surg. 2008;122(4):1089–94.
27. Lister G. Reconstruction of the hypoplastic thumb. Clin Orthop Relat Res. 1985;195:52–65.
28. Smith P, et al. Blauth II thumb hypoplasia: a management algorithm for the unstable metacarpophalangeal joint. J Hand Surg Eur Vol. 2012;37(8):745–50.
29. Vacher C, et al. Congenital thumb hypoplasia. Clinical study of twenty patients. Ann Chir Main Memb Super. 1997;16(4):316–25.

Thumb Hypoplasia: Genesia, Pollicization

14

Giorgio Pajardi, Elisa Rosanda, and Chiara Parolo

Abstract

Congenital malformation of the thumb is one of the most important problems in congenital disease. The hypoplastic thumb is characterized by a variable degree of bony and soft tissue inadequacy. It may occur alone or as part of a multiple congenital anomaly syndrome. Depending on degree of hypoplasia, the nonsurgical or surgical treatment differs. Every treatment, usually, starts very early in the childhood to improve brain plasticity.

In case of surgical management, the primary goal is to improve or restore pincer grip. In general when the hypoplastic thumb lacks basilar joint stability or is absent, the hand is best treated by politicization of the index finger. When hypoplasia is less severe, surgical strategy includes first web deepening, MP ligamentoplasty, opponensplasty, and tendon transfer.

G. Pajardi
Department of Hand Surgery and Rehabilitation, S. Giuseppe Hospital IRCCS MultiMedica, Milan University, Milan, Italy
e-mail: gpajardi@centrostudimano.it

E. Rosanda (✉) · C. Parolo
Milan, Italy
e-mail: elisa.rosanda@multimedica.it; chiara.parolo@multimedica.it

Keywords

Congenital hand deformities · Thumb hypoplasia · Pollicization · First web deepening · Opponensplasty · Tendon transfer

Congenital malformation of the thumb is one of the most important problems in congenital disease. The thumb has unique characteristics despite of long fingers. The CMC joint, the intrinsic and extrinsic muscles, the vascularization, and innervation make it the most important finger in the hand with the capability of opposition that differentiates human from the other species.

The hypoplastic thumb is characterized by a variable degree of bony and soft tissue inadequacy. There are several definitions of hypoplastic thumb: A thumb is considered to be underdeveloped if deficiency of any one or all structures is present [1]. Congenital hypoplastic thumb is defined as a short, underdeveloped thumb with deficient or absent intrinsic muscles with or without deficient extrinsic musculoskeletal structures [2]. The thumb is considered hypoplastic when its tip does not reach the midway point of the proximal phalanx of the index finger.

Depending on degree of hypoplasia, the nonsurgical or surgical treatment differs. In general, when the hypoplastic thumb lacks basilar joint stability or is absent, the hand is best treated by politicization of the index finger. When hypopla-

G. Pajardi (ed.), *Pediatric Hand Surgery*, https://doi.org/10.1007/978-3-031-30984-7_14

sia is less severe, the thumb should be retained and reconstructed.

Treatments, usually, starts very early in the childhood. The pollicization is performed at about 1 year of age. This is preferred because by 6 months the infant begins to move the thumb voluntarily, by 9 months the thumb gains its independence and mobility from the palm whereas by 1 year of age, it becomes a crucial portion of hand function [3]. Than younger surgery takes advantage of brain plasticity and ease of incorporation into daily activities.

14.1 Epidemiology

The exact incidence of thumb hypoplasia is difficult to determine because of the large number of upper limb malformations, which contain some type of thumb deficiency. Kozin reported that the rate of birth anomalies is about 1% to 2%; of these about 10% occur in the upper extremity [4]. Entin [5] reported a 16% incidence of thumb hypoplasia among Canadian patients whereas Flatt [6] published an 11.2% incidence of thumb abnormalities and a 3.6% incidence of thumb hypoplasia or aplasia.

14.2 Associated Conditions

Thumb hypoplasia can occur isolated or in the context of other diseases. The presence of associated congenital anomalies and syndromes should be investigated with the aid of a geneticist.

More common association include:

- Holt Horam syndrome.
- VACTERL associations: vertebral abnormalities, anal atresia, cardiac abnormalities, tracheo esophageal fistula and/or esophageal atresia, renal agenesis and dysplasia, and limb defects.
- TAR SYNDROME (thrombocytopenia-absent radius): does not result in thumb hypoplasia but instead leads to a flat broad thumb.
- Fanconi anemia.
- CHARGE syndrome (coloboma of the eye, heart defects, atresia of the nasal choanae, retardation of growth and/or development, genital and/or urinary abnormalities, and ear abnormalities and deafness).

14.3 Classification

Muller described the first classification of thumb hypoplasia in 1937, subsequent modification done by Blauth, Buck-Gramcko and Manske has improved the classification.

Nowadays, the accepted classification is the modified Blauth classification that is categorized into five general types or grades.

This classification is used not only to describe the degree of hypoplasia but also to predict physical findings and guide treatment.

A type I hypoplastic thumb is stable with good overall function but slightly smaller than a typical thumb. Both intrinsic and extrinsic muscles are present.

In type II and type III, there is a narrowing of the thumb index web space, aplasia/hypoplasia of thenar muscles, and instability of the thumb metacarpophalangeal (MCP) joint. In type II, thumbs have intrinsic muscle aplasia/hypoplasia whereas type III thumbs have intrinsic and extrinsic muscle aplasia/hypoplasia.

Manske et al. [7] sub-classified type III thumbs into A or B based on the condition of the carpometacarpal (CMC) joint. The distinction is that the type IIIA thumb has a stable CMC joint. Type IIIB has severely underdeveloped CMC joint unstable.

Type IV deficiency is a floating thumb, in which a rudimentary digit is connected to the hand by only skin and a neurovascular bundle. Type V deficiency is a complete absence of the thumb (Fig. 14.1).

14.4 Indications

In severe grade of hypoplasia, from type IV to type V, the indication is the pollicization of the index finger.

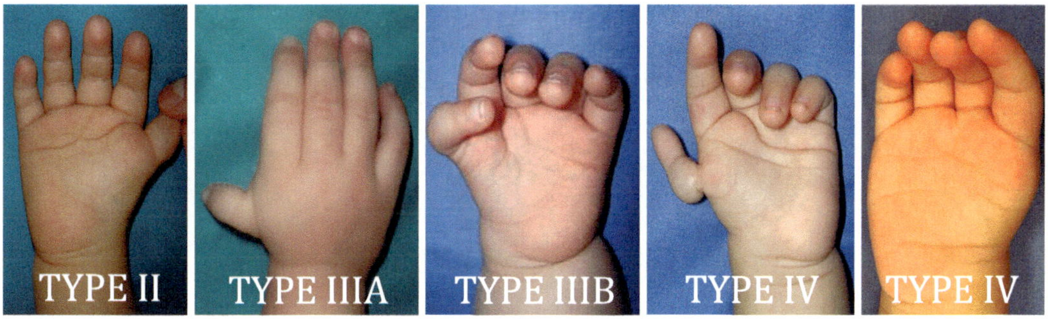

Fig. 14.1 Grades of thumb hypoplasia from grade II onwards

Although in the last years there are some controversial for the indication in Blauth IIIB, index finger pollicization remains the ideal reconstruction also in this grade of hypoplasia.

Pollicization is also indicated in other congenital diseases as mirror hand, macrodactyly, multifingered hand and some traumatic cases.

The patient has to be healthy and able to tolerate general anesthesia. Must be investigated for any associated syndrome and disease. The surgery is not appropriate for children with several central nervous system deficiencies.

Must be discussed with parents the expected functional results: a stiff index finger will make a stiff neo thumb [8].

14.5 Techniques

The current technique of pollicization represents a consolidation of contributions from surgeons over the last 100 years [9–11].

The procedure was first described by Littler in 1952, modified by Buck-Gramcko in 1971 and then many surgeons refined the technique to improve appearance and function.

In the literature, the most discussed items include skin incision, positioning and fixation of the metacarpal head, rebalancing of intrinsic muscles and extensor tendons.

There isn't a perfect technique but every surgeon prefers the one in his hands is better.

The goals are to provide ample access to the index for pollicization, to reconstruct the first web space, recreate a functional new thumb with a good opponent position.

The pollicization requires a stepwise approach. Some of the critical points are:

1. Adequate design of the skin incision to allow easy index finger transposition and creation of an adequate thumb-index web space. This allows avoiding scar in the web space and preventing a contracture.
2. Preservation and reinsertion of intrinsic muscles in order to ensure thumb adduction and abduction,
3. Epiphysiodesis of the grow plate of metacarpal to prevent excessive growth of the base of the pollicized index finger,
4. extension of the MCP joint to avoid future thumb hyperextension,
5. fixation of the new thumb in opposition [12].

Our personal technique based on Buck-Gramcko technique modified by Foucher [13].

In this procedure, there' s a modification of the skin incision, rebalancing of extensor tendons, and bone fixation (Fig. 14.2).

The surgery starts with the children placed in a supine position under general anesthesia. A brachial plexus axillar block is performed to avoid pain during operation and in the early postoperatory period. A pediatric tourniquet is placed on the upper arm. Preoperative antibiotic prophylaxis is administered routinely.

The limb is gently exsanguinated to allow better visualization of the digital vessels.

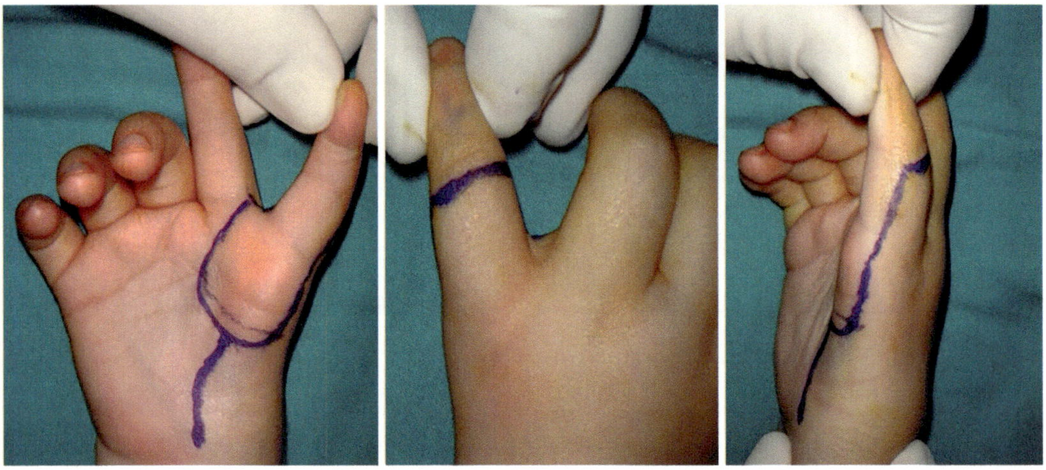

Fig. 14.2 Buck-Gramcko technique modified by Foucher: skin incision

In children with a type IV or IIIB thumb hypoplasia, the incision wraps around the base of nonfunctional thumb. The extra digit is then removed with bone, tendon, nail, and neurovascular bundle are cauterized. In case of presence of hypoplastic thenar muscle, this is detached and preserve to restore thenar eminence.

The palmar skin is incised first and the flap is raised distally. Neurovascular bundles are identified and isolated from common digital vessels and nerves to the index-long web space and radial side of index finger. Additional dissection could be necessary in case of arterial variations. The distal arterial bifurcation is identified and its contribution to the long finger is ligated. Proximal microdissection is necessary to further separate the proper digital nerves to easier translation of the finger. To prevent inadvertent vessel injury could be helpful the use of surgical loop.

The first annular pulley of the index finger is identified and incised to allow mobilization of index finger and prevent buckling of the flexor tendons after the digit is shortened. The intermetacarpal ligament is identified and divided.

The dorsal incision extends transversely across the PIP joint. The dorsal flap is sharply elevated with the conservation of as many dorsal veins as possible. The veins are then followed proximally to allow good exposure of extensor tendons until MCP joint. The index extensor tendons are isolated and cut at the MCPJ. Then are splitted proximally until PIP joint into two bundle. This procedure creates new tendons for the reinsertion of intrinsic muscle.

The pollicization proceeds with the identification, isolation, and mobilization of the first dorsal and palmar interossei muscles. They are released distally with a portion of aponeurosis in preparation for suture fixation and reinsertion. Beware to isolate carefully the tendons from collateral ligaments to avoid damage of the metacarpophalangeal joint.

Once all of the soft tissues are adequately dissected and prepared, the entire metacarpal bone is exposed.

Removing of the diaphysis metacarpal bone shortens the index finger. With the soft tissues retracted, two osteotomies through metaphyseal portion are performed in a perpendicular direction. The distal cut is directly through the physis using a fine blade. In this step, it is important to preserve the periosteal because it gives stability to the new CMC joint. Then it is performed the epiphysiodesis through physeal ablation to prevent unwanted growth of the new thumb.

The base and the head of the metacarpal bone are fixed into hyperextension position with a mini or micro mitek anchor. This position is made to rectify the discrepancy between index metacarpophalangeal joint that hyperextend and normal thumb carpometacarpal joint that does not hyperextend.

Many authors prefer to give the right position and fix the new joint with a Kirschner wire. Usually, we prefer to avoid that to allow early rehabilitation program. The correct position is reached by suturing the intrinsic muscle, tendons, and skin. Just in older children, the fixation with k wire could give more stability at the joint.

Next step is the reinsertion of intrinsic muscles and extensor tendons. The palmar and dorsal interossei muscles are sutured at the ulnar and radial bands, respectively. In this way, the palmar interossei muscles become the new adductor pollicis and the dorsal one the new abductor of the thumb. The proximal portion of extensor tendon is reattached to the central part of extensor complex to be new extensor pollicis longus.

This rebalancing gives a stable and good position to the thumb: about 45 degrees of abduction and 135 degrees of pronation.

Once the index finger has been secured in the new position is important to ensure hemostasis control to avoid bleeding and hematoma formation.

The final closure of the skin is performed with rotation of the volar part of the flap to cover the first web space. This allows avoiding scar in the first web space and giving more stability to the thumb. Any redundant skin is excised (Fig. 14.3).

The procedure is completed. The tourniquet is deflated. Any persistent bleeding, ischemia or venous congestion must be investigated before making the dressing. The upper extremity is immobilized with a well-padded long arm cast with the thumb in an opposition.

The child is admitted overnight and the arm is elevated to promote venous drainage. Ten days later, the cast and the dressing are removed under sedation and replaced with removable split. From now start the rehabilitation program.

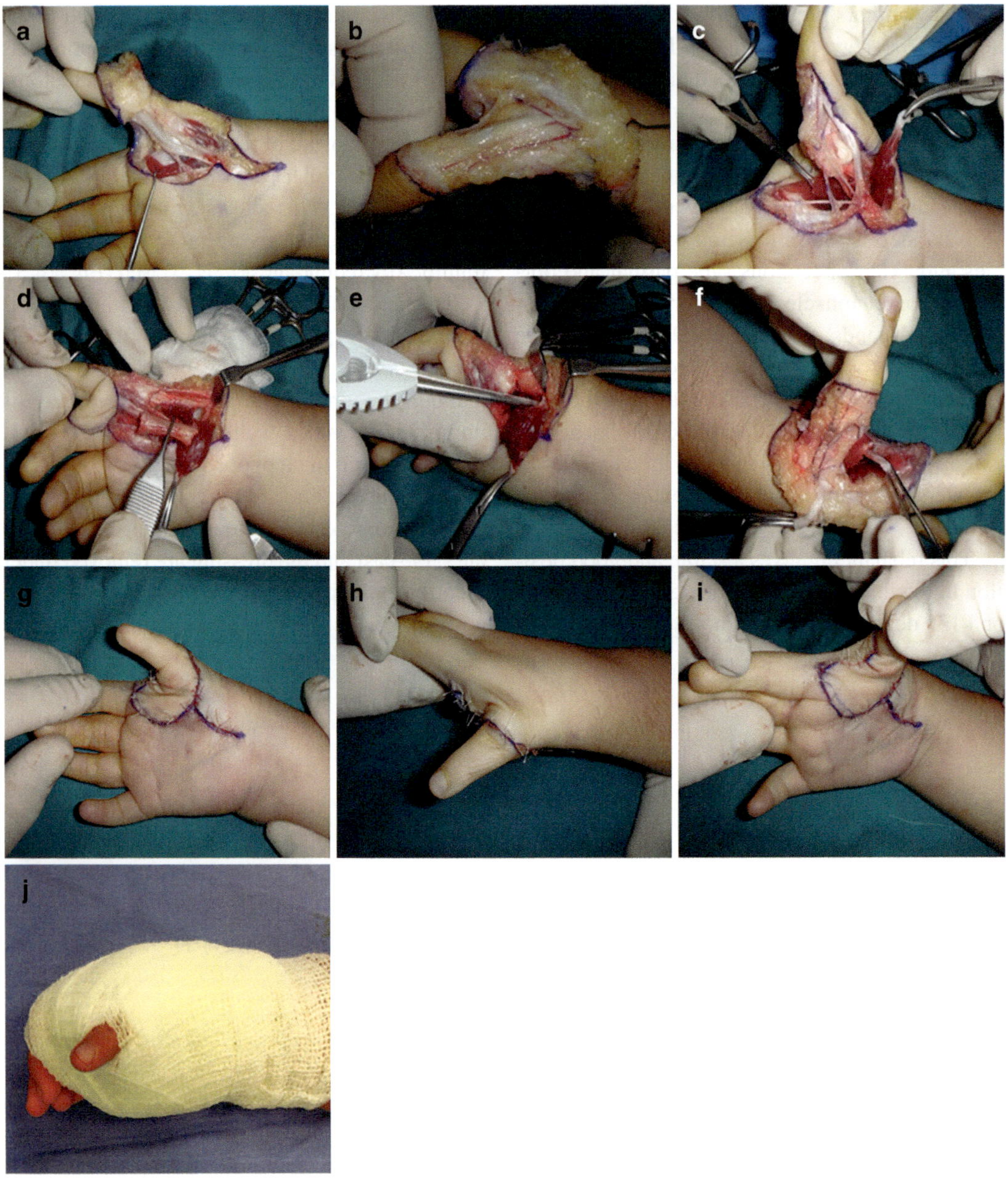

Fig. 14.3 Pollicization technique: (**a**) isolation of the index finger, including the neurovascular bundles, tendons, and soft tissue attachments. (**b**) Isolation of dorsal veins and extensor tendons. (**c**) Detached interossei muscles and reserved for later reconstruction. (**d**) Isolated metacarpal bone (**e**). Fixation with anchor base and head of metacarpal bone. (**f**) Reinsertion interossei muscles. (**g–i**) Final skin suture. (**j**) Dressing and cast

14.6 Complications and Outcomes

The common complications are wound dehiscence and maceration, necrosis of distal part of the flap. Infection and hematomas are rare. Vascular compromise can occur but is extremely rare and can happen if the dissection will not respect the neurovascular bundle.

Long-term complications are: keloid or hypertrophic scar, insufficient first web space, excess of length caused for ablation's failure growth

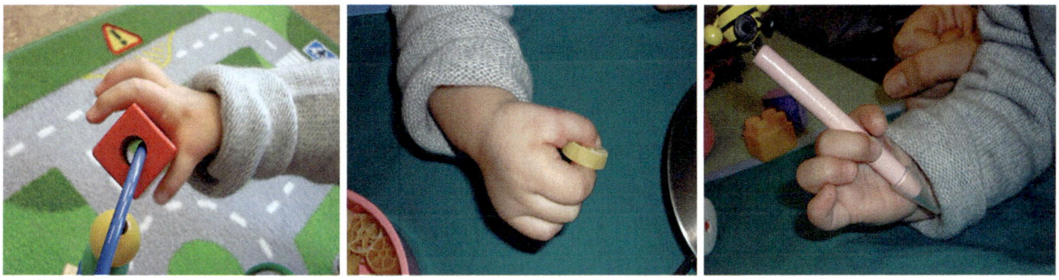

Fig. 14.4 Pollicization results

plate, hyperextension of MCP joint, malrotation of the thumb, stiffness or instability, lack of opposition.

Sometimes this result needs a second surgery as revision of first web space, tenolysis, epiphysiodesis and osteotomy of metacarpal, rotational osteotomy, and opposition transfer [14].

The results following pollicization are dependent on the status of index finger and its surrounding musculature. Pollicization of index finger provides a better result in isolated thumb hypoplasia compared with patients with a hypoplastic or absent radius [15].

A mobile index finger transferred to the thumb position provides stability for grasp and mobility for fine pinch. A stiff index finger, however, provides a stable thumb for gross grasp but will not be nimble enough to participate in pinch [16].

Pollicization is one of the most beautiful procedures in congenital disease but is a relatively uncommon procedure that requires considerable repetition to gain adequate experience. The surgeon must be expert to reach the best result and avoid dramatic complications (Fig. 14.4).

References

1. Upton J III. Hypoplastic or absent thumb. In: Mathes S, Hentz V, editors. Plastic surgery, vol. 8. Amsterdam: Saunders; 2006. p. 323–67.
2. Rayan G. Congenital thumb hypoplasia. J Okla State Med Assoc. 1995;87:546–50.
3. Edgerton M, Snyder G, Webb W. Surgical treatment of congenital thumb deformities (including impact of correction). J Bone Joint Surg. 1965;47(8):1453–74.
4. Kozin SH. Upper-extremity congenital anomalies. J Bone Joint Surg. 2003;85:1564–76.
5. Entin M. Congenital anomalies of the upper extremity. Surg Clin N Am. 1960;40:497.
6. Flatt A. The care of congenital hand anomalies. St. Louis: CV Mosby; 1977. p. 55–79.
7. Manske PR, McCaroll HR Jr, James MA. Type IIA hypoplastic thumb. J Hand Surg. 1995;20A:246–53.
8. Manske PR, Rotman MB, Dailey LA. Long-term functional results after pollicization for the congenitally deficient thumb. J Hand Surg Am. 1992;17(6):1064–72.
9. Buck-Gramcko D. Pollicization of the index finger: method and results in aplasia and hypoplasia of the thumb. J Bone Joint Surg Am. 1971;53(8):1605–17.
10. Littler JW. On making a thumb: one hundred years of surgical effort. J Hand Surg Am. 1976;1(1):35–51.
11. McCarroll HR. Congenital anomalies: a 25-year overview. J Hand Surg Am. 2000;25(6):1007–37.
12. McDonald TJ, James MA, McCarroll HR, Redlin H. Reconstruction of the type IIIA hypoplastic thumb. Tech Hand Up Extrem Surg. 2008;12(2):79–84.
13. Foucher G, Medina J, Loréa P, Pivato G, Szabó Z. Pollicization in congenital differences. Handchir Mikrochir Plast Chir. 2004;36:146–51.
14. Kozin SH, Zlotolow DA. Common pediatric congenital conditions of the hand. Plast Reconstr Surg. 2015;136(2):241e–57e.
15. Kozin SH, Weiss AA, Webber JB, Betz RR, Clancy M, Steel HH. Functional results after index finger pollicization for congenital aplasia or hypoplasia of the thumb. J Hand Surg Am. 1992;17:880–4.
16. Kozin SH. Pollicization: the concept, technical details, and outcome. Clinics Orthop Surg. 2012;4(1):18–35.

15 Radial Longitudinal Deficiency: Classification and Surgical Technique

Steven E. R. Hovius, Martijn Baas, and Christianne A. van Nieuwenhoven

Abstract

Radial longitudinal deficiencies comprise a spectrum of anomalies that require type-specific surgical or conservative treatments. This chapter reports our experience of over 300 arms. Multiple corrections have been described, in general a treatment algorithm should start with stabilisation of the wrist before specific corrections are made to improve hand function, such as a pollicisation or an opponens plasty. If indicated, lengthening of the forearm or cosmetic corrections can be performed, although one must consider that these corrections could jeopardise obtained wrist stabilisation and hand function. Partial recurrence of the radial deviation of the wrist is commonly reported, however, this does not necessarily lead to inability. Inability seems to be mostly affected by overall hand function.

Keywords

Radial longitudinal deficiency
Epidemiology · Classification · Surgical management · Outcomes

15.1 Radial Longitudinal Deficiency and Syndromes

Radial longitudinal deficiency (RLD) exhibits a wide spectrum of radial anomalies of the upper limb, ranging from thumb hypoplasia to a completely absent radius, humeral and shoulder anomalies. It is the most common longitudinal failure of formation with a prevalence estimated between 1 in 15,000–25,000 live births [1, 2]. RLD is also one of the congenital upper limb anomalies that most frequently present with associated anomalies, some of which have major surgical implications or can be life-threatening [3].

The most frequently associated syndromes/associations include VACTERL association, Holt–Oram syndrome, Thrombocytopenia absent radius (TAR) syndrome, Fanconi anaemia and Duane-Radial Ray syndrome [4]. However, the differential diagnosis for radial longitudinal

S. E. R. Hovius (✉)
The Xpert Clinics, Rotterdam, The Netherlands

Radboudumc University Medical Center, Nijmegen, The Netherlands
e-mail: s.hovius@xpertclinic.nl; steven.hovius@radboudumc.nl

M. Baas
Department of Plastic and Reconstructive Surgery, Amsterdam University Medical Center, Amsterdam, The Netherlands
e-mail: m.baas@erasmusmc.nl

C. A. van Nieuwenhoven
Department of Plastic and Reconstructive Surgery and Hand Surgery, Erasmus University Medical Center, Rotterdam, The Netherlands
e-mail: c.vannieuwenhoven@erasmusmc.nl

G. Pajardi (ed.), *Pediatric Hand Surgery*, https://doi.org/10.1007/978-3-031-30984-7_15

Table 15.1 RLD syndromes and their associated anomalies and suggested diagnostics

Syndrome	Associated anomalies	Recommended diagnostics
Holt–Oram syndrome	Cardiac anomalies	Echocardiogram Complete blood count Abdominal/renal ultrasound Radiographs of the spine Chromosome breakage test
	Vertebral anomalies	
Fanconi anaemia	Blood Dyscrasias	
	Ear anomalies, deafness, facial anomalies	
	Renal anomalies	
TAR syndrome	Thrombocytopenia, present in the first months of life	
	Cardiac anomalies	
	Renal anomalies	
VACTERL syndrome	Vertebral anomalies	
	Anal atresia	
	Cardiac anomalies	
	Tracheoesophageal fistula/oesophageal atresia	
	Renal anomalies	

defects extends to over 30 syndromes and associations [5].

In patients with multiple severe anomalies, the RLD will be one of the last anomalies to be (surgically) addressed. However, in our practice, it occurs that the hand surgeon is the first to be consulted in a patient who, after a thorough examination, appears to have additional congenital anomalies. Therefore, the surgeon dealing with RLD should be well aware of the spectrum of anomalies that can present with RLD. Furthermore, there are numerous anomalies that could influence the per-operative condition of the patient, e.g. thrombocytopenia in TAR syndrome or tracheomalacia in VACTERL patients which might not be noticed till the first sleep induction by the anaesthesiologist. Thus, thorough clinical examination is warranted (Table 15.1) and paediatricians and/or geneticists should be consulted when multiple congenital anomalies are present [6].

15.2 Presentation

Patients with RLD can present at the outpatient clinic with a variation of malformations in the upper limb (Table 15.2). The mildest form is hypoplasia of the thumb with or without stiffness of the radial-sided fingers. Patients may only present because of the hypoplastic thenar musculature. The most severe forms of RLD can affect both entire arms with complete absence of the radius, humeral and shoulder deformities. The time of presentation depends on the severity of the anomaly and the general development of the child: in mild anomalies, the first signs might be the aberrant employment of the hand when the child starts to grasp small objects or even at a moment when the child finds problems with writing. This is in contrast with cases with severe anomalies which are referred directly postnatally or even prenatally.

Table 15.2 Clinical presentation of radial longitudinal deficiencies can include

Hypoplastic or absent thumb, sometimes radial polydactyly
Absent, hypoplastic or stiff fingers predominantly on the radial side of the hand
Radial deviation of the wrist
Agenesis or hypoplasia of scaphoid, trapezium, trapezoid and lunate
Agenesis or hypoplasia of the radius
Growth deficit of the ulna with or without bowing
Growth deficit of the humerus
Hypoplastic gleno-humeral development
High prevalence of bilateral occurrence, although contralateral anomalies can be minor

Commonly, patients present with unilateral complaints but have bilateral anomalies at physical examination. Left – right differences can occur randomly, but also predisposition for left-sided anomalies have been described in Holt-Oram syndrome [7].

15.3 Function

Like Flatt pointed out, RLD is an abnormal hand joined to a poor limb by a bad wrist [8]. The functional deficit depends on the bilateral or unilateral occurrence of RLD, the quality and strength of the thumb and remaining digits, radial deviation of the wrist and the length of the forearm. Patients who are affected bilaterally have a bad upper limb function in terms of washing, dressing, feeding, in essence most activities of daily life. However, they compensate very well by using alternative methods to achieve their activities in daily life. Unilateral cases use the affected limb mainly as an aid. Depending on the stiffness of the fingers either the index and the middle finger or the ring finger and the little finger are used for a scissors grip. In a very young child, hand function analysis is not well established, while in an older child, hand function analysis should be included in decision-making.

15.4 Classification

To establish a treatment algorithm, it is useful to classify the observed anomalies. In current literature, the most accepted classification scheme is the modified Bayne and Klug classification (Table 15.3) [9, 10]. The modified Bayne and Klug classification takes into account the developmental defects in the thumb, the carpus, both the proximal and the distal radius, and the humerus. Based on the observed defects, the limb is classified in a range from Type N, including just a hypoplastic thumb or absent thumb, to Type 5 which would include an absent radius and hypoplasia of the proximal humerus and glenoid (Fig. 15.1).

The type N RLD only comprises thumb hypoplasia or the total absence of the thumb. The severity of thumb hypoplasia or aplasia does not necessarily correlate with the severity of other radial defects, for example patients with TAR syndrome often have thumbs. Therefore, the thumb is a separate entity in the classification but the severity of thumb hypoplasia does not differentiate between any of the other RLD types in the classification. The severity of hypoplasia of the thumb does influence the surgical algorithm regarding opposition plasty or pollicisation and should therefore be thoroughly evaluated.

Type 0 RLD comprises of either carpal bone defects or proximal radial defects such as radioulnar synostosis or congenital radial head dislocation or easy subluxation. The distal radius is normally developed in Type 0 RLD. Differentiation between a Type N or Type 0 RLD might not be possible at the first consultation, as the radial carpal bones will start ossifying at the age of 4–6 years, with complete ossification at 12–14 years. Before ossification, only radial deviation of the wrist without distal radial anomalies indicates carpal bone defects. However, radial deviation is not a formal component of the modified Bayne classification.

Table 15.3 The modified Bayne and Klug classification for RLD

Type	Thumb	Carpal bones	Distal radius	Proximal radius	Humerus
N	Absent or Hypoplastic	Normal	Normal	Normal	Normal
0	Absent or Hypoplastic	Absent, hypoplasia or coalition	Normal	Normal, radioulnar synostosis, radial head dislocation	Normal
1	Absent or Hypoplastic	Absent, hypoplasia or coalition	>2 mm shorter than ulna	Normal, radioulnar synostosis, radial head dislocation	Normal
2	Absent or Hypoplastic	Absent, hypoplasia or coalition	Hypoplasia	Hypoplasia	Normal
3	Absent or Hypoplastic	Absent, hypoplasia or coalition	Physis absent	Hypoplasia	Normal
4	Absent or Hypoplastic	Absent, hypoplasia or coalition	Absent	Absent	Normal
5	Absent or Hypoplastic	Absent, hypoplasia or coalition	Absent	Absent	Abnormal glenoid and proximal humerus

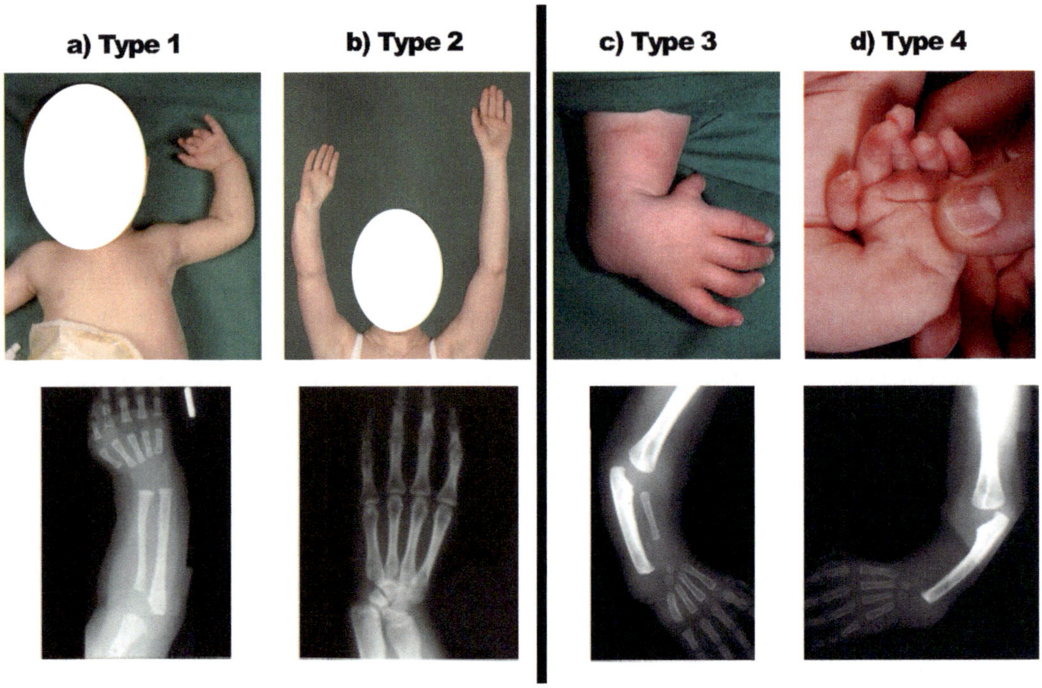

Fig. 15.1 (**a**) Type 1: radius >2mm shorter with deviation of the wrist. (**b**) Type 2: adult with absent and hypoplastic carpal bones and short radius. (**c**) Type 3: very short radius with absent physis and hypoplastic thumb and carpus. (**d**) Type 4: absent radius and hypoplastic thumb and hypoplstic and absent carpal bones

Types 1 to 3 are defined by increasing severity of radial hypoplasia, with a minimum difference of 2 mm shortening of the distal radius compared to the ulna in Type 1. When the proximal radius is also hypoplastic, it is considered a Type 2 RLD. Lastly, when there is no physis of the distal radius, the anomaly is classified as a Type 3 RLD.

Types 4 and 5 are both defined by a completely absent radius and, in Type 5, also proximal hypoplasia of the humerus and glenoid co-exist. It is noteworthy that also in less severe RLD, the humerus might be shorter as compared to healthy individuals. However, this hypoplasia is different to the humeral anomalies observed in Type 5 RLD [10].

Alternative to the modified Bayne and Klug classification, Simo Vilkki published his severity grading, which focuses more on the quality and range of motion of the remaining digits, the wrist and the elbow joint (Table 15.4) [11]. Although this severity grading has not been psychometrically validated, it has been used as a predictor for less favourable outcomes of RLD surgery [12]. The Vilkki severity grading scores the Hand, Wrist radial deviation and Proximal deficits (WHP) (Table 15.3). Higher points reflect the severity of the condition. A separate chapter in this book written by Simo Vilkki will be provided on longitudinal radial deficiency containing a different treatment algorithm.

Table 15.4 Vilkki HWP severity grading

		Severity points
HAND	Useful thumb	−2
	Stiff MCP II-V, flexion <45 degrees	1/digit
	Stiff or camptodactylic PIP II-V, extension deficit >20 degrees	1/digit
	Absence of digit or ray II-V	2/ray
	Syndactyly between digits II-III	1
	Ulnar pinching pattern	1
WRIST	Mild radial deviation (10–30 degrees)	2
	Moderate radial deviation (30–60 degrees)	4
	Severe radial deviation (60–90 degrees)	6
	Extreme radial deviation (>90 degrees)	8
	Ulna bow 20–40 degrees	1
	Ulna bow >40 degrees	2
	Neglected early splinting (start >6 months)	2
PROXIMAL	Elbow extension deficit >15 degrees	1
	Elbow flexion: Weak active 60–80 degrees	2
	Below 60 degrees	3
	No active flexion	4
	Shoulder abduction or flexion <120 degrees	3
	Intercalary bone defect, major shoulder instability	6
Total maximum		30 (max 10 points/domain

15.5 Treatment

The treatment options for RLD comprise conservative methods, surgical correction or a combination of both. Conservative methods of treatment should start early, if possible, a few days after birth. Both splinting and soft tissue manipulation by the parents have been described. Splinting however in very small children is cumbersome. Therefore, we advise frequent manipulation and stretching of the wrist instead of splinting to overcome as much of the radial deviation as possible before starting surgical correction of the wrist, or continuing with correction of the thumb. Many surgical corrections have been described; our surgical algorithm has four aims (Table 15.5).

Table 15.5 The aims of surgery

1. To stabilise the wrist on the distal end of the ulna, without further compromising the growth potential
2. To improve hand functions like prehension, grip and pinch strength
3. To increase the overall length of the forearm, without comprising hand function
4. To create a better appearance, without compromising hand function

Contraindications for surgery are seriously associated congenital differences. If possible, they should be corrected first. Next, the patient should be able to gain functional benefit from the correction. For instance, in patients with severe congenital differences or severe mental or other physical disabilities, we choose not to operate the RLD. Lastly, a stiff elbow is a contraindication since positioning of the hand in line with the ulna will prohibit moving the hand to the face [13, 14]. Note however that the elbow tends to become less stiff, thus this contraindication should be reevaluated over time.

Relative contraindications are Types I and II RLD according to Bayne and adolescents or adults who present with a primary, untreated, RLD. These patients are used to their deformity and do rather well in activities in daily living and their wish is mostly to be more socially accepted. However, correcting their deformity could jeopardise their hand function. Furthermore, a stiff wrist in radial deviation with stiff fingers is a relative contraindication for centralisation because the forearm will be short as the distal physis of the ulna will be damaged; and the wrist and fingers will not improve in function as they are stiff. To minimise the risk for range of motion loss, growth potential and complications due to extended surgery in RLD correction, some congenital hand surgery centres advocate to only do a soft tissue release and a bilobed flap for coverage [15].

15.6 Surgical Algorithm

Over the years, we developed a treatment algorithm based on a series comprising 308 arms (see Table 15.6). Treatment options will be discussed based on the type of deformity according to the Bayne and Klug classification.

15.6.1 Type N–0

The treatment for hypoplastic thumbs is described in a different chapter. However, the type N anomaly can be contralateral to a more severe RLD. In these cases, a personalised surgical planning should be made, taking into consideration the dexterity and the motor development of the child together with the general condition and the wish of the parents. In our practice, we would first do soft tissue distraction and wrist stabilisation and subsequently evaluate which side comes first to correct or create a thumb. In general, we would do the (supposed) dominant hand first. If possible, this enables the operated hand to train more when the contralateral side is treated [16]. The dominant hand however needs about 4–6 years to become obvious while treatment in our unit mostly starts much earlier.

15.6.2 Type I–II

In Types I and II, the distal radius is hypoplastic and the wrist is more radially deviated than normal wrists. Typically, the wrist can be passively corrected to central but it is not possible to ulnar deviate the wrist. In type II the radial deviation can become quite extensive with growth due to a growth deficit of the distal end of the radius in relation to the ulna. In most cases, Type I RLD does not require surgical intervention. In Type II RLD, often a tendon rebalancing with or without a wrist stabilisation is performed. Soft tissue distraction is seldom needed prior to wrist stabilisation in these cases. However, if soft tissue manipulation did not result in any correction of radial deviation and the radial deviation cannot be redressed, it can well be considered.

In the growing child, length discrepancies between radius and ulna in Type II RLD are difficult to correct. Non-vascularised bone grafts have been used, but the lengthened radius will always be too short as it doesn't have enough growth potential compared to the ulna. Vascularised bone with a growth plate does have this growth potential. Both proximal fibula and metatarsal phalangeal joint transfers have been described [17–22].

Table 15.6 Arms treated in our centre, according to the modified Bayne and Klug classification

Type	Arms
N	24
0	111
1	32
2	13
3	21
4	104
5	1
Not classifiable	2
Total	**308**

15.6.3 Type III–V

Treatment of radial deviation in RLD Types III–V is most challenging and has been extensively studied [13, 23–33]. At the Department of Plastic and Reconstructive Surgery of the Erasmus University Medical Center Rotterdam, children with these anomalies have been treated from 1972 onwards. Before 1987 arthrodesis of the wrist was mostly performed [34, 35]. Since 1987, the wrists in radial dysplasia Type III or IV were stabilised with as much preservation of the carpus and soft tissues as possible, using a modified Bayne's technique [30]. Our current algorithm is presented in Table 15.7.

Table 15.7 Treatment algorithm in Types III–V RLD

1. Preoperative manipulation and splinting to decrease radial deviation
2. Soft tissue distraction
3. Wrist stabilisation with or without ulna osteotomy
4. Pollicisation or opposition plasty
5. Forearm lengthening
Treatment starts in the first year, if no contra-indications exist

In the earlier days, during wrist stabilisation procedures the distal ulna was often shaved, carpal bones were partially excised, tightness of soft tissues could be difficult to overcome, and wrist mobility could be severely impaired. Several authors have tried to overcome the same problems by pre-treatment with distraction [36–41] to facilitate stabilisation. Therefore, we started to distract from 1993 onwards at our department before stabilisation of the wrist.

15.7 Distraction of the Soft Tissues at Wrist Level

Since 1993, we used an external device, a modified Orthofix external distractor (EBI Medical Systems, Inc., Parsipanny, NJ) for distraction of the soft tissues at wrist level. The external distractor was modified with a longer body for distraction. Using an open technique, the pins are manually inserted at the radial side, and placed in the distal ulna (two pins), and in the second and third metacarpal (two pins). Initially, the fixator was placed at the ulnar side. However, the pins are inclined to be pulled out by the forces during distraction. Great forces are needed to reposition the wrist on the distal end of the ulna, thus pushing seems better than pulling. Furthermore, the deformation is mainly on the radial side therefore distraction seems logical on the pathologic side when using a uni- or biplanar external fixator. Soft tissue distraction is carried out by the parents (if possible once or twice daily half turns, resulting in approximately 0.25–0.5 mm per day). When the proximal carpal configuration is distracted distally to the distal end of the ulna in preferably a central position, distraction is stopped. The main complication was the loosening of pins with or without pin track infection. The fixator is maintained about 4 weeks after completion of the distraction before the wrist stabilisation procedure is performed preserving mobility at wrist level (Fig. 15.2).

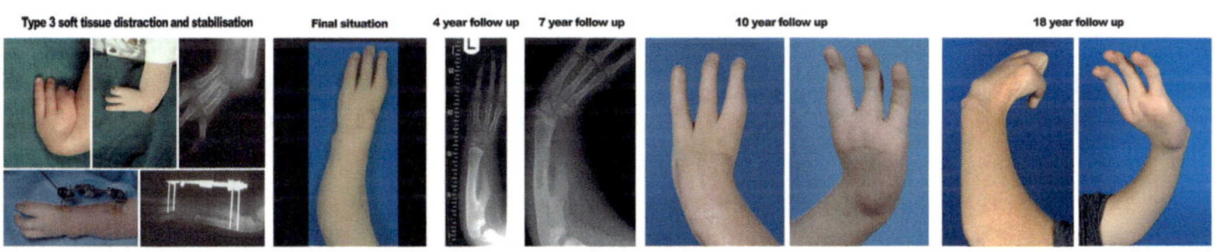

Fig. 15.2 Long term follow-up from early manipulation of the hand, soft tissue distraction, stabilisation of the wrist, Xrays and pictures of the distal forearm and hand show an increase in radial deviation over 18 year follow up

15.8 Wrist Stabilisation

In this chapter, we will use the term wrist stabilisation. This has been done to prevent misunderstanding with the terms centralisation and radialisation.

Centralisation has been popularised by Douglas Lamb [42]. In centralisation, an ulnocarpal arthrodesis is performed following soft tissue release. In this technique, a slot is created in the carpus following which the distal end of the ulna is shaved and inserted into the slot.

The term radialisation is introduced by Buck-Gramcko [43]. The main difference in his technique is that he preserves the pseudo-wrist. Following thorough release of the soft tissues and capsule, the distal end of the ulna is shaved as well as the proximal carpus. The carpus is shifted more to the ulnar side thus the distal end of the ulna is subsequently more radial. If possible, the tight radial structures are transposed to the ulnar side.

In our unit, the treatment of longitudinal radial deficiency and especially the repositioning of the wrist can be divided in the period before distraction and after distraction.

Before distraction, radial and ulnar skin incisions were used, and a bilobed flap according to Evans [26, 44] was performed. The pseudo capsule was extensively released in a circular manner. Furthermore, in Bayne's technique [30] the remnants of the radial muscles should be transposed to the ulnar side. In a number of cases, these remnants were mostly inactive and very fibrotic, and therefore were not transposed. If necessary carpal bone (mostly partial lunate) was excised, the distal ulna was 'shaved', and/or osteotomy of the ulna was performed in severe bowing. Shortening of the extensor carpi ulnaris was performed in all wrists together with tightening of the ulnar capsule.

From 1993 onwards, following distraction, it was not necessary to perform an Evans bilobed transposition flap anymore because of an adequate soft tissue cover. Also, it was hardly necessary to partially or totally excise carpal bones and shave the distal ulna as was nearly always performed before distraction.

15.9 Pollicisation

Pollicisation is described extensively in a different chapter; thus, we will only emphasise our indications. There is no consensus when a pollicisation should be performed in RLD. Usually, pollicisation is performed in the hand with severe hypoplastic or absent thumbs with relatively normal forearms. In some cultures, the emphasis is more towards maintaining the hypoplastic first digit and attempts are made to reconstruct the hypoplastic thumb. In general, if a patient has a scissor grip between the two most ulnar digits, pollicisation might not be feasible because the pollicised index finger-mostly stiff will not be used. Furthermore, in severely hypoplastic or absent radial bones, the indication for pollicisation can be debated. In these cases, the new 'thumbs' are very weak in strength in contrast to the pollicised index fingers in the four-fingered hand without forearm problems [45]. Therefore, our indication for pollicisation in RLD Types III and IV is when the index and middle finger are used as scissors grip, together with the wish of the parents and/or child depending on their age. When the index and the middle finger are used, the position of the index finger changes in time with pronation of the index finger itself and widening of the 'second' web, obtaining a thumb like position. Seemingly, the index finger is already represented in the brain as a thumb, making incorporation of the pollicised index finger practicable to the child. In bilateral RLD Types III and IV with a radial scissors grip, the pollicisation's do better as in the unilateral cases as the need to use them is more urgent. A typical result of pollicisation is presented in Fig. 15.3.

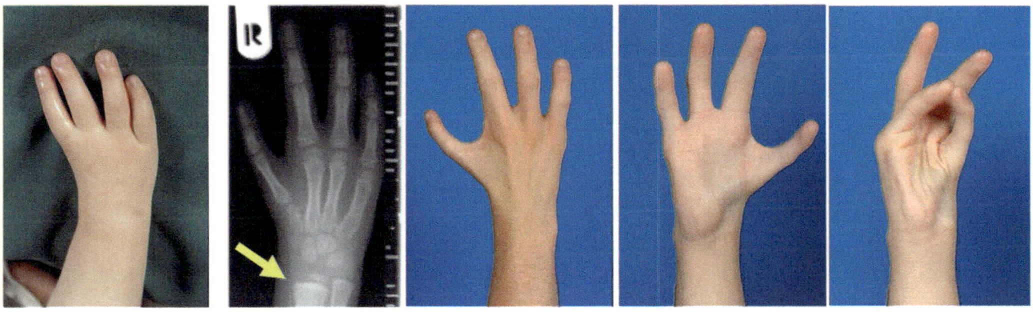

Fig. 15.3 Results of pollicisation of the contralateral hand of the same patient as in Fig. 15.2

15.10 Ulnar Bone Distraction in RLD

The goals of forearm distraction lengthening are to improve aesthetic appearance and to increase function. With lengthening of the forearm, the affected arm can function more optimally in space, precluding abnormal elbow and shoulder function. Since we have used distraction however growth of the ulna has been far better than before distraction, indicating that the pressure on the distal ulnar growth plate is less leading to less growth disturbance in an already diminished growing ulna because of the disease. The indication to lengthen the ulna has therefore become less.

Several elongation techniques have been reported, however, in series with mixed diagnosis, using different devices, gaining from 2 to 13 cm in ulnar length [10, 14, 46–48]. Peterson e.a. reported the experience with Ilizarov lengthening in a homogenous group of patients with radial longitudinal deficiency [48]. The average gain of forearm length reported was 4.4 cm, with a mean lengthening index of 9 weeks per cm. Pin site infection was mentioned for all cases, with additional complications as delayed union and recurrence of radial deviation.

We have used ulnar callus distraction in motivated children (and parents) with Types III and IV RLD, we have distracted the ulna in 15% of our patients.

The start of distraction varied from age 10–22 years old. We mainly used an Orthofix uniplanar device especially developed for us for the younger children, due to the extreme forces needed to lengthen the ulna substantially. In the older children, the normally available devices were used. Distraction took 6 months to 18 months depending on the number of problems encountered and if the patient could endure the whole process. Length was gained from 4 to 13 centimetres (average 8 cm) (Fig. 15.4). A lengthening of 4 cm is insufficient as the length discrepancy between the forearms is still large. Nearly every patient had pin-track infections. We used special pins covered with hydroxyapatite to ensure a better fixation in the bone. This did indeed result in less loosening. Early union was encountered, but rare. Non-union occurred in two cases leading to necessitate a free fibular flap in one and a vascularised transfer of the remnant radius in the other. In both cases, union was achieved. Neurologic deficits or vascular problems were not encountered, probably because of the slow rate of distraction. After distraction, the ulna is usually fixated using plates and screws to prevent fractures. We have encountered a fracture in one patient without plate and screw fixation of the distracted ulna.

Following distraction fingers and elbow can become stiffer. The slow rate of distraction however provides ample time to diminish stiffness. If the growth plate of the distal end of the ulna was

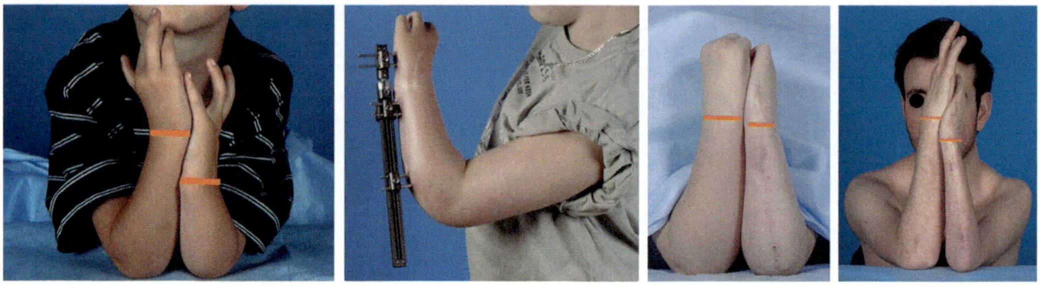

Fig. 15.4 Results of ulnar bone distraction of the same patient as in Fig. 15.2

intact before bone distraction, it stayed intact even after long-term distraction.

It is also common with increased lengthening that radial deviation increases. It is the reason why the device is also fixed to the metacarpal bones.

15.11 Outcomes in RLD Treatment

15.11.1 Function, Participation and Activity

As discussed, the optimal treatment for RLD is patient and anomaly specific. Therefore, treatment-specific long-term outcome data is sparse. However, multiple studies have used the International Classification of Function, Disability and Health context to objectify disabilities in RLD cases [12, 49–51]. In general, all studies describe little or no limitations on the activity and participation levels of RLD patients. This observation was explained by the fact that children adapt well to their physical limitations over time.

Although stabilisation of the wrist is one of the main objectives in the correction of RLD, long-term data suggest that radial angulation is not the most important factor for activity or self-perceived disability. It is even suggested that there is no difference in patients who did or did not undergo stabilisation of the wrist. Considering the retrospective nature of the study, the possible bias by indication and the limited patients included, these results should be interpreted with great care. The questionnaires used are also non-specific. However, the consensus should be not to strive for an anatomical position of the wrist, but rather to strive for a position that does not restrict the employability of the hand [12, 49].

Rather than radial deviation of the wrist, studies based on the ICF model suggest that range of motion of the digits and wrist may be more important to activity and participation. Furthermore, in adults, grip strength, key pinch, forearm length and elbow motion also seemed to be more important. Unfortunately, not all of these deficits can be addressed, e.g. elbow motion can often be compromised by elbow movement restrictions which can be part of the RLD spectrum of anomalies. Furthermore, lengthening the forearm can cause subluxation of the wrist which then would compromise wrist range of motion. In practice, detailed evaluation of the patient's limitations in activity is the only option to prioritise one operative goal over another.

The appearance of the arm was studied by multiple authors using questionnaires or VAS scales. Overall, patients rate their arm at a level of 25–50% on a VAS scale from best to worst aesthetic outcome. Furthermore, patients indicated that they have very low expectations of improvement of appearance of their limb by surgery [12, 32, 49, 50].

15.11.2 Surgical Versus Non-surgical Treatment

Few studies directly compare non-surgical treatment with centralisation or radialisation. Kotwal et al. described in their retrospective review a population of 446 patients, of which 109 were not operated and 202 had a centralisation and 107 a radialisation [52]. Strength was more than three times as much in the operated group. Appearance and patient-reported outcome scored better in the operated group. Recurrence of radial deviation (>35°wrist) in the operated group occurred in 15% ($n = 46$), while recurrence of ulnar bowing occurred in 22% (Early reoperations occurred in 6.5% ($n = 20$) and late reoperations in 10% ($n = 31$). Reoperations occurred 2.4 times more in the centralisation group.

Murphy et al. performed a meta-review in 2017 consisting of 12 selected articles [53].

Non-surgical patients with RLD had 84° radial deviation at long-term follow-up and a 'wrist' active motion of 61° which was better than most patients after surgery. In these patients, ulnar length was predicted to be 64% of normal. Soft tissue release only had a modest decrease in radial deviation when compared with non-operated patients. Soft tissue distraction with either centralisation or radialisation achieved 16° radial deviation, while radialisation maintained better active 'wrist' function of 46° and ulnar length when compared with centralisation.

When microvascular second metatarsophalangeal joint transfer was performed 'wrist' active motion was 83°, with good ulnar length when compared to other surgical techniques, but with more radial deviation (28°).

Little data is available on soft tissue distraction prior to wrist stabilisation of RLD. Dana et al. describe a visible recurrence of the radial deformity in seven out of eight patients [54]. Furthermore, Manske et al. reported their long-term follow-up data comparing wrist stabilisation with wrist stabilisation after soft tissue distraction. Based on 13 limbs, they conclude that although soft tissue distraction facilitates wrist stabilisation it might not contribute to less recurrence of radial deviation or volar subluxation. On the contrary, these parameters were slightly worse than the non-distraction group. Nevertheless, the authors continue to use soft tissue distraction to facilitate wrist stabilisation [55].

In our experience, fewer secondary corrections were needed since the introduction of distraction. Also, the growth plate of the distal end of the ulna was preserved in all soft tissue distraction patients- except one with partial fusion- with subsequent wrist stabilisation at long-term follow-up. Growth in patients who didn't have later ulnar bone distraction was 75% of the normal length, compared to approximately 50% in the patients who did not have soft tissue distraction prior to wrist stabilisation. A few dislocations were encountered at long-term follow-up, this occurred with or without prior soft tissue distraction.

15.11.3 Pollicisation in RLD Patients

Pollicisation outcomes in patients with RLD are far less optimal in patients with RLD as compared to isolated thumb hypoplasia. Many articles have reported on their results following pollicisation. Only a few functional data are compared with normative comparable age data of thumb function. This is important because when pollicisation's are compared with the other side outcome can be far better as the other side is very often not normal [45]. Extensive evaluation of the pollicisation range of motion revealed that overall the range of motion is about 20–95 percent of the healthy thumb range of motion, whereas the strength is 13–77%. In severe RLD patients (Types III and IV), especially flexion in the MP joint and opposition range of motion were significantly less. Furthermore, all strength measurements (such as Grip strength, Pinch strength and Key Pinch) are significantly lower in severe RLD patients. In severe RLD, 62% required additional abductor digiti quinti opponens plasty (Huber transfer) to correct opposition range of motion and strength. It seems therefore logical to aim for more stability in the transposed index by creating a stable base by fixation instead of a hypermobile pseudo-CMC1 joint. Even though range of motion and strength measurements are significantly different to normal, patients and their parents are satisfied with function and appearance of the pollicised index finger, regardless of the severity of the RLD.

15.11.4 Residual Ulnar Growth and Distraction Osteogenesis

The residual ulnar growth is different for operated and non-operated patients. In a study of 124 affected limb (mainly type IV), non-surgically treated patients attained 64% of the normal ulnar length at a mean age of 8 years, whereas the operated group attained 48–58% of normal ulnar length at a mean age of 9.8 years, depending on the surgical technique [56]. Ulna lengthening of as much as 7.0 cm or 75% of the preoperative length has been described [46]. Distraction is a lengthy procedure that took a mean duration of 204 days in this study. Recurrence of radial deviation and ulnar bowing is frequent and can nullify the ulnar length obtained during distraction. Furthermore, over-distraction can result in poor consolidation and cases in whom a fibula interposition graft was required have been described. As mentioned afore in our experience, distraction time varied from 6 to 18 months with a gained length from 4 to 13 centimetres (average 8 cm).

15.12 Conclusion

Radial longitudinal deficiency exhibits a spectrum of both bone and soft tissue malformations, ranging from thumb hypoplasia to radial agenesis with or without humeral involvement. Surgically corrected patients are often more satisfied than conservatively treated patients. However, the surgical algorithm should first focus on which patients not to operate, such as patients with a stiff elbow or stiff wrists in radial deviation with camptodactyly of the fingers, as overtreatment can further impair wrist motion, residual ulnar growth and can cause stiffer fingers. Growth of the forearm can be preserved by using soft tissue distraction before wrist positioning. Considering wrist positioning procedures, radialisation has better results than centralisation in terms of growth and wrist function. Recurrence rates of radial deviation are high in the growing limb.

Pollicisation is a useful adduct in the treatment of RLD, but should not be performed in patients who develop an ulnar grip pattern. Overall, a pollicised thumb functions less in RLD patients when compared to the four-fingered hand.

Ulnar lengthening should be used selectively, as it can induce recurrence of radial deviation. To my opinion, it should not be used if less than 5cm lengthening can be obtained.

References

1. Ekblom AG, Laurell T, Arner M. Epidemiology of congenital upper limb anomalies in Stockholm, Sweden, 1997 to 2007: application of the Oberg, Manske, and Tonkin classification. J Hand Surg Am. 2014;39(2):237–48.
2. Vasluian E, van der Sluis CK, van Essen AJ, et al. Birth prevalence for congenital limb defects in the northern Netherlands: a 30-year population-based study. BMC Musculoskelet Disord. 2013;14:323.
3. Wall LB, Ezaki M, Oishi SN. Management of congenital radial longitudinal deficiency: controversies and current concepts. Plast Reconstr Surg. 2013;132(1):122–8.
4. de Graaff E, Kozin SH. Genetics of radial deficiencies. J Bone Joint Surg Am. 2009;91(Suppl 4):81–6.
5. Baas M, Stubbs AP, van Zessen DB, et al. Identification of associated genes and diseases in patients with congenital upper-limb anomalies: a novel application of the OMT classification. J Hand Surg Am. 2017;42(7):533–545 e534.
6. Colen DL, Lin IC, Levin LS, Chang B. Radial longitudinal deficiency: recent developments, controversies, and an evidence-based guide to treatment. J Hand Surg Am. 2017;42(7):546–63.
7. Sulaiman FA, Nishimoto S, Murphy GR, et al. Tbx5 buffers inherent left/right asymmetry ensuring symmetric forelimb formation. PLoS Genet. 2016;12(12):e1006521.
8. Skerik SK, Flatt AE. The anatomy of congenital radial dysplasia. Its surgical and functional implications. Clin Orthop Relat Res. 1969;66:125–43.
9. James MA, McCarroll HR Jr, Manske PR. The spectrum of radial longitudinal deficiency: a modified classification. J Hand Surg Am. 1999;24(6):1145–55.
10. Goldfarb CA, Manske PR, Busa R, Mills J, Carter P, Ezaki M. Upper-extremity phocomelia reexamined: a longitudinal dysplasia. J Bone Joint Surg Am. 2005;87(12):2639–48.

11. Vilkki SK. Severity grading in radial dysplasia. J Hand Surg Eur. 2014;39(9):977–83.
12. Ekblom AG, Dahlin LB, Rosberg HE, Wiig M, Werner M, Arner M. Hand function in children with radial longitudinal deficiency. BMC Musculoskelet Disord. 2013;14:116.
13. Buck-Gramcko D. Radialization as a new treatment for radial club hand. J Hand Surg. 1985;10A(6 Pt 2):964–8.
14. Tonkin MA, Nanchahal J. An approach to the management of radial longitudinal deficiency. Ann Acad Med Singap. 1995;24(4 Suppl):101–7.
15. Ezaki M. Challenging the dogma: a straight wrist should be the goal in radial dysplasia. J Hand Surg Eur. 2021;46(1):14–20.
16. Ardon MS, Selles RW, Hovius SE, et al. Stronger relation between impairment and manual capacity in the non-dominant hand than the dominant hand in congenital hand differences; implications for surgical and therapeutic interventions. J Hand Ther. 2014;27(3):201–7; quiz 208
17. Morsy M, Parry JA, Moran SL. Vascularized second metatarsophalangeal joint transfer for salvage of failed centralization in Radial longitudinal deficiency: case report. Ann Plast Surg. 2017;78(2):195–7.
18. Yang J, Qin B, Li P, Fu G, Xiang J, Gu L. Vascularized proximal fibular epiphyseal transfer for Bayne and Klug type III radial longitudinal deficiency in children. Plast Reconstr Surg. 2015;135(1):157e–66e.
19. de Jong JP, Moran SL, Vilkki SK. Changing paradigms in the treatment of radial club hand: microvascular joint transfer for correction of radial deviation and preservation of long-term growth. Clin Orthop Surg. 2012;4(1):36–44.
20. Innocenti M, Delcroix L, Manfrini M, Ceruso M, Capanna R. Vascularized proximal fibular epiphyseal transfer for distal radial reconstruction. J Bone Joint Surg Am. 2005;87 Suppl 1(Pt 2):237–46.
21. Innocenti M, Delcroix L, Manfrini M, Ceruso M, Capanna R. Vascularized proximal fibular epiphyseal transfer for distal radial reconstruction. J Bone Joint Surg Am. 2004;86-A(7):1504–11.
22. Vilkki SK. Distraction and microvascular epiphysis transfer for radial club hand. J Hand Surg Br. 1998;23(4):445–52.
23. Tsuyuguchi Y, Yukioka M, Kawabata H, Kawai H, Ono K. Radial ray deficiency. J Pediatr Orthop. 1987;7(6):699–704.
24. Watson HK, Beebe RD, Cruz NI. A centralization procedure for radial clubhand. J Hand Surg. 1984;9A(4):541–7.
25. Pickford MA, Scheker LR. Distraction lengthening of the ulna in radial club hand using the Ilizarov technique. J Hand Surg. 1998;23B(2):186–91.
26. Pilz SM, Muradin MS, Van der Meulen JJ, Hovius SE. Evaluation of five different incisions for correction of radial dysplasia. J Hand Surg. 1998;23B(2):183–5.
27. Manske PR, McCarroll HRJ, Swanson K. Centralization of the radial club hand: an ulnar surgical approach. J Hand Surg. 1981;6A(5):423–33.
28. Manske PR, McCarroll HR Jr. Radial club hand. In: Buck-Gramcko, editor. Congenital malformations of the hand and forearm. London: Churchill Livingstone; 1998. p. 433–48.
29. Glossop ND, Flatt AE. Opening versus closing wedge osteotomy of the curved ulna in radial clubhand. J Hand Surg. 1995;20A(1):133–43.
30. Bayne LG, Klug MS. Long-term review of the surgical treatment of radial deficiencies. J Hand Surg. 1987;12A(2):169–79.
31. Damore E, Kozin SH, Thoder JJ, Porter S. The recurrence of deformity after surgical centralization for radial clubhand. J Hand Surg. 2000;25A(4):745–51.
32. Goldfarb CA, Klepps SJ, Dailey LA, Manske PR. Functional outcome after centralization for radius dysplasia. J Hand Surg. 2002;27A(1):118–24.
33. Geck MJ, Dorey F, Lawrence JF, Johnson MK. Congenital radius deficiency: radiographic outcome and survivorship analysis. J Hand Surg. 1999;24A(6):1132–44.
34. Lamb D. The treatment of radial club hand. Absent radius, aplasia of the radius, hypoplasia of the radius, radial paraxial hemimelia. Hand. 1972;4(1):22–30.
35. Lamb DW. Radial club hand. A continuing study of sixty-eight patients with one hundred and seventeen club hands. J Bone Joint Surg. 1977;59A(1):1–13.
36. Kessler I. Centralisation of the radial club hand by gradual distraction. J Hand Surg. 1989;14B(1):37–42.
37. Tonkin MA. Radial longitudinal deficiency (radial dysplasia, radial clubhand). In: Green DP, Hotchkiss RN, Pederson WC, editors. Green's operative hand surgery. 4th ed. Philadelphia, PA: Churchill Livingstone; 1999. p. 344–58.
38. Nanchahal J, Tonkin MA. Pre-operative distraction lengthening for radial longitudinal deficiency. J Hand Surg. 1996;21B(1):103–7.
39. Paley D, Herzenberg JE. Distraction treatment of the forearm. In: Buck-Gramcko, editor. Congenital malformations of the hand and forearm. London: Churchill Livingstone; 1998. p. 73–118.
40. Seitz WH Jr. Distraction lengthening in the hand and upper extremity. In: Green DP, Hotchkiss RN, Pederson WC, editors. Green's operative hand surgery. 4th ed. Philadelphia, PA: Churchill Livingstone; 1999. p. 619–35.
41. Catagni MA, Szabo RM, Cattaneo R. Preliminary experience with Ilizarov method in late reconstruction of radial hemimelia. J Hand Surg. 1993;18A(2):316–21.
42. Lamb DW. The treatment of longitudinal radial deficiency. Prosthetics Orthot Int. 1991;15(2):100–3.
43. Buck-Gramcko D. Radialization as a new treatment for radial club hand. J Hand Surg Am. 1985;10(6 Pt 2):964–8.
44. Evans DM, Gateley DR, Lewis JS. The use of a bilobed flap in the correction of radial club hand. J Hand Surg Br. 1995;20B(3):333–7.
45. de Kraker M, Selles RW, van Vooren J, Stam HJ, Hovius SE. Outcome after pollicization: comparison of patients with mild and severe longitudinal radial deficiency. Plast Reconstr Surg. 2013;131(4):544e–51e.

46. Farr S, Petje G, Sadoghi P, Ganger R, Grill F, Girsch W. Radiographic early to midterm results of distraction osteogenesis in radial longitudinal deficiency. J Hand Surg Am. 2012;37(11):2313–9.
47. Yoshida K, Kawabata H, Wada M. Growth of the ulna after repeated bone lengthening in radial longitudinal deficiency. J Pediatr Orthop. 2011;31(6):674–8.
48. Peterson BM, McCarroll HR Jr, James MA. Distraction lengthening of the ulna in children with radial longitudinal deficiency. J Hand Surg Am. 2007;32(9):1402–7.
49. Ekblom AG, Dahlin LB, Rosberg HE, Wiig M, Werner M, Arner M. Hand function in adults with radial longitudinal deficiency. J Bone Joint Surg Am. 2014;96(14):1178–84.
50. Holtslag I, van Wijk I, Hartog H, van der Molen AM, van der Sluis C. Long-term functional outcome of patients with longitudinal radial deficiency: cross-sectional evaluation of function, activity and participation. Disabil Rehabil. 2013;35(16):1401–7.
51. Buffart LM, Roebroeck ME, Janssen WG, et al. Hand function and activity performance of children with longitudinal radial deficiency. J Bone Joint Surg Am. 2008;90(11):2408–15.
52. Kotwal PP, Varshney MK, Soral A. Comparison of surgical treatment and nonoperative management for radial longitudinal deficiency. J Hand Surg Eur Vol. 2012;37(2):161–9.
53. Murphy GRF, Logan MPO, Smith G, Sivakumar B, Smith P. Correction of "wrist" deformity in radial dysplasia: a systematic review and meta-analysis. J Bone Joint Surg Am. 2017;99(24):2120–6.
54. Dana C, Auregan JC, Salon A, Guero S, Glorion C, Pannier S. Recurrence of radial bowing after soft tissue distraction and subsequent radialization for radial longitudinal deficiency. J Hand Surg Am. 2012;37(10):2082–7.
55. Manske MC, Wall LB, Steffen JA, Goldfarb CA. The effect of soft tissue distraction on deformity recurrence after centralization for radial longitudinal deficiency. J Hand Surg Am. 2014;39(5):895–901.
56. Sestero AM, Van Heest A, Agel J. Ulnar growth patterns in radial longitudinal deficiency. J Hand Surg Am. 2006;31(6):960–7.

Progressive Bone Distraction Lengthening in the Treatment of Congenital Malformations of the Upper Limb

16

Mario Paracuollo, Chiara Novelli, Giulietta Proserpio, Keit Young, and Giorgio Pajardi

Abstract

Congenital deficiencies and developmental deformities of the upper extremity often present deformities that include, to variable degrees, shortening and angulation of forearm, metacarpal o phalanx. The need for lengthening is mandatory when these deformities affect upper limb ability in bilateral manipulation and when they impede hand function. Common indications for bone lengthening include radial or ulnar longitudinal deficiency, multiple hereditary exostosis, brachymetacarpia, metacarpal sinostosis, symbrachydactyly, and posttraumatic growth arrest. The normal rate of distraction lengthening is about 1 mm/day for each bone in the upper extremity. When planning a lengthening procedure to the upper limb, the surgeon must be aware of the correct indications, the duration of the procedure—about 3 to 6 to 9 months, the demand of contemporaneous intense kinesiotherapy and also about possible complications. Complications are quite frequent; common complications are pins infection, pins rupture, and pins disruption; also delay in callus formation could happen, and sometimes it requires the need of a bone graft. The authors believe that the functional, cosmetic, and psychological benefits of upper limb lengthening outweigh the highly demanding procedure, in terms of surgical skill and patient and family collaboration.

Keywords

Bone distraction lengthening · Congenital deformities · Radial club hand Brachymetacarpia · Callus formation

M. Paracuollo (✉)
Milan University, Milan, Italy

Department of Hand Surgery, C.T.O. Hospital, Naples, Italy

C. Novelli · G. Proserpio · K. Young · G. Pajardi
Department of Hand Surgery and Rehabilitation, S. Giuseppe Hospital IRCCS MultiMedica, Milan University, Milan, Italy
e-mail: chiara.novelli@multimedica.it; gpajardi@centrostudimano.it

16.1 Historical Perspective

In 1902, Codivilla performed the first femoral lengthening procedure; as chief of the Rizzoli Institute in Bologna, he performed traction through a nail introduced into the calcaneum and, while a plaster cast maintained traction, renewed

G. Pajardi (ed.), *Pediatric Hand Surgery*, https://doi.org/10.1007/978-3-031-30984-7_16

plasters allowed for further "stages" of lengthening [1]. Putti, his assistant, further developed this work [2]. One of the pioneers in applying lengthening to upper limb and especially to the hand was Matev [3–8]. The first case of congenital malformation correction with bone distraction lengthening (BDL) was published by Kessler et al. in 1977 [9, 10]. Further indications for BDL in congenital malformations and in post-traumatic growth problems were developed by Ilizarov [11–17], Wagner [18], Monticelli [19–21], and De Bastani [22].

16.2 Indications

Malformations in which moderate bone lengthening could provide functional and cosmetic improvement is a potential indication for "Progressive bone distraction lengthening" (PBDL). Typically, young patients adapt to their disability by using different patterns of prehension, as such not all deformities need correction and function must never be compromised for the purpose of cosmesis. The amount of scaring and fibrosis should be considered when a "cosmetic" correction is planned. Similarly, elongation of a stiff finger for the purpose of cosmesis is inappropriate and may hamper the function [23, 24].

A cosmetic prosthetic device may be more appropriate; however, if the patient's appearance is greatly improved without added scar, the absence of sensibility could be functionally disturbing for the child. Functional prostheses may have a place in some cases of malformation, especially in some cultural backgrounds in order to hide the deformity, but have little place in unilateral agenesia. A combination of PBDL to fit a below-elbow myoelectric prostheses was used by Seitz et al. in a case of phocomelia [25–28]. In the hand, the prosthesis is rarely superior to PBDL, but a simple rigid arm compared to a mobile and unique thumb (even longer) could be proposed as a temporary or definitive help for function [29].

Among all of the techniques of restoring hand skeleton length, we count the following ones:

- Toe transfer: could provide, in one stage, a major lengthening with a good sensibility but Hodest mobility; despite some hypoplasia grades, symbrachydactyly with a unique thumb remains an excellent indication to this procedure [30–33]. According to our point of view, such an operation has to be performed early, before development of the pinch patter, or in any case within 5 years old [34, 35]. Congenital band syndrome with thumb amputation represents a perfect indication for reconstruction, but in this case, the limit of age is less relevant and, even if the integration is not total, the function is usually improved and the mobility is better because of normal tendons [36]. The major contraindications to the procedure are an associated foot malformation (absent toe) and parental decisions.
- Vascularized bone and epiphyseal transfer: Tsai treated forearm deformities with vascularized fibular epiphyseal transfer, but only few of them had shown persistent growth [37]. In case of both thumb hypoplasia and monodactylous type symbrachydactyly a good choice would be a vascularized epiphysis toe transfer combined with PBDL for the thumb [38, 39].
- Distal bone grafting: a free non-vascularized toe phalanx transfer is a simple one-stage procedure useful in case of "empty skin pouch" in case of transverse deficiency or symbrachydactyly, as well as in Blauth stage IIIB thumb hypoplasia with absent first carpo-metacarpal joint in order to provide better stabilization [40–43]. The mobility of the reconstructed joint is unpredictable as well as the length of the finger, which could be corrected by secondary PBDL. Goldberg and Watson showed that if the periosteum and the capsulo-ligamentous complex are preserved, some growth could be expected, at least when the operation is performed before 2 years of age [44].
- One-stage lengthening: osteotomy, liberation and perioperative distraction of the two fragments with a laminar-spreader is a recognized procedure [45]. However, the length obtained is less than with progressive distraction and the procedure is burdened by higher rate of complications compared with PBDL [46, 47].
- On-top plasty: an island composite transfer is a time-honored technique for both thumb and finger lengthening, especially indicated

for congenital band syndrome [48]. The amount of lengthening depends on the transferred stump and some loss has to be expected because of the palmar vessels shortness [49]. Ogino has compared single-stage lengthening with on-top plasty and PBDL the latter giving the greatest lengthening (12–13 mm) compared with one-stage and on-top (2–10 mm and 3–17 mm, respectively), as well as single-stage lengthening has demonstrated a higher rate of complications (malunion, bone graft collapse or resorptions, and delayed union caused by extensive liberation) [46].

PBDL can be performed at variable levels (radius, ulna, carpus, metacarpus, and phalanx), depending on the type of malformations (Table 16.1).

Patient age is a matter of debate. Matev proposed a lower limit of 8 years, and Kessler presented a series of 11 malformations treated by the PBDL procedure between five and 11 years old [6, 9]. Nowadays, the minimum surgical age for PBDL is 11 months, but the deciding factor is the quantity of bone to lengthen. One must consider the appropriate distance from the epiphysis to fix the four Kirschner-wires (K-wires) to distract the osteotomy-site. According to Smith and Greene, a "chondrotomy" is possible in the same way [29]. Another relevant local factor is the pliability of the distal skin in order to avoid soft tissue damage. With respect to forearm bone discrepancy, the beginning of PBDL should be combined with the clinical or radiological evidence of radial head subluxation [60].

Table 16.1 Type of malformations in which the progressive distraction bone lengthening has been used

Forearm:
• Radial deficiency or hemimelia, thrombocytopenia absent radius syndrome [50]
• Thumb hypoplasia
• Ulnar deficiency
• Multiple hereditary exostosis (Raimondo, Cheng) [16, 51–55], multiple enchondromatosis (Raimondo) [16, 56–58], dyschondrosteosis (Cheng) [51], phocomelia (Seitz) [26], Madelung's deformity [59]
• Hand:
• Brachydactyly, brachymetacarpy, and brachyphalangy.
• Symbrachydactyly, with insufficient length of the ulnar or radial ray, insufficient joint stability (lengthening-translocation), insufficient first web (lengthening-translocation-ray amputaion), amniotic band syndrome (either thumb or fingers)
• Metacarpal synostosis, central polydactyly, cleft hands short thumb with delta phalanx
• Apert syndrome (Upton, Pensler)

16.3 Operative Technique

The principle is to lengthen through a longitudinal dorsal or a lateral incision, minimal dissection, and protection of structures (neurovascular structures and tendons); four bicortical pins or K-wires are introduced proximally and distally in relation to the selected site of bone section and assembled with the external construct. Either a monolateral external fixation or a circular Ilizarov instead of an Ilizarov hybrid fixation could be used for bony distraction; circular fixation enables the use of wires instead of screws thus making fixation of the soft tissues less bulky, while a monolateral Exfix is a less heavy and demanding device for the young patient. Finally, the bone is cut according to the technique selected; the osteotomy is performed percutaneously by pre-drilling the bone prior to using the frame and then completed with an osteotome. In the forearm, the preferred levels for osteotomy are the distal radial metaphysis and the proximal ulnar metaphysis just distal to the coronoid process, but some prefer to perform a bifocal distal-proximal osteotomy of the ulna [61].

In case of ulna hypoplasia with dislocation of radial head, first, the ulna is lengthened, then the radial head is progressively reduced and, finally if required the radius is elongated.

After a period of rest of typically 5–7 days, the first distraction is performed by the surgeon and demonstrated to the relatives, explaining also the rhythm of lengthening with its potential pitfalls and complications. The initial distraction is generally 0.75 mm per day or 1.0 mm per day, divided into three to four turns of 0.25 mm elongation in order to prevent nerve damages and obtain a near continuous distraction. Typically, the amount of lengthening per day is fragmented, avoiding any turn before sleeping in order to avoid child suffering. Follow-up visits are performed from once a week to once a month. X-ray controls are performed depending on which the rate of elongation should be reduced or even suspended for a while, according to the development of the bone regeneration.

When the desired length is obtained, a "stabilization" phase of variable length is instituted, especially in cases with a high percentage of lengthening of significantly tight soft tissues. The premature removal of the apparatus can lead to deformity or post-removal fracture of the regenerate. Secondary surgery (bone graft, web deepening, hardware removal) is performed according to the indication.

Rehabilitation, either formal or with games, is useful, including physiotherapists and occupational therapists. After bone healing, if some joint stiffness remains, dynamic splinting may be necessary as well as scar compression in case of hypertrophic scaring.

16.4 Technical Variations

Multiple devices have been developed and several alternatives of PBDL exist through the monocortical to multiple-level osteotomy, the hemicallotasis, and the combined epiphysiodesis plus distraction osteogenesis; however, it is mandatory to [22]:

- minimize the approach and preserve vascularization
- preserve the periosteum hence a longitudinal incision)
- perform a transverse corticotomy
- maintain a delay before lengthening, allowing for early callus formation (from 5 to 10 days, according to the bone)
- -use a slow pace of lengthening (up to 1 mm/day, four times a day), and
- maintain the fixation until solid bone healing is obtained (with visible trabeculation)

Preservation of the medullary canal, as proposed by Ilizarov, is possible in the forearm but not practical in the small bones of the hand. The literature does not demonstrate the superiority of medullary canal integrity in bone healing [62, 63].

Some authors propose a combined approach of external fixation and elastic stable intramedullary nailing (ESIN) in order to speed up the lengthening time in the forearm, to improve the healing index, and to prevent regenerate fractures after external fixator (ExFix) removal [61].

16.5 Technical Problems According to the Applications of PBDL

- Forearm Lengthening: The purpose of this procedure is to correct a forearm about 60% shorter than the normal and, if possible, to adjust the bowing, especially by using an Ilizarov Exfix. When performed, the mean lengthening in the literature varies from 2.4 to 8.1 cm, with a distraction time of 11–12 weeks and a treatment time of 8 months (total treatment time per lengthening - "lengthening index" of 1.3 month per centimetre) [16, 17, 26, 51, 64–67]. The radial club hand is the main indication, allowing a redistribution of soft tissue, retracted on radial side, and facilitating centralization or radialization of the wrist without carpal bone resection [68–73]. Other indications mentioned in the literature are; ulnar deficiency, multiple exostosis, and multiple enchondromatosis [16, 51–58]. In ulnar deficiency, Bayne type II with a short proximal ulna, it is possible to lengthen the forearm and build a one-bone forearm of acceptable length and good stability; the entire radius could be transferred on the proximal fragment of the cubitus, at the same time correcting the bowing [69, 70]. Good improvement in cosmesis is generally achieved [74, 75] (Figs. 16.1, 16.2, 16.3, and 16.4).
- First Metacarpal: The strength of the adductor explains some angulation with closure of the first web; this could happen during the PBDL if the stability of the ExFix is not strong enough, or later when the device is removed, after "supposed" bone healing [3, 5, 76]. This could be avoided by using a double-frame

device with perforating K-wires and insertion of a longitudinal K-wire, which also helps to prevent MPJ flexion deformity in case of the short first phalanx. A second stage is frequently necessary to deepen the first web, though when possible PBDL should be performed at the first phalanx level to avoid this deepening. In case of a combined second ray defect, could be suggested to faster the PBDL, than resect the second ray and its metacarpal and use the finger-bone-bank as a graft to fill the defect, in order to obtain a better pinch with the third ray. In case of a hypoplastic thumb Blauth type III, when reconstruction is elected, a secondary thumb lengthening could be necessary to maintain functional length. In case of short thumb, short fingers and narrow first web, a good choice may be to lengthen the second ray, then at a second step the distal part is translocated onto the third ray and the remaining second ray is proximally sacrificed to deepen the web a provide a "relative" lengthening of the thumb [8, 77–79].

- Other Metacarpals: Metacarpal PBDL is an option mainly in cases of contraindications or impossibility of the transfer. It is usually better to lengthen an ulnar metacarpal to provide a huge web and ulnar support during pinch;

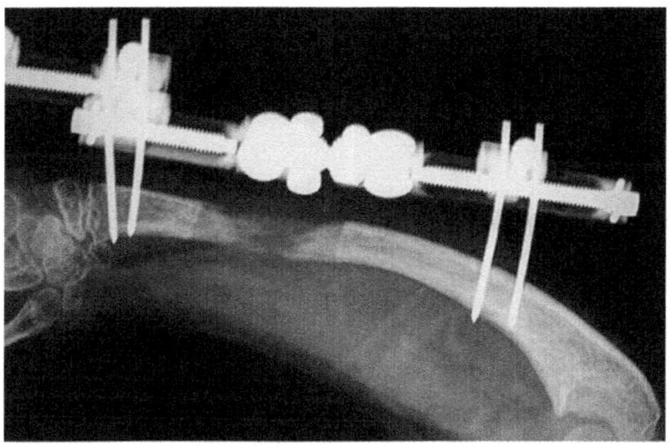

Fig. 16.1 Radial club hand—callotasis

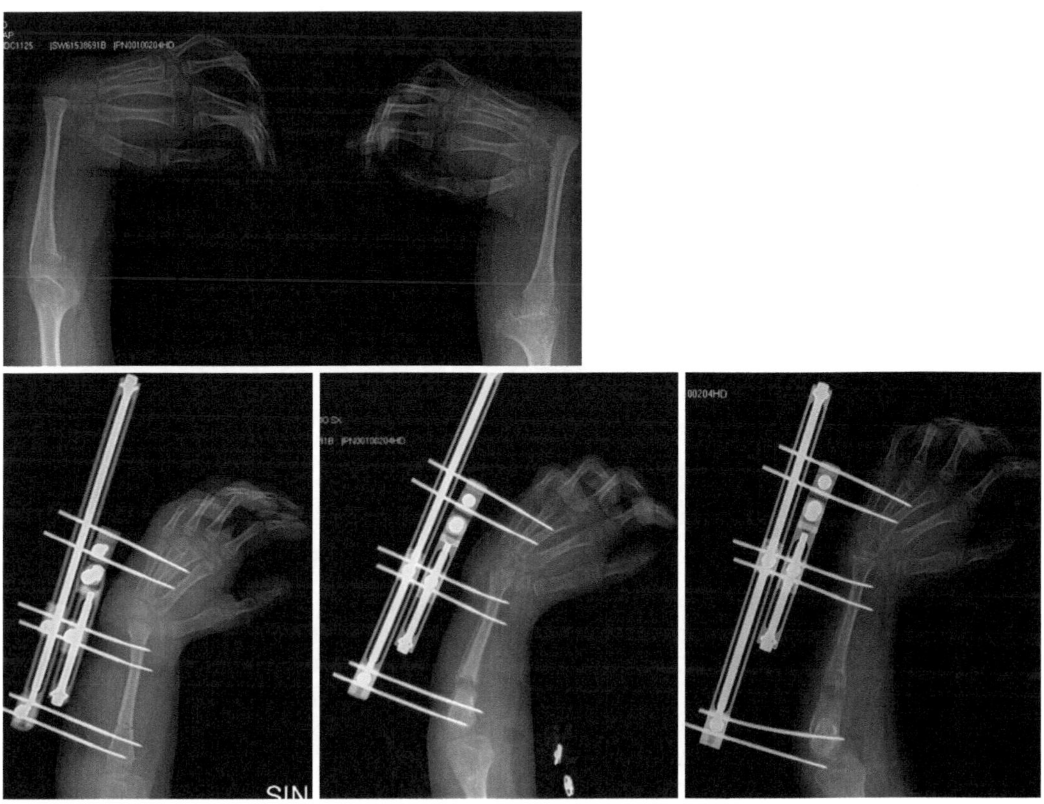

Fig. 16.2 Radial club hand. Radius length pre-op: 7.13 mm; post-op: 96.42 mm

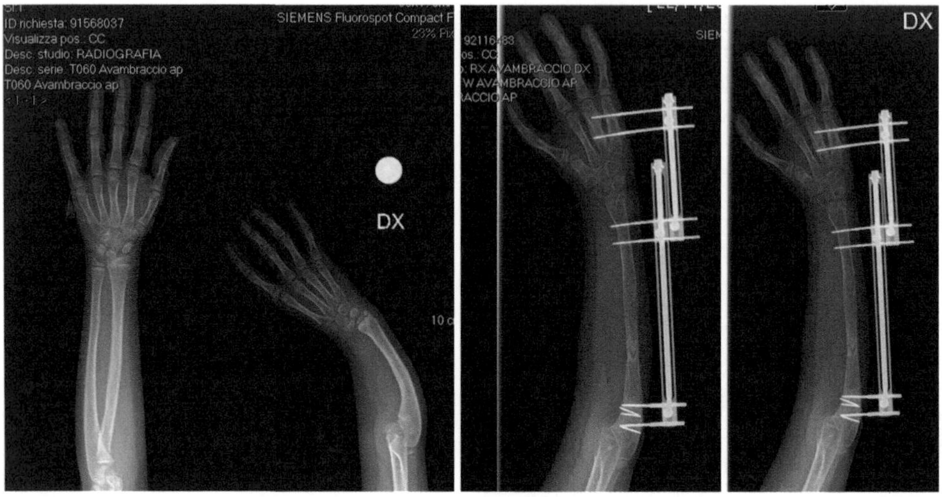

Fig. 16.3 Radial club hand. Radius length pre-op: 113.1 mm; post-op: 174.2 mm

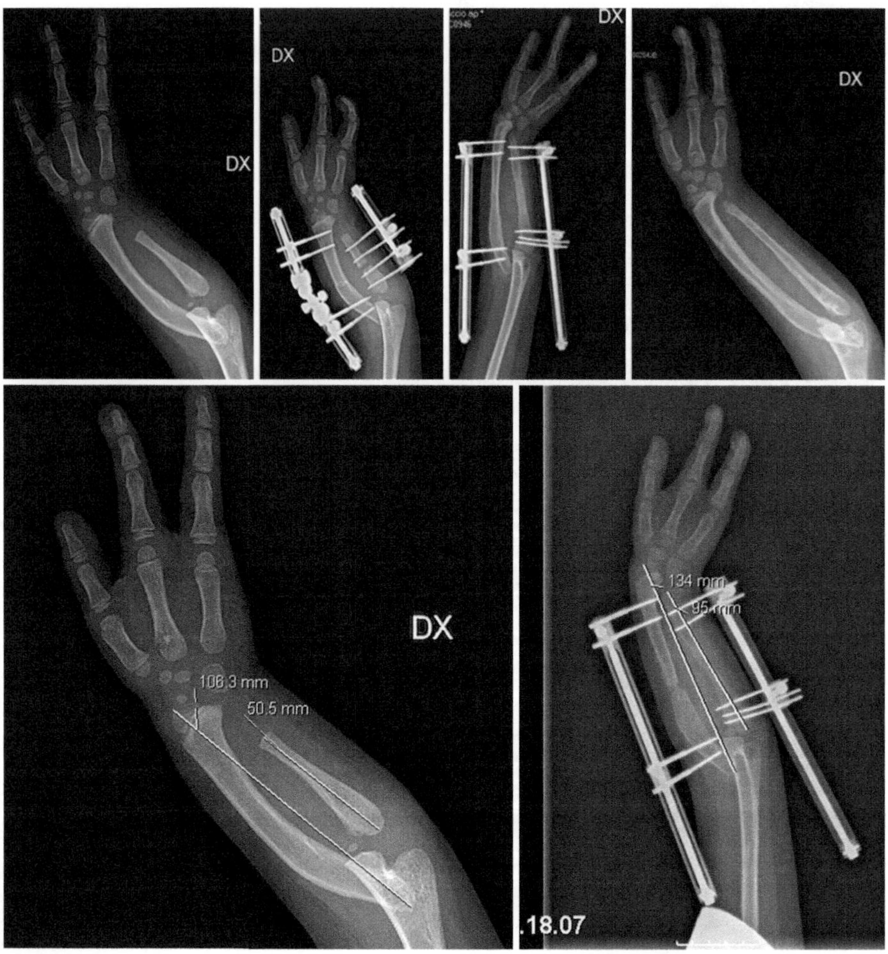

Fig. 16.4 Ulnar club hand—callotasis and duble ExFix change. Radius length pre-op: 106.3 mm; post-op: 134 mm. Ulna length pre-op: 50.5 mm; post-op: 95 mm

however, in malformations with limited thumb motion, a more radial metacarpal is selected to obtain a pinch. Further indications are, isolated brachymetacarpy and associated with metacarpal synostosis [46, 80–83] (Figs. 16.5 and 16.6).

- Metacarpal Synostosis: PBDL is necessary to correct asymmetric U and Y-shaped synostoses, as well as a K-shaped fourth–fifth metacarpals synostosis in order to correct the "notching" of the convergent short fifth ray with fourth. The PBDL allows for correction

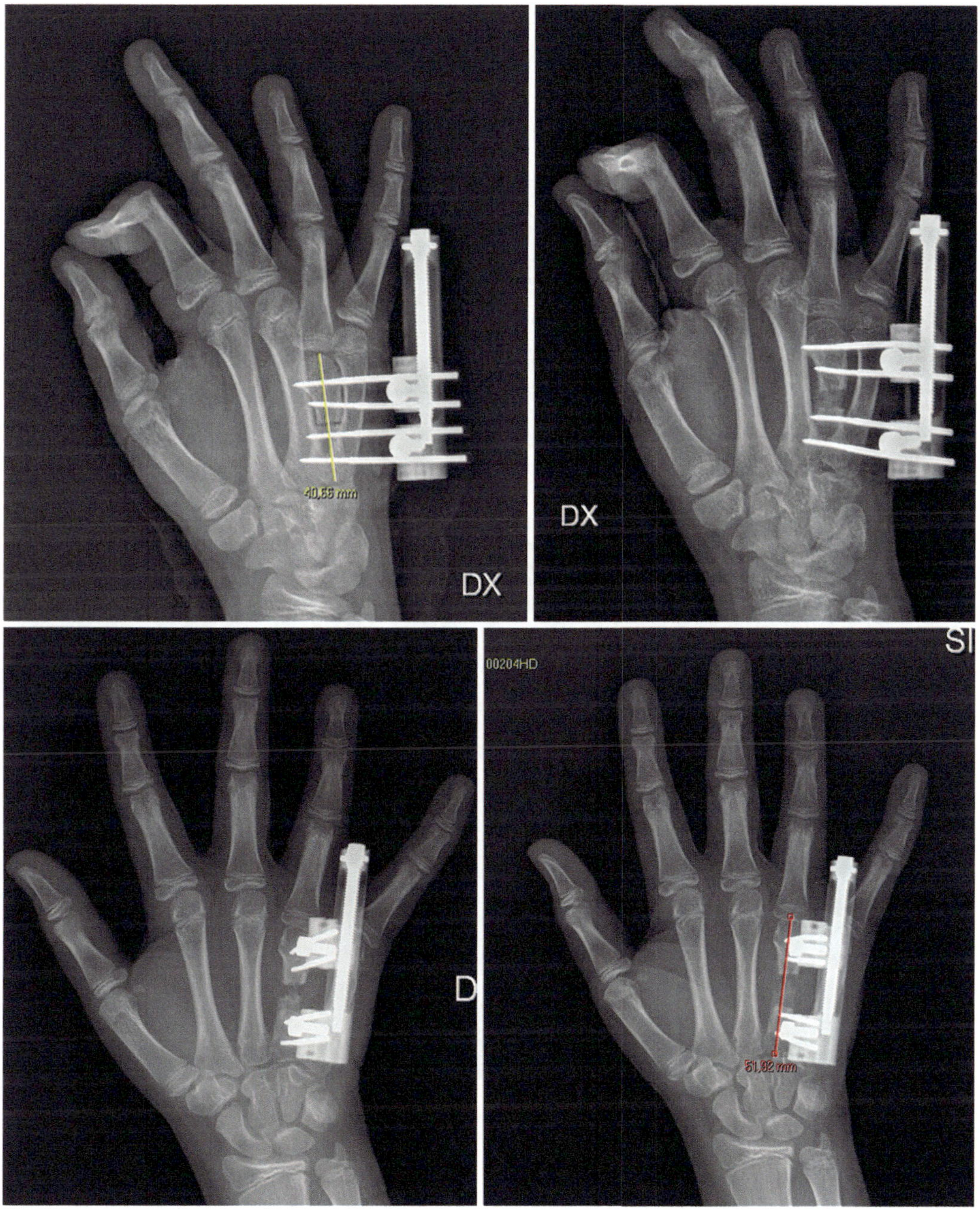

Fig. 16.5 Brachymetacarpy—50 days Lengthening; 1.3 cm gain

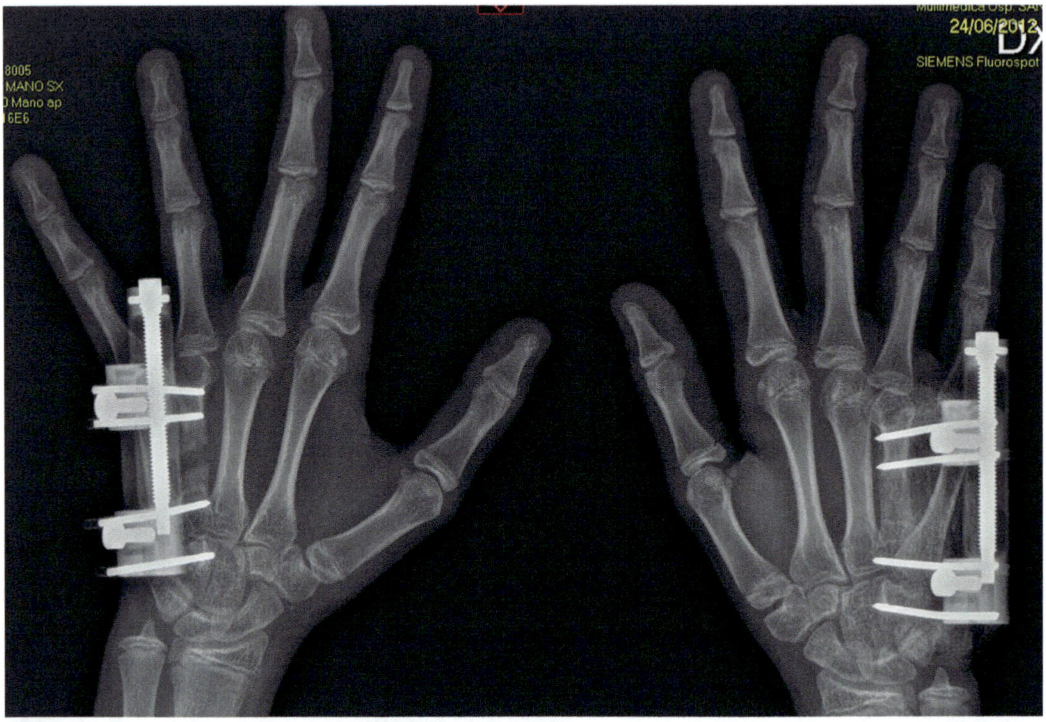

Fig. 16.6 Bilateral Brachymetacarpy—callotasis

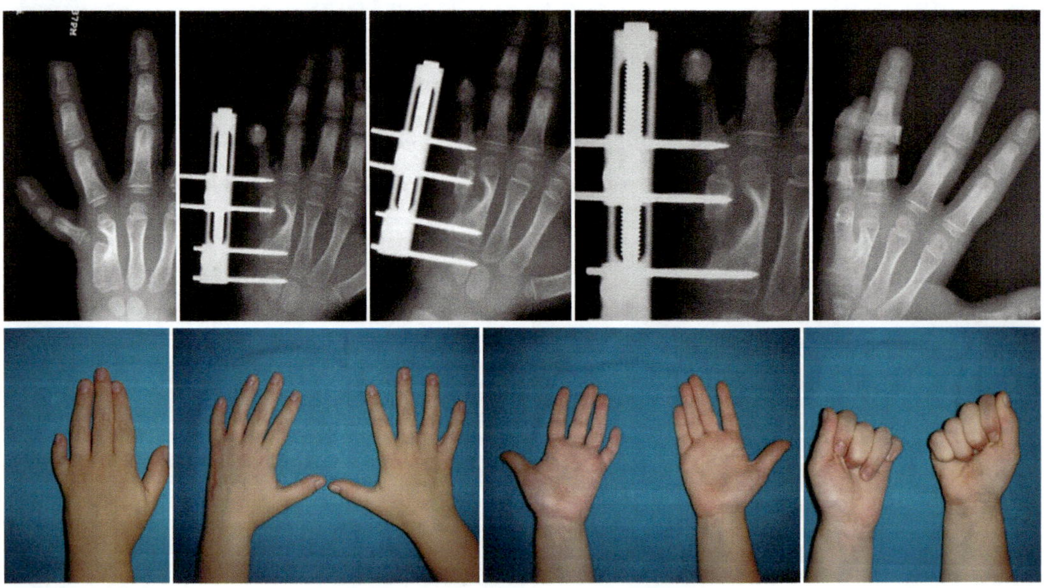

Fig. 16.7 Metacarpal synostosis in a 6-year-old child—callotasis

of the full-blow deformity rebalancing the metacarpal in a 6-year-old child - callotasis length, re-establishing the MPJ flexion, and correcting the adduction. On the fifth metacarpal, a double-frame device could allow a "differential" distraction to correct the obliquity of the epiphysis [84, 85] (Figs. 16.7, 16.8).

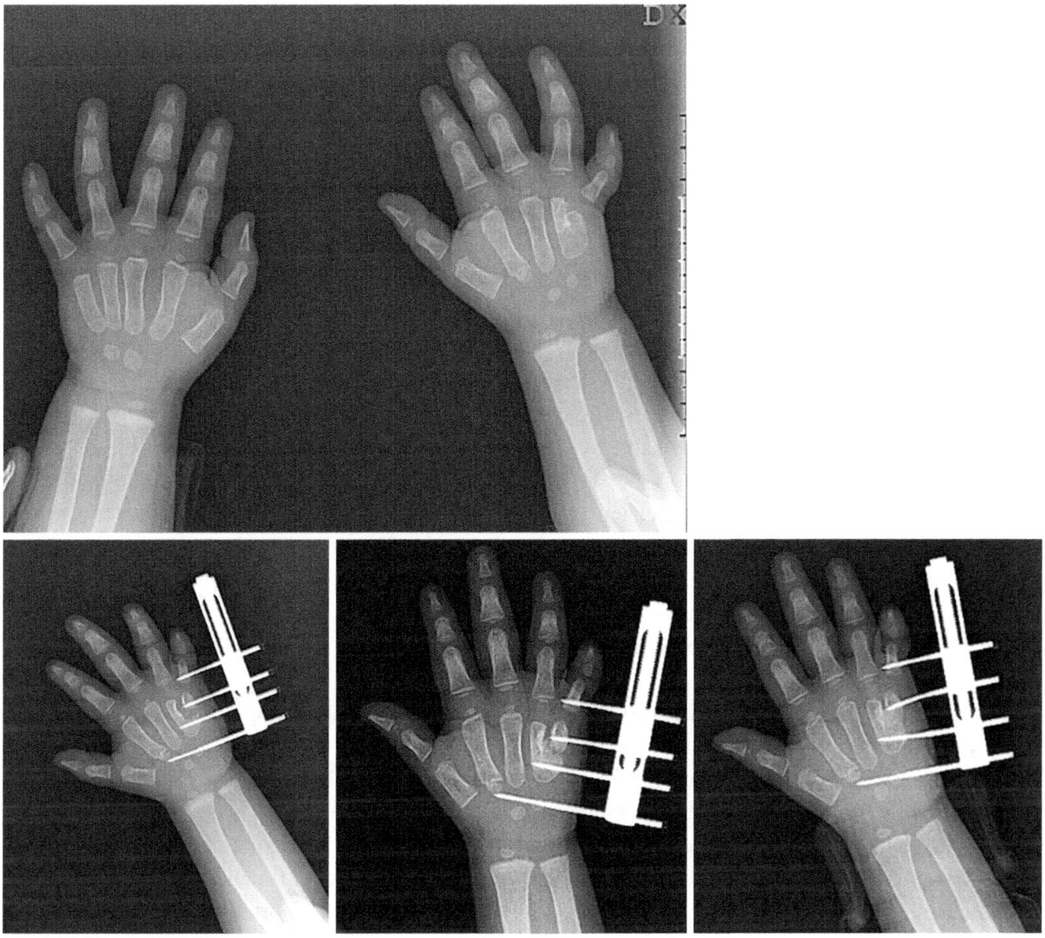

Fig. 16.8 Metacarpal synostosis in a 4-year-old child—callotasis

- Phalangeal: PBDL could be a surgical option in case of a stiff first interphalangeal joint with insufficient muscles and an evident lack of opposition. A delta phalanx could be corrected and lengthened at the same time, and even the distal phalanx could be the site of PBDL to correct a Kirner deformity [81, 86].

16.6 Complications

Complications are rare. Below they are summarized according to each technical step.

- Poor pin placement could cause unstable fixation, neurovascular injuries, and stiffness due to tendon impingement; a small incision is advisable to insert the pins.
- Epiphyseal injury is a major complication in very young babies that could be related to direct injury either by k-wire or by dissection; prevention occurs through limited dissection and careful placement of the pins with perioperative fluoroscan control, if necessary.
- Pin track infection is a common complication that could be minimized by keeping the apparatus clean with hydrogen peroxide for the first week and then alcohol solution, and dressing the pins by antiseptic-soaked dressings. If the infection is not controlled by several days of local treatment, the pin should be removed and replaced at another insertion

site. It is advisable to preserve approximately 0.5 cm between the device and the skin in order to avoid skin ulceration and facilitate cleaning of the pin sites [9, 26, 27, 87].

- Pain in common and can be difficult to manage in young patients, despite analgesics; the incidence is lower in slow-pace PBDL and avoiding the distraction before going to bed. Occasionally the lengthening has to be slowed or even stopped for a short time.
- Skin blanching or breakdown are rare complications in congenital cases, but typically occur in cases of fast PBDL; in case of insufficient quality of distal skin, a flap is advisable before attempting the lengthening.
- Distraction neuropathies cause transient sensory disturbance and require removal of pins or PBDL slowing; in their experimental work, Ippolito et al. found some definite changes in the myelin sheath after 8% of lengthening [47, 88–90].
- Early bone healing is more a theoretical risk, unless the PBDL is not performed properly (e.g., in reverse) or the pace of lengthening is too slow or stopped for too long; in patients with an excellent callus on the radiographs, lengthening speed could be increased [91].
- Loss of length can occur either by mechanical failure of the material or during the bone grafting or the translocation; later it may be related to pseudoarthrosis, malunion, or osteomyelitis.
- Mechanical failure of the device, generally avoided by weekly examinations.
- Callus deformation is seen when the ExFix is removed too early after callotasis; a particular site of risk is the first metacarpal, where the adductor is a strong deforming force [91].
- Delayed healing after callotasis could require a bone graft and a further stabilization by osteosynthesis or external fixation; a delay of more than 2 months after stopping the PBDL, waiting for bone healing, is an acceptable limit in children [51].
- Joint deformity is a particular risk that should be managed by placing an axial K-wire to prevent fragment tilting or flexed-extensive deformity.
- Stiffness is attributable to several factors, such as the congenital deformity itself (as in the radial club hand), prolonged use of the device impeding finger motion, tendon adhesion and intrinsic muscles fibrosis, which may occur in extensive PBDL. Prevention focuses on early mobilization of all joints (not blocked by the PBDL) with hand physiotherapists and if required temporarily ceasing lengthening [51].

Globally, at the forearm level, the complication rate is higher than in the hand but much lower than in the lower limb; however, the rate decreases depending on the expertise of the surgeon and the engagement and education of the caregivers [92, 93].

16.7 Conclusions

The upper limb has different alignment requirements from those in the lower limb, and moderate discrepancies in forearm length do not usually produce a significant functional deficit. However, the combination of shortening and angular deformities can reduce the ability to carry out simple activities of daily living. A deficiency in forearm length reduces the volume of space available for the hand and may cause functional and cosmetic problems; a relative discrepancy between the length of the radius and ulna not only causes shortening of the forearm but may result in subluxation of proximal and/or distal joints and limitations of prono-supination. Further soft-tissue contractures may worsen the range of movement and dexterity of the limb [60].

Full restoration of forearm length is not considered a requirement for a successful outcome, as the mobility of the shoulder can compensate for residual deformity; instead the lengthening should be sufficient to improve function and appearance, minimizing the risk of increasing complications (delayed non-union, pin-site infections, and Sudek syndrome).

PBDL has a place in the treatment of congenital hand and forearm malformations, particularly given its advantages, such as simplicity of execution and efficacy of lengthening. However, this technique deserves a leaning curve and all of the details need to be mastered to provide the expected final functional and cosmetic outcomes.

References

1. Codivilla A. On the means of lengthening, in the lower limbs, the muscles and tissues which are shortened through deformity. 1904. Clin Orthop Relat Res. 1994;(301):4–9.
2. Putti V. The operative lengthening of the femur. 1921. Clin Orthop Relat Res. 1990;250:4–7.
3. Matev IB. Thumb reconstruction through metacarpal bone lengthening. J Hand Surg Am. 1980;5(5):482–7.
4. Matev IB. Thumb reconstruction after amputation at the interphalangeal joint by gradual lengthening of the proximal phalanx. A case report. Hand. 1979;11(3):302–5.
5. Matev IB. Thumb reconstruction in children through metacarpal lengthening. Plast Reconstr Surg. 1979;64(5):665–9.
6. Matev IB. The bone-lenghtening method in hand reconstruction: twenty years's experience. J Hand Surg Am. 1989;14(2 Pt 2):376–8.
7. Matev IB. Thumb metacarpal lengthening. Tech Hand Up Extrem Surg. 2003;7(4):157–63.
8. Foucher G, Hultgren T, Merle M, Braun JM. Matev's digit lengthening technic. Apropos of 20 cases. Ann Chir Main. 1988;7(3):210–6.
9. Kessler I, Baruch A, Hecht O. Experience with distraction lengthening of digital rays in congenital anomalies. J Hand Surg Am. 1977;2(5):394–401.
10. Kessler I, Hecht O, Baruch A. Distraction-lengthening of digital rays in the management of the injured hand. J Bone Joint Surg Am. 1979;61(1):83–7.
11. Ilizarov GA. Basic principles of transosseous compression and distraction osteosynthesis. Ortop Travmatol Protez. 1971;32(11):7–15.
12. Ilizarov GA, Deviatov AA, Trokhova VG. Surgical lengthening of the shortened lower extremities. Vestn Khir Im I I Grek. 1972;108:100–3.
13. Ilizarov GA. The possibilities offered by our method for lengthening various segments in upper and lower limbs. Basic Life Sci. 1988;48:323–4.
14. Ilizarov GA. The tension-stress effect on the genesis and growth of tissues: part II. The influence of the rate and frequency of distraction. Clin Orthop Relat Res. 1989;239:263–85.
15. Messina A. The Ilizarov method for lengthening and correction of the ulna in radial club hand. Ann Chir Main. 1988;7:238–46.
16. Raimondo RA, Skaggs DL, Rosenwasser MP, Dick HM. Lengthening of pediatric forearm deformities using the Ilizarov technique: functional and cosmetic results. J Hand Surg Am. 1999;24:331–8.
17. Villa A, Paley D, Catagni MA, Bell D, Cattaneo R. Lengthening of the forearm by the Ilizarov technique. Clin Orthop. 1990;250:125–37.
18. Wagner H. Operative lengthening of the femur. Clin Orthop Relat Res. 1978;136:125–42.
19. Monticelli G, Spinelli R. Distraction epiphysiolysis as a method of limb lengthening. I. Experimental study. Clin Orthop Relat Res. 1981;(154):254–61.
20. Monticelli G, Spinelli R, Bonucci E. Distraction epiphysiolysis as a method of limb lengthening. II. Morphologic investigations. Clin Orthop Relat Res. 1981;154:262–73.
21. Monticelli G, Spinelli R. Distraction epiphysiolysis as a method of limb lengthening. III Clinical applications. Clin Orthop Relat Res. 1981;154:274–85.
22. De Bastani G, Aldegheri R, Renzi-Brivio L, Trivella G. Limb lengthening by callus distraction (callotasis). J Pediatr Orthop. 1987;7(2):129–34.
23. Cowen NJ, Loftus JM. Distraction augmentation manoplasty: technique for lengthening digits or entire hands. Orthop Rev. 1978;7:45–53.
24. Cowen NJ. Surgical management of the hypoplastic hand. In: Cowen NJ, editor. Practical hand sugery. Miami, Symposia Specialties; 1980.
25. Seitz WH, Dobyns JH. Digital lengthening. With emphasis on distraction osteogenesis in the upper limb. Hand Clin. 1993;9(4):699–706.
26. Seitz WH, Froimson AI. Callotasis lengthening in the upper extremity: indication, techniques and pitfalls. J Hand Surg Am. 1991;16(5):932–9.
27. Seitz WH, Froimson AI. Digital lengthening using the callotasis technique. Orthopedics. 1995;18(2):129–38.
28. Seitz WH, Shimko P, Patterson RW. Long-term results of callus distraction-lengthening in the hand and upper extremity for traumatic and congenital skeletal deficienties. J Bone Joint Surg Am. 2010;92(Suppl 2):47–58.
29. Smith AA, Greene TL. Preliminary soft tissue distraction in congenital forearm deficiency. J Hand Surg Am. 1995;20(3):420–4.
30. Foucher G, Medina J, Navarro R, Nagel D. Toe transfer in congenital hand malfomations. J Reconstr Microsurg. 2001;17(1):1–7.
31. Papadogeorgou EV, Soucacos PN. Treatment alternatives of congenital hand differences with thumb hypoplasia involvement. Microsurgery. 2008;28(2):121–30.
32. Netscher DT, Lewis EV. Technique of nonvascularized toe phalangeal transfer and distraction lengthening in the treatment of multiple digit symbrachydactyly. Tech Hand Up Extrem Surg. 2008;12(2):114–20.

33. Dautel G, Barbary S. Second toe transfer in congenital hand differences. Chir Main. 2008;27(Suppl 1):D48–61.
34. Foucher G. Toe transplantation in congenital malformations of the hand. Bull Acad Natl Med. 1997;181(8):1737–45.
35. Pajardi G, Lamas C, Medina J, Foucher G. Progressive bone distraction lengthening in the treatment of congenital malformations of the hand. Tech Hand Up Extrem Surg. 2000;4(4):262–71.
36. Chiu DTW, Patel A, Sakamoto S, Chu A. The impact of microsurgery on congenital hand anomalies associated with amniotic band syndrome. Plast Reconstr Surg Glob Open. 2018;6(4):e1657.
37. Tsai TM, Ludwig L, Tonkin M. Vascularized fibular epiphyseal transfer. A clinical study. Clin Orthop Relat Res. 1986;210:228–34.
38. Foucher G, Sammut D, Citron N. Free vascularized toe-joint transfer in hand reconstruction: a series of 25 patients. J Reconstr Micrusurg. 1990;6(3):201–7.
39. Hierner R, Berger AK. Long-term results after vascularised joint transfer for finger joint reconstruction. J Plast Reconstr Aesthet Surg. 2008;61(11):1338–46.
40. Buck-Gramcko D, Pereira JA. Proximal toe phalanx transplantation for bony stabilization and lengthening of partially aplastic digits. Ann Chir Memb Super. 1990;9(2):107–18.
41. Buck-Gramcko D. The role of nonvascularized toe phalanx transplantation. Hand Clin. 1990;6(4):643–59.
42. Buck-Gramcko D. Progress in the treatment of congenital malformations of the hand. World J Surg. 1990;14(6):715–24.
43. Carroll RE, Green DP. Reconstruction of hypoplastic digits using toe phalanges. J Bone Joint Surg Am. 1975;57A:727–32.
44. Goldberd NH, Watson HK. Composite toe (phalanx and epiphysis) transfers in the reconstruction of the aphalangic hand. J Hand Surg Am. 1982;7(5):454–9.
45. Fultz CW, Lester DK, Hunter JM. Single stage lengthening by intercalary bone graft in patients with congenital hand deformities. J Hand Surg Br. 1986;11(1):40–6.
46. Ogino T, Kato H, Ishii S, Usui M. Digital lengthening in congenital hand deformities. J Hand Surg Br. 1994;19:120–9.
47. Pajardi G. Gli allungamenti ossei nelle malformazioni confenite dell'arto superiore. Riv Ital. Chir Plastica. 1992;(suppl 24):215–9.
48. Panattoni LB, Ebersole GM, Cavadas PC. Microvascular "on-top-plasty": an alternative for thumb reconstruction in constriction band syndrome. Int J Orthopl Surg. 2018;1(1):18–26.
49. Kumar B, Bhat AK, Acharya AM. The use of composite tissue spare parts to restore tripod hand function in post-traumatic and congenital hand deficiency. Hand Surg. 2015;20(3):380–5.
50. Catagni MA, Szabo RM, Cattaneo R. Preliminary experience with Ilizarov method in late reconstruction of radial hemimelia. J Hand Surg Am. 1993;18:316–21.
51. Cheng JCY. Distraction lengthening of the forearm. J Hand Surg Br. 1991;16:441–5.
52. Burgess RC, Cates H. Deformities of the forearm in patients who have multiple cartilaginous exostosis. J Bone Joint Surg Am. 1993;75-A:13–8.
53. Dahl MT. The gradual correction of forearm deformities in multiple hereditary exostoses. Hand Clin. 1993;9:707–18.
54. Pritchett JW. Lengthening the ulna in patients with hereditary multiple exostoses. J Bone Joint Surg (Br). 1986;68-B:561–5.
55. Akita S, Murase T, Yoenobu K, et al. Long-term results of surgery for forearm deformities in patients with multiple cartilaginous exostoses. J Bone Joint Surg Am 2007; 89-A:1993–1999.
56. Peterson HA. Deformities and problems of the forearm in children with multiple hereditary osteochondromata. J Pediatr Orthop. 1994;14:92–100.
57. Fogel GR, McElfresh EC, Peterson HA, Wicklund PT. Management of deformities of the forearm in multiple hereditary osteochondromas. J Bone Joint Surg[Am]. 1984;66-A:670–80.
58. Masada K, Tsuyuguchi Y, Kawai H, et al. Operations for forearm deformity caused by multiple osteochondromas. J Bone Joint Surg (Br). 1989;71-B:24–9.
59. Houshian S, Schrøder HA, Weeth R. Correction of Madelung's deformity by the Ilizarov technique. J Bone Joint Surg (Br). 2004;86-B:536–40.
60. Hill RA, Ibrahim T, Mann HA, Siapkara A. Forearm lengthening by distraction osteogenesis in childre. A report of 22 cases. J Bone Joint Surg (Br). 2011;93-B(11):1550–5.
61. Jager T, Popkov D, Lascombes P, Popkov A, Journeau P. Elastic intramedullary nailing as a complement to Ilizarov's method for forearm lengthening: a comparative pediatric prospective study. Ortho Trauma Surg Res. 2012;98(4):376–82.
62. Frierson M, Ibrahim K, Boles M, Bote H, Ganey T. Distraction osteogenesis: a comparison of corticotomy techniques. Clin Ortop. 1994;301:19–24.
63. Seitz WH. Distraction lengthening in hand and upper extremity. Green's Operative Hand Surgery, 6th ed.
64. Abe M, Shirai H, Okamoto M, Onomura T. Lengthening of the forearm by callus distraction. J Hand Surg Br. 1996;21(2):151–63.
65. Klein C, Ferrari V, Deroussen F, Juvet-Segarra M, Gouron R. Forearm lengthening and prosthetic management in children with transverse congenital forearm deficiency. Hand Surg Rehab. 2019;38(2):129–34.
66. Launay F, Pesenti S. Forearm lengthening: management of elbow and wrist. J Child Orthop. 2016;10:593–5.
67. Mader K, Gausepohl T, Pennig D. Shortening and deformity of radius and ulna in children: correction of axis and length by callus distraction. J Pediatr Orthop B. 2003;12:183–91.
68. Kawabata H, Shibata T, Masatomi T, Yasui N. Residual deformity in congenital radial club hands after previous centralisation of the wrist: ulnar length-

ening and correction by Ilizarov method. J Bone Joint Surg Br. 1998;80(5):762–5.
69. Prokopovich VS. Aligning of length of the forearm bones in the congenital club hand in children. Orthop Traumatol. 1980;1:51–3.
70. Takagi T, Seki A, Mochida J, Takayama S. Bone lengthening of the radius with temporary external fixation of the wrist for mild radial club hand. J Plast Reconstr Aesth Surg. 2014;67(12):1688–93.
71. Pickford MA, Scheker LR. Distraction lengthening of the ulna in radial club hand using the Ilizarov technique. J Hand Surg Br. 1998;23:186–91.
72. Huang SC, Kuo KN. Differential lengthening of the radius and ulna using the Ilizarov method. J Pediatr Orthop. 1998;18:370–3.
73. Peterson BM, McCarroll HR Jr, James MA. Distraction lengthening of the ulna in children with radial longitudinal deficiency. J Hand Surg Am. 2007;32:1402–7.
74. Peterson HA. The ulnius: a one-bone forearm in children. J Pediatr Orthop Br. 2008;17:95–101.
75. Senes F, Catena N. Correction of forearm deformities in congenital ulnar club hand: one-bone forearm. J Hand Surg. 2012 Jan;37(1):159–64.
76. Moy OJ, Peimer CA, Sherwin FS. Reconstruction of traumatic or congenital amputaion of the thumb by distraction-lengthening. Hand Clin. 1992;8(1):57–62.
77. Foucher M, Lamas C, Mir X. Reconstrucciòn digital segun tecnica de Matev. Estudios de 45 casos. Rev Iber Cir Mano. 2000;27:31–9.
78. Kessler I. Transposition lengthening of a digit ray after multiple amputations of fingers. Hand. 1976;8:176.
79. Hu W, Gasnier P, Le Nen D, Kerfant N, Boloorchi A. Description of an original conservative method for the surgical management of the Blauth IIIb thumb hypoplasia: "relative lengthening - thumb stabilization". Ann Chir Plast Esthet. 2012 Aug;57(4):342–9.
80. Smith RJ, Gumley GJ. Metacarpal distraction lengthening. Hand Clin. 1985;1:417–29.
81. Houshian S, Ipsen T. Metacarpal and phalangeal lengthening by callus distraction. J Hand Surg Br. 2001;26(1):13–6.
82. Matsuno T, Ishida O, Sunagawa T, Ichikawa M, Ikuta Y, Ochi M. Bone lengthening for congenital differences of the hands and digits in children. J Hand Surg. 2004;28(4):712–9.
83. Dhalla R, Strecker W, Manskel PR. A comparison of two technique for digital distraction lengthening in skeletally immature patients. J Hand Surg. 2001;26(4):603–10.
84. Horii E, Miura T, Nakamura R, Nakao E, Kato H. Surgical treatment of congenital metacarpal synostosis of the ring and little fingers. J Hand Surg Br. 1998;23(5):691–4.
85. Buck-Gramcko D, Wood VE. The treatment of metacarpal synostosis. J Hand Surg. 1993;18(4):565–81.
86. Norat F, Dreant N, Lebreton E, Magalon G. Clinodactylies: delta phalanx and Kirner deformity. Chir Main. 2008;27(Suppl 1):S165–73.
87. Caton J. Traitement des inégalités de longueur des membres inférieurs et des sujets de petite taille chez l'enfant et l'adolescent. Rev Chir Orthop. 1991;77(Suppl 1):31–80.
88. Ippolito E, Peretti G, Belloci M, et al. Histology and ultrastructure of arteries, veins and peripheral nerves during limb lengthening. Clin Orthop. 1994;308:54–62.
89. Huang K, Zeng Y, Xia H, Liu C. Alterations in the biorheological features of some soft tissues after limb lengthening. Biorheology. 1998;35(4–5):355–63.
90. Yokota A, Doi M, Ohtsuka H, Abe M. Nerve conduction and microanatomy in the rabbit sciatic nerve after gradual limb lengthening - distraction neurogenesis. J Orthop Res. 2003;21(1):36–43.
91. Pensler JM, Carrol NC, Cheng LF. Distraction osteogenesis in the hand. Plast Reconstr Surg. 1998;102(1):92–5.
92. Dahl MT, Gulli B, Berg T. Complications of limb lengthening: a learning curve. Clin Orthop. 1994;301:10–8.
93. Dahl MT. Upper-extremity lengthening. In Gupta A, Kay SPG, Scheker LR. The growing hand: diagnosis and management of the upper extremity in children; Mosby LTD 2000; 108: 1049–1057.

Radial Club Hand: Microvascular Reconstruction

17

Simo K. Vilkki

Abstract

With microvascular reconstruction, it is possible to add an autogenous growing bone and joint unit for radial club hand stabilization. The reconstructive procedure is carried out at ages between 3 and 6 years. As a first step, the hand is aligned to optimal position with a slow soft tissue distraction. The microvascular bone and joint transfer is done after 2 months distraction period. The graft includes subtotal second metatarsal bone with MTP-joint and proximal toe phalanx. The distractor, as an ex-fix, is continued until sound bone healing or about additional 2 months. Thereafter the reconstructed wrist is protected during 1 month with a long plaster cast followed by 3 months of splinting period. Good results can be obtained when graft alignment is optimal, graft survival is good and growth continues. Achieved wrist motion and stability depends on available muscles of the forearm. The wrist motion is clearly superior compared with centralization or radialization. The range of active motion is weaker to extension or maximally 30° while flexion to 60–80° is commonly achieved. Forearm length is retarded in radial club hand. This technique will ensure the natural ulna growth or about 70% of normal ulna length. Pollicization can be performed 1 year later when it is feasible. In long term, hand alignment remains good until age 11, however, in adolescence the ulna has greater growth potential than transferred metatarsal bone and some radial deviation may slowly occur. Therefore, secondary alignment correction may be needed or ulna growth distally can be stopped before puberty.

Keywords

Radial club hand · Aplasia radii
Microvascular reconstruction · Soft tissue distraction · MTP-joint graft · Joint transfer
Wrist reconstruction · Failed centralization

17.1 Introduction

17.1.1 General Principles before Operative Treatment

Conservative measures in early management of radial dysplasia child are most important readily after the birth and should be continued until operative treatment becomes indicated to keep the wrist supple. Adequate splinting and manipulative exercises are mandatory and useful.

Supplementary Information The online version contains supplementary material available at https://doi.org/10.1007/978-3-031-30984-7_17.

S. K. Vilkki (✉)
Department of Hand and Microsurgery, Tampere University Hospital, Tampere, Finland
e-mail: simo@vilkki.fi

G. Pajardi (ed.), *Pediatric Hand Surgery*, https://doi.org/10.1007/978-3-031-30984-7_17

17.1.2 Hand Quality

In order to be able to compare different patients and their treatment results all defects and functional limitations of the radial club hand extremity must be carefully evaluated and recorded.

Overall hand quality can be evaluated using radial dysplasia severity grading (eTable 17.1) [1]. That is important before setting indications on which treatment method should be chosen for a certain radial club extremity. Mild and moderate severities or severity index (S.I.) below 17 is usually suitable for microvascular reconstruction using a second toe-ray graft (subtotal MT bone + MTP-joint + proximal phalanx). Very high severity (S.I. over 20) in radial dysplasia extremity means commonly that there is a poor muscle power and the ability to control wrist extension may remain unsatisfactory. Additionally, severe fixed wrist deformity is more challenging in aligning the hand. Traditionally, a complete lack of elbow flexion force has been a contraindication for wrist alignment, because the hand is probably not reaching the mouth anymore. The better the hand quality (low severity index), the greater the indication for microvascular wrist reconstruction is considered (Fig. 17.1).

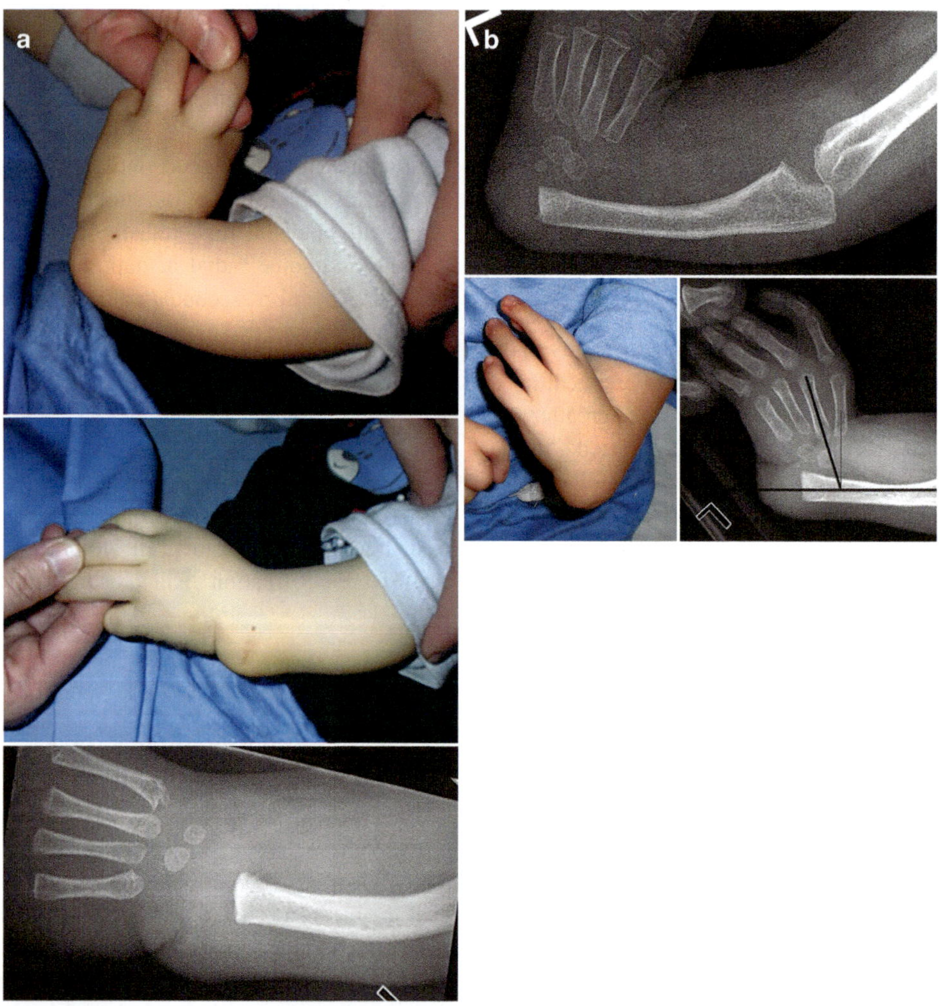

Fig. 17.1 (**a**) Mild severity and easy hand alignment passively. The hand quality was good and severity index was 4 (very mild). (**b**) A poor-quality hand with fixed deformity. Severity index was 22 (severe). Observe: X-ray should be taken pulling the hand to the end-point with moderate force when assessing the wrist tightness

17.1.3 Indications and Prerequisites for Microvascular Reconstruction

Radial club hands with Bayne–Klug types III and IV are candidates for microvascular wrist reconstruction. In types I and II, other less invasive methods should be used. Recommended age for the procedure is between 3 and 6 years.

When there has been a previous surgical attempt, the age can be higher (up to age 10 years) because a very good indication for microvascular wrist reconstruction is a failed centralization/radialization extremity [2] (Morsy et al). A previous procedure may have worsened the growth of distal ulna. This means that the growth balance between the transferred MTP-joint graft and distal ulna will be more optimal compared to intact distal ulna. Special circumstances may apply patients with TAR syndrome as the anatomy may be different at wrist and proximal hand due to the existence of a good thumb ray. An MRI study should be done in those cases preoperatively to understand the better anatomy of the wrist.

A prerequisite for the complex wrist reconstruction procedure is a good family cooperation. Especially distraction period and long healing time with distractor in place will need perfect cooperation and good understanding from the parents. Suboptimal psychological factors and social circumstances will play a role during the long-standing treatment period and may affect the success of treatment.

Other important prerequisites are that the treating team has experience in distraction, microsurgical culture is well adopted in the treating hospital and there is experience in toe-to-hand transfer for children among the treating team (Table 17.1).

Table 17.1 Steps in microvascular reconstruction of radial club hand

1.	Early continuous splinting from birth
2.	Slow (2 months) soft tissue distraction at age 3
3.	Stabilizing microvascular MTP II -joint transfer
4.	Primary healing time (2 months) with distractor in place!
5.	Protection of the graft during six postoperative months
6.	Pollicization usually 1 year after wrist correction

17.2 Distraction

17.2.1 General Principles and Choice of Distractor

Soft tissue distraction needs experience and patience. Special attention and understanding are needed for choosing distractor type, pin positioning, primary alignment, distraction speed, and control of distraction during advancement. Additionally, possible complications need to be overcome. The author has used a unilateral distractor (Fig. 17.2.) on ulnar side of hand and forearm, because it enables the operative procedure on the radial side of the wrist and forearm. Important in choosing the distractor is that it is lightweight, it does not bother the child too much and the daily distraction procedure must be easy to perform by parents. The modules with three pins, at distal and proximal part in the distractor, should be adjustable to allow necessary freedom at the time of assembly. A clearly visible mm scale on the longitudinal bar is very helpful for precise control of the advancement of distraction and preventing from accidental misunderstanding. The longitudinal bar length in distraction varies with age and forearm size. A common bar length is 150 mm at the age of 3 years. Three pins are safe at both ends and a pin brakeage is very rare. A pin site infection, which sometimes occurs, seldom makes problems with all three pins simultaneously.

17.2.2 Pin Positioning

Distal pins at hand metacarpal (MC) bones should include always the stable part of the hand skeleton. That means that MC II and III are included. When only two ulnar metacarpals are included, the distraction easily happens at wrong level or at CMC IV-V joint level, being simultaneously less effective at the wrist level. The pins at metacarpals are not allowed to disturb distal epiphyseal growth zones. Also, the base of the second metacarpal must be left without pin. Preferably one of the pins can be inserted into ulnar part of carpal bones. Three pins with diameter 1½-2 mm are used and they are inserted

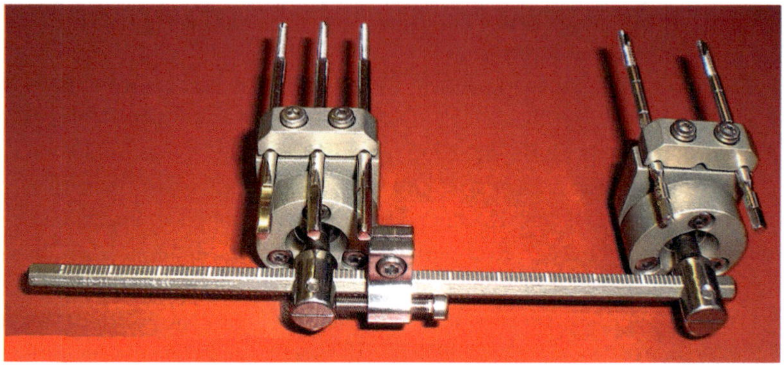

Fig. 17.2 Unilateral distractor with a clear millimeter scale. Ball joints at both ends are practical in primary alignment

from ulnar or dorso-ulnar side. When pins are inserted, the finger extensors are carefully protected.

Proximal pins with diameter 3 mm are positioned from dorso-ulnar side into proximal ulna starting about 30 mm from olecranon. Cubital joint is carefully protected, and pin positioning is checked with perioperative X-ray fluoroscopy.

Pin alignment must be planned with a possibility to align the distal pins parallel with proximal pins when the hand is aligned accordingly to almost straight position in P-A view. Wrist is kept in a neutral position to eliminate the flexion tendency.

17.2.3 Distractor Alignment

Distractor is placed on dorso-ulnar aspect of the wrist and forearm. Then it is not a problem for the child and not on the way when the second phase operation is actual.

The transport of the hand will occur to distal direction somewhat dorsally and ulnarly. Therefore, longitudinal bar alignment in P-A view should deviate mildly ulnarly and in side-view parallel or mildly dorsally compared with distal ulna (Fig. 17.3). The surgeon can use moderate manipulating force to straighten the wrist during assembly to achieve good initial alignment. An axillary block at the end of the operation can be done for pain control. The timetable for distraction is planned for 60 days and the speed of distraction can be 1 mm per day during the first 7 days but thereafter only ½ mm a day.

17.2.4 Advancement of Distraction

It is important to teach the parents carefully to observe and control distractor function. What really happens should be measured. Distance of distal and proximal pins and their inclinations should be continuously observed. The knobs or screws used for distraction may need special attention as they may move by themselves during the child's activities due to vibration. After daily distraction procedure, the distraction screw is regularly taped to prevent unwanted motion. Active finger motion exercises are continuously encouraged throughout the whole treatment period.

X-ray controls for distraction advancement are performed every 3 weeks or when especially needed. When problems with hand or distraction alignment are noticed at first control, then it is wise to improve the hand position and change the pin inclinations to optimum. This requires general anesthesia and operation theatre circumstances.

During long-standing distraction, there is a need to take care of pin sites. Shower is allowed daily to keep the pin sites clean. The use of 1% hydrogen peroxide with soft cleaning sticks to remove the crusts is useful in preventing from infectious complications. Other distractor-related complications may be a pain due to too fast progress or sometimes a fracture of delicate metacarpal bone due to torsion forces between the pins. Also, pain from a pin site infection is a possibility and needs attention and treatment. The patient may have unexpected trauma when falling or catching

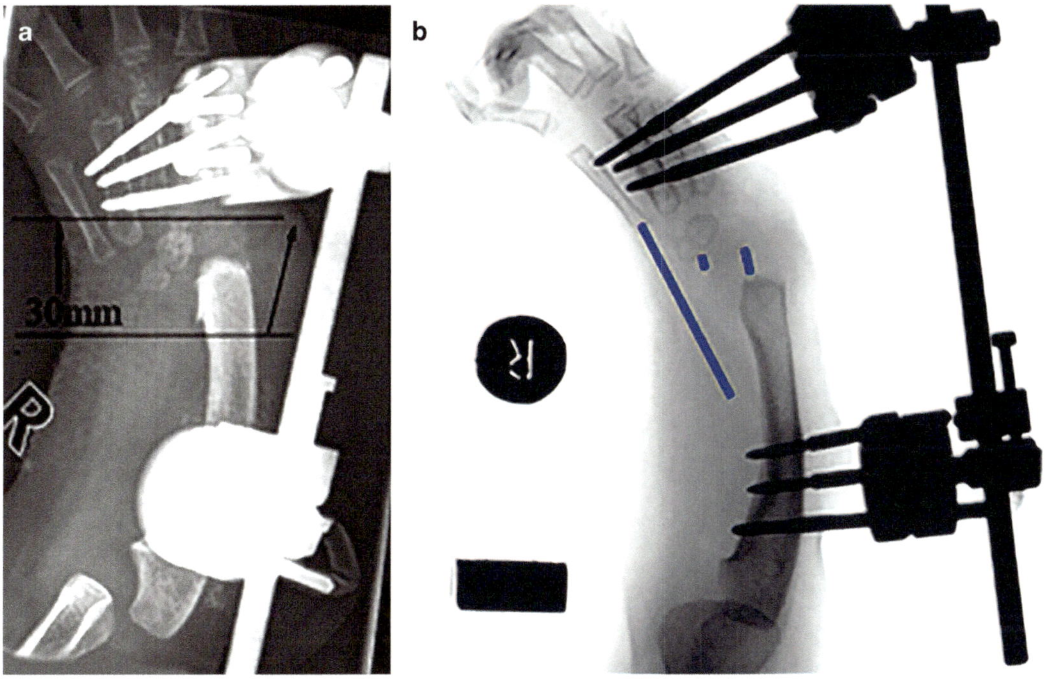

Fig. 17.3 (**a**) Distractor alignment at the beginning. Observe cartilage overlapping! Planned distraction will take about 60 days with the speed of 0.5 mm per day. (**b**) Alignment after distraction of one month. Long blue line is the length estimated for the graft. Short blue marks show remaining overlapping of carpal and ulna head cartilages which must be eliminated with further distraction

the device against other objects. Therefore, a special bandage or light bag-like coverage of the extremity under distraction may be used when child is out and playing.

17.2.5 How Much to Distract or Where is the Goal of Distraction?

There is commonly a need for 25 to 30 mms of distraction after primary alignment. The graft length (MT bone + PP) at foot can be measured from X-ray image and it varies at age 3 from 40 to 55 mm's in length. Note: MT-bone base (1 cm part) is left at foot. The space at wrist needed for the graft should be about 45–50 mm (Fig 17.4a–c). In the beginning, carpal bones and distal ulna are partly overlapping. After 15–20 mm's distraction, carpal bones have moved on top of distal ulna. Usually, there will be space enough and the hand alignment has become corrected when the distance between visible carpal bones and visible distal ulna is 15 mm (Fig. 17.4c). At the same time, the skin contour on ulnar border of the wrist is stretched out.

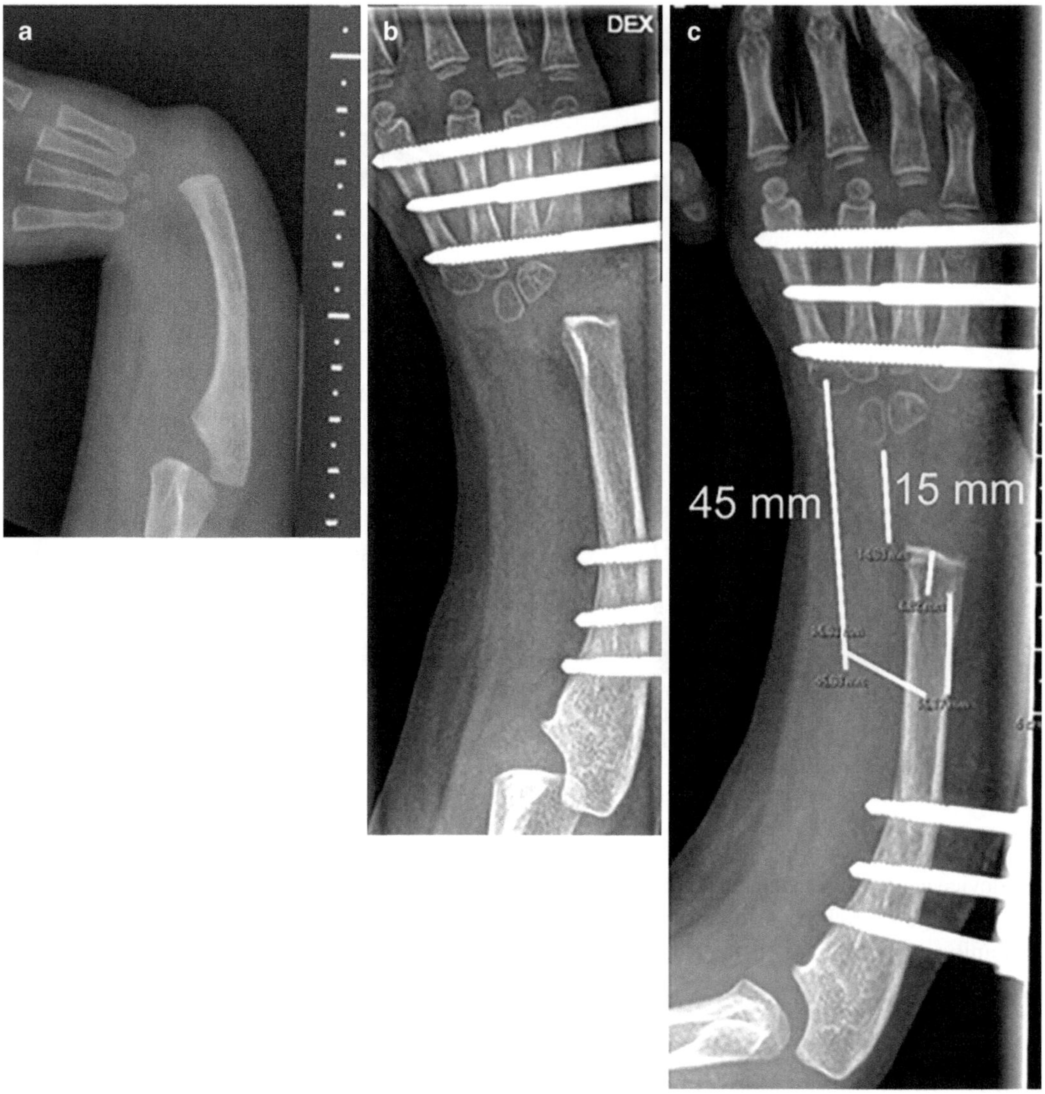

Fig 17.4 (**a**) Initial X-ray. (**b**) Distraction in progress. (**c**) Situation when enough space for the graft has been created

17.3 Operative Treatment. Microvascular Wrist Reconstruction

17.3.1 Goal of Operation

A non-supported hand, due to lack of radius, will enable pathologic hand position or radial deviation. There is a need to reconstruct the radial half of the wrist with sound tissue unit which can stabilize the non-supported hand and is able to grow.

A MTP-II joint graft from the foot provides a unit with growing metatarsal bone together with a joint. It will enable the growth and can immediately prevent from deformity as supporting structure. It also can enable a controlled wrist motion. The growth of a microvascular epiphyseal bone transfer was first studied experimentally in a dog model [3]. Clinically first series using MTP-II joint transfer for radial club hand was published in 1998 [4].

17.3.2 Anesthesia

Pediatric anesthesia suitable for long-lasting tissue transfer is needed [5]. Two teams operating simultaneously at hand and foot are considered necessary. Anesthesia time is often long with about 7–10-h duration and has been managed with special approach combining a continuous axillary plexus block and general anesthesia. This method decreases the need for strong sedation and pain medication when axillary block is effective.

17.3.3 Foot Dissection and Raising the MTP II-Joint Graft Flap

Previous principles of toe transfer in pediatric patients [6, 7] can be followed. Special rules necessary in joint transfer are few: Ipsilateral foot serves as donor. Minimum of skin from the foot can be taken with the toe (Fig. 17.5). Primary closure without skin graft is essential for donor site and leaves the foot without problems. Another appreciated factor is that the base of second metatarsal is left in place, so that integrity of transversal tarsal arch is not destroyed. During dissection, just the structures necessary for joint graft are carefully identified. Dorsal vein system, two dorsal metatarsal nerves which innervate the MTP-joint, extensor tendons, and first dorsal metatarsal artery are located on dorsal side of the foot. On plantar side, the flexor tendons and plantar metatarsal artery in space between II and III metatarsal bones are necessary structures. Plantar nerves are not included because the distal part of the toe is not used in the transfer. After the bone is osteotomized near the base of metatarsal bone, the toe can be slightly lifted and separated gently from attached side structures and underlying adductor hallucis muscle, which is carefully preserved. Then the dissection of arteries is continued proximally until dorsalis pedis artery to ensure longer pedicle. The main parts of interos-

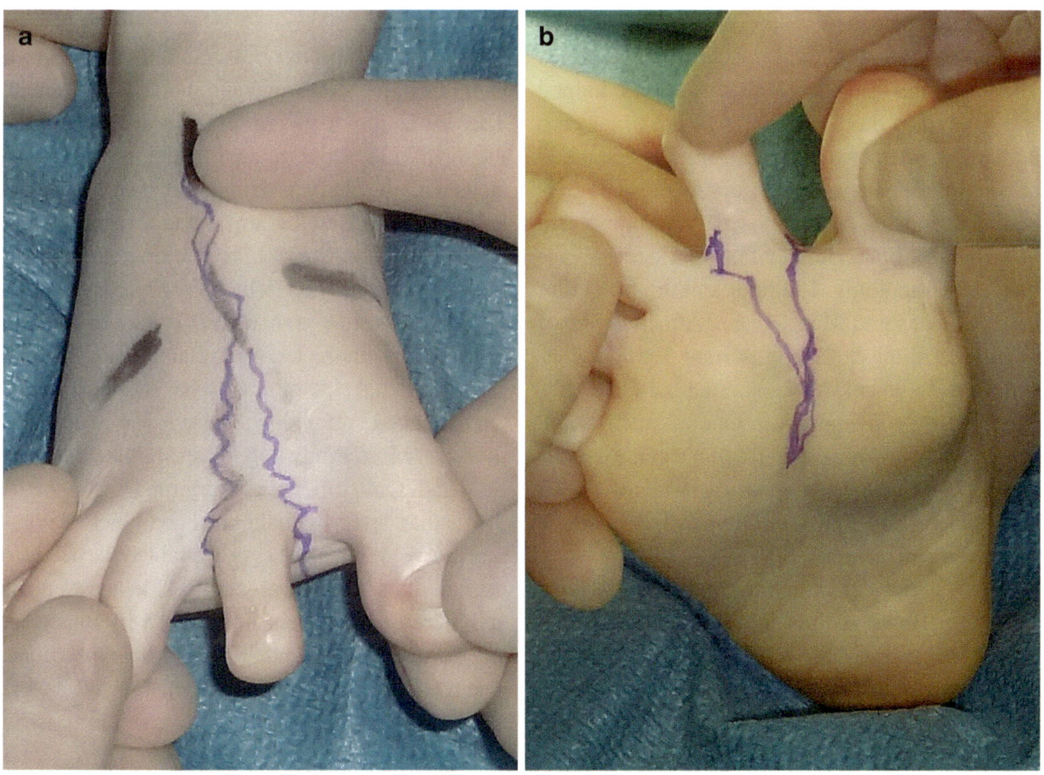

Fig. 17.5 (**a**) Fast zig zag incisions are used, and narrow skin area is taken with the graft. (**b**) Plantar view of the plan

seous muscles on both sides of the metatarsal bone are kept intact so that the network of blood vessels for the bone is minimally disturbed. Extensor tendons attached to the graft (at base of proximal phalanx) are taken with long tails and so are toe flexor tendons. Usually when toe-graft is otherwise prepared free, the artery and vein pedicle is left still in continuity. Tourniquet is discontinued, and toe-graft circulation is checked for possible bleeders and left in peace for 20 min before continuing.

17.3.4 Final Preparation of MTP-II Graft

This is done after the final separation of vascular pedicles separately on the hand table.

The graft distal portion or intermediate phalanx and distal phalanx with the nail must be removed. The skin of toe is saved creating a fillet flap by incising it from dorsal fibular side longitudinally and releasing the skin flaps so that they can cover the joint from tibial side. The flexor tendons are attached to the distal bones to be amputated and they will lose their insertions. Therefore, flexor tendon ends distally are looped and sutured to the flexor sheet of proximal phalanx to provide new firm insertion. The distal end of proximal phalanx is then opened, cartilage is removed, and raw bone exposed. At proximal end of metatarsal bone, the raw bone surface is available after osteotomy. The final length of the joint graft is measured (Fig. 17.6). Attachments of interosseous muscles are important during reconstruction. To be able to reconstruct the ulnar (fibular) interosseous muscle, a tendon graft should be attached at this point to ulnar interosseous insertion because it is impossible when the graft is in place. The joint stability will depend on active dynamization of all four sides of the joint: extensor tendon, flexor tendon, and both interossei forces. However, it is seldom possible to find more than two to three useful muscle units for the transfer during recipient side preparation.

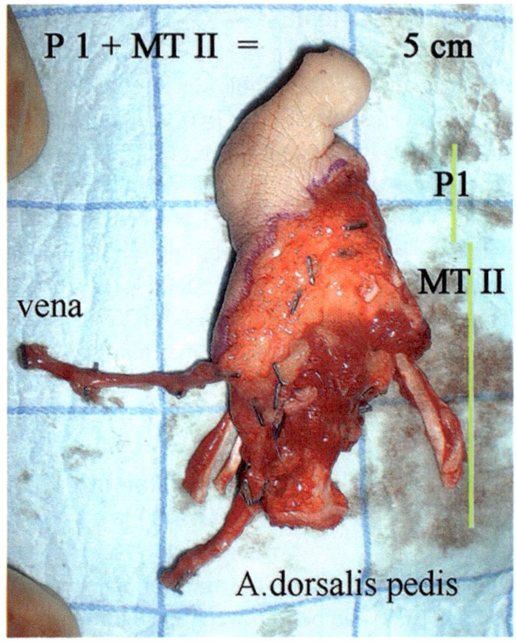

Fig 17.6 A readymade toe MTP-II joint graft

17.3.5 Wrist Recipient Site Preparation

Preoperatively the existing arteries are localized using Doppler ultrasound and marked on the skin. The distraction device is kept in place throughout the operation. Longitudinal radial zig-zag incisions with distal and proximal transverse incisions are used. The distal forearm is widely opened with large developed flaps. It is readily important to identify cephalic vein, which is very constant and suitable for vein connection. It is situated nearby or together with the large combined radial-median nerve on radial side of wrist. The antebrachial fascia is opened and widely excised from the operative area. Mostly only hypoplastic radial artery can be found. Quite often the artery on volar aspect is the median artery with the median branch of common nerve. When neither is available, one needs to use the ulnar artery with end-to-side anastomosis and therefore it is identified. Next very important step is to release the radial tight muscle insertions. The tendons going to finger extensors and flexors are identified and protected. All remaining tight tissue on radial aspect of the wrist is separated from wrist bones and proximal part of the hand. This tissue represents abnormally developed, scarred, and contracted existing parts of ECRL, ECRB, FCR, BR, and APL. During the release, the visible muscle units are separated and marked as possible muscles for the transfer. It would be necessary to find at least three such units (Fig. 17.7).

Under fluoroscopy , the base of II metacarpal bone and the epiphyseal area of ulna is identified and marked with injection needles (Fig. 17.8a). By this means, the epiphysis of ulna can be protected and the right level for the graft localized. The space for the graft is automatically created when adequate and complete release to radial side contracted and scarred muscles are done. Preparation of distal and proximal connection site: Distally MC II basal cortex with cartilage is removed, and raw bone exposed. Proximally the ulna cortex is opened about 6–8 mms proximally from visible bone of distal ulna. A 3–4 mm thick

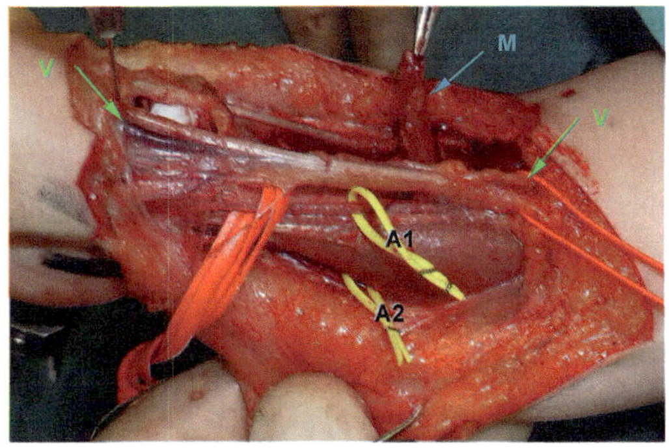

Fig. 17.7 Recipient site. Radial side of the wrist and forearm exposed. The yellow bands are marking median artery A1 and ulnar artery A2. Green piles are marking the vein with the main nerve. One visible muscle unit for transfer is marked with blue pile

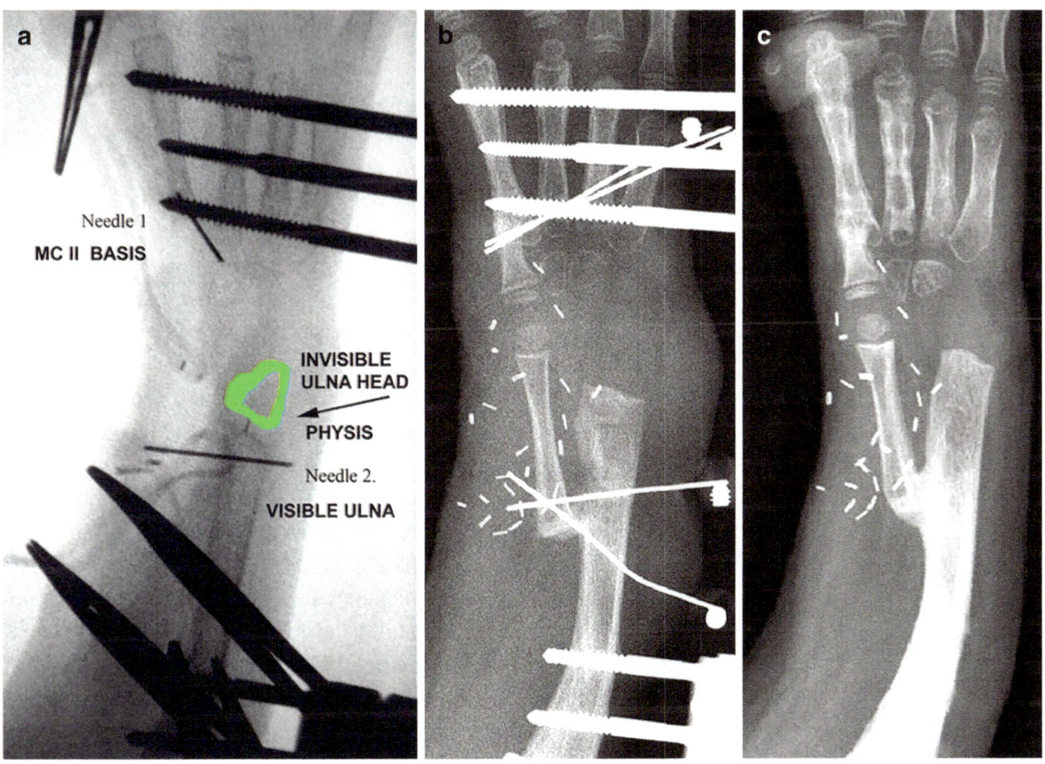

Fig. 17.8 (**a**) Both osteosynthesis sites marked with injection needles. Invisible ulnar head (green area) and distal ulnar epiphysis on its proximal side must be protected. (**b**) X-ray postoperatively showing good alignment of the transferred joint graft. Observe thin K-wires drilled through the forearm and proximal hand. (**c**) Well-united graft 4 months postoperatively

and 20 mm long bone flap with proximally intact periosteum is created with a sharp chisel and turned out as a platform radially [8]. To allow the metatarsal graft to become aligned parallel with ulna, some parts of radial wrist column cartilage (usually scaphoid and trapezoideum) can be removed to add space for the joint. The length between ready-prepared base of the MC II and the created bony platform at ulna is measured. At this point, the distractor can be still adjusted with 1–2 mm additional lengthening when necessary.

17.3.6 Reconstruction of the Radial Half of the Wrist with MTP-II-Joint Graft

The reconstruction continues with placing the joint graft between two created raw bone sites, MC II base and bony radial platform created on radial aspect of distal ulna (Fig. 17.8.). The MTP-joint position should be kept in slight 10–15° flexion for the better initial stability and aligning the joint with the wrist position. The graft is placed dorsal side pointing dorsally. Both graft ends are fixed with two 0.6 mm K-wires to keep it in optimum position (Fig. 17.8b). Those 4 K-wires can be drilled through the opposite side of forearm leaving them visible and protected (Fig. 17.9). Reconstructed wrist is immediately checked with fluoroscopy and graft position is improved when necessary. The toe extensor-, flexor- and two interosseal-tendons are then connected with tendon muscle units which were found during dissection. At least the detached muscle mass is divided into two parts. Best muscle force should be given to extensor side and less to flexor side. Both interosseous insertions are activated when possible.

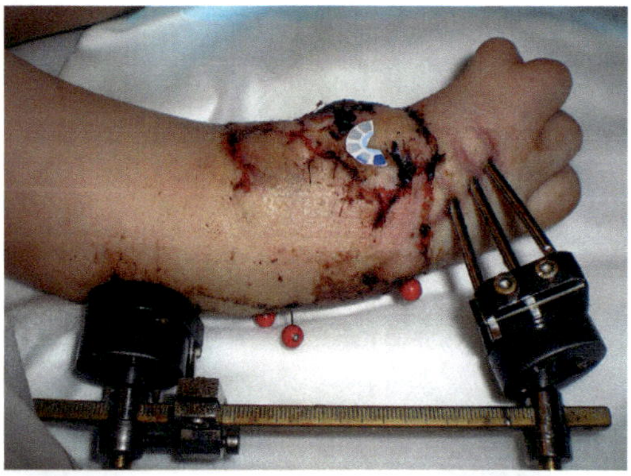

Fig. 17.9 Situation 5 days postoperatively shows a good color of the filleted toe-skin. Skin temperature indicator is used for flap monitoring. Red balls are protecting the K-wires on ulnar skin. Their removal is very simple at 4 weeks

Microsurgical part must be done using operative microscope: Artery, usually dorsalis pedis, is connected either end-to-end with median artery or end-to-side with ulnar artery. Also, a piece or about ¼ of the radial dorsal part of the common nerve is connected to two tiny dorsal toe nerves.

The fillet flap of toe skin usually covers the joint and transferred graft only partly.

Dorsal forearm skin distally is usually loose on the ulnar aspect of the wrist and allows, when separated distally with transverse incision and undermined, a mild shift to radial direction. Additionally, some split skin graft is often necessary to help in wound coverage.

17.4 Postoperative Treatment

17.4.1 Early Postoperative Care

The graft circulation, which sometimes starts slowly, becomes improved when patient is awake and fluid balance has become corrected. Patient is followed at intensive care unit or recovery room for the first night observing the flap skin color, temperature, and turgor. The skin over the graft swells during the first postoperative night when the hemodynamics is normalized with adequate fluid substitution. Pain is eliminated using a continuous axillary plexus catheter for the first 3–4 days. Patient is kept in bed rest for about 5 days postoperatively and the graft condition is monitored continuously (Fig. 17.9.). Dressing changes at wrist are done daily. On the sixth postoperative day, the foot dressing change is performed and a below knee walking plaster cast is placed for 4 weeks and walking exercises started. Patient is sent home on the 7th–9th day after operation. Next X-ray control is done at 4 weeks and the small K-wires can be pulled out from ulnar border of the wrist and forearm very easily (no anesthesia required). The foot has healed and walking with normal shoes are permitted.

17.4.2 Distractor Removal

Sound protection of the reconstructed wrist is needed for 6 months. The distractor remains in place for next 8–9 weeks postoperatively. During that time, the bone will heal and consolidate at both graft ends when the graft survival and circulation has continued normally. The removal of distractor is done after 2 months under general anesthesia. When there is any doubt of consolidation, then the fixation pins can be left inside the plaster to maintain further stability. A long plaster cast from MCP- level to axilla is used with elbow joint in 90° flexion. That plaster is continued for 1 month. Finger motion is encouraged. At 3 months postoperatively, a volar regular splint is continued for the next 3 months. The child is encouraged to use the hand daily and wrist extension exercises are started and continued intermittently without the splint.

17.4.3 Pollicization

In good quality hands, the lack of functional thumb can be treated with pollicization 6–12 months after joint stabilization. When the pinching pattern has been in between index and middle finger the useful thumb can be created using common techniques. When there exist some remnants of red-colored toe-pulp type skin, its removal or need for other scar correction, can be combined to pollicization.

17.5 Results

The wrist motion depends on the quality of forearm muscles and wrist extension tends to be generally weaker than flexion. When the treatment period is over, the child can usually keep the hand easily in neutral position and the flexion will improve and the range of wrist motion is commonly between 60 and 90°. The fingers may have more stiffness in early postoperative period due to distraction, but their motion will return to preoperative level during postoperative treatment period. The hand alignment is very good or even overcorrected to mild ulnar deviation. The transferred MT-bone will hypertrophy during the first 2 years. The scars will improve in the same time period.

17.5.1 Early Prognosis

During the following 6–8 years or at age 4–11, the hand alignment and hand usage will be common without problems (Fig. 17.10). A straight and mobile wrist has been achieved in good quality forearms. A slow return to mild radial deviation will happen because metatarsal arm at the end of distal Y-form ulna has lower growth pace than distal ulna arm. The ulna growth is usually at the level of intact ulna for these patients. Due to malformation, ulna length will remain commonly about 1/3 less compared to normal side or normal percentile at same age.

17.5.2 Long-Term Results

Long-term results using microsurgical techniques were published in 2008 [9] (Vilkki). In 19 cases followed 11 years in mean, the total wrist motion was 83° in mean and clearly superior to other published series [10] (Murphy et al. 2017). Also, the forearm (ulna) growth did follow the natural pace or gave about 67% of the length compared to normal ulna length (Fig. 17.11). So, the technique does not deteriorate the ulna growth. Hand alignment or radial deviation was 28° in mean. There were, however, some wrists where the metatarsal bone graft deviated too much, and attention has been paid that the Y-fork should never deviate more than 40° during the growth period.

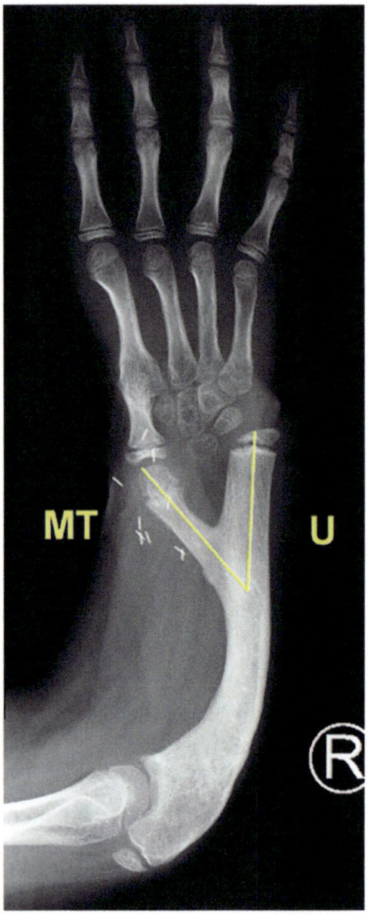

Fig. 17.10 Good growth balance at Y-fork arms during the growth. MT-arm length 45.5 mm and Ulna-arm length 44.0 mm. Total Ulna length 130 mm. X-ray taken at about 10 years of age and almost 8 years postoperatively.

17.5.3 Donor Side Morbidity

The foot development has been good in long term after second ray removal. Very few complaints have been reported and most patients consider their operated foot as normal (Fig. 17.12). It is important that during primary operation the web space can be closed without skin grafts. Therefore, only minimum of skin has been taken with the graft.

17.5.4 Observations on the Results

17.5.4.1 The Metatarsal: Distal Ulna Ratio

The balance [11] in two forks at Y-form ulna is slowly changing with the growth and age. Due to overcorrection, there will be some ulnar deviation of the wrist axis after the transfer and it slowly will turn into mild radial deviation at adolescence. This may sometimes be an indication for secondary correction at the age of 12–15 years.

17.5.4.2 MTP-II Joint Alignment and Stability

There has appeared a tendency for MTP-joint subluxation in some extremities. That will affect the result allowing more radial deviation. This was learnt during long-term follow-up study and more attention has been paid thereafter to primary operation. It is important to reconstruct all possible stabilizing forces around the joint. A slight flexion at the joint graft will further provide better stability in the beginning. Possible reasons for later developing instability are collected in Table 17.2.

17.5.4.3 Necessity for Long-Term Follow-Up

Especially after age 11, the continuous observation on development of wrist alignment and MTP-joint stability is important. During adolescence, the second faster growth spurt may change the wrist axis to turn slowly into radial deviation. At that period from 11 to 15 years, a keen follow-up is mandatory. The tendency for the change to radial deviation can be eliminated by performing an epiphyseodesis at distal ulna. Alternatively, when the ultimate length of forearm is important, a reoperation to correct the malalignment may be needed in some cases. That salvage operation can be accomplished with a **joint transport** technique (Fig. 17.13). It requires an osteotomy at the base of metatarsal graft and use of secondary dis-

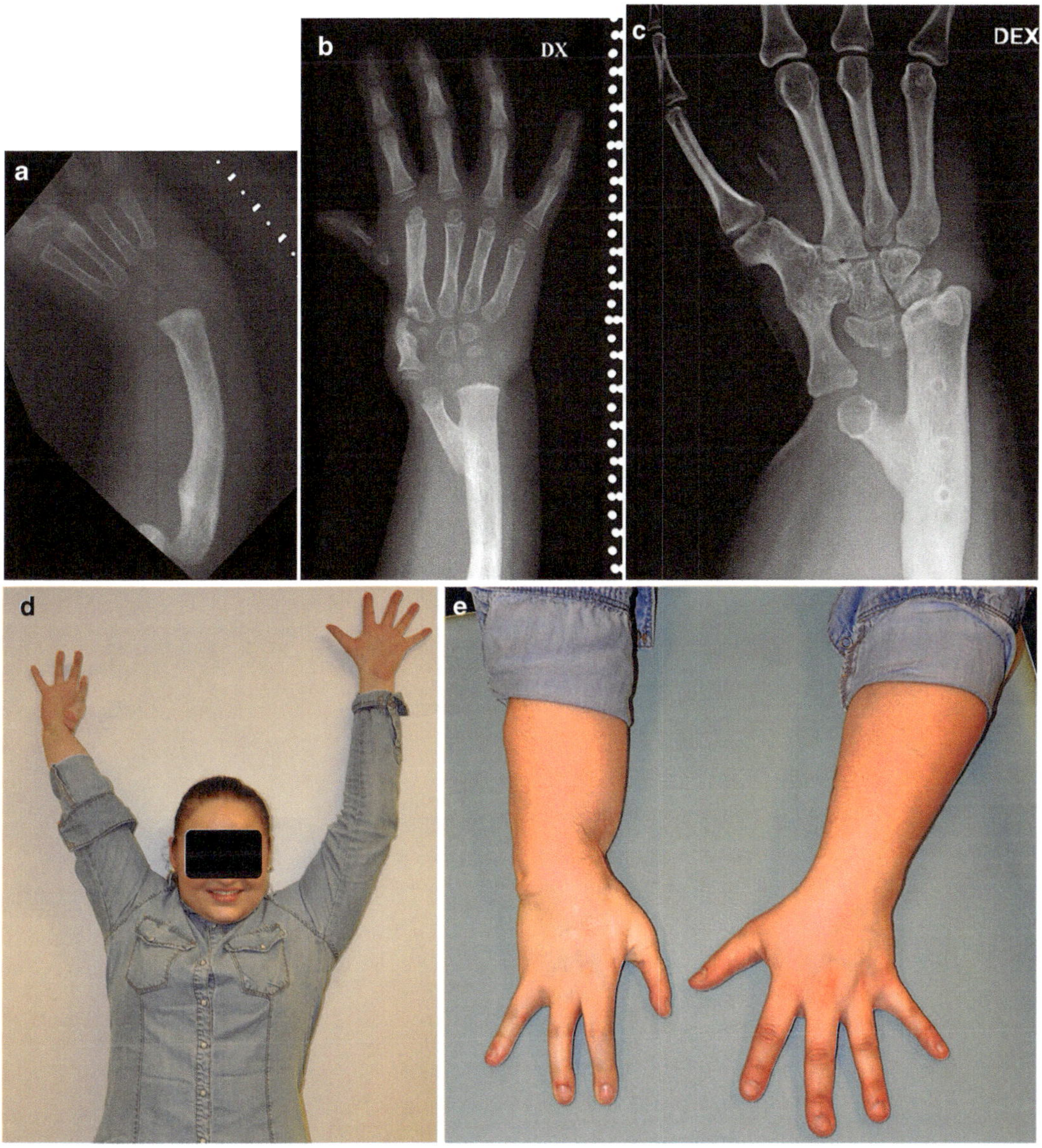

Fig 17.11 A long-term result: Wrist reconstruction was done at age 15 months. Pollicization at age 3 years and corrective ulna osteotomy at age 14 years. (**a**–**c**) X-ray series taken at 1 year, 3 years, and 26 years. (**d**, **e**) The Patient at age 26. Good wrist mobility from 20-degree extension to 70-degree flexion. Her profession is a nurse (video 17.1)

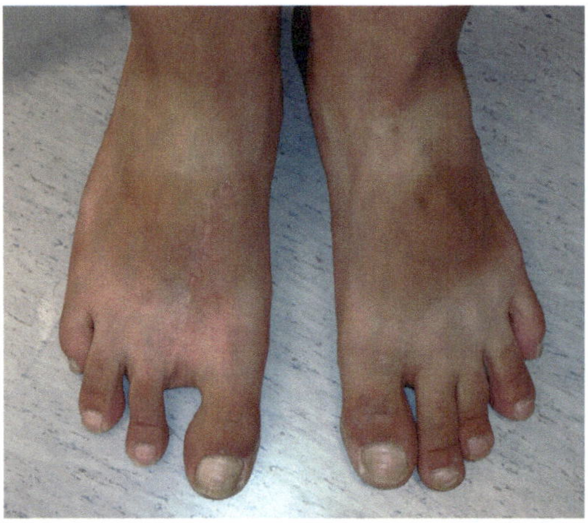

Fig. 17.12 "No problems at the donor foot postoperatively. Second ray removed from the right foot. Also the scar has remained minimal when a fast Zig-Zag incision was used. Compare Figure Fig. 17.5a"

Table 17.2 Possible reasons for malalignment and instability

1.	Primary malalignment of the graft
	• Too much deviation of MT-branch. Below 40° is acceptable
	• Joint graft in hyperextension
2.	Primary lack of external muscle power around the joint because of difficulty to reconstruct normal dynamic stabilizers of the MTP-joint. Often not enough tendons to be transferred
3.	Secondarily malalignment due to a poor metatarsal bone growth, leading to wrong balance at Y-fork during the growth
4.	Secondary instability at MTP-II joint

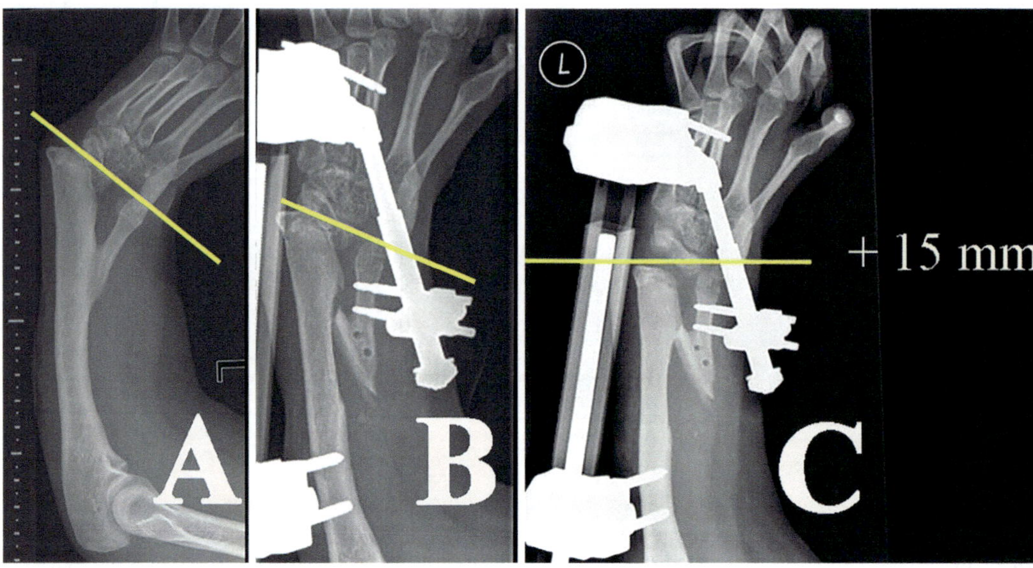

Fig 17.13 (a–c) X-ray series of a salvage procedure to correct wrist motion axis and alignment. Secondary distraction after detachment of the proximal graft end with longitudinal osteotomy. Joint transport will happen easily using double distractors. A small separate fixator is attached between two pins inserted at metatarsal bone and one distal hand pin together with larger distractor

traction. The metatarsal becomes elongated during distraction and it easily consolidates spontaneously with new bone formation. Selection and need for secondary procedures as well as timing are made individually.

17.6 General Remarks about Microvascular Reconstruction of Radial Club Hand

17.6.1 Positive Remarks

Microvascular reconstruction with MTP-II joint transfer has some advantages over conventional methods. The approach is less traumatic to epiphysis of distal ulna. It allows a natural growth of ulna as it would typically happen in radial dysplasia. However, it cannot normalize the forearm length, which will commonly remain clearly subnormal in Types II–IV of radial dysplasia. In author's series, relative ulna length (RUL) has been in mean 67%.

The wrist-like active extension-flexion mobility has regularly been superior compared to centralization or radialization series. A common range of total active motion (TAM), which is easily achieved, has been between 75 and 100° and in long-term study was in mean 83%.

Cosmetic appearance is greatly improved with corrected wrist stability (Fig. 17.14).

The donor site morbidity remains commonly very low after second toe ray removal. It is comparable with typical toe-to-hand transfer.

17.6.2 Negative Remarks

There is a slow tendency to partial recurrence of radial deviation at adolescence. This is because metatarsal bone growth is slower than distal ulna growth during the second growth spurt after age 11 years.

Secondary subluxation at transferred MTP-joint due to inadequate stabilizing muscle force can in some lower quality hands deteriorate the result. Therefore, this reconstruction is not recommended for low-quality extremities with very high severity index.

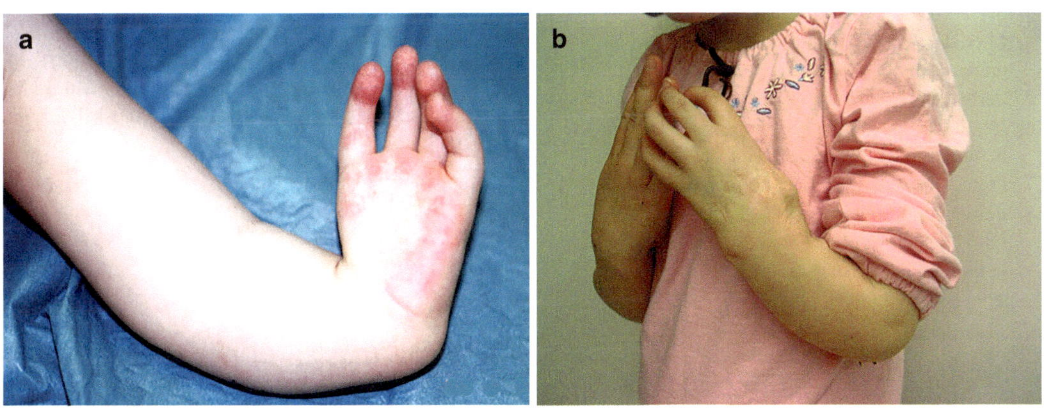

Fig. 17.14 (**a**) An example of a severely deviating radial club hand that was operated at age 2 years with vascularized MTP-II joint transfer. Severity Index was mild or 6 p. (**b**) The treated forearm at age 6 years

17.7 Conclusion

The microvascular option using MTP-II ray for reconstruction of radial dysplasia

types III and IV is providing a stabilization of radial club hand with growing bone and movable joint unit. It is giving good results during the first decade of life, but it may need further treatment when second growth spurt in adolescence is actual. However, the demand for secondary corrections has remained low in author's series. Alternatively, an epiphyseodesis of distal ulna at age 11–12 years or a salvage procedure with joint transport more distally at a later stage can be used for further correction. Good motion at the wrist is appreciated by patients [12]. Donor site morbidity is commonly considered minimal. The treatment cannot overcome commonly appearing limb length discrepancy in unilateral cases (Table 17.3).

Table 17.3 Main principles for successful microvascular reconstruction

1.	Treat from the birth with continuous stretching and splinting
2.	Before any operation check the quality of involved extremity using severity grading.
3.	Distract slowly to full correction to allow some overcorrection
4.	Microsurgical skill and treatment culture is the prerequisite for success
5.	Perfect alignment of the graft is mandatory
6.	Healing of the graft at both ends must be complete before disassembly of distractor
7.	Protect the graft during first 6 months
8.	Pollicization, when feasible, is done 1 year after joint transfer
9.	Follow-up is necessary through the growth period and especially important before adolescence

References

1. Vilkki SK. Severity grading in radial dysplasia. J Hand Surg Eur Vol. 2014;39(9):977–83.
2. Morsy M, Parry JA, Moran SL. Vascularized second metatarsophalangeal joint transfer for salvage of failed centralization in radial longitudinal deficiency: case report. Ann Plast Surg. 2017;78:195–7.
3. Nettelblad H, Randolph MA, Weiland AJ. Free microvascular epiphyseal-plate transplantation. An experimental study in dogs. J Bone Joint Surg Am. 1984;66(9):1421–30.
4. Vilkki SK. Distraction and microvascular epiphysis transfer for radial club hand. J Hand Surg Br. 1998;23:445–52.
5. Inberg P, Kassila M, Vilkki S, Neuvonen P. Anaesthesia for microvascular surgery in children: a combination of general anaesthesia and axillary plexus block. Acta Anaesthesiol Scand. 1995;39:518–22.
6. Vilkki SK. Advances in microsurgical reconstruction of the congenitally adactylous hand. Clin Orthop Relat Res. 1995;314:45–58.
7. Vilkki SK. Vascularized joint transfer for radial club hand. Tech Hand Up Extrem Surg. 1998;2:126–37.
8. Vilkki SK. Radial Club hand: wrist distraction and joint transplantation. In: EFORT textbook: surgical techniques in Orthopaedics and traumatology 55.370-C-10. Amsterdam: Elsevier; 2001. p. 5p.
9. Vilkki SK. Vascularized metatarsophalangeal joint transfer for radial hypoplasia. Semin Plast Surg. 2008;22:195–212.
10. Murphy GRF, et al. Correction of "wrist" deformity in radial dysplasia: a systematic review and meta-analysis. J Bone Joint Surg Am. 2017;99:2120–6.
11. Vilkki SK, Paavilainen P, et al. Vascularized second metatarsophalangeal joint transfer for radial deficiency—an update. J Hand Surg. 2018;43(9):907–18.
12. Ekblom, et al. Hand function in children with radial longitudinal deficiency. BMC Musculoskel Disord. 2013;14:116–29.

18 Metacarpal Synostosis

Anna M. Acosta and Terry R. Light

Abstract

Metacarpal synostosis is an uncommon hand anomaly that may occur in isolation (ring-small metacarpal) or in connection with a congenital syndrome (Apert, Ellis–van Creveld). It has been hypothesized to be sporadically inherited via x-linked recessive or autosomal dominant traits and is possibly linked to a genetic abnormality in the FGF16 gene. This hand difference likely forms during the first 4–8 weeks of gestation during rapid development of the upper limb.

Children are most often evaluated due to parental concerns regarding a deviated finger, most commonly the small finger that is abducted from the hand. Radiographic examination can confirm the diagnosis of metacarpal synostosis. Treatment is guided by symptoms and digital function. Operative treatments involving osteotomy and bone graft interposition. Though multiple techniques address deformity and length discrepancy, affected digits may remain hypoplastic and stiff and may benefit from amputation.

Keywords

Metacarpal synostosis · Apert syndrome · Ellis–van Creveld · Bone Graft · Osteotomy

18.1 Introduction

Metacarpal synostosis is an uncommon congenital anomaly of the hand characterized by a partial or complete fusion of the metacarpals [1]. The incidence of metacarpal synostosis has been variously estimated to be 0.02%, 0.07% [2], 0.002 [3], and 0.007 [4]. The first recorded documentation of metacarpal synostosis was an 1827 drawing depicting fusion of metacarpals in a German publication [5, 6]. Metacarpal synostosis has been referred to as absent fifth metacarpal [3], syndactyly type V [7], bilateral ulnar thumbs [8], congenital metacarpal malformation [9], and fifth ray anomaly [10].

Though metacarpal synostosis may occur between any adjacent two rays, it is most commonly observed as fusion between the ring and small finger metacarpals [5, 6, 11–14]. Metacarpal synostosis may occur in isolation or in association with other anomalies including central polydactyly, radial deficiency, ulnar deficiency, cleft hand, and Apert syndrome [5–6, 11–12, 15].

Hands with metacarpal synostosis have one of two common appearances. The first is a seemingly normal hand with fingers that are deviated in the coronal plane from the normal resting

A. M. Acosta
MemorialCare Miller Children's & Women's Hospital Long Beach, Long Beach, CA, USA

T. R. Light (✉)
Loyola University Stritch School of Medicine, Maywood, IL, USA
e-mail: tlight@lumc.edu

G. Pajardi (ed.), *Pediatric Hand Surgery*, https://doi.org/10.1007/978-3-031-30984-7_18

alignment of the hand. The digits cannot be straightened out with manipulation. Abutment of the proximal phalanx bases at the metacarpophalangeal joints (MCPs) of the neighboring fingers causes the splaying deformity. The second, less common appearance, is an overly broad or wide palm due to metacarpal shaft deviation with associated adduction of the involved finger. The clinical and radiographic appearance of the hands guides classification and treatment strategies. Surgical correction of metacarpal synostosis aims to alter bony structure to allow for soft tissue realignment across the metacarpophalangeal joints. Correction of metacarpal synostosis can be challenging, with early technically success in some patients eroded by recurrence of deformity

18.2 Genetics

Metacarpal synostosis may occur in isolation or in association with other hand anomalies. Early German literature suggested a familial inheritance pattern for cases of metacarpal synostosis [5]. More recent literature has suggested a sporadic inheritance patterns, x-linked recessive, or autosomal dominant, for most cases of isolated metacarpal synostosis [1, 2, 5, 16]. The most common presentation of isolated metacarpal synostosis involves the ring and small finger metacarpals. Jamsheer et al. [1] reported on two unrelated patients with a sporadic presentation of ring-small metacarpal synostosis. Through exome DNA sequencing, they found a genetic nonsense mutation on chromosome Xq21.1 in exome 3 of the FGF16 gene associated with X-linked recessive mutations. Thus, they hypothesized that X-linked recessive FGF16 mutations may be a novel cause of isolated metacarpal synostosis [1]. Other authors have noted this anomaly to be more prevalent in males supporting the likelihood of an x-linked recessive inheritance pattern. Females are more likely to be genetic carriers [5]. Robinow et al. [7] published a case report on a family with 4 members diagnosed with syndactyly type V, syndactyly with metacarpal and metatarsal synostosis. His study of this family suggested a sporadic mutation in the first individual affected (mother), proceeding into the following generation as an autosomal dominant trait to three of her four children.

Metacarpal synostosis may also present as part of a syndrome. Gottschalk et al. [2] detailed syndromes involving carpal coalitions and metacarpal synostosis. Ellis–van Creveld syndrome is a rare disorder of chondro-ectodermal dysplasia that presents as a short-limbed dwarfism. Hands of individuals with Ellis–van Creveld syndrome may demonstrate metacarpal synostosis, clinodactyly, capito-hamate coalition, or postaxial polydactyly [15]. It is an autosomal recessive disorder effecting the EVC1 and EVC2 genes on chromosome 4p16 [2]. Half of Ellis–van Crevald syndrome patients also show abnormalities in the cardiac system, skin, nails, hair, and teeth.

Although uncommon, the most frequent syndrome associated with metacarpal synostosis is Apert Syndrome. Acrocephalosyndactyly, or Apert syndrome, is an autosomal dominant disorder characterized by craniofacial malformations and complex complicated syndactyly of the hands [17]. Metacarpal synostosis in patients with Apert syndrome is different from synostosis noted in isolated cases. The Apert hand synostosis involves the proximal portion of the ring and small finger metacarpals, however, the small finger is not held in an abducted position as it is in isolated cases [17] (Fig. 18.1). Dao et al. [17] determined that approximately 77% of their Apert syndrome patients demonstrated ring-small metacarpal synostosis. They noted that because not all synostoses were ossified at birth the synostosis may not always be visible initially on radiographic examination. Because the synostosis is only evident later in childhood, one can infer that a synchondrosis or synfibrosis presents at birth later ossifies. The authors also observed that the small finger in patients with Apert syndrome tended to be the most "normal" digit in these hands. They suggested that it was beneficial to resect the synostosis bridge between the ring-small metacarpal synostosis to increase the mobility of the small finger carpometacarpal join thereby enhancing the ability of the small finger to reach the thumb [17].

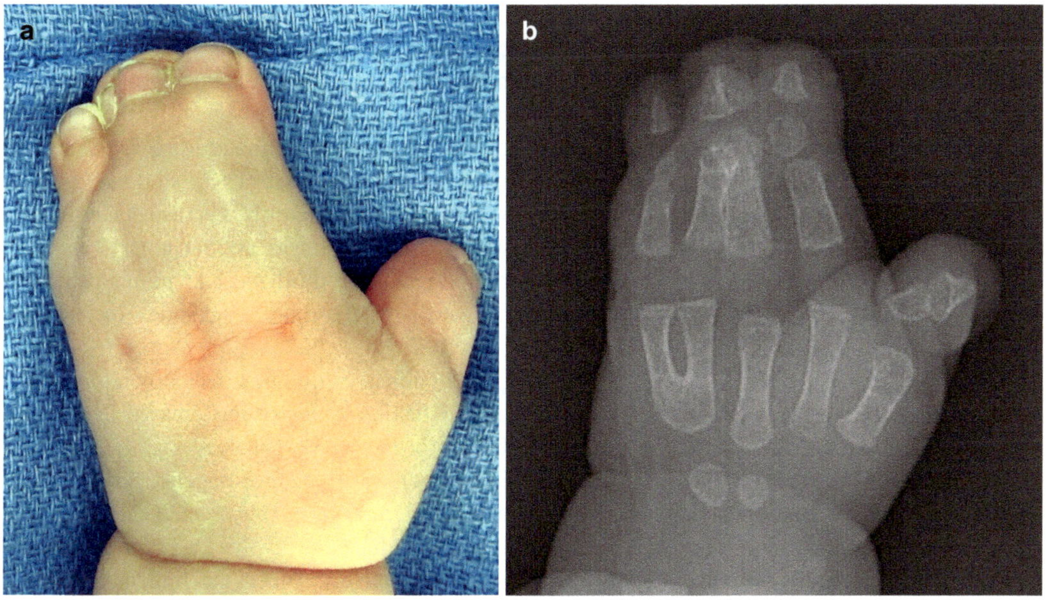

Fig. 18.1 (**a**, **b**) (**a**) Clinical photograph of a hand in a patient with Apert syndrome. (**b**) Radiograph of a hand in a patient with Apert syndrome demonstrating complex complicated syndactyly with metacarpal synostosis

18.3 Embryology

Upper limb embryologic development occurs between the fourth and eighth week of gestation. At week 4, the upper limb bud begins to develop, at week 5, the hand plate is present, at week 7, interdigital apoptosis and chondrification of middle phalanges occur, and at week 8, wrist and carpal inter-zones are created. Most congenital hand anomalies occur during weeks 4 and 8 of gestation during the rapid development of the upper limb [18]. Most authors have felt that metacarpal synostosis was secondary to a failure of differentiation during limb bud development. Other authors have challenged this theory citing similarities between the hands of metacarpal synostosis and limb longitudinal deficiencies as evidence that this condition is due to a failure of formation.

Dermatoglyphics is the study of hand and foot skin ridge patterns. Temtamy and McKusick [16] studied the dermatoglyphics in the hands of patients with syndactyly and in the hands of patients with metacarpal synostosis. The authors found abnormalities in the patterns of digital triradii c and d in patients with metacarpal synostosis similar to the abnormalities in patients with syndactyly. Miura [12] reviewed 14 patient cases with metacarpal synostosis using hand pattern profiles and dermatoglyphics. Miura also concluding that the differences in patients with metacarpal synostosis were similar to those of patients with syndactyly of the ring and small fingers. They concluded that metacarpal synostosis should be classified as failure of separation/differentiation (as syndactyly is classified) rather than as a failure of formation or longitudinal deficiency.

Ogino and Kato [4] reviewed nine cases of metacarpal synostosis. They found characteristics common to the hands of patients with ring-small metacarpal synostosis and shared with the hands of patients with ulnar longitudinal deficiency. Patients with ring-small metacarpal synostosis tended to have a relatively small, small finger with hypoplastic hypothenar musculature and generalized hypoplasia of the hand. Citing prior studies of longitudinal deficiency, Ogino and Kato hypothesized that this limb hypoplasia seen in metacarpal synostosis may also be related to a deficit in mesenchymal cells in the developing limb bud. However, in their study, they had one patient without hypoplasia of the ulnar side of the hand, leading them to consider an alternate explanation of the failure of induction of the digital rays in the hand plate, as previously hypothesized by Miura [12] and Temtamy and McKusick [16].

18.4 Clinical Exam

Metacarpal synostosis may not be apparent at birth. Parents often seek evaluation because the small finger is "growing crooked". Most will have detected a deviation of the small finger from the rest of the hand over time. They may observe the child having difficulty with the finger becoming caught or what they perceive as an awkward grasping pattern, as the finger remains deviated or scissors over the neighboring finger as the hand is closed. Parents often comment that there seems to be an "absent knuckle" when the short small finger is compared to the contralateral side [19] (Fig. 18.2)

Synostosis involving the ring and small metacarpals is the most common pattern of involvement. Sixty to eighty percent of these children have bilateral hand involvement [5]. Synostosis of the middle and ring metacarpals is the second most common pattern. These children present with the divergence of the two fingers, a radially deviated middle finger and an ulnarly deviated ring finger. The third most common pattern is synostosis of the thumb and index metacarpals (Fig. 18.3).

On clinical exam, the affected hand may lack digital flexion or extension creases [5]. Active flexion of the fingers involved may be restricted in addition to splaying of fingers apart from one another [1, 5, 12, 20]. The affected child is unable to fully adduct the involved fingers either passively or actively. When the fingers are flexed into a clenched fist, they may scissor over the adjacent finger [21].

In the ring-small metacarpal synostosis, the small finger may be hypoplastic and abducted from the ring finger. Muira [12] attributed the finger abduction phenomenon to be secondary to both bony and soft tissue developmental differ-

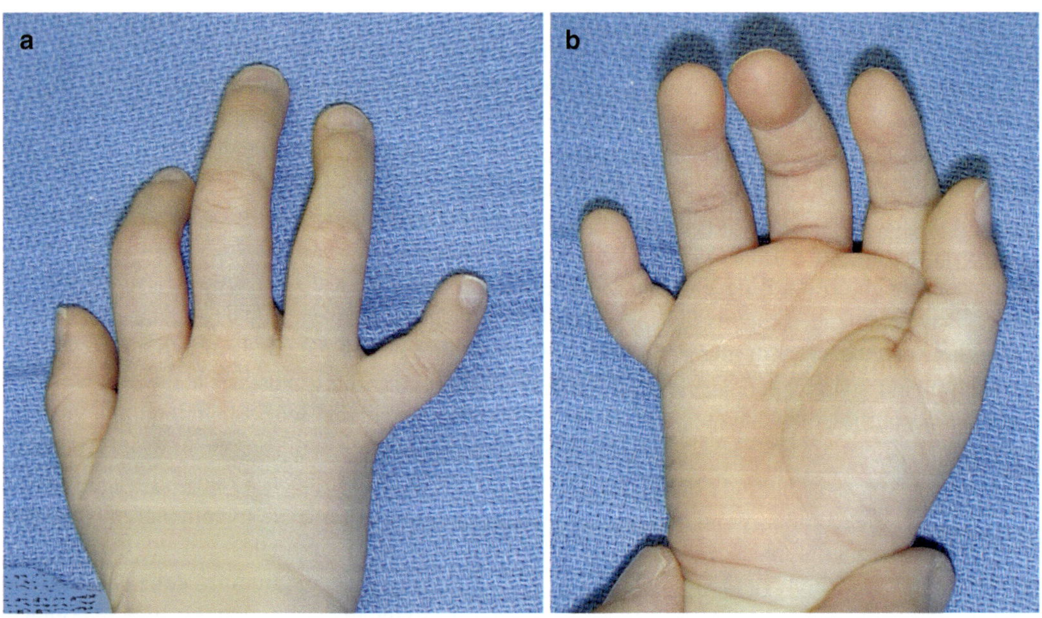

Fig. 18.2 (**a**, **b**) Clinical photograph of a hand with isolated ring-small finger metacarpal synostosis. (**a**) dorsal (**b**) volar

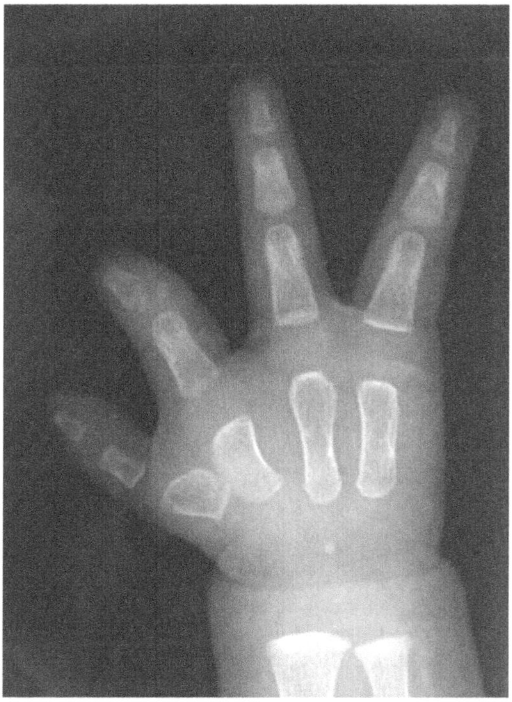

Fig. 18.3 Thumb-index metacarpal synostosis

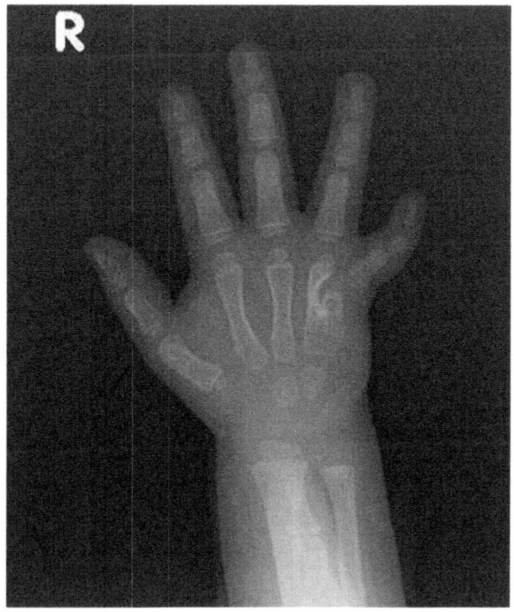

Fig. 18.4 Radiograph of hand with isolated ring-small finger metacarpal synostosis with compression of head of small finger metacarpal

ences. He found that intrinsic muscles were displaced palmarward to the synostosis. When the metacarpal heads converge distally, the proximal phalangeal bases on the adjacent fingers abut resulting in static deviation. The normally central tracking extrinsic flexors and extensor tendons are then forced to track eccentrically as the finger deviates and the space between the metacarpal heads is narrowed. This creates a secondary dynamic abduction force across the metacarpophalangeal joints, further deviating the finger.

As the metacarpal heads converge distally, the physeal orientation in the distal metacarpal becomes convergent with the adjacent metacarpal metaphysis/shaft leading to altered bone development. Buck-Gramcko hypothesized that associated small finger hypoplasia may be secondary to the pressure applied by the adjacent finger metacarpal [5, 14, 20] (Fig. 18.4). In line with the Hueter-Volkman principles, compression across the metacarpal epiphysis may cause retardation of longitudinal growth of the bone. Buck-Gramko described hypoplastic changes to progress over the first few years of life but reported minimal change after the age of 4 years [5].

18.5 Radiographic Exam

Radiographic examination of the hand will confirm the clinical examination and will establish the diagnosis of metacarpal synostosis.

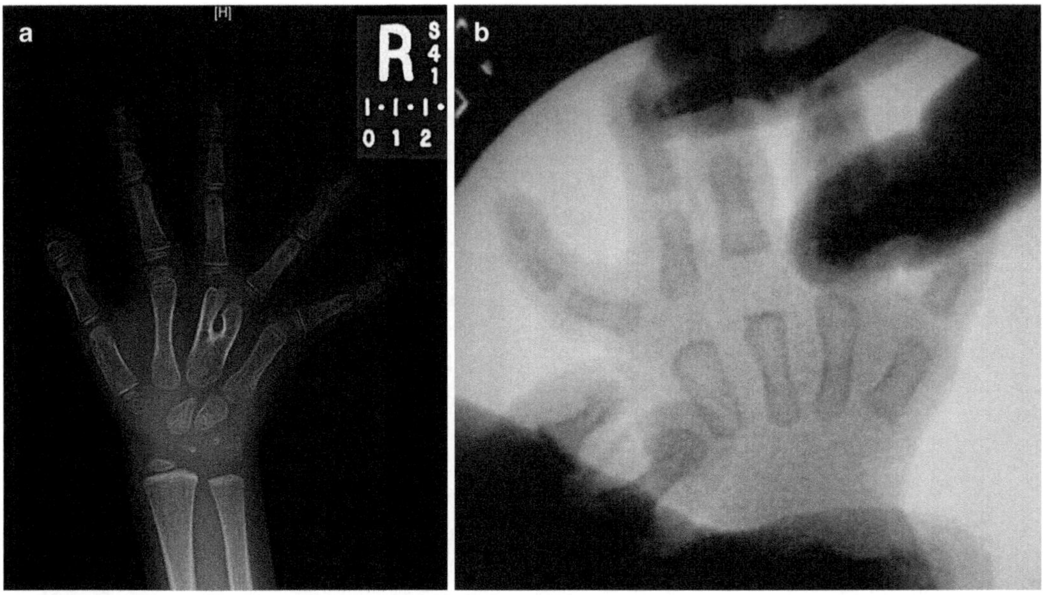

Fig. 18.5 (**a**, **b**) (**a**) Partial metacarpal synostosis of the middle and ring finger. (**b**) Complete metacarpal synostosis (expanded metacarpal head)

Synostosis, when present, is invariably present proximally at the base of the metacarpals. Fusion between the metacarpals may be partial or may extend the entire length of the involved rays in a complete synostosis. The metacarpal head may take the form of a single expanded head or as two distinct heads (Fig. 18.5). The metacarpal shafts may deviate, converge, or run parallel to one another (Fig. 18.6). The converging metacarpals may appear hypoplastic and the physis abnormal secondary to compression of the neighboring metacarpal cortex. The proximal phalanx of the adjacent fingers will often abut at the base causing deviation of the phalanges at the metacarpophalangeal joint (Fig. 18.7).

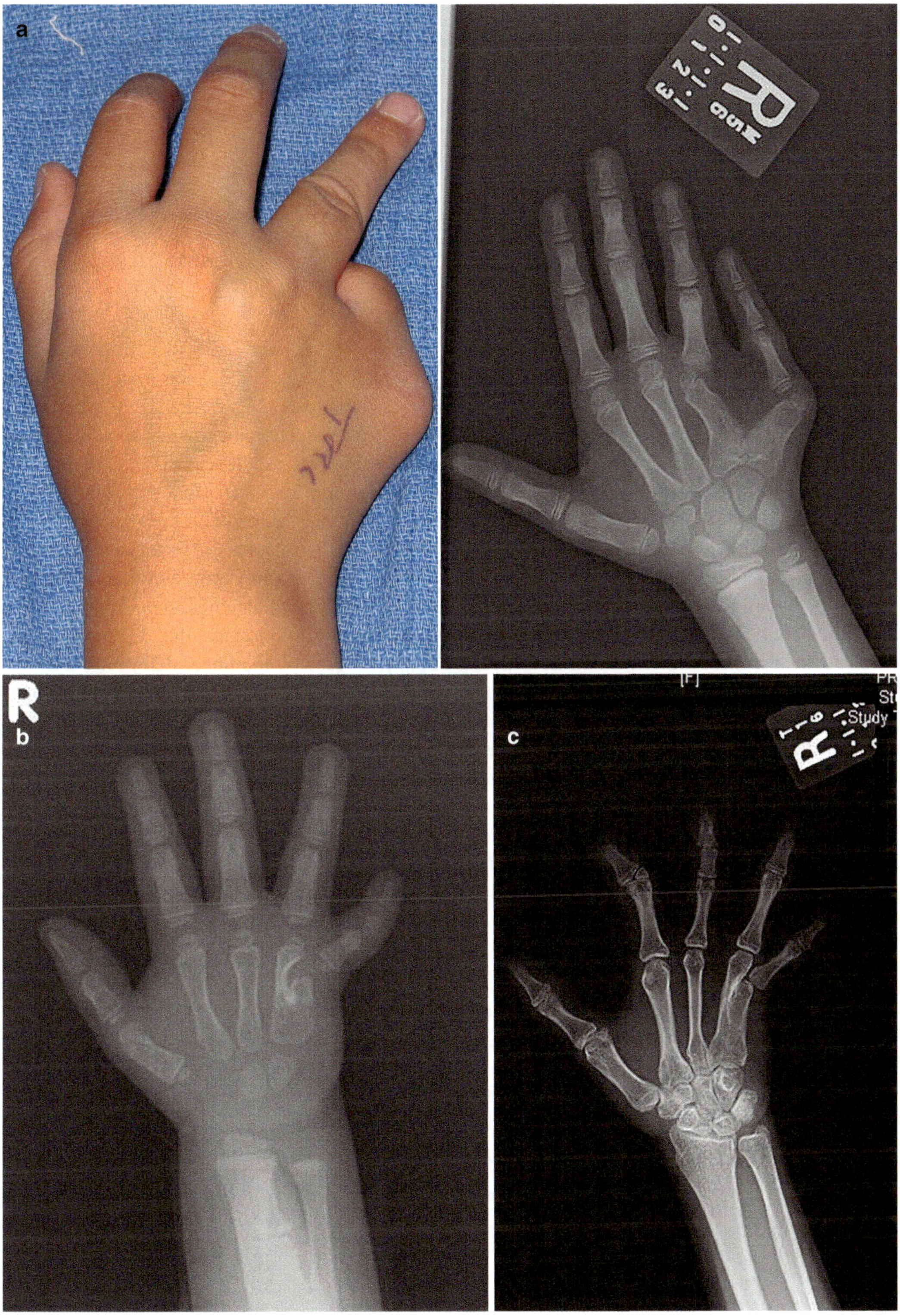

Fig. 18.6 (**a**–**c**): Ring-small finger metacarpal synostosis with deviating (**a**), converging (**b**), and close parallel (**c**) metacarpal shafts. Resultant adduction (**a**) or abduction (**b**, **c**) of the small finger at the MCP

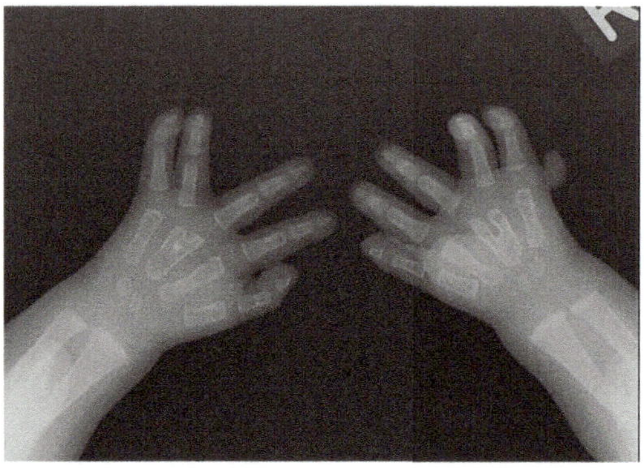

Fig. 18.7 Radiograph of bilateral hand middle-ring finger metacarpal synostosis. Phalangeal abutment at the base of proximal phalanx' of middle and ring fingers causing splaying deformity

18.6 Classification

In 1993, Buck-Gramcko and Wood [5] proposed a simple classification system for metacarpal synostosis after evaluating 109 patients with 152 involved hands. They described three different anatomic types of metacarpal synostosis (Table 18.1). Type I involves coalition at the base of the metacarpal only with minimal deformity or growth disturbance. Type II hands have a synostosis that extends up to half of the length of the metacarpal shaft. The small finger is often small, short, and ulnarly deviated. Type III hands include a synostosis that extends along more than half of the length of the metacarpal. Type III hands were subdivided into two groups. Type IIIA hands have a synostosis of greater than 50% of the metacarpal shaft length but possess a separate metacarpophalangeal joint for each digit. Type IIIB hands have a metacarpal synostosis of more than 50% of the metacarpal length and the involved digits share a common metacarpophalangeal joint, creating a digit termed a "super digit" by Wood [22]. In 2001, Foucher et al. [6] presented a new classification system for metacarpal synostosis (Fig. 18.8). They argued that though the Buck-Gramcko and Wood classification system was simple and easy to use, it failed to address the characteristics that would determine surgical treatment. They observed 36 patients with metacarpal synostosis over a 24-year period and proposed an "easy-to-remember" classification system based on the shape of the synostosis, the direction of the epiphysis growth, the finger deformity, webbing and hypoplasia of the metacarpal bone (Table 18.2).

Table 18.1 Buck-Gramcko and Wood [5] classification of metacarpal synostosis

Type I	Synostosis at the base of the metacarpals with minimal growth disturbance
Type II	Synostosis involving <50% of the metacarpal shafts
Type III	Synostosis involving >50% of the metacarpal shafts
IIIa	Separate metacarpophalangeal joint for each digit
IIIb	Common metacarpophalangeal joint for both digits, "super digit"

In 2014, Liu et al [23] proposed a third classification system for metacarpal synostosis. Liu reported difficulty classifying every patient with ring-small metacarpal synostosis using either the Buck-Gramcko/Wood Classification or the Foucher classifications. Liu's aim was to create a treatment-oriented system that focused on the most common metacarpal synostosis, ring-small metacarpal synostosis. They evaluated 20 hands in 13 patients with ring-small synostosis treated over a 20-year period. Their classification system was defined by the inter-metacarpal angle (IMA) and the degree of shortening of the small finger ray. They proposed treatments based on their classification (Table 18.3).

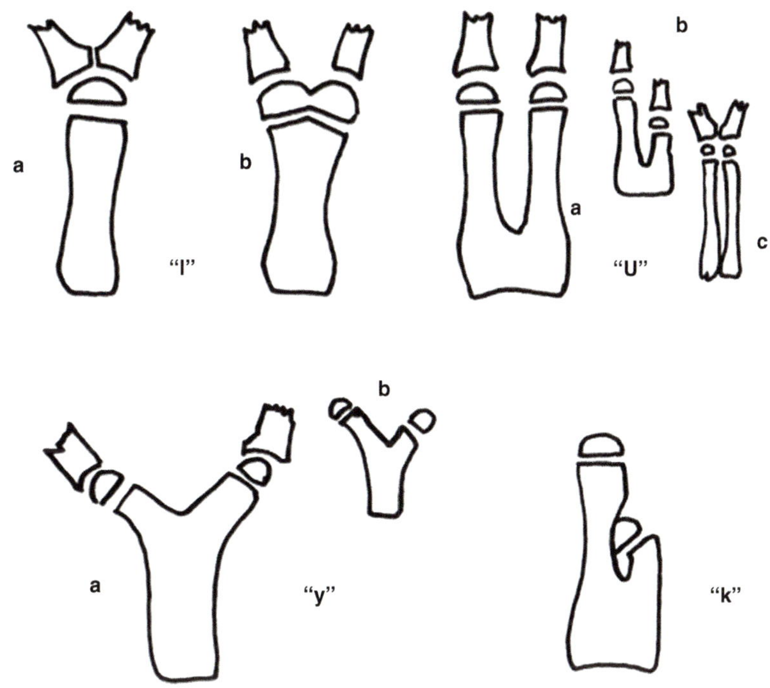

Fig. 18.8 Foucher et al. [6] classification picture diagram. Permissions pending

Table 18.2 Foucher et al. [6] classification of metacarpal synostosis

Shape	Deformity	Description
I-shaped		Single enlarged metacarpal
	Id	Two *distinct metacarpophalangeal joints*
	If	Single (fused) metacarpophalangeal joint for two fingers
U-shaped		Parallel epiphysis and synostosis at metacarpal base
	Us	Symmetric metacarpal lengths
	Ua	Asymmetric metacarpal lengths
	Ut	Tightly fused metacarpals
Y-shaped		Divergent epiphysis
	Ys	Symmetric metacarpal lengths
	Ya	Asymmetric metacarpal lengths
K-shaped		Converging metacarpals and short fifth metacarpal, fingers diverge, or shaped like parentheses with or without webbing

Table 18.3 Liu et al. [23] classification for fourth-fifth metacarpal synostosis

Type	Description of Deformity
Type A1	Narrow IMA *without* severe shortening of the fifth ray, no/mild deformity
A2	Narrow IMA, *with* severe shortening of the fifth ray, no/mild deformity
Type B1	Wide IMA, *without* severe shortening of the fifth ray, wide palm; wide fourth web; bony prominence on ulnar palm; poor abduction of the small finger
B2	Wide IMA, *with* severe shortening of fifth ray, wide palm; wide fourth web; bony prominence on ulnar palm; poor abduction of the small finger
Type C1	Reverse IMA, *without* severe shortening of fifth ray, narrow palm; abduction deformity of the little finger
C2	Reverse IMA, *with* severe shortening of fifth ray, narrow palm; abduction deformity of the little finger

18.7 Treatment

Treatment of metacarpal synostosis is guided by patient function and family preferences. The severity of deformity is not the sole consideration when making treatment decisions. Treatments options range from observation to reconstruction to amputation. Many patients with metacarpal synostosis have satisfactory hand function with minimal or no digital malalignment. Buck-Gramcko observed that many deformities stabilize around 4 years of age [5].

Amputation may be considered in patients with a stiff or nonfunctioning digit that inhibits hand function. Yuan et al. [24] published a case report of a 4-year-old with a ring-small metacarpal synostosis and Y-shaped deformity. Though the authors suggested amputation based on the fingers' interference with hand function, the family declined this treatment.

Surgical treatment of metacarpal synostosis is guided by the severity and shape of the deformity as well as the specific metacarpals involved. All techniques involve osteotomy of the conjoined metacarpals and interposition of a spacer fashioned to realign the metacarpal heads into a more normal anatomic relationship. Bony realignment may reposition the metacarpal epiphysis into an uninhibited position and improve the balance of intrinsic and extrinsic muscles across the metacarpal heads. Repositioning the metacarpal head improves the mechanical axis of the musculotendinous units crossing the joint and allows the digit to rest in a more anatomic orientation without abutment against the adjacent digit [11] (Fig. 18.9). Ueba and Seto [15] recommended

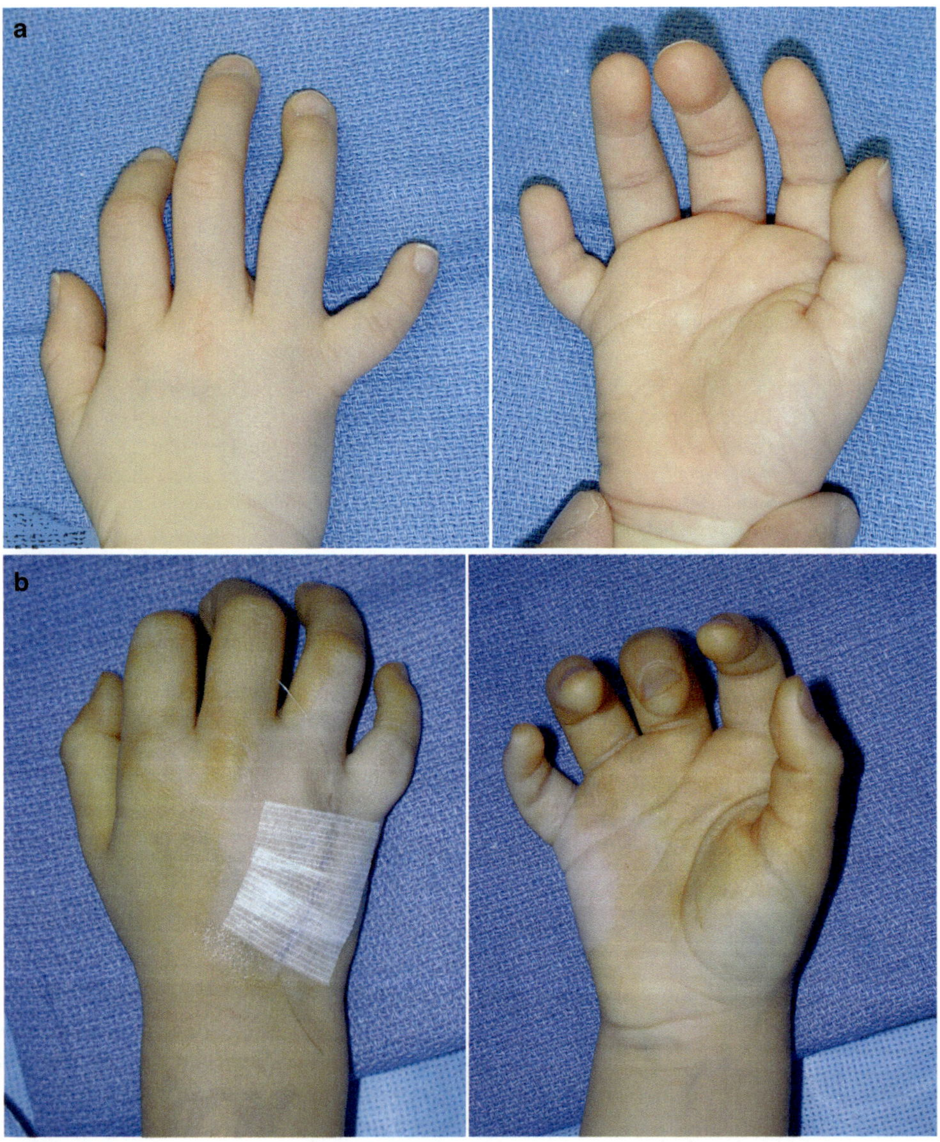

Fig. 18.9 (**a**, **b**) Pre (**a**) and post (**b**) operative clinical photographs demonstrating "splaying deformity" and correction after metacarpal synostosis widening osteotomy with bone graft interposition

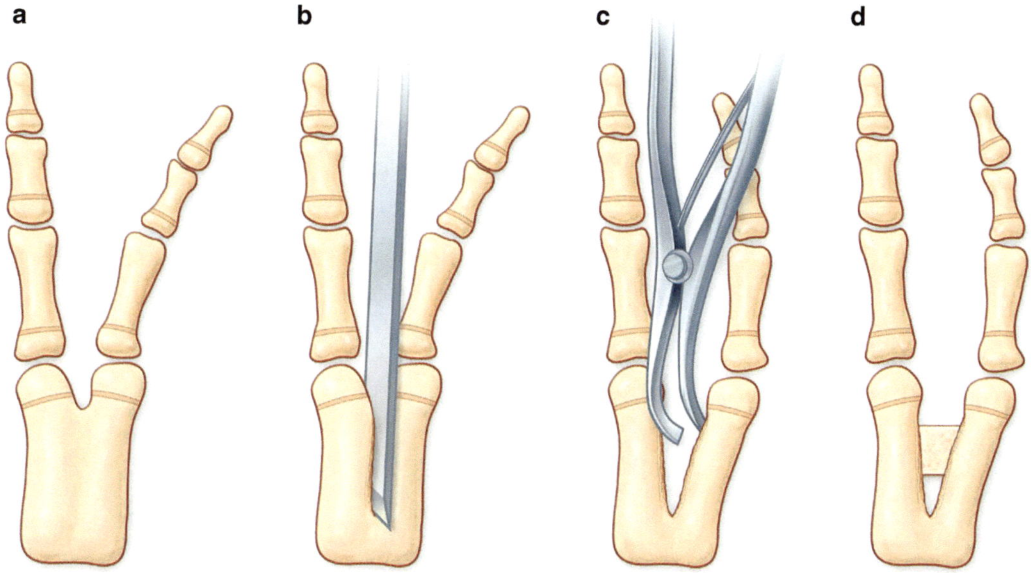

Fig. 18.10 Metacarpal synostosis osteotomy with graft interposition. (**a**) Metacarpal synostosis with abduction of small finger. (**b**) Longitudinal osteotomy of synostosis does not penetrate carpo-metaarapl joint. (**c**) Lamina spreader increases space between metacarpal diaphyses and gradually realigns small finger small metacarpal. (**d**) Metacarpal spread is secured with bone graft substitute block. Reproduced from [11]

surgical correction of metacarpal synostosis before the age of 2 years. In patients with splaying deformity, they stressed that if the metacarpal is not osteotomized early, the growth would be permanently impaired secondary to compression of the epiphysis by the adjacent metacarpal. Early surgical correction may improve orientation and facilitate opposition when the small finger metacarpal is involved. In contrast, Ueba and Seto warned that surgical correction of these small bones in young children is technically challenging and increases the risk of physeal injury [15].

Several surgical techniques have been described that address either middle-ring or ring-small metacarpal synostosis. In 1981, Hikosaka and Yabe [25] described an osteotomy of the synostosis with interposition of an iliac crest bone autograft spacer. In 1988, Iwaswa et al. [26] described an osteotomy with interposition of a costal cartilage autograft spacer. Both of these techniques demonstrated the positive effect of widening the space between the metacarpals and repositioning the metacarpal heads in synostoses causing splaying deformity of the fingers (Fig. 18.10). Both of these procedures, however, required a remote donor site to obtain the spacer.

In 1988, Muira [12] described the correction of metacarpal synostosis with an osteotomy and interposition of a silicone spacer. He hypothesized that the silicone would permit independent carpometacarpal motion and could obviate the need to harvest bone graft from the iliac crest of a skeletally immature child. Although the technique corrected the deformity and avoided the donor site morbidity of bone block harvest, follow-up demonstrated re-synostosis of the metacarpal bases [12, 15, 22].

Gottschalk et al. [11] advocated a longitudinal osteotomy of metacarpal synostoses with interposition of a synthetic bone block. They fashioned a spacer from a bone substitute, coralline hydroxyapatite, which mimics the porosity of cancellous bone (Fig. 18.11). They achieved deformity correction and realignment of the metacarpal shafts while avoiding donor site morbidity.

Although these techniques corrected digital splaying deformity, none addressed digital length discrepancy. Hooper and Lamb [20] attempted to address this issue when they described a technique of an oblique osteotomy in the small finger metacarpal. The osteotomy was based from prox-

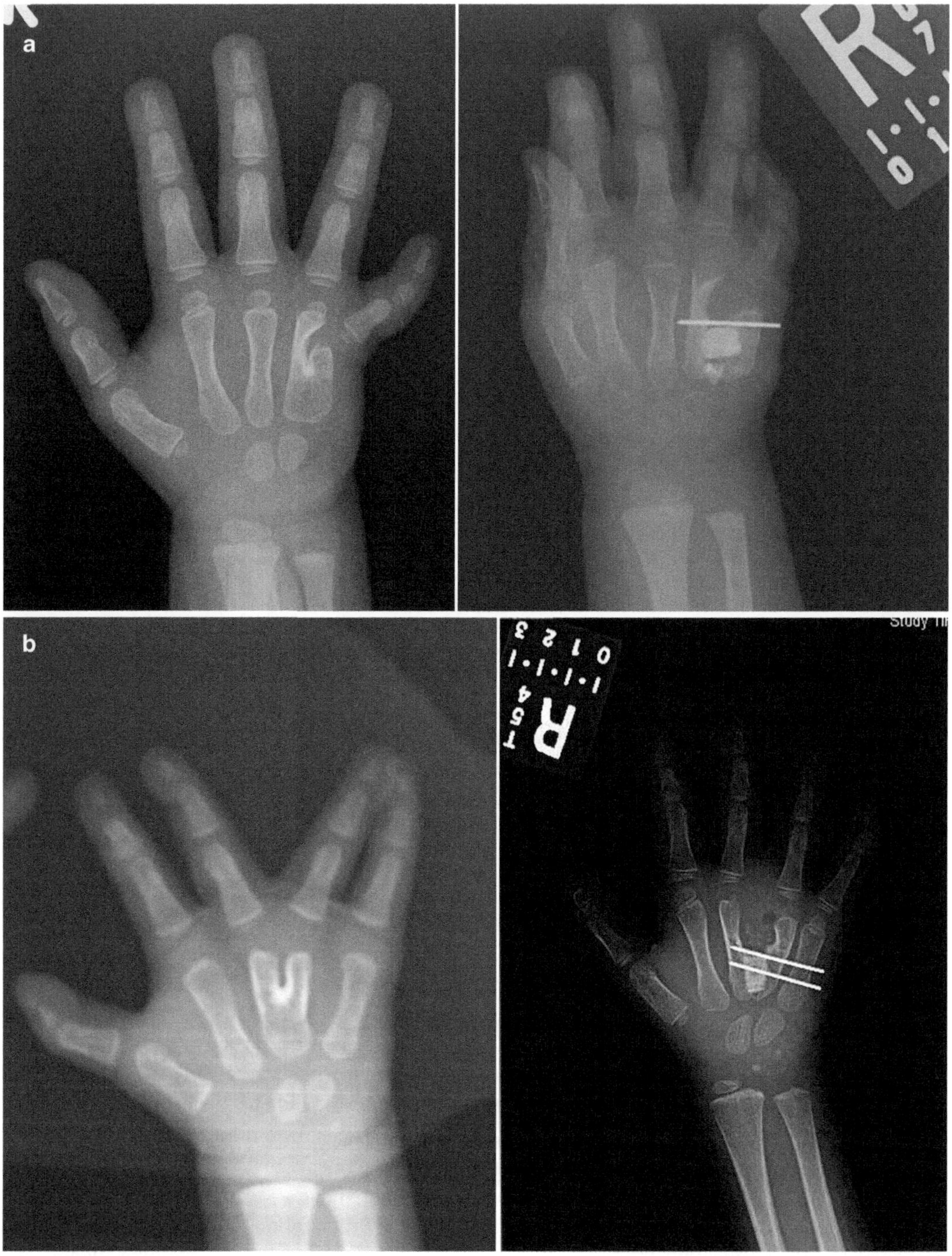

Fig. 18.11 (**a**, **b**) Ring-small (**a**) and middle-ring (**b**) finger metacarpal widening osteotomy with interposition of bone substitute graft spacer [11]

imal radial to distal ulnar in the small finger metacarpal shaft. The metacarpal was then wedged open radially while maintaining ulnar bony contact, resulting in the straightening of the small metacarpal shaft and realignment in parallel the ring metacarpal. This effectively addressed the digital splaying deformity but final results failed to substantially lengthen the metacarpal as they had intended.

In 2004, Jianmongkol et al. [14] proposed a single-stage technique for both deformity correction and lengthening of the metacarpal. They described a double osteotomy coupling a longitudinal osteotomy through the metacarpal synostosis with an oblique-transverse osteotomy through the metaphyseal base of the shortened metacarpal. Two bone graft spacers were inserted, one between the metacarpals for correction of angular deformity and one at the base of the shortened metacarpal providing length.

While some authors devoted their work to address metacarpal synostoses with splaying deformity, others focused on metacarpal synostoses with finger adduction deformity. In 2000, Yamamoto et al. [27] described an osteotomy in metacarpal synostosis with diverging metacarpals and finger adduction. Their technique involved an osteotomy of the synostosis which included the harvest of a wedge-shaped bone block from the synostosis bifurcation. An opening wedge osteotomy was then performed ulnarly on the small finger metacarpal shaft, leaving the radial cortex intact to maintain the stability of the osteotomy. The harvested wedge was then repositioned into the opening wedge osteotomy of the small finger metacarpal, realigning the small and ring finger metacarpal shafts. The repositioning of the metacarpals into a more parallel position allowed for realignment of the adducted digit and a slight increase in the length of the shortened metacarpal shaft. This technique allowed deformity correction without the addition of surgical site morbidity from autograft bone block harvest.

Kawabata et al. [28] described a technique of hemi-callotasis designed to correct both finger adduction deformity and the digital length discrepancy. This technique was based upon the treatments proposed by Paneva-Holevick and Yankov in 1980 and De Bastiani in 1987, which demonstrated the ability to lengthen callous 1 mm/day using rigid external fixation. Kawabata based the osteotomy of the small finger metacarpal on Fowler's technique for tibial valgus correction. In Kawabata's technique, a transverse osteotomy of the small finger metacarpal shaft was performed preserving an intact radial cortex to maintain the osteotomy site stability. The metacarpal was lengthened 1 mm/day using a mini monolateral external fixator on the ulnar side of the bone in an opening wedge technique. Kawabata achieved both deformity correction and lengthening of the small finger metacarpal, permitting rebalancing of the abductor digiti minimi force and resulting correction of the finger adduction deformity.

In 1993, Buck-Gramcko and Wood [5] detailed their technique for the treatment of middle-ring and ring-small metacarpal synostoses. Like others, their technique employed the use of synostosis osteotomies and bone graft interposition. Their goal was to convert a Type II or III synostosis into a Type I (refer to Table 18.1 for Buck-Gramcko and Wood classification). In addition, they suggested the possible need for correction of the soft tissues after altering bony alignment. They recommended soft tissue reconstruction to include the possible release or reconstruction of the inter-metacarpal ligament and/or reconstruction of the collateral ligaments of the metacarpophalangeal joint.

Buck-Gramcko and Wood [5] also discussed treatment for complicated deformities such as thumb-index metacarpal synostosis. They hypothesized that if treated early, realignment and independent thumb motion may be possible. The surgical procedure included the shifting or transferring of tendons and reconstruction of the collateral ligaments to achieve appropriate thumb function and opposition. Deepening of the first web space with local skin flaps or a large dorsal rotational flap was identified as an essential step. The authors recognized that in cases in which the division of the thumb-index metacarpal synostosis would result in a hypoplastic, functionless thumb; that thumb ablation and index pollicization might be a preferable treatment.

18.8 Complications

Many hands with metacarpal synostosis have metacarpophalangeal joint stiffness, metacarpal deformity, and in some instances a hypoplastic nonfunctioning digit. Surgical treatment of the metacarpal deformity will not correct the hypoplastic nature of the digit nor resolve metacarpophalangeal joint stiffness (Fig. 18.12). Surgical treatment may result in physeal arrest or osteonecrosis of the metacarpal head. This risk might be greater in small hands.

Recurrence of the metacarpal deformity and renewed splaying of digits has also been reported with long-term follow-up. Re-synostosis of the metacarpal bases is expected after widening osteotomy but has not shown to adversely affect hand function. Re-convergence of metacarpals is more likely after middle-ring synostosis osteotomy than after ring-small synostosis osteotomy.

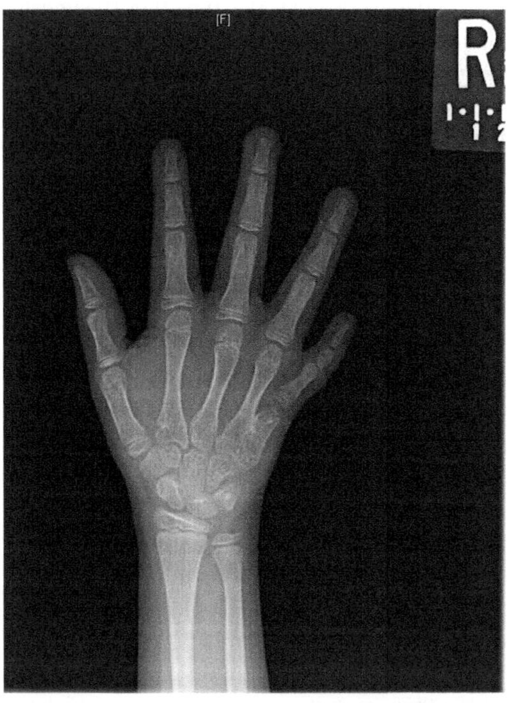

Fig. 18.12 Follow-up radiograph status post-ring-small finger metacarpal synostosis osteotomy with graft interposition demonstrating continued shortening of the small finger metacarpal and hypoplasia

18.9 Summary

Metacarpal synostosis is an uncommon hand anomaly that may occur in isolation (ring-small metacarpal) or in connection with a congenital syndrome (Apert, Ellis-van Creveld). It has been hypothesized to be sporadically inherited via x-linked recessive or autosomal dominant traits and is possibly linked to a genetic abnormality in the FGF16 gene. This hand difference likely forms during the first 4–8 weeks of gestation during rapid development of the upper limb.

Children are most often evaluated due to parental concerns regarding a deviated finger, most commonly the small finger that is abducted from the hand. Radiographic examination can confirm the diagnosis of metacarpal synostosis. Treatment is guided by symptoms and digital function. Operative treatments involving osteotomy and bone graft interposition have been described in multiple variations. Though multiple techniques address deformity and length discrepancy, the affected digits may remain hypoplastic and stiff. Patients with nonfunctioning, stiff, or painful digits may benefit from amputation. Complications with surgical correction of metacarpal synostosis can include physeal arrest, osteonecrosis of the metacarpal head, and recurrence of the deformity. Patients with metacarpal synostosis are able to lead full and active lives regardless of their deformity.

References

1. Jamsheer A, Zemojtel T, Kolanczyk M, Stricker S, Hecht J, Krawitz P, Doelken SC, Glazar R, Socha M, Mundlos S. Whole exome sequencing identifies FGF16 nonsense mutations as the cause of X-linked recessive metacarpal 4/5 fusion. J Med Genet. 2013;50:579–84.
2. Gottchalk MB, Danilevich M, Gottschalk HP. Carpal coalitions and metacarpal synostoses: a review. Hand. 2016;11(3):271–7.
3. Buckwalter JA, Flatt AE, Shurr DG, Dryer RF, Blair WF. The absent fifth metacarpal. J Hand Surg Am. 1981;6:364–7.
4. Ogino T, Kato H. Clinical features and treatment of congenital fusion of the small and ring finger metacarpals. J Hand Surg Am. 1993;18A:995–1003.

5. Buck-Gramcko D, Wood VE. The treatment of metacarpal synostosis. J Hand Surg Am. 1993;18A:565–81.
6. Foucher G, Navarro R, Medina J, Khouri RK. Metacarpal synostosis: a simple classification and a new treatment technique. Plast Reconstr Surg. 2001;108(5):1225–31.
7. Robinow M, Johnson GF, Broock GJ. Syndactyly type V. Am J Med Genet. 1982;11:475–82.
8. Harvey FJ. Bilateral ulnar “thumbs”. Hand. 1979;11(1):95–7.
9. Deliss L. Congenital metacarpal malformation. Hand. 1977;9(3):275–8.
10. Gomez RJ. An unusual carpal coalition associated with fifth ray anomalies in the hand. J Hand Surg Br. 1998;23B(4):537–8.
11. Gottschalk HP, Bednar MS, Moor M, Light TR. Metacarpal synostosis: treatment with a longitudinal osteotomy and bone graft substitute interposition. J Hand Surg Am. 2012;37A:2074–81.
12. Miura T. Congenital synostosis between the fourth and fifth metacarpal bones. J Hand Surg Am. 1988;13A:83–8.
13. Yildirim S, Akan M, Akoz T. Phalangeal osteotomy for the treatment of metacarpal synostosis: a case report. Hand Surg. 2003;8(1):87–91.
14. Jianmongkol S, Thammaroj T, Vipulakorn K. Congenital metacarpal synostosis treated by double bone blocks technique: a case report from Thailand. Hand Surg. 2005;10(1):131–4.
15. Ueba Y, Seto Y. Congenital metacarpal synostosis treated by longitudinal osteotomy and placement of a silicone wedge. Handchir Mikrockir Plast Chir. 1997;29:297–302.
16. Tetamy S, McKusick V. The genetics of hand malformations. Birth Defects Orig Artic Ser. 1978;14(3):1–619.
17. Dao KD, Shin AY, Kelley S, Wood VE. Synostosis of the ring-small finger metacarpal in Apert acrosyndactyly hands: incidence and treatment. J Pediatr Ortho. 2001;21:502–7.
18. Kozin SH. Embryology of the upper extremity. In: Wolfe S, editor. Greens operative hand surgery. 7th ed. Philadelphia, PA: Elsevier; 2017. p. 1208–16.
19. Waters PM, Bae DS. Radioulnar and metacarpal synostosis. In: Pediatric hand and upper limb surgery. Philadelphia, PA: Lippincott Williams and Wilkins; 2012. p. p161–5.
20. Hooper G, Lamb DW. Congenital fusion of the little and ring finger metacarpal bones. Hand. 1983;15(2):207–11.
21. Horii E, Miura T, Nakamura R, Nakao E, Kato H. Surgical treatment of congenital metacarpal synostosis of the ring and little fingers. J Hand Surg Br. 1998;23B(5):691–4.
22. Wood VE. Super digit. Hand Clin. 1990;6(4):673–84.
23. Liu B, Zhao JH, Tian W, Chen SL, Li C, Zhu J. Isolated ring-little finger metacarpal synostosis: a new classification system and treatment strategy. J Hand Surg Am. 2014;39(1):83–90.
24. Yuan C, Gou S, OuYang Y. Congenital metacarpal malformation: fifth metacarpal complete absence or fourth and fifth metacarpal synostosis. ANZ J Surg. 2010;80:663–4.
25. Hikosaka H, Yabe Y. Treatment for fourth and fifth metacarpal synostosis with abduction deformity of the little finger. Seikeigeka. 1981;32:1682–4.
26. Iwasawa M, Hayashi R, Matsuo K, Hirose T. The use of costal cartilage as a spacer in the treatment of congenital metacarpal fusion. Eur J Plast Surg. 1988;11:138–40.
27. Yamamoto N, Endo T, Nakayama Y. Congenital synostosis of the fourth and fifth metacarpals treated by free bone grafting from the fusion site. Plast Reconstr Surg. 2000;105(5):1747–50.
28. Kawabata H, Yasui N, Che YH, Hirooka A. Treatment for congenital synostosis of the fourth and fifth metacarpals with the hemicallotasis technique. Plast Reconstr Surg. 1997;99(7):2061–5.

Epidermolysis Bullosa

19

Chiara Novelli, Chirara Parolo, Veronica Fasoli, and Giorgio Pajardi

Abstract

Recessive dystrophic epidermolysis bullosa (RDEB) is a congenital disease caused by a mutation in the *COL7A1* gene, it causes several systemic and acral dysfunctions. The affected patients frequently show hand contractures and pseudosyndactyly. Although multiple treatments exist that can improve the hand malformations, there are currently still no radical cures for this disease because of its high recurrence rate. The surgical treatment aims to increase hand function and finally ameliorate patients' quality of life, despite recurrence of the disease is something certain. A correct surgical procedure should always be associated with correct postoperative skin dressings and splinting. Hand function is normally substantially improved after the complete release of pseudosyndactyly and achievement of favorable digital web spaces. Recurrence takes place normally in 2–4 years, getting worsen with the increasing age of the patients. In conclusion, surgical correction followed by skin dressing changes is an effective approach to improving mitten-hand malformations in RDEB patients.

Keywords

Recessive dystrophic epidermolysis bullosa · Hand deformity · Surgical management · Wound dressing · Postoperative splinting

19.1 Definition and Classification

Epidermolysis bullosa (EB) is a rare genetic disorder characterized by skin fragility and susceptibility to rubbing, determining the formation of blistering and shearing lesions, spontaneously or even due to the mildest trauma, such as gentle pressure or friction. In particular, the term "Epidermolysis Bullosa" (EB) includes a heterogeneous group of hereditary diseases that can be divided into four major subtypes: EB simplex (EBS), junctional (JEB), dystrophic (DEB), and Kindler syndrome (KS).

Some of these are very slight, with a little affection of the skin that resolves spontaneously during growth; some others are very severe and can cause death during intrauterine development or neonatal age. Subtypes are determined by several factors including the level of skin cleavage, phenotype, mode of inheritance, and molecular

C. Novelli (✉) · C. Parolo · V. Fasoli
Milan, Italy
e-mail: chiara.novelli@multimedica.it; chiara.parolo@multimedica.it

G. Pajardi
Department of Hand Surgery and Rehabilitation, S. Giuseppe Hospital IRCCS MultiMedica, Milan University, Milan, Italy
e-mail: gpajardi@centrostudimano.it

G. Pajardi (ed.), *Pediatric Hand Surgery*, https://doi.org/10.1007/978-3-031-30984-7_19

origin. Generally speaking, EBS encompasses all subtypes of EB and it is characterized by mechanical fragility and blisters confined to the epidermis within the basal keratinocytes. JEB includes all subtypes with blisters formation within the lamina lucida of the skin basement membrane. DEB patients have blisters formation in the superficial papillary dermis, at the level of the anchoring fibrils. KS patients have blisters formation in multiple levels within or beneath the basement membrane.

In addition to the manifestations of skin and mucous membranes, EB can affect multiple body systems, causing several functional deficiencies. For example, the typical hand deformities that develop in recessive DEB (RDEB), due to reduced or absent collagen VII, have a devastating impact on the quality of life of patients and include the following: adduction contracture of the thumb; pseudosyndactyly of the digits; flexion contractures of the interphalangeal (IP), metacarpophalangeal (MCP), and wrist joints; less frequently, extension contractures of the MCP joints from dorsal scarring. The "mitten" deformity develops when the hand becomes encased in an epidermal cocoon. All structures in the hand may be affected: cutaneous involvement results in dermal fibrosis, pseudosyndactyly, contractures, atrophic finger and thumb tips, nail loss (due to subungual blistering lesions), and dermal cocooning. Musculotendinous involvement may result in shortening of the flexor tendons and intrinsic muscle contractures. Articular involvement produces stiff, subluxed, or even destroyed joints in older patients. Generalized osteoporosis and thinned, wedge-shaped distal phalanges may also be found. With each episode of relatively minor trauma to the hand, ulceration produces fibrinous adhesions and scarring, which results in the obliteration of web spaces, progressing to the fingertips and causing pseudosyndactyly. The same process occurs in the first web space, initially causing an adduction contracture. This condition may also progress until the thumb is no longer independent. A grading system may be used to describe adduction deformity of the first web space and pseudosyndactyly.

The severity of the disease is mainly determined by the particular form of the disease from which the patient suffers, but it is useful to broadly categorize the disease into the "nonscarring" and "scarring" (dystrophic) types. Pearson in 1971 first classified the different aspects of EB. Furthermore, in 1989 the first United Meeting on diagnosis and classification of congenital EB took place. In 2002, the second United International Meeting on the classification and diagnosis of EB changed the classification system. In particular, it has been attempted to simplify as much as possible the classification of EB, to reduce the numerous subclassification present in literature, even if with poor results (in the official classification there are ten types of EB). At first, they eliminate clinical aspects with a rare incidence or that cannot be considered as a separate clinical identity. Thus, more than 14 classes have been erased. Most eponyms have been erased in order to have the lowest number of categories. Nevertheless, some of them, as for example Weber–Cockaine disease or Hallopeau–Siemens syndromes, can not be abolished, because the names are of simple and direct approach and claim immediate images of clinical conditions well-known by the general physician all over the world. The removal of this eponyms could add further misunderstanding and moreover could even reduce the number of confirmed diagnosis.

The new categorization suggests to classify the patients affected by EB in three main groups, based on microbiological observation of the skin lesion and especially on the ultrastructural level of the cleavage in cutaneous area, utilizing finally the same criterion used by Pearson. The first group includes EB simplex (EBS), in which the cleavage area and consequently the site of formation of blisters is inside the epidermal layer. Generally, the hands are affected, but heal without significant scary tissue. The second group includes Junctional EB (JEB), in which the cleavage and the blisters formation happens exactly on the surface of the basal lamina, at the dermal–epidermal junction; also, this form doesn't cause considerable scar. Finally, Dystrophic or

Dermolytic EB (DEB) is characterized by blisters formation below the basal lamina. Due to the depth of these lesions, wounds healing causes the formation of retractile scars.

Inside the three main groups, there are further kinds of group with typical different characteristics.

In April 2019, some leading experts met in London, UK, to review the relevant data and to revise the system of classification of these disorders, considering in particular epidermolysis bullosa (EB), and focusing on the molecular etiology whenever possible. EB is the prototypic group of disorders with SF, defined by blistering from minimal mechanical trauma with disruption at the dermo-epidermal junction. The four major classical EB types are EB simplex (EBS), junctional EB (JEB), dystrophic EB (DEB), and Kindler EB (KEB). Other disorders with skin fragility, where blisters are only a minor part of the clinical picture or are not seen because skin cleavage is very superficial, are classified as separate categories. These include peeling skin disorders, erosive disorders, hyperkeratotic disorders, and connective tissue disorders with skin fragility. Because of the possible similar skin manifestations, these “EB-related” disorders should be considered in the differential diagnosis.

The proposed system is strictly clinically oriented. The classification of patients with skin fragility begins at the bedside and is based on personal and family history, as well as the presence or absence of specific clinical features. Only later on in the diagnostic process patients will be further classified based on specific molecular findings.

The transmission of this pathology is inherited through an autosomic dominant mode for the EBS and autosomic recessive mode for the JEB. The DEB is autosomic dominant in some subtypes and autosomic recessive in the Hallopeau–Siemens. In particular, mutations in the same gene may be inherited in an autosomal dominant or recessive manner and may result in distinct clinical phenotypes (e.g., KRT5, KRT14, PLEC, COL17A1, or COL7A1). On the other hand, in DEB and EBS, similar phenotypes may be either dominant or recessive or may be caused by mutations in different genes (e.g., COL7A1, KRT5, KRT14, PLEC, DST, EXPH5, or KLHL24). Prenatal testing and diagnosis have been available for more than two decades. Owing to the recessive nature of RDEB, unfortunately, parent’s carrier status is generally unknown, and such testing is rarely suggested. For all these reasons, the EB molecular classification is still complex.

Eisen (1966) and Bauer (1980) suggested that the pathology should be referred to a lesion of the gene which coded for a collagenases. More recent studies of 1991 and others demonstrated definitively that RDEB is linked to multiple different mutations in chromosome 3p21 of the COL7A1 gene that codes for type VII collagen. Type VII collagen composes the building block of anchoring fibrils proteins of the epidermal basement membrane. An abnormal type of this anchorin protein results in presence of blistering below the basal lamina, due to a defect of cellular adherence. Molecular biology represents the only possible field to achieve the remedy of the pathology, because it is only by a substitution of the affected gene by a healed one that we can cure the disease. Even though a classification based only on molecular aspects has been proposed, actually molecular data don’t seem to be enough to create a correct and detailed classification. The acknowledgment possessed till now still not match perfectly with the different phenotypes of the disease, so that it is still so difficult to create a valid molecular classification.

19.2 Systemic Compromission

RDEB is the clinical condition requiring the most significant care and medical assistance: in fact, almost each part of the body could be affected and progressively damaged by the pathology.

Hands involvement is almost certain. As previously said, little patient hands appear closed with fist, with flexed adducted thumb, often with partial or complete obliteration of the first web. The interdigital webs also progressively diminish, with a process that is called pseudosyndactylization of the long fingers. Commonly nails are lost and sometimes the distal phalanx appears reabsorbed. Although the deformity results only from soft tissue contracture, secondary capsular and joint retraction, associated to tendon shortening, is a common finding.

Blistering lesions, frequently ulcerated, could be found in every district characterized by an epithelial layer, especially in skin regions more exposed to rubbing, as well as loss of cutaneous annexes and sometimes scarring alopecia.

Unfortunately, it is common to find blistering lesions also in all the gastrointestinal tract. Oral and perioral blisters lead to microstomia; the esophageous mucosa is commonly affected by lesions and frequently presents scaring circumferential stenosis; perianal blisters and fissuring lead equally to stenosis and consequently to fecal retention. Such findings lead to a malnutrition clinical picture resulting in the delay of growth, caused by the pain in feeding and defecation. Moreover, at the level of the intestinal tract, there is a reduction in the minimal rate of protein absorption across the affected mucous tissue.

In severe cases, also eye mucosa can be involved, with painful cheratitis, or sometimes symblepharon.

Generally, a varying degree of anemia is noticed, possibly due to the association of malnutrition and frequent and continuous bleeding.

The high rate of development of skin cancerous lesions in these patients can not be forgotten. It is well-known that patients affected with RDEB are exposed to a major risk of generating squamocellular carcinoma especially in the third and fourth decades. Other forms of EB (SEB, JEB) show an incidence of this pathology that can be related to the normal population. On the other side, patients affected with RDEB show 6% of probability to develop cancerous lesions at age of 20, 21% at 25 years, and 53% at 35 years. Therefore, it is mandatory, particularly after the first two decades of life, an accurate monitoring of every change of the aspect, size, or color of all the skin lesions, for example, any ulcer which delay in healing or an abnormal thickness of the skin. It is in fact well-known that these patients do not have a really prolonged expectance of survival and the most frequent causes of death are infections, anemia, multi-organ failures following malnutrition, but also skin carcinomas.

19.3 Treatment

As previously said, hands are one of the most common affected sites within this pathology. The frequent use of the hand, in fact, exposes this district to recurrent and repeated trauma; moreover, even minor modifications in hand anatomy (e.g., narrowing of the first web) can result in a significant functional impairment that could be initially compensated by the baby, but tend to progress in disabilities affecting a child's most common daily activities.

It goes therefore without saying, that we should pursue a treatment as soon as the baby loses independence in hand movements and manipulation, due to the formation of the before mentioned "cocoon deformity".

Conservative treatments are preferred to invasive approaches in case of mild to moderate deformities. Stretching exercises, protective and web retaining gloves, as well as splinting can help delay the comparison of first symptoms and disease progression. Unfortunately, patients often refer to a specialist when the disease has become severely debilitating and hand functions are already compromised. At this stage, the management is unequivocally a surgical treatment.

Generally, surgery occurs when the patient is very young; the mean age of the first surgery in fact is around 1–3 years. Young patients are usually operated under general anesthesia. In patients older than 14, a regional block can be proposed, especially for dressing. Anesthetic procedure is a delicate step and for this reason, well-trained anesthetic specialist and nursing teams are required for these patients.

At first, any adhesive dressing can be used, because it is a further cause of lesion. Moreover, these babies present a small and fragile subcutaneous vascular system that lies beyond a very thick skin, due to scary tissue. For these reasons, the intravenous canulation procedure is very difficult. Also, endotracheal intubation requires a particular attention because of the already-mentioned microstomya and the delicate oral mucosa.

There is not an univocal opinion about the use of tourniquet. Some authors consider it useless and only a source of further trauma. According to other author's experience, a careful installation of the tourniquet, avoiding any pressure point directly on the skin and reducing the pressure value, contributes to minimize blood loss and to reduce operative time.

Surgery begins with the degloving of the hand; afterward the opening of the first interdigital web until the muscular level, associated sometimes at the release of the adductor pollicis brevis. Later the release of the palmar crease, with the stretching of the metacarpo-phalangeal joint, of the proximal interphalangeal joint and, if possible, of the distal interphalangeal joint, always avoiding tendons exposure and areolar tissue. K wires are inserted longitudinally to keep the fingers extended for the first 2 weeks and then they are removed in the first change of dressing in sedation (Fig. 19.1).

Further medications are done until the hand is quite rehepitelized and the patient can tolerate the change of dressing without any sedation (Fig. 19.2).

Since the morbidity caused by tissue withdrawal at the donor site often outmatches the advantages at the receiving site obtained after surgery, waiting for a spontaneous healing is often the best course of action. Many covering solutions have been proposed in different scientific works, most of them having already been tested in burn surgery. In our center, we used many of the proposed solutions, all presenting potentialities, as well as limits. Keratinocyte laminae could be for instance a valuable instrument, at least theoretically. Compared to skin graft surgery, which has the problem of the availability of sufficient tissue from our patients, the use of keratinocyte laminae poses no limitations in

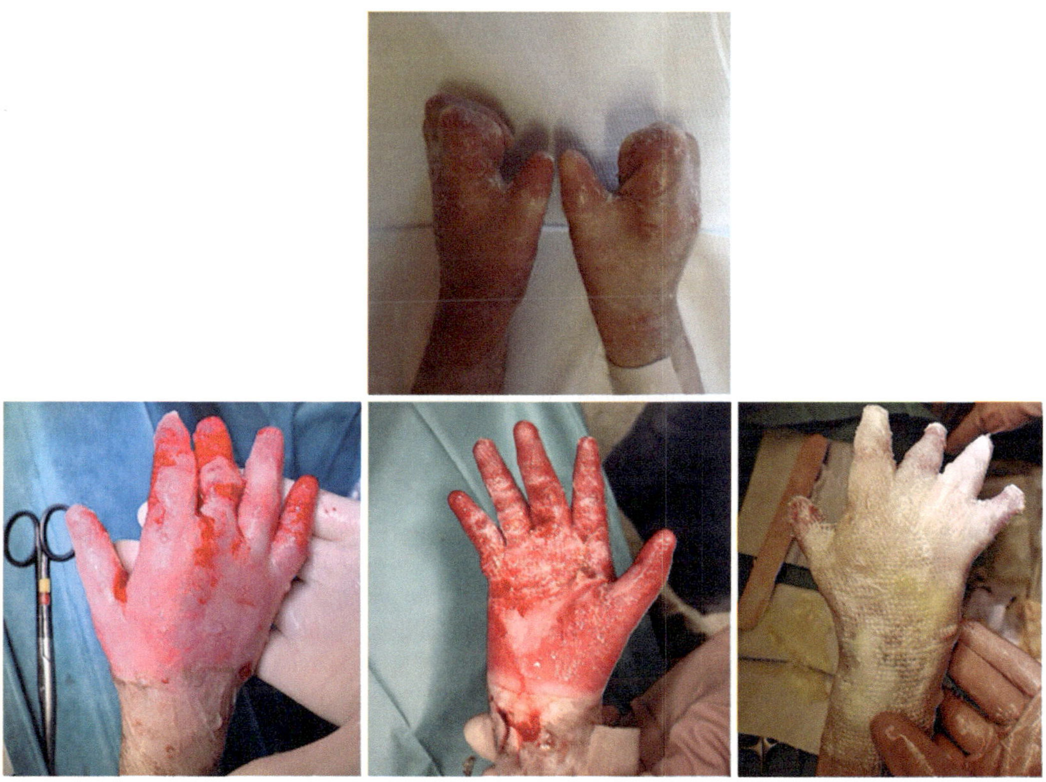

Fig. 19.1 Case 1. Preoperative image showing "cocoon hand deformity" of both hands in a patient with EB and results obtained after its subsequent surgical treatment and dressing

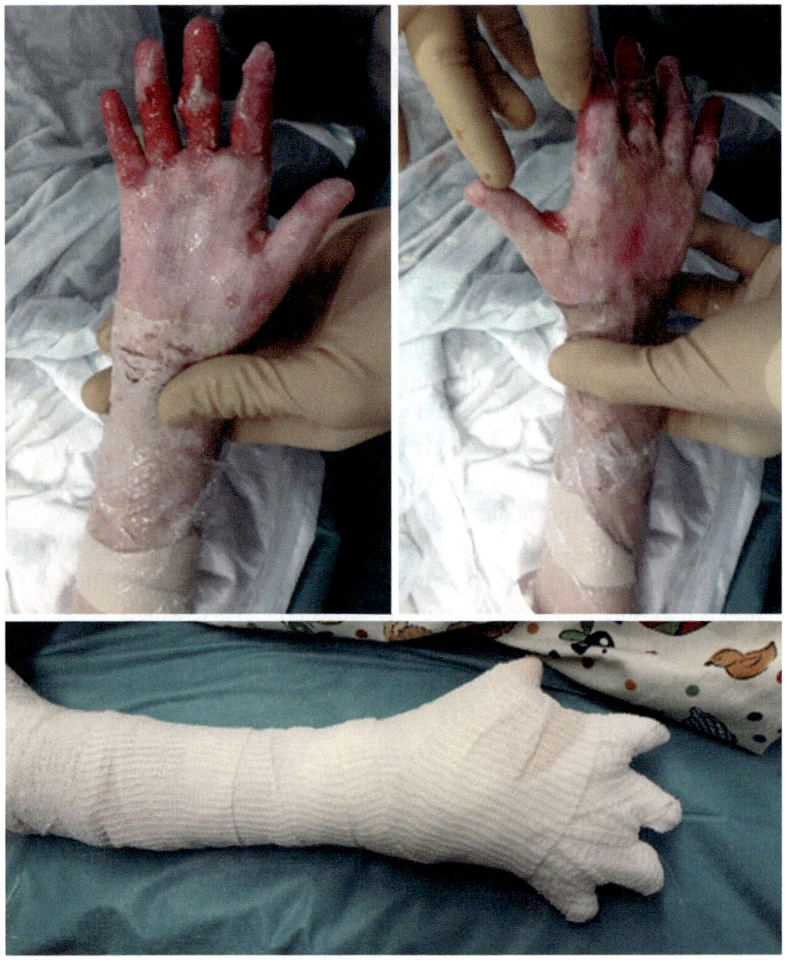

Fig. 19.2 Case 1. Postoperative images 2 weeks after surgery. Dressing is changed and re-epithelialization process has begun

terms of quantity. Moreover, skin grafts from our patients are often poor in terms of quality and present the same fragility as the receiving site. On the other hand, the extreme vulnerability of keratinocyte laminae definitely represents a limitation to its use.

The operation ends with the application of dynamic splint, which consists in a thermoplastic material. The splint is used to exercise an extension traction on the long fingers and thumb; elastic bands are connected by one side to the splint and on the other side anchored to each digital segment, through a transversal Kirschner wire which has previously been passed through the last phalanx. This last procedure in our experience seems to be the key in improving the surgical results, and mostly increasing the relapse-free interval. The splint in fact allows progressive distension of the fingers without employing an excessive forced extension during surgery. The latter could cause tendons exposure, which could not be covered due to the poverty of available grafts. Moreover, the application of the dynamic splint allows a good performance of dressing during the postoperative period, reducing the action on the finger and so preserving the granulating tissue, and reducing pain.

Dressing is delayed as far as possible in order to favor a leaded spontaneous wound healing. Only in case of infection dressing could be anticipated, although, on the contrary on what could be thought, these episodes are extremely rare.

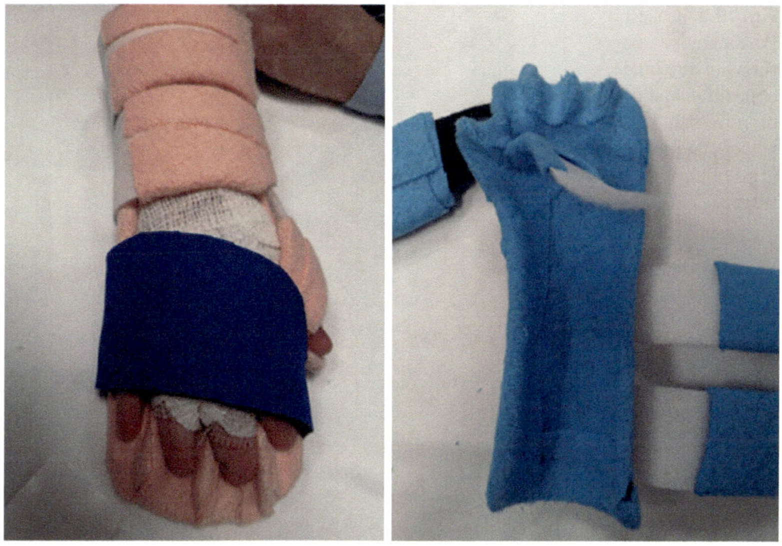

Fig. 19.3 Static splint is used after surgery to provide a passive stretch maintaining the optimal position of fingers. Later on splint is recommended also overnight

Routinely bandage is removed at the 15th, 30th, and 45th days postoperative. During the last period, it is possible to let the hand free from bandage and to begin active rehabilitation even before removing the dynamic splint.

Rehabilitation must begin early: intraoperative positioning of the splint can be considered the first physiotherapeutic step. The aim of rehabilitation program is to fight the retraction tendency of the scars, that is enhanced by the pathophysiology of the disease, but also taking care of the fragility of the newborn cutaneous tissue, because of the risk to cause new skin lesions. The opened hand position gained with surgery is first maintained by a valve splint. When all the wounds are healed and the status of the skin allows it, the splint is substituted with a dorsal static splint eventually converted in dynamic with a progressive traction on each finger, to maintain the extension strength. This splint can be modified according to the different adaptations of the new anatomical feature of the hand (Fig. 19.3).

As previously said, EB is characterized by frequent relapses. Surgical results should be considered "unsatisfactory" when relapse occurs within 2 years from the first surgery, "good" if it occurs within 2–4 years and "excellent" after 4 or more years. At relapse, a second operation results necessary. However, the concept itself of "relapse" is difficult to understand in this particular pathology. A deviation in flexion of the fourth and fifth finger is quite common, but this condition is absolutely compatible with a reasonable functioning hand; on the contrary, even a slight restriction of the first interdigital space can hinder the use of the hand itself, due to the impossibility of grasping large objects. Surgeon should pay attention to follow the evolution of the pathology, intervening only according to the demands of the patients and not aiming to maintain categorically the hand opened. This last behavior risks to lead to an increased and unjustified number of surgical procedures in the patient history (Fig. 19.4).

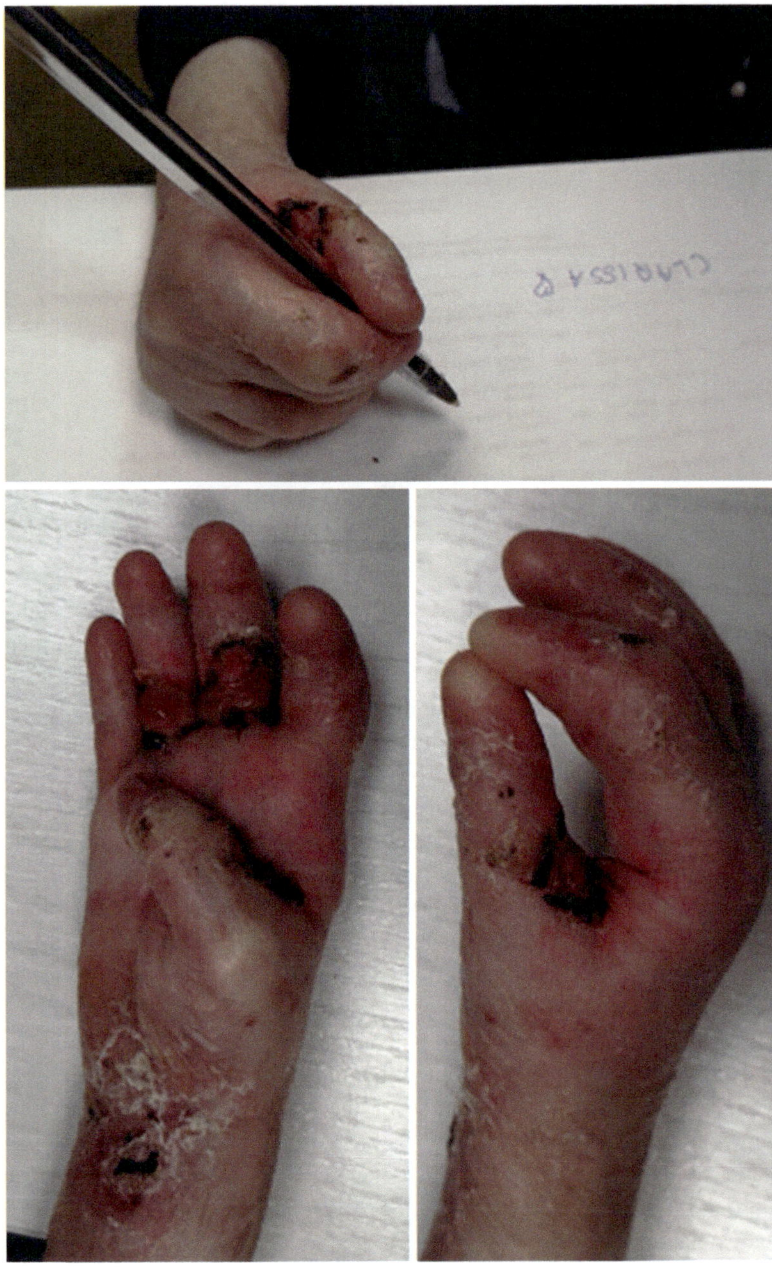

Fig. 19.4 Case 1. Postoperative images showing maximal opposition and full range of movement both in power and precision grips obtained after surgery

19.4 Natural History

The clinical features and complications of different forms of EB often change and evolve over time and this is important in order to recognize the different subtypes and anticipate the clinical course and related problems. Natural history of the disease partly reflects different stages in child's growth. However, certain subtypes of EB have a natural evolution with varying degrees of severity in which specific clinical signs can be observed or disappeared over time.

Distinguishing the major subtypes of EB in the neonatal period considering only clinical features is extremely unreliable and this highlights the need for rapid and accurate laboratory diagnosis. Blistering lesions in babies often have a predilection for the extremities and around the diaper area, but, as the child grows up, the pattern of blistering will usually become more characteristic of its subtype. For example, in localized EBS blisters will form predominantly on feet, whereas in intermediate or severe DEB subtypes, fragility will become more marked over bony prominences, such as the knees and elbows. While babies with severe JEB may have relatively little skin blisters at birth, over the first few months the characteristic granulation tissue affecting the face, ears, and distal digits becomes more prominent and distinctive. In KEB, early childhood blistering lesions resolve as photosensitivity and progressive poikiloderma become more evident.

Some sequelae of EB are irreversible and progressive, for example, skin and oral mucosal scarring or nail loss in DEB; therefore, they tend to become more marked with age. In severe EBS, infants have very severe and extensive skin blisters and this subtype can have a lethal course. However, the course of disease improves over time, such that adults may have very limited blisters confined largely to acral sites. The clinical features of EBS with mottled pigmentation also change over time, often with blistering improving throughout childhood, paralleled by the development of the characteristic pigmentary changes unrelated to previous sites of blistering and punctate palmoplantar keratoses. Intermediate EBS with KLHL24 mutations is notable for its severe skin loss at birth which gets better with age, and also by the development of cardiomyopathy in early adulthood. Similarly, in EBS with PLEC mutations, SF is accompanied by the onset of progressive muscular dystrophy at any point between infancy and adulthood and has also been associated with cardiomyopathy.

The extent and pattern of blistering may vary in distinct forms of EB. For example, RDEB inversa usually comprises intermediate severity of generalized blisters early in life, but later, in childhood to adulthood, the sites of predilection become markedly flexural. Pruriginosa DEB also evolves over time, with the development of prurigo-like nodules and linear lesions on the lower legs initially, spreading generally more proximally and also onto the arms. The onset of specific pruriginosa features may be extremely delayed, with onset in late adulthood.

Similarly, the distribution of localized pretibial DEB evolves with age. In late-onset JEB, SF tends to start in mid-childhood with progressive scleroderma-like atrophy and nail changes developing subsequently. A number of cases of severe JEB in infancy have been associated with spontaneous improvement and longer-term survival; in such cases, LAMB3 mutations, resulting in a truncated but partially functional b3 laminin chain, have been postulated to result in an intermediate clinical picture.

The mechanisms behind the distinct patterns of distribution and their fluctuation over time in different subtypes of EB are not fully understood, but likely reflect specific genetic consequences at a protein level. Further elucidation of genotype–phenotype correlation in EB-causing genes as well as other genetic modifiers, may provide some clarification in time.

In addition to disease-specific natural history, EB may be accompanied by many secondary complications that develop over time and often depend on the general severity of the EB type, as well as environmental and confounding factors, such as bacterial colonization. For example, anemia, reduced bone mineral density, renal impairment, progressive skin contractures, and the development of squamous cell carcinoma are all potential complications of severe RDEB and their onset depends on interindividual variability.

Revisions of the EB classification is closely linked to scientific developments in diagnostic and research and should be a useful tool for researchers and clinicians dealing with patients with EB (for counseling, prognostication, follow-up, and screening for complications). Emerging therapeutic options and clinical trials open new perspectives and underscore the importance of molecular genetics and genotype–phenotype correlations to predict therapeutic options for precision medicine.

EB-associated proteins have distinct roles in assuring the mechanical stability of the cells and adhesion, as well as structural and functional particularities (e.g., laminin 332, integrin a6b4 87, or collagen XVII 88 in controlling keratinocyte stemness). Yet, there are common pathogenetic mechanisms, such as chronic tissue damage and inflammation, that apply to all/several types of EB.

Some therapeutic principles, like induction of read through of PTC mutations, RNA-based therapies (e.g., antisense oligonucleotides for exon skipping 93), or modulation of protein misfolding, may be applied for different genes/proteins, under the premise of knowledge of individual mutations and their consequences. Therefore, subclassification of EB and SF disorders based on the molecular defect, and stratification of mutations for precision medicine is a tempting challenge for the future.

19.5 Conclusions

Several surgical approaches have been proposed in the literature for congenital EB and they all differ for the extension of the surgical technique. Various scientific works have proposed large skin graft obtained from lower limbs, with successive frequent dressings and heavy immobilization (also in plaster). The results of such techniques seem not to be better both in early postoperative period and in long-term controls when compared to less invasive scheme.

Since EB is a pathology that limits dramatically the quality of life of the patient and reduces his lifespan, a more physiologic approach should be preferred.

The final goal is to grant patients some level of independence in their personal life, making them capable of satisfying their primary needs by at least carrying out gross movements with their hands.

Further Reading

Bauer E. The role of skin collagenase in epidermolysis bullosa. J Invest Dermatol. 1962;39:551.

Campiglio GL, Pajardi G, Rafanelli G. A new protocol for the treatment of hand deformities in recessive dystrophic epidermolysis bullosa (13 cases). Ann Chir Main Memb Super. 1997;16(2):91–100.

Christiano AM, Amano S, Uitto J, et al. Premature termination codon mutations in the type VII collagen gene in recessive dystrophic epidermolysis bullosa result in nonsense-mediated mRNA decay and absence of functional protein. J Invest Dermatol. 1997;109(3):390.

Cuono C, Finseth F. Epidermolysis bullosa: current concepts and management of the advanced hand deformity. Plast Reconstr Surg. 1978;62:280.

Donati L, Klinger M, Campiglio GL. Wound healing: an up to date. In: Moody F, Montorsi W, Montorsi M, editors. Advances in surgery. New York: Raven Press; 1991.

Donati L, Magliacani G, Bormioli M, et al. Clinical experience with keratinocytes grafts. Burns. 1992;18:S19–26.

Eisen A. Human skin collagenase: relationships to the pathogenesis of epidermolysis bullosa dystrophica. J Invest Dermatol. 1969;52:449.

Fine JD, Eady RA, Bauer EA, et al. Revised classification system for inherited epidermolysis bullosa: report of the second international consensus meeting on diagnosis and classification of epidermolysis bullosa. J Am Acad Dermatol. 2000;42(6):1051.

Gipson M. Squamous cell carcinoma in epidermolysis bullosa dystrophica. Hand. 1975;7:179.

Glicenstein J, Mariani D, Haddad R. The hand in recessive dystrophic epidermolysis bullosa. Hand Clin. 2000;16(4):637.

Greider JL Jr, Flatt A. Care of the hand in recessive epidermolysis bullosa. Plast Reconstr Surg. 1983;72(2):222.

James I, Wark H. Airway management during anesthesia in patients with epidermolysis bullosa dystrophica. Anesthesiology. 1982;56:323.

Kelly R, Koff H, Rothaus K, et al. Brachial plexus anesthesia in eight patient with recessive dystrophic epidermolysis bullosa. Anesth Analg. 1987;66:1318.

Ladd A, Kibele A, Gibbons S. Surgical treatment and post-operative splinting of recessive dystrophic epidermolysis bullosa. J Hand Surg. 1996;21:888.

Mallipeddi R. Epidermolysis bullosa and cancer. Clin Exp Dermatol. 2002;27(8):616.

Pajardi G, Signorini M, Rafanelli G, Donati L. L'epidermolisi bollosa congenita, nostro protocollo nel trattamento globale dell'arto superiore.

Parente MG, Chung LC, Ryynanen J, et al. Human type VII collagen: cDNA cloning and chromosomal mapping of the gene. Proc Natl Acad Sci U S A. 1991;88:6931–5.

Pearson RW, Fitzpatrick T. Dermatology in general medicine. New York: McGraw Hill; 1971.

Uitto J, Pukkinen L, Chistiano AM. The molecular basis of the dystrophic forms of epidermolysis bullosa. In: Fine JD, Bauer EA, McGuire J, et al., editors. Epidermolysis bullosa: clinical, epidemiologic and laboratory advances and the findings of the national Epidermolysis Bullosa Registry. Baltimore: Johns Hopkins University Press; 1999.

Weber F, Bauer JW, Sepp N, et al. Squamous cell carcinoma in junctional and dystrophic epidermolysis bullosa. Acta Derm Venereol. 2001;81(3):189.

Arthrogryposis: Introduction and Classification

20

Olga Agranovich

Abstract

Arthrogryposis is a heterogeneous condition defined as multiple congenital contractures in two or more different areas of the body. Amyoplasia is the most common form of arthrogryposis occurring in about 1/10,000 live births. It presents a sporadic condition. The incidence of upper limb deformities due to amyoplasia is high (72–84.8%). The patients with amyoplasia have typical deformities of upper extremities: the shoulder joints are held in adduction, the elbow joints—in extension (less often in flexion), the wrists—in flexion, the thumbs adducted, and the fingers' joints—in varying degrees of flexion. The muscles are either absent, reduced in size, or replaced by fibrous or adipose tissue. The classification of upper limbs deformities is based on the level of spinal cord injury. All deformities are divided into two groups (differ from each other by the level of damage of the spinal cord and range of passive and active motion in all joints of the upper limb): isolated forms and complex forms (the latter present amyoplasia in combination with other pathology—obstetric palsy, cerebral disorders, and congenital hand anomalies).

Keywords

Arthrogryposis · Multiple congenital contractures · Upper limb · Spinal cord

The term arthrogryposis is used to describe a very heterogeneous group of affected individuals who are recognized in the newborn period as having multiple congenital contractures that affect two or more different areas of the body [1].

The incidence of arthrogryposis is about 1/3000 pregnancies [2]. Of these children, about 1/3 primarily have limbs affected, 1/3 have limbs plus other body areas affected with normal intelligence, and 1/3 have central nervous system dysfunction (in the past, half of these would die at birth or in the first year). Over 400 specific genetic abnormalities (including gene mutations and chromosomal abnormalities, deletions, and duplications) have been associated with multiple congenital joint contractures [3–6]. The joint contractures are secondary to a lack of motion during fetal life. Multiple processes can lead to a lack of fetal limb movement, including muscle abnormalities, nerve anomalies, a restricted intrauterine space, vascular insufficiency, and maternal illness, but often the course of this pathology remains unknown [7].

Amyoplasia is the most common form of arthrogryposis occurring in about 1/10,000 live births and presents a sporadic condition [3, 4]. The incidence of upper limb deformities due to

O. Agranovich (✉)
Arthrogryposis, Federal State Budgetary Institution the Turner Scientific Research Institute for Children's Orthopedics Under the Ministry of Health of the Russian Federation, St. Petersburg, Moscow, Russia

G. Pajardi (ed.), *Pediatric Hand Surgery*, https://doi.org/10.1007/978-3-031-30984-7_20

amyoplasia is high (72–84.8%) [3, 8, 9]. Gibson and Urs examined 114 patients with arthrogryposis and found out that the wrist was most commonly affected (32%), closely followed by the hand (26%), elbow (25%), and shoulder (19%) [8, 9].

20.1 Classification of Upper Limbs Deformities Due to Amyoplasia

The patients with amyoplasia have typical deformities of upper limbs: the shoulder joints are held in adduction, the elbow joints—in extension (less often in flexion), the wrists—in flexion, the thumbs adducted and the fingers' joints—in varying degrees of flexion. The muscles are either absent, reduced in size, or replaced by fibrous or adipose tissue [10]. In 84% of the cases, patients with arthrogryposis have deformities of both upper extremities [11].

The goals of treatment of upper limb deformities are to achieve independent function sufficient for self-feeding and peroneal care [7]. In less severe cases, it is possible to restore upper limb function up to normal, in more severe cases, some improvement of self-service can be achieved. The degree of success depends on the level of spinal cord injury and severity of pathology.

The classification of upper limbs deformities is based on the level of spinal cord injury (in modification of Brown et al. [12]). All deformities are divided into two groups (differ from each other by the level of damage of the spinal cord and range of passive and active motion in all joints of upper limb).

- Isolated forms: type 1 (C6-C7), type 2 (partial C5, C6-C7), type 3 (C5-Th1), and type 4 (C6) (Table 20.1).
- Complex forms (present amyoplasia in combination with other pathology): obstetric palsy, cerebral disorders, and congenital hand anomalies (symbrachydactyly, ectrodactyly, polydactyly).

Table 20.1 Variants of upper limb deformities due to amyoplasia linking with the level of spinal cord injury

	C6	C6-C7	C5-C7	C5-Th1
Shoulder			+[a]	+
Elbow	+	+	+	+
Wrist		+	+	+
Hand		±	+	+
Rotation deformities			+	+
Self-ability problems	±	±	±	+

± Possible functional insufficiency in upper limb or segment

[a] + Obligatory functional insufficiency in upper limb or segment

20.2 Isolated Forms of Upper Limb Deformities Due to Amyoplasia

20.2.1 Type 1: Level of Spinal Cord Injury: C6-C7

20.2.1.1 Clinical Picture

Shoulder—full passive movement, active movement is totally or moderately limited (abduction ≥70°), the muscles of shoulder girdle are normal or moderately hypoplastic.

Elbow—full or moderately limited passive movement, active movement limited or absent, active supination is limited.

Wrist—full or limited passive movement, active flexion is preserved, active extension is limited or absent.

Hand—a good hand function, fingers contractures are rare, sometimes limitation of thumb abduction may be seen.

Prognosis of treatment is good (Fig. 20.1).

20.2.2 Type 2: Level of Spinal Cord Injury: Partial C5, C6-C7

20.2.2.1 Clinical Picture

Shoulder—passive movement is fully or partially limited, active movement limited (abduction 30–45°), the shoulder-girdle muscles are hypoplastic.

Elbow—fully or moderately limited passive movement, active movement is severely limited or absent, active supination is absent.

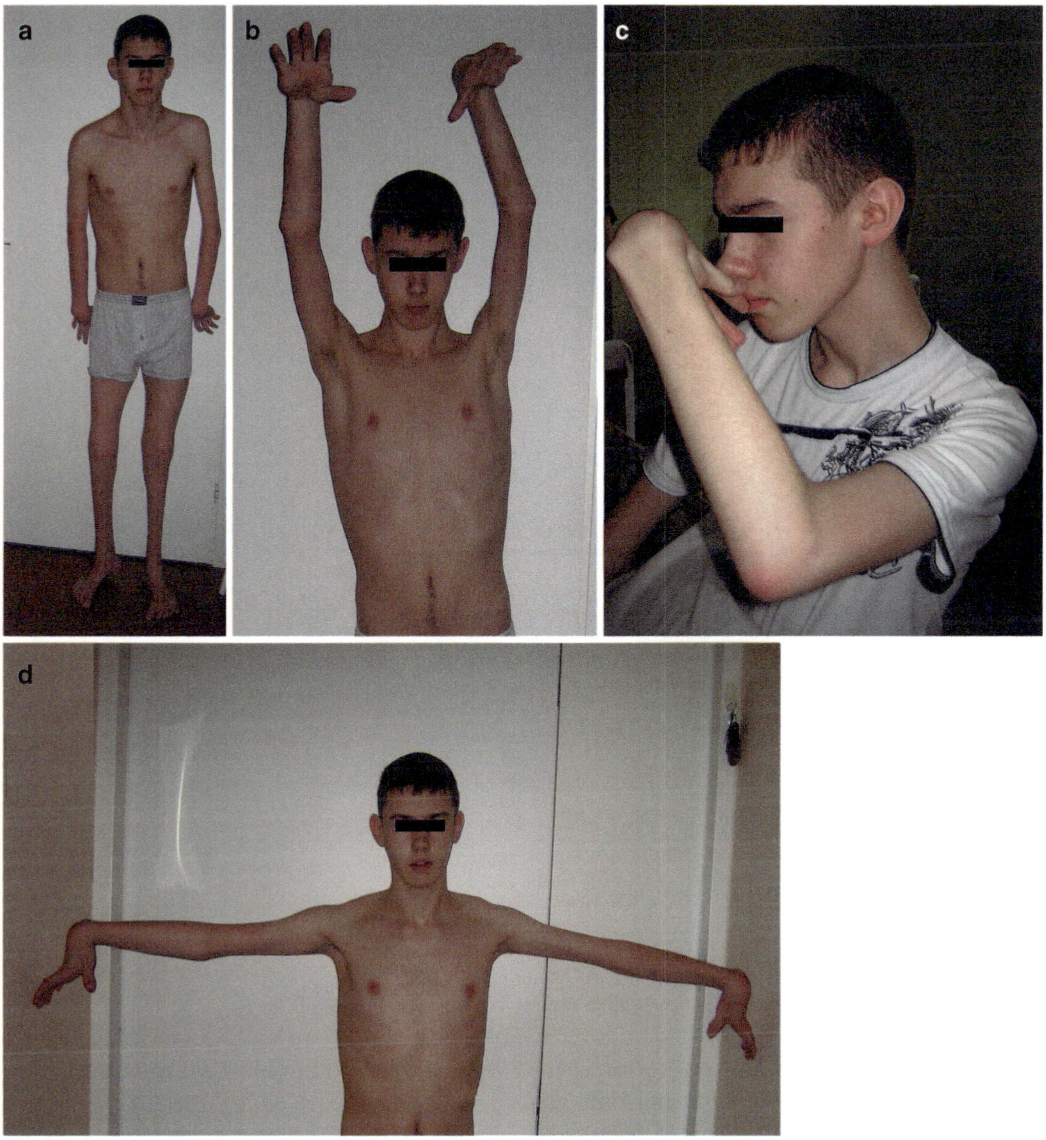

Fig. 20.1 Upper limb deformities in patient with level C6-C7. Clinical picture (**a**–**d**)

Wrist—flexion contracture with ulnar deviation, passive movement is moderately limited, active flexion is limited, active extension is limited or absent.

Hand—a good or moderately limited hand function, sometimes fingers contractures and thumb-in-palm are present.

Prognosis of treatment is good or satisfactory (Fig. 20.2).

20.2.3 Type 3: Level of Spinal Cord Injury: C5-Th1

20.2.3.1 Clinical Picture

Shoulder—passive movement is limited, active movement is absent or severely limited (abduction 10–30°), shoulder-girdle muscles are hypoplastic or aplastic, and internal rotation of upper extremity is limited.

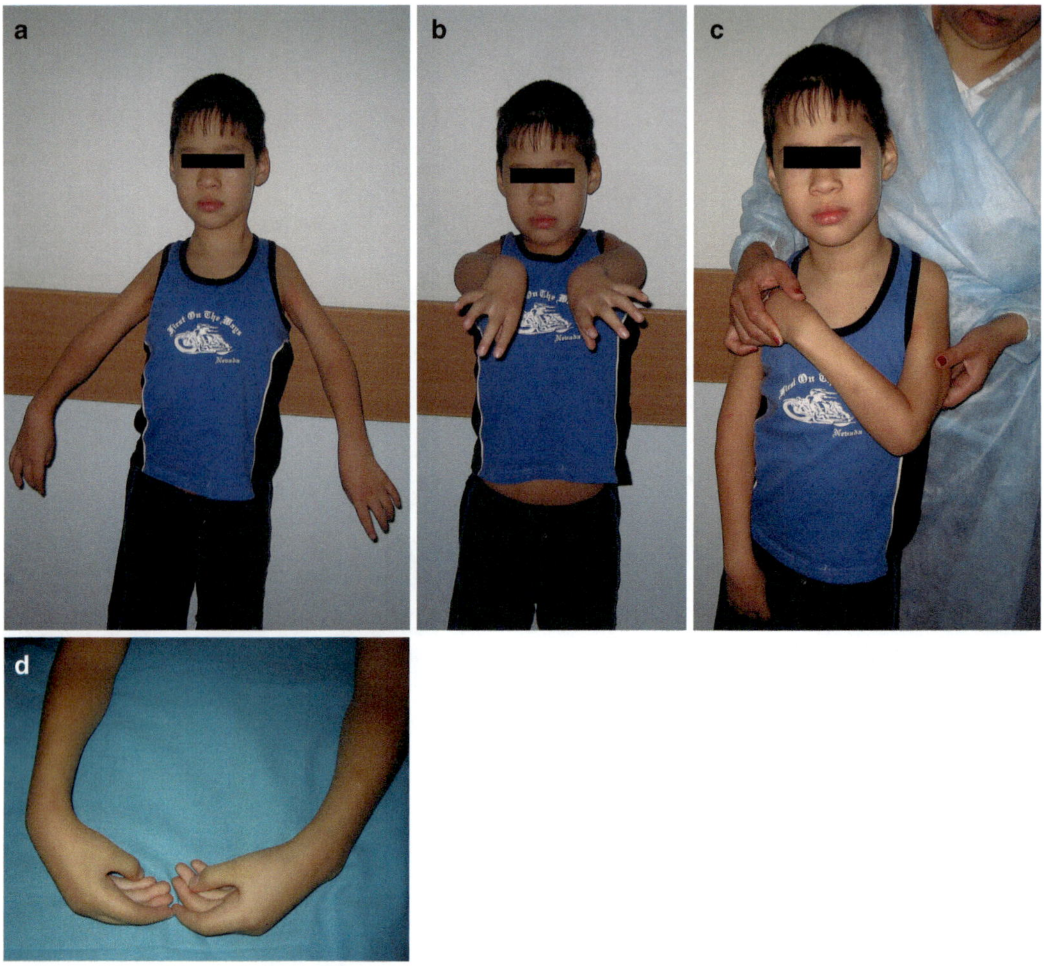

Fig. 20.2 Upper limb deformities in patient with level C5-C7. Clinical picture (**a**–**d**)

Elbow—extension or flexion contracture, passive movement is severely or moderately limited, active movement is severely limited or absent, and active supination is absent.

Wrist—flexion contracture with ulnar deviation or hand in the middle position, passive movement is severely limited or absent, active flexion is severely limited or absent, and active extension is absent.

Hand—function is poor or absent, flexion fingers contractures, symphalangia, thumb-in-palm symptom is present.

Prognosis of treatment is satisfactory or poor (Fig. 20.3).

20.2.4 Type 4: Level of Spinal Cord Injury: C6

20.2.4.1 Clinical Picture

Shoulder—full passive movement is present, active movement is full or moderately limited, and shoulder-girdle muscles are preserved or moderately hypoplastic.

Elbow—passive flexion is severely limited or preserved, active extension is preserved, and active flexion is moderately or severely limited.

Wrist—contractures are absent.

Hand—function is good and fingers contractures are absent.

Prognosis of treatment is good (Fig. 20.4).

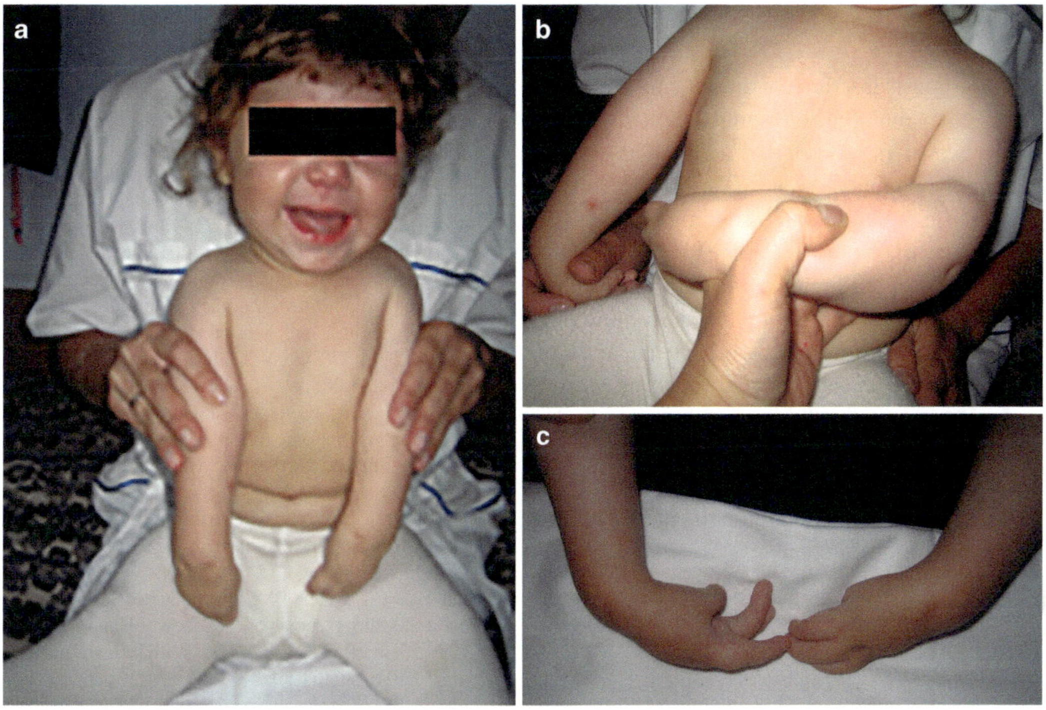

Fig. 20.3 Upper limb deformities in patient with level C5-Th1. Clinical picture (**a**–**c**)

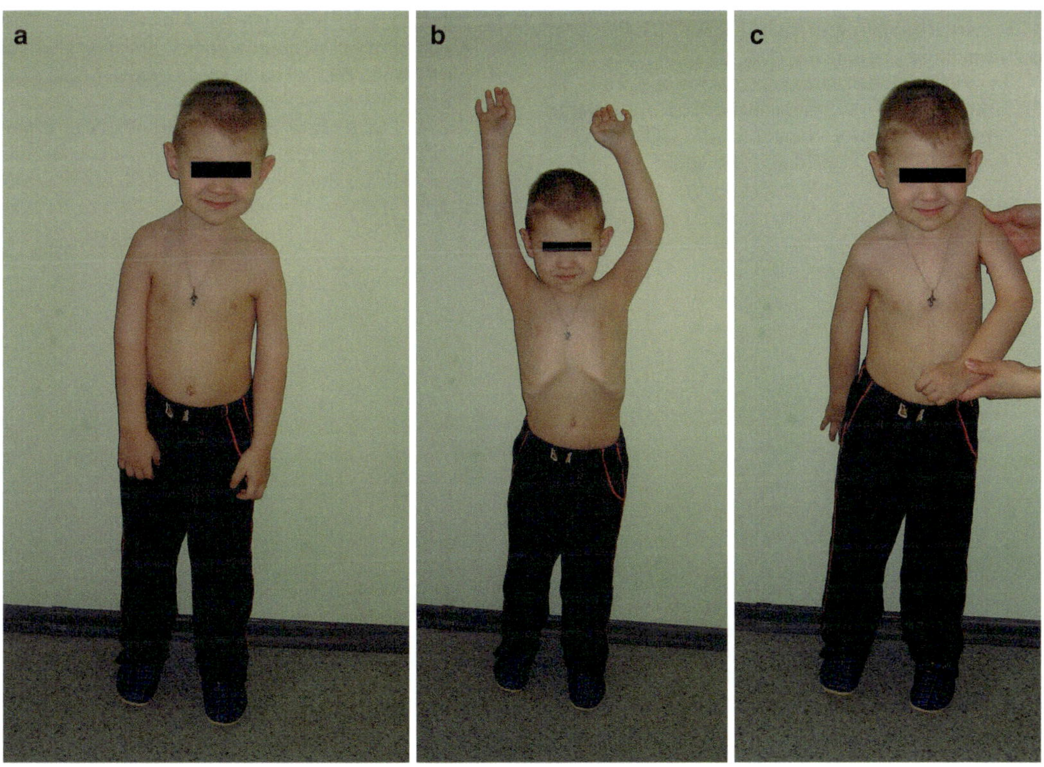

Fig. 20.4 Upper limb deformities in patient with level C6. Clinical picture (**a**–**c**)

20.3 Summary

Arthrogryposis is a rare condition, which is characterized by multiple congenital contractures that affect two or more different areas of the body. The most common type of arthrogryposis is amyoplasia. It is a sporadic condition, which has a frequency of one in 10,000 live births. The classification of upper limbs deformities is based on the level of spinal cord injury. All deformities are divided into two groups based on the level of damage of the spinal cord and range of passive and active motion in all joints of the upper limb.

Correct diagnosis of the type of upper limb deformity in patients with amyoplasia may allow for selection of the optimal treatment and for the prediction of the outcome.

References

1. Bamshad M, Van Heest AE, Pleasure D. Arthrogryposis: a review and update. J Bone Joint Surg Am. 2009;91(Suppl 4):40–6. https://doi.org/10.2106/JBJS.I.00281.
2. Lowry RB, Sibbald B, Bedard T, Hall JG. Prevalence of multiple congenital contractures including arthrogryposis multiplex congenita in Alberta, Canada, and a strategy for classification and coding. Birth Defects Res A Clin Mol Teratol. 2010;88(12):1057–61. https://doi.org/10.1002/bdra.20738.
3. Hall JG, Aldinger KA, Tanaka KI. Amyoplasia revisited. Am J Med Genet A. 2014;164A(3):700–30. https://doi.org/10.1002/ajmg.a.36395.
4. Hall JG, Kiefer J. Arthrogryposis as a syndrome: gene ontology analysis. Mol Syndromol. 2016;7:101–9. https://doi.org/10.1159/00044661.
5. Hall JG, Reed SD, Driscoll EP. Amyoplasia: a common sporadic condition with congenital contractures. Am J Med Genet. 1983;15:571–90. PMID: 6614047. https://doi.org/10.1002/ajmg.1320150407.
6. Hall JG. Arthrogryposis (multiple congenital contractures): diagnostic approach to etiology, classification, genetics, and general principles. Eur J Med Genet. 2014;57(8):464–72. https://doi.org/10.1016/j.ejmg.2014.03.008.
7. Kozin SH. Arthrogryposis. In: Green D, Hotchkiss R, Pederson W, Wolfe S, editors. Green's operative hand surgery. 5th ed. New York: Churchill Livingstone; 2005.
8. Gibson DA, Urs NDK. Arthrogryposis multiplex congenita. J Bone Joint Surg. 1970;52B:483–93. PMID:5455080.
9. Van Heest A, Waters PM, Simmons BP. Surgical treatment of arthrogryposis of the elbow. J Hand Surg Am. 1998;23(6):1063–70. PMID: 9848560. https://doi.org/10.1016/S0363-5023(98)80017-8.
10. Mennen U. Arthrogryposis multiplex congenita: functional classification and the AMC disc-o-gram. J Hand Surg Br. 2004;29(4):363–7. PMID:15234501. https://doi.org/10.1016/j.jhsb.2004.02.007.
11. Sells JM, Jaffe KM, Hall JG. Amyoplasia, the most common type of arthrogryposis: the potential for good outcome. Pediatrics. 1996;97(2):225–31. PMID:8584382.
12. Brown LM, Robson MJ, Sharrard WJ. The pathophysiology of arthrogryposis multiplex congenita neurologica. J Bone Joint Surg Br. 1980;62(3):291–6. PMID: 7410459.

21 Thumb in Arthrogryposis

Chiara Novelli, Giulietta Proserpio, and Giorgio Pajardi

Abstract

Arthrogryposis is a congenital disorder, a set of conditions of different aetiologies that are characterized by joint stiffness and contractures affecting at least two different areas of the body. Thumb in arthrogryposis is clasped with a flexion adduction deformity. It is characterized by deficiency of thumb extensors, flexion contracture of the metacarpophalangeal joint with possible instability, narrowing of the first web space due to different contractures of the web structures and lack of skin. Thumb function, its position, its length, its stability and its strength are essential for a proper grip. The loss of these features due to contracture in arthrogryposis reduces significantly patients' function and dexterity. Manipulation of the deformities starting soon after birth can improve the range of motion, which, if surgery needs to be done, makes the operation less extensive. Release of structures that are contracted, skin correction, gain of stability, good position and, if possible, replacement of structures that are weak or absent are the aim of the surgical treatment.

Keywords

Thumb · Arthrogryposis · Thumb contracture Thumb correction · First web contracture · First web release

Arthrogryposis is a descriptive term used to describe a host of clinical conditions resulting in nonprogressive multiple congenital joint contractures [1]. Once arthrogryposis was considered a distinct diagnosis for multiple joint contracture, it is now understood that arthrogryposis is a description of a heterogeneous group of some 300 different conditions with a variety of aetiologies including gene mutations [2].

The term arthrogryposis derives from the Greek words *arthros* (joint) and *grypon* (hooked), and it was coined by Rosencrantz [3]. In 1923, Stern used the term arthrogryposis multiplex congenita to describe the observed multiple joint involvement at birth [4]. Then the term amyoplasia appeared (literally, "a" means no, "myo" means muscle, "plasia" means development); it was created by Sheldon underling the thought that the primary cause for the condition was poor foetal muscle development [5].

C. Novelli (✉) · G. Proserpio
Milan, Italy
e-mail: chiara.novelli@multimedica.it

G. Pajardi
Department of Hand Surgery and Rehabilitation, S. Giuseppe Hospital IRCCS MultiMedica, Milan University, Milan, Italy
e-mail: gpajardi@centrostudimano.it

G. Pajardi (ed.), *Pediatric Hand Surgery*, https://doi.org/10.1007/978-3-031-30984-7_21

All forms are associated with foetal akinesia; in most cases, joint development is normal during embryogenesis, but at a certain moment, there is a movement decrease. Foetal movements are crucial to the correct development of joints; a reduction leads to contracture. An early onset of akinesia and the severity of contracture are related, as demonstrated in several in vivo studies [6, 7]. All factors that reduce foetal movements are involved in arthrogryposis, and its aetiology is multifactorial. Possible causes of akinesia include myopathic processes, neuropathic processes, neuromuscular endplate abnormalities, abnormalities of connective tissue, limitations of in utero space, maternal illness, maternal exposures, compromise of blood supply to placenta and foetus, metabolic disturbances and epigenetic disorders like part of complex syndromes [8].

In utero decreased movement leads to an increase of connective tissue around the joints that limits the joint movement, and it increases the contractures [9], muscle atrophy of the muscles associated with the joint due to disuse and abnormal joint surfaces that appear more squared.

Thumb in arthrogryposis is in palm with a narrow first web and soft tissue and muscle contractures (Fig. 21.1). The problems associated with joint contractures are a lack of skin, short tendons, joint stiffness with instability and weak muscles [10]. Particularly thumb is characterized by deficiency of the extensors (Fig. 21.2), flexion contracture of the metacarpophalangeal joint that can be also instable, skin deficiency of the first web and narrowing of the first web space due to variable combinations of contracture of the web structures. Also flexor pollicis longus can present a contracture. Thenar muscles are hypoplastic with fibrosis. Grasp and pinch are limited or absent by the severity of these deformities.

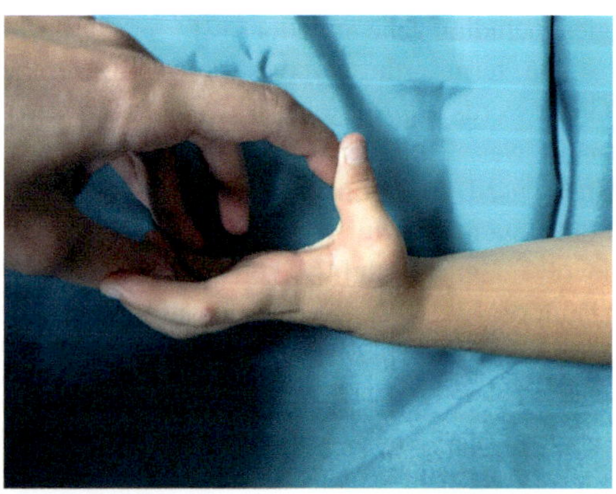

Fig. 21.1 Typical aspect of thumb in arthrogryposis

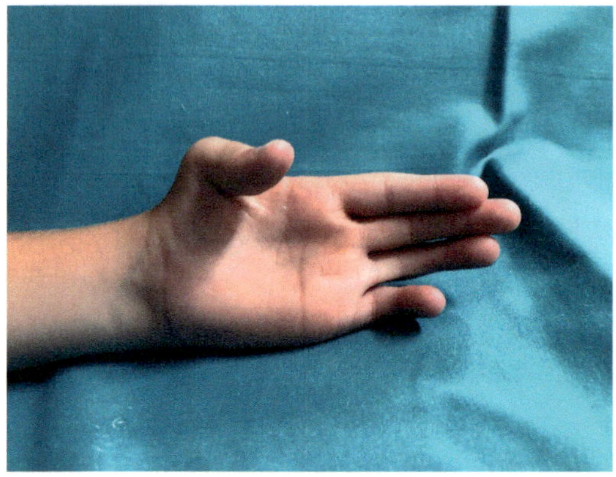

Fig. 21.2 Lack of extension

Goal of treatment is to improve thumb mobility and function in order to increase independence with activities of daily living. Occupational and physical therapies are essential components of treatment, and they begin at a very young age. Surgery became important when poor results are achieved with physiotherapy. Every treatment, surgical and nonoperative, must be tailored to each patient. A realistic family and patient expectation is also essential because it is not possible to restore a normal digital motion; function can just be improved [11]. For the assessment, hand X-rays are required.

First approach with thumb in palm is a gentle manipulation and stretching since birth, repeating them a lot of times during the day. The use of customized splints to continue stretching and maintain results during the night is also indicated. Free use of the upper limbs during the day is essential to allow children to explore and find their own way of managing activities. Parents need the support of trained hand therapists to learn the correct way of manipulating and stretching the thumb. Occupational therapists can assist in providing orthoses or adaptive equipment to support some activities, especially as children get older.

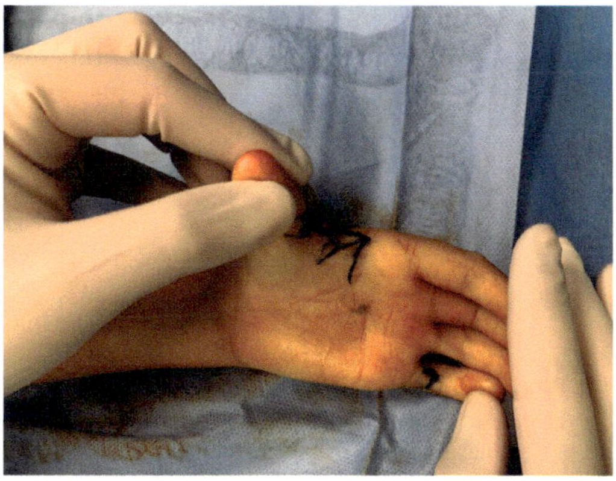

Fig. 21.3 Skin drawing

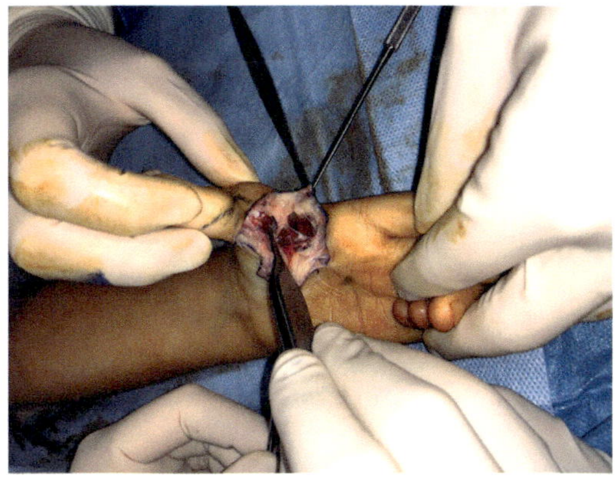

Fig. 21.4 Muscle release

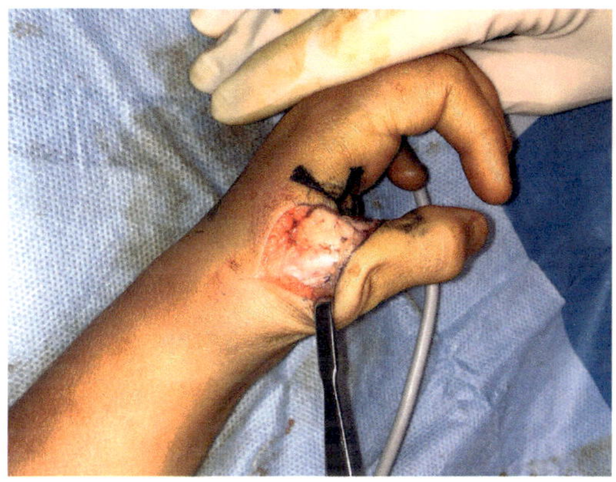

Fig. 21.5 Extensor tendon correction

If adequate progress is not achieved, surgery becomes necessary. Timing of surgery is controversial, but early management is recommended to have a minimal impact on child development. Surgery should be done before contractures become more fixed and joint surface anatomy and joint congruity change, making joint movement more difficult and limited. With time also intra-articular adhesions increase, preventing normal gliding surfaces; the skin becomes less pliable, further preventing normal joint movement [12].

The techniques of reconstruction of clasped thumb in arthrogryposis have not been widely discussed in the literature.

The aims of thumb correction are to release the narrow web structures, to augment the skin of the first web and to obtain extension and stabilization of the metacarpophalangeal joint. Different techniques of skin flaps have been described for skin augmentation of the narrow web, using of four-flap z-plasties [13] or a local flap [14, 15] (Fig. 21.3).

After web skin incision, the tight fascia of the first dorsal interosseous and adductor pollicis have to be released. When adductor release alone does not allow proper thumb positioning, also the thenar muscles must be released (Fig. 21.4). An incision is made next the thenar crease, and the origin of the thenar muscles is released after first identifying and protecting the motor branch of the median nerve. A Kirshner fixation of the metacarpophalangeal joint can be done for correct skin and thumb position healing. When there is an instability of the metacarpophalangeal joint, a chondrodesis can be performed [16], and sometimes also an opponensplasty is needed.

If the flexor pollicis longus is tight and prevents thumb abduction, a lengthening at the musculotendinous junction can be performed with attention to not weaken the function.

After muscle and soft tissue release, a careful examination can reveal the status of active thumb extension. In some cases, extensor pollicis longus function is present. However, in some cases, the extensor pollicis longus is poor or absent, and it has to be treated to avoid recurrence of thumb deformity. Sometimes, this tendon can be plicated (Fig. 21.5); otherwise a tendon transfer can

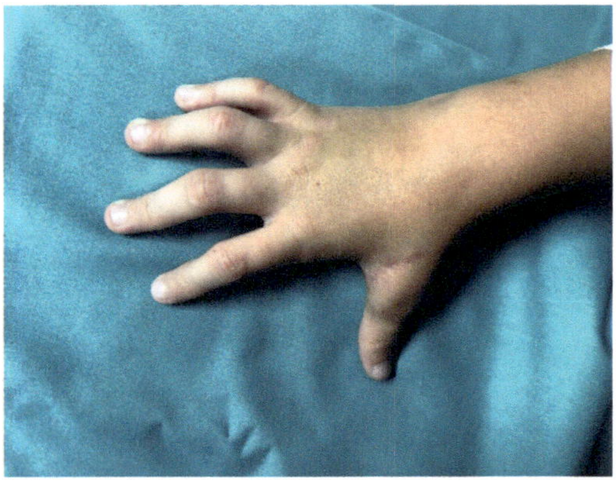

Fig. 21.6 Follow-up

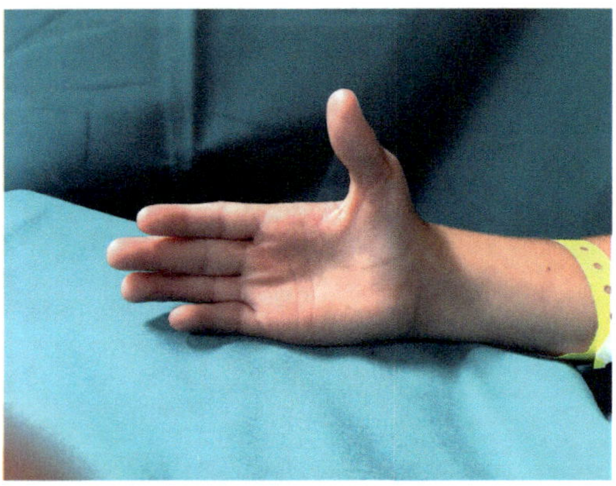

Fig. 21.7 Improvement in thumb extension

be considered to increase extensor power [17]. Unfortunately, in many cases, no adequate tendon is available for transfer.

After skin healing and Kirshner wire removal, physiotherapy and splinting are essential. The risk of recurrence or development of worse contractures is high without a correct postoperative protocol compliance.

Thumb in arthrogryposis treatment is a challenge to the hand surgeon and therapist. An early non-operative approach with manipulation and splints is necessary and can avoid surgery. Surgery becomes indicated when an adequate progress is not achieved. Its aim is to improve thumb position (Fig. 21.6) and function (Fig. 21.7) to allow patient independence.

References

1. Bamshad M, Van Heest AE, Pleasure D. Arthrogryposis: a review and update. J Bone Joint Surg Am. 2009;91(Suppl 4):40–6.
2. Bevan WP, Hall JG, Bamshad M, Staheli LT, Jaffe KM, Song K. Arthrogryposis multiplex congenita (amyoplasia): an orthopaedic perspective. J Pediatr Orthop. 2007;2:594–600.
3. Rosencranz E. Uber kongenitale kontrakturen der oberen extremitöten. Z Orthop Chir. 1905;14:52–62.
4. Stern WG. Arthrogryposis multiplex congenita. J Am Med Assoc. 1923;8:1507–10.
5. Sheldon W. Amyoplasia congenita: multiple congenital articular rigidity: arthrogryposis multiplex congenita. Arch Dis Child. 1932;7:117.
6. Moessinger AC. Fetal akinesia deformation sequence: an animal model. Pediatrics. 1983;72:857–63.
7. Hall JG, Opitz JM, Reynolds JF. Analysis of Pena Shokeir phenotype. Am J Med Genet. 1986;25:99–117.
8. Hall JG. Arthrogryposis (multiple congenital contractures): diagnostic approach to etiology, classification, genetics, and general principles. Eur J Med Genet. 2014;57:464–72.
9. Swinyard CA. Concepts of multiple congenital contractures (arthrogryposis) in man and animals. Teratology. 1982;25:247–59.
10. Lester R. Problems with the upper limb in arthrogryposis. J Child Orthop. 2015;9:473–6.
11. Waters PM, Bae DS. Hand and upper limb surgery: a practical guide. Philadelphia: LWW; 2012. p. 237–44.
12. Mennen U, Van Heest A, Ezaki MB, Tonkin M, Gericke G. Arthrogryposis multiplex congenita. J Hand Surg Br. 2005;30:468–74.
13. Broadbent TR, Woolf RM. Flexion-adduction deformity of the thumb-congenital clasped thumb. Plast Reconstr Surg. 1964;34:612–6.
14. Abdel-Ghani H. Modified dorsal rotation advancement flap for release of the thumb web space. J Hand Surg Br. 2006;31:226–9.
15. Ezaki MB, Oishi SN. Index rotation flap for palmar thumb release in arthrogryposis. Tech Hand Up Extrem Surg. 2010;14:38–40.
16. McCarroll HR, Manske PR. The windblown hand: correction of the complex clasped thumb deformity. Hand Clin. 1992;8:147–59.
17. Oishi SN, Agranovich O, Pajardi GE, Novelli C, Baindurashvili AG, Trofimova SI, Abdel-Ghani H, Kochenova E, Proserpio G, Jester A, Yilmaz G, Senaran H, Kose O, Butler L. Treatment of the upper extremity contracture/deformities. J Pediatr Orthop. 2017;37:S9–S15.

Vascular Malformations

22

Luciana Marzella and Piero di Giuseppe

Abstract

Vascular malformations (VMs) are a complex and multifactorial conditions that can involve any area of the body for which diagnosis and treatment often require a multidisciplinary approach. VMs are congenital anomalies that are subdivided into numerous categories grouped into arterious, venous, capillary lesions or a combination of all of these. There is much confusion surrounding these little known malformations; this is due mainly to the presence of numerous and varied classifications. Misclassifications or incorrect diagnoses are common and are usually due to the limited experience of clinicians or radiologists involved in the diagnosis and management of vascular malformations; recognizing a vascular malformation and appropriately classifying it are essential for optimal patient care and require solid knowledge and experience. The origin of vascular malformations is a genetic defect that, in many associated syndromes, is inherited in an autosomal recessive manner, while in the non-inherited forms, it is a random genetic defect.

Although embolization and sclerotherapy are helpful in other districts, they should be avoided in the hand because of the high failure rate and sequela; that is why surgical treatment is the best choice for the hand.

Keywords

Vascular malformations · Sclerotherapy · Embolization · Arteriovenous · Haemangioma

22.1 Introduction

Congenital Vascular Malformation is a malformed vessel that results from developmental arrest during embryogenesis and presents at birth as an inborn vascular defect and continues to grow at a rate that is proportional to the growth rate of the body, regardless of its type [1].

Vascular malformations (VMs) are a complex and multifactorial conditions that can involve any area of the body for which diagnosis and treatment often require a multidisciplinary approach [2].

VM can involve any vessel in any organ or tissue, in a non-schaematic manner. This characteristic explains the need for accurate diagnosis in order to plan appropriate treatment based on the type of malformation, site (superficial or deep, localized or infiltrating) and extension (limited or extended), tissue involvement and, lastly, the haemodynamic effects of the VM [3].

L. Marzella (✉)
Hand Surgery Unit, IRCCS Galeazzi-Sant'Ambrogio GSD, Milan, Italy

P. di Giuseppe
Columbus Clinic Center, Milan, Italy
e-mail: chirurgiadellamano@fastwebnet.it

G. Pajardi (ed.), *Pediatric Hand Surgery*, https://doi.org/10.1007/978-3-031-30984-7_22

22.2 Epidemiology

Confusion in terminology and classification has influenced epidemiologic data. Haemangioma is still confused with some venous malformations and syndromic or mixed vascular malformations which are reported as distinctly different entities in the literature.

VMs are rare anomalies that can involve all areas of the body; the upper limb accounts for 30–60% of cases [2, 4–6]. Fifty percent of lesions are diagnosed within the first 2 years from birth, but minor forms, although present at birth, often go unnoticed until adolescence or adulthood when trauma or hormonal alteration stimulates cellular proliferation, causing the lesions to become more evident [2, 7–9].

In our personal experience, based on more than 220 cases of surgically treated VMs of the hand, the distribution was different because VMs represented 49% of cases, arterovenous malformations (AVMs) 36%, while lymphatic malformations (LMs) and combined lymphovenous malformations (LVMs) 13.20% and others 2.40%.

22.3 Classifications

Vascular malformations (VMs) are congenital anomalies that are subdivided into numerous categories [4, 7, 8] grouped into arterious, venous, capillary lesions or a combination of all of these. There is much confusion surrounding these little known malformations; this is due mainly to the presence of numerous and varied classifications [2].

The first classification was presented in 1863 by Rudolph Virchow, who divided angiomas into three categories: angioma "symplex", angioma "cavernosum" and angioma "racemosus" [2, 10]. In 1964, Malan and Puglionisi proposed dividing vascular malformations into two large groups of congenital malformations: dysplasia (normal formation with structural deviations) and hamartoma (abnormal development of normal tissue in a determined area of the body) [2, 7, 8]. The first real classification of congenital vascular malformations to achieve general consensus was the Mulliken's classification of 1982 [2, 11]. For the first time, a clear distinction was made between vascular tumours, the most representative of which is haemangioma, and real vascular malformations. This classification supplied the framework for all classifications to follow: the Hamburg classification of 1988 [3], modified in 1993 [2, 12], and the ISSVA (International Society for the Study of Vascular Anomalies) classification of 1996 [2, 13], further modified in 2014 [2]. This is an articulated classification made up of various appendixes simplified into a table (Table 22.1).

Based on angiographic features, vascular malformations are distinguished as high or low flow depending on the presence or absence of a haemodynamically significant arterial axle [2, 14]. The existence of so many classifications that fail to meet with universal agreement clearly shows vascular malformations to be a complex subject for which a multifactorial approach is needed that takes into account the site of the anomaly [2]. Misclassifications or incorrect diagnoses are common and are usually due to the limited experience of clinicians or radiologists involved in the diagnosis and management of vascular malformations. The use of an inappropriate imaging modality (e.g. CT instead of MRI) and poor image quality can also contribute to this clinical dilemma [13]. The most common misdiagnosis or misconception is the use of the term haemangioma to mean venous malformations. This misconception can easily lead to incorrect triaging and mistreatment. For example, patients are commonly treated with steroids because of the interpretation of a haemangioma lesion on the imaging study [13]. Another common mistake is calling the malformation an AVM although all clinical and radiologic findings are characteristic of a low-flow vascular anomaly. Therefore, recognizing a vascular malformation and appropri-

Table 22.1 ISSVA classification of vascular anomalies ©2014 International Society for the Study of Vascular Anomalies available at "issva.org/classification" accessed 29th October 2017

Vascular tumours			Vascular malformations	
Benign	Locally aggressive	Malignant	Simple	Combined
Infantile haemangioma	Kaposiform haemangioendothelioma	Angiosarcoma	Capillary malformation (C)	CVM and CLM
Congenital haemangioma	Retiform haemangioendothelioma	Epithelioid haemangioendothelioma	Lymphatic malformation (LM)	LVM and CLVM
Tufted haemangioma	PILA (papillary intralymphatic angioendothelioma) and Dabska tumour		Venous malformation (VM)	CAVM
Spindle-cell haemangioma	Composite haemangioendothelioma		Arteriovenous malformation (AVM)	CLAVM
Epithelioid haemangioma	Kaposi sarcoma		Arteriovenous fistula	
Pyogenic granuloma				

ately classifying it are essential for optimal patient care and require solid knowledge and experience [13].

22.4 Aetiology and Embryology

Poor knowledge still today leads the population to consider vascular malformations something caused by a mother's unsatisfied cravings during pregnancy. In fact, they are known as birthmark. Several factors have been identified, some proven and others strongly involved: genetic and chromosomal abnormalities, mother's age, damaging chemical compound and infections (cytomegalic inclusion disease, herpes virus and toxoplasmosis). Thalidomide and other drugs, as well as alcohol, tobacco and cocaine abuse, have all been identified as causes of birth defects [15]. Some maternal diseases and exposures have also been associated with birth defects. These include endemic goitre, diabetes, thyroid disease, tuberculosis and hypoxia [15–18].

Vascular malformations have an incidence of 1.2% [13] and can involve all areas of the body with upper limb incidence between 30% and 60% [4–6]. Fifty percent of lesions are identified within the first 2 years of life, but minor forms, although present at birth, often go unnoticed until adolescence or adulthood when trauma or hormonal alteration stimulate cellular proliferation, causing them to be more evident [7–9]. In fact, a 2012 study revealed the presence of androgen, oestrogen and growth hormone receptors in the malformations [19].

The origin of vascular malformations is a genetic defect that, in many associated syndromes, is inherited in an autosomal recessive manner, while in the non-inherited forms, it is a random genetic defect. Gene mutations of some vascular malformations have been identified, thatis, lymphatic mutations concern PIK3CA [20]. Somatic activating mutations in GNAQ and GNA11 are associated with congenital haemangioma [21]. Endothelial cells in capillary malformations are enriched for somatic GNAQ mutations [22]. Somatic mutations in MAP2K1 are a common cause of extracranial arteriovenous shunting malformation (AVM) [23].

The mutation of these genes results from developmental errors during embryogenesis. Angiogenesis takes place in two stages [15] as follows:

1. Reticular stage: angioblasts and primitive vascular cells evolve by forming a primitive vascular network.
2. Truncular stage: certain areas of the primitive capillary network regress while others evolve into mature vessels.

Genetic anomalies can involve both the stages so we can have the following:

1. Reticular vascular malformations (true vascular malformations): primitive vascular regression defect, areas of multiple dysplastic vessels of small and medium calibre localized anywhere in the body, can be extensive and infiltrate tissue.
2. Truncular vascular malformations (vascular anomalies): a defect of main vessels, aplasia, hypoplasia, dilatations, hyperplasia, aneurisms and fistulas.

22.5 Diagnosis

VMs are present at birth, may be visible or become evident later, may be superficial and localized to one small area or represent an extensive malformation of the deep tissue.

VMs may involve any vessel and any tissue. This fundamental characteristic explains why the clinical profile can vary, especially for extratruncular VM.

Vascular malformations may appear either as a predominant lesion (e.g. VM, LM, AVM) or as a mixed anomaly comprising various VMs [24].

Truncular malformations of the upper limb are quite rare, while extratruncular malformations are more common.

A medical examination is sufficient in most cases to establish diagnosis. Nevertheless, instrumental investigations are necessary to better define extension, tissue involvement and characteristics, especially in combined vascular malformations.

VMs may present as solitary or multiple lesions, either superficial and localized or deep and extensively infiltrative. VMs can cause pain, and when the lesions involve the muscle, nerve or bone, they may be complicated by specific secondary symptoms (Fig. 22.1).

VMs in the upper extremities are easily collapsed when the arm is elevated to allow venous drainage.

LMs are generally asymptomatic, until complications develop (e.g. lymphatic leakage, intralesional bleeding, infection) or functional impairment occurs.

Local hyperthermia, a thrill and bruit that are the hallmarks of AVM often match visibly dilated veins. Ischaemic changes and ulceration of the skin can develop distal to the shunt, often with intractable pain and intermittent bleeding. Distal gangrene is likely if arterial insufficiency is severe. Combined or syndromic VMs are less common in the hand and appear as a particular picture that associates aspects of the various components of the malformation.

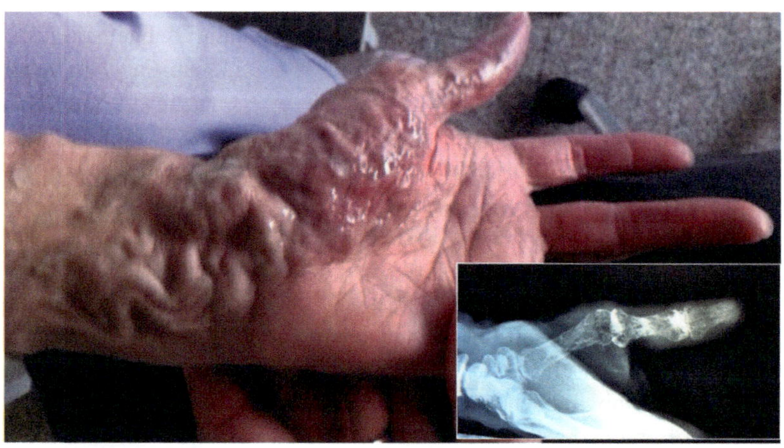

Fig. 22.1 AV vascular malformation infiltrating the thenar muscles, showing dilated drainage veins and ischaemic distal phalanx. X-ray shows bone involvement

22.6 Haemangioma

The term haemangioma is often used erroneously. Mulliken published an article in 2011 showing that out of 320 papers examined, 71.3% (228) erroneously used the word haemangioma. Patients whose lesions were mislabelled were more likely to receive improper treatment (20.6%) compared with those whose lesions were designated using the International Society for the Study of Vascular Anomalies terminology [25]. The article concluded with the affirmation: "Haemangioma continues to be commonly misused to describe any type of vascular anomaly, and terminological imprecision is prevalent among both medical and surgical fields. Inaccurate designation of the vascular anomaly is associated with an increased risk of erroneous management". Haemangiomas are among the most common benign tumours in children, appearing in 7–10% of infants [26, 27]. Approximately, 30% of haemangiomas are present at birth, with the remainder becoming evident within the first 4 weeks of life [27, 28]. Clinically, they are characterized by a period of rapid growth followed by a static period and, eventually, slow involution. Histologically, haemangiomas show endothelial cell proliferation, which is accelerated during the rapid growth phase [27]. Patients with congenital haemangioma are surgically treated in cases of abnormal growth with signs of nerve or joint compression which could cause permanent damage during growth or in the presence of ulceration (Fig. 22.2).

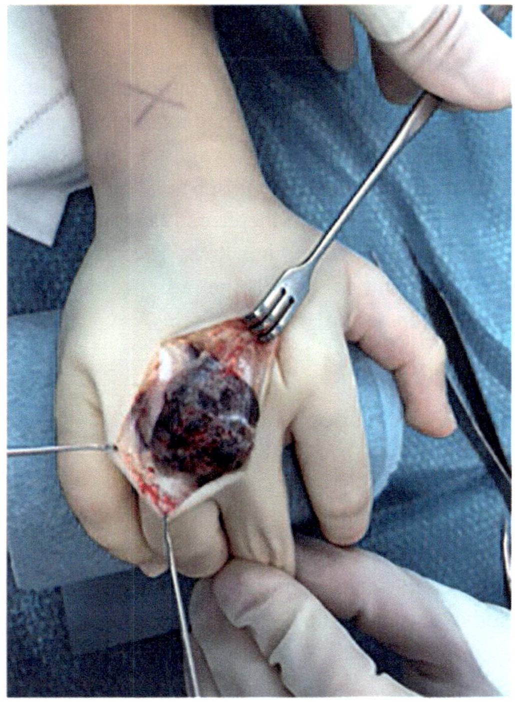

Fig. 22.2 Haemangioma in a 4-year-old child

22.7 Imaging

Radiography, ultrasonography (US), CT (computed tomography) and MRI (magnetic resonance imaging) are usually performed to confirm the suspected diagnosis, to determine the extent of the vascular anomaly and to search for associated abnormalities [29, 30].

22.7.1 Echo-Doppler

The first exam is echography associated with a Doppler, which enables to diagnose richly vascularized formations. In this way, it is possible to identify the presence or absence of flow within the detected mass and therefore classify the malformation as low or high flow. The absence of flow can point us towards the presence of vascular deficiencies or lymphatic forms.

22.7.2 Magnetic Resonance Angiography (MRA)

MRA is an indirect, noninvasive, operator-dependent exam. Results are influenced by the number of scans, exposure time and thickness and extension of field, as well as the experience of the radiologist. MRA supplies images of the malformation, site and extension in tissue and represents the elective exam for the venous and lymphovenous vascular malformations, as seen in Fig. 22.3.

22.7.3 Angiography

Angiography is a direct, invasive exam with possible complications (infection, vessel breakage, ischaemic pain, intolerance to contrast medium, shock). It requires hospital or day hospital admission that affects overall costs. Angiography helps to focalize the vascular malformation nidus inside an arteriovenous malformation.

The evolution of angiography is the video-digital-angiography, elective for complex hidden arteriovenous malformations (Fig. 22.4).

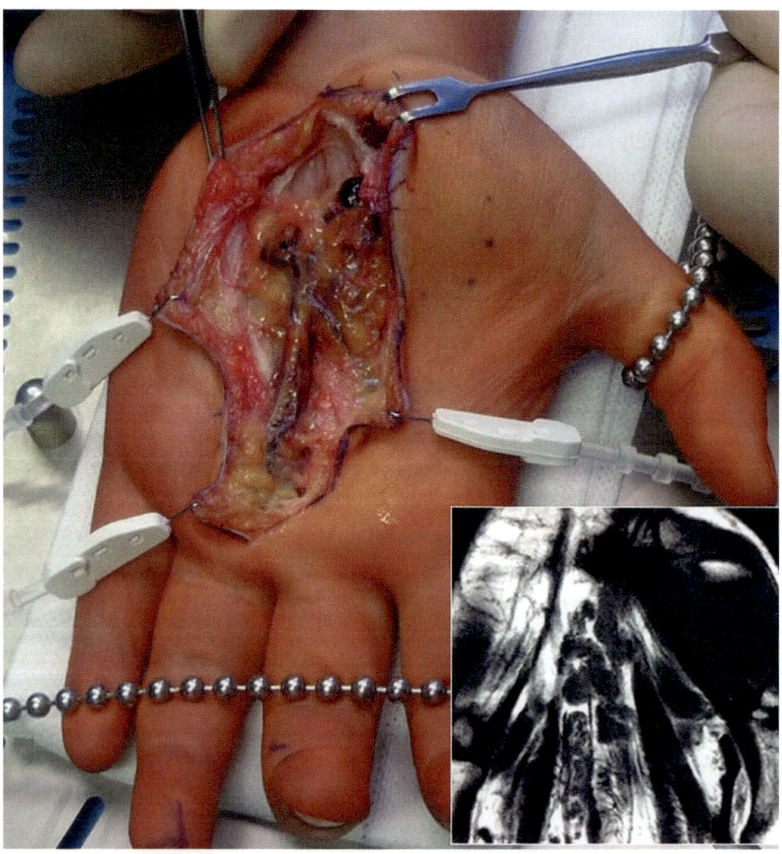

Fig. 22.3 Venous malformation in the palm of an 18-year-old woman, detected with a MRI in the presence of a unclear clinical picture

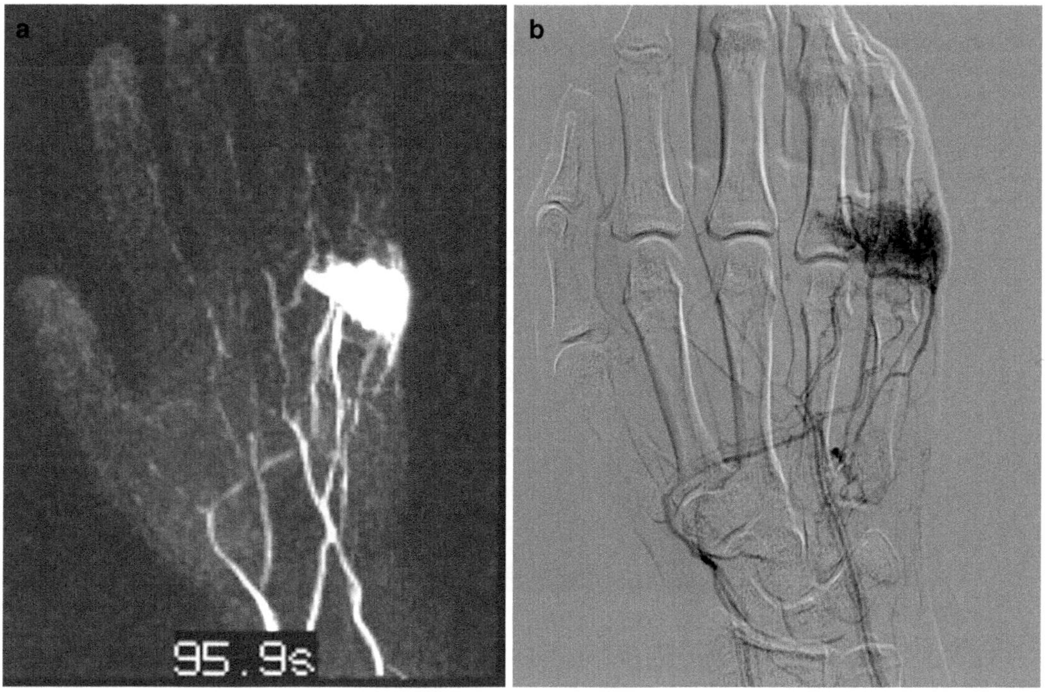

Fig. 22.4 VM in a 26-year-old woman: (**a**) AngioMRI and (**b**) arteriography

22.7.4 Lymphoscintigraphy

This is an elective exam for lymphatic forms, enabling identification of site and spread. It is invasive because of the radioactive contrast medium so its use is limited.

22.8 Treatment Principles

For compressible lesions, such as lymphatic and venous VM, tailored compressive dressings can be worn to provide symptomatic relief and alleviate pain, heaviness and dragging secondary to limb distension [31]. In some patients, this also provides some improvement in aesthetic appearance. Sclerotherapy and embolization, which are very common in other districts, should be avoided in the hand, because of the high failure rate and sequelae, and should be limited in superficial proximal forms performed by a skilled radiologist [32]. Commonly used sclerosing agents include alcohol or sodium tetradecyl sulphate, ethanol and ethibloc ([Johnson and Johnson] a combination of amino acids, ethanol and contrast agents) [10, 31, 33]. Some surgeons prefer sodium tetradecyl sulphate for small superficial lesions; 100% ethanol is used for larger and deeper VMs [10]. Administration of ethanol directly into the lesion can be very painful; therefore most procedures are performed under general anaesthesia. Potential complications include necrosis of the overlying skin and nerve injury due to extravasation. In rare cases, post-inflammatory hyper-pigmentation and infection can occur in the presence of ulceration [33].

Arterious embolization can be considered during angiography for arteriovenous malformations (AVMs), but this procedure can be extremely risky especially for distal portions of the hand due to the high risk of ischaemia; it is therefore used as a first step treatment to reduce the mass to prepare it for surgery [15] (Fig. 22.5).

Indications for surgical treatment are pain, intralesional thrombosis, bleeding, nerve compression, recurrent infection, functional disability, overgrowth and compartment syndrome. Incomplete resection and diffuse lesions can

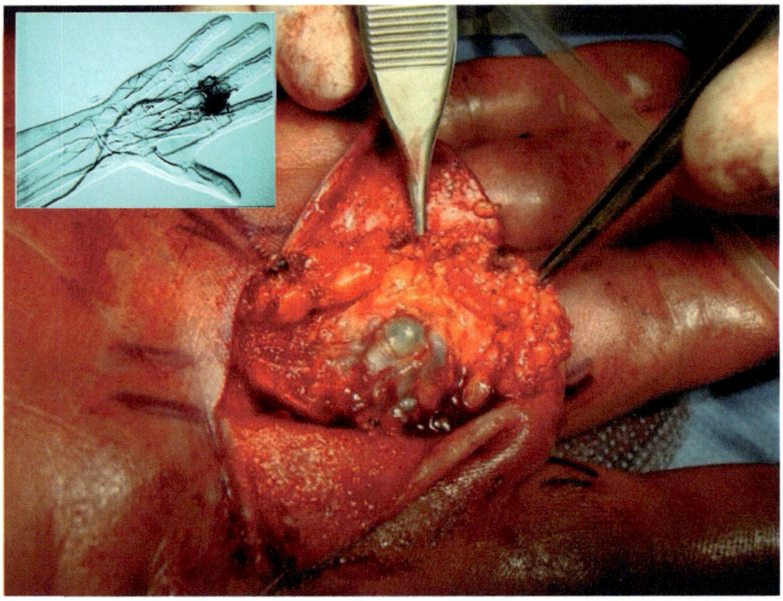

Fig. 22.5 Arteriovenous malformation limited to the distal palm of a 23-year-old man. Signs of previous proximal embolization are evident in the angiography image

cause recurrence [34]. In cases of massive lesions, limb amputation or ray resection may be indicated [27, 35]. Of all the vascular malformations, high-flow-type lesions exhibit the poorest prognosis. Following some authors despite early and aggressive multistaged excision and microvascular reconstruction, 90% of patients require major amputation to alleviate pain and chronic ulceration [35].

The surgeon should avoid performing intraneural dissection as first approach [27] and capsulectomies when excising the lesion. Bleeding, pain, oedema, CRPS (complex regional pain syndrome), wound dehiscence and, of course, recurrence are possible complications.

22.9 Surgical Treatment

Radical surgical excision remains the only definitive cure for certain vascular malformations, but it can be associated with high morbidity. On the other hand, incomplete resection of the malformed tissue often results in a high risk of recurrence. Recurrence following treatment remains a significant problem for all embryologically immature extratruncular lesions, and the potential for recurrence should never be underestimated [24].

Particularly when dealing with the hand, the challenge is to obtain a good equilibrium between radical excision and prevention of recurrence, complications and functional impairment. This is the approach that we call "functionally radical excision".

We follow the indications of conservative surgery proposed by Belov [24] and a diagnostic and therapeutic programme tailored for each patient (Fig. 22.6).

A multidisciplinary approach is a well-defined surgical plan in a delimited area, under tourniquet control, with step-by-step procedures, and when possible, avoid returning to the same operative field unless absolutely necessary, in which case wait sufficiently for tissue to stabilize and avoid intraneural or articular procedures.

In VM of the hand, *tissue involvement* is the most important feature because of the presence of highly functional, complex components confined to a small space [36].

In VM, *skin* is thinned by compression while fat tissue is extensively involved. This allows a subdermal dissection to preserve skin flaps and reduce bleeding (skin sparing technique). In

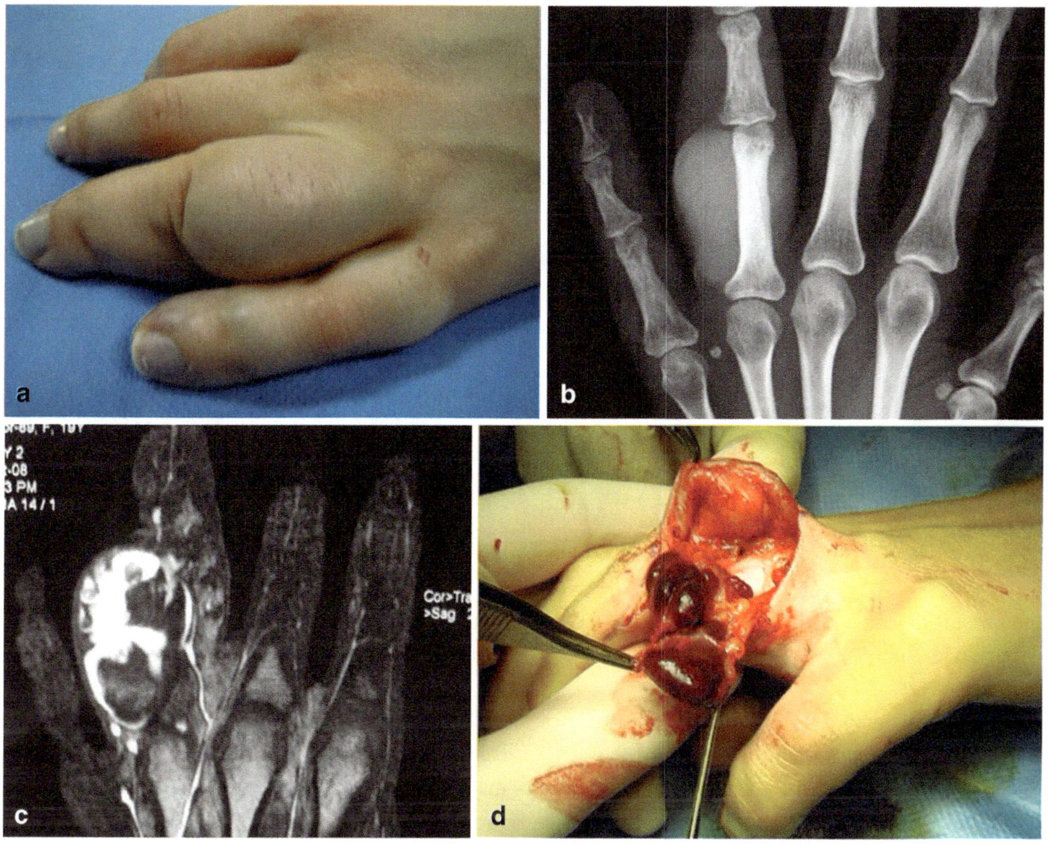

Fig. 22.6 (**a**) Clinical picture of a venous malformations in a 20-year-old woman. (**b**) X-ray shows bone compression deformity. (**c**) MRI shows expansive mass. (**d**) Operative aspect of venous malformed tissue

AVMs, subcutaneous tissue is involved and skin is damaged by ischaemia or direct invasion [24, 36].

Three points have been noted in our experience regarding skin as follows:

- As skin has a "passive motor function" and scars can hamper movements, the choice of skin incisions is a very important point in surgical planning. Mapping the lesions and drawing incisions help to avoid scar contracture.
- When not damaged, flaps undermined at the subdermal plane survive and allow good coverage avoiding grafts or distant flaps.
- In LVM, skin can be excised following some patterns together with the malformed tissue [36].

Other than the skin, the involvement of nerves and bones is the greatest challenge in this kind of surgery:

Bone can be affected in low- (venous) or high- (arteriovenous) flow malformations. Radiography and haemodynamic evaluation help to decide on treating with surgery alone or a combined sclerotherapy and surgical approach.

Joint instability can be due to direct bone or ligament involvement. In case of severe PIP (proximal interphalangeal) or DIP (distal interphalangeal) joint instability, temporary immobilization with K wires is recommended [36].

Nerves: Here the choice is to limit surgery to surrounding malformed vessels, thus avoiding entering the nerve. Pain and impaired nerve function are the main complaints, and external decompression is the first procedure used to reduce symptoms [35, 36].

The use of a microscope permits a more precise dissection and avoids lesions to the epineurium. Internal neurolysis is a risky procedure and

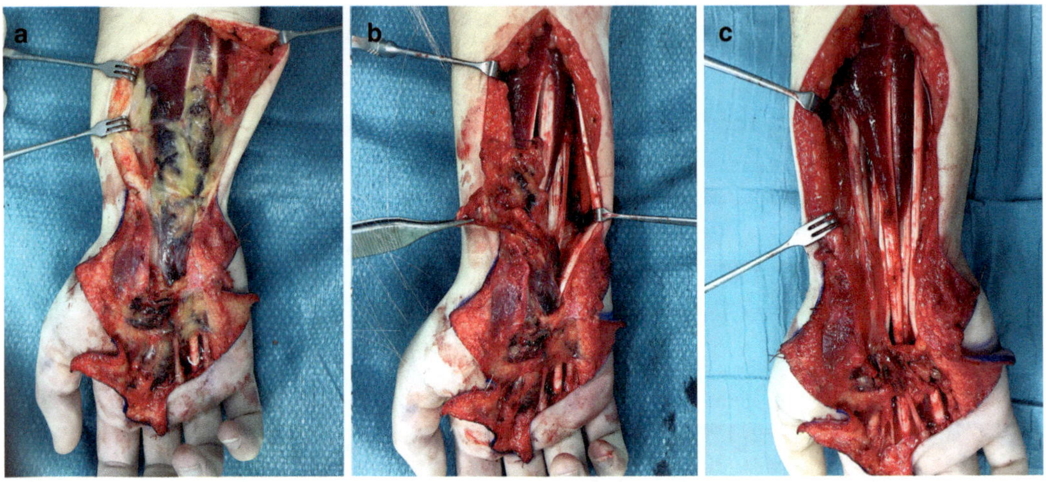

Fig. 22.7 (**a**) Intraoperative image of a VM involving all tissues in the wrist; (**b**) no evidence of tendon involvement during surgery; (**c**) complete excision of the VM

may result in nerve resection and grafting. In our experience such a procedure has never been performed.

In case of nerve damage, repair by suture or graft should be performed immediately.

Tendons are never affected while synovia is commonly involved.

In some cases, we observed involvement of tendon sheets just like in rheumatoid arthritis while tendons were almost completely undamaged (Fig. 22.7). Synovectomy is a safe and effective operation and permits to remove malformed tissue around tendons [36].

Muscles are widely and frequently involved, and their partial or total excision is often the only way to obtain significant reduction of the VM mass.

In cases in which it is necessary to resect groups of muscles, it is possible to perform secondary palliative procedures.

When a single expendable distal muscle is involved, total resection is the procedure of choice. When an important muscle or group of muscles are infiltrated, partial resection should be considered. Here also it is possible to combine sclerotherapy prior to surgery, to reduce the malformed mass in AVMs.

Multiple forearm muscles are often infiltrated or present sclerosis following previous operations or other treatments. In such cases, an individual analysis of residual function and healthy muscles, considering symptoms and haemodynamic findings, can provide guidelines for surgery. Excision of flexor carpi ulnaris if palmaris longus and flexor carpi radialis are preserved, or resection of a mass inside flexor digitorum superficialis, thus weakening its function, if flexor digitorum profundus is spared, can be proposed [36].

22.10 Complications

Distal ischaemia and skin necrosis or nerve damage are the main complications that Belov's principles of functionally radical surgery aim to prevent.

Haematomas and partial skin necrosis are generally minor sequelae and do not affect the final result. The use of tourniquet, drains and appropriate postoperative dressing reduce these risks.

Our surgical approach is conservative, but sometimes, in the presence of massive AVMs, amputation is unavoidable.

Extensive tissue involvement and damage secondary to treatments, particularly in children, can induce muscle retraction, progressive bone deformation and joint stiffness that require secondary surgery.

22.11 Syndromic Forms

In syndromic forms, vascular malformations are associated with general disorders. The forms that involve the hand and upper limb are Maffucci syndrome, Klippel-Trenaunay syndrome, Park-Weber syndrome, Proteus syndrome and Cloves syndrome.

22.11.1 Maffucci Syndrome (MS)

Maffucci syndrome is a rare congenital disorder characterized by multiple central cartilaginous tumours (enchondromas) in association with cutaneous spindle cell haemangiomas. Patients with MS have a high incidence of malignant transformation [37]. MS was first described in 1881 as differential diagnosis with Ollier's syndrome, which is a simple multiple enchondromatosis. Treatment of MS is surgical excision of enchondromas and vascular malformations.

22.11.2 Klippel-Trenaunay Syndrome (KTS)

Clinical features are (1) port-wine stains that may be localized to a relatively small area or involve the lateral aspect of one or more extremities; (2) limb hypertrophy or gigantism, presenting with an extremity that is longer and larger in circumference than the unaffected limb; (3) large clusters of varicose veins extending throughout the entire extremity; and (4) large lateral venous collector called the vena marginalis lateralis [15]. Most of these patients can be treated by compression and sclerotherapy and by sleeping in Trendelenburg position. However, some patients have pain, venous ulceration, venous thrombosis and pulmonary embolism that do not respond to conservative measures and need to be treated aggressively. It is important to stop bleeding that may sometimes be copious [27].

22.11.3 Park-Weber Syndrome (PKWS)

PKWS is often confused with KTS. Clinical features are capillary venous malformations that involve upper or lower limb, arteriovenous shunts and anomalies and hypertrophy of bones and tissues.

22.11.4 Proteus Syndrome (PS)

Proteus syndrome is a mosaic, progressive overgrowth disorder involving vessels, skin and skeleton and caused by a somatic activating mutation in AKT1 [38, 39].

Proteus syndrome appears with localized macrosomia, congenital lipomatosis and slow flow vascular malformations, connective tissue nevus and epidermal nevus. There are usually some manifestations at birth. The vascular abnormalities that have been reported in Proteus syndrome are capillary and slow-flow venous malformation [38–40].

Patients with Proteus syndrome have a high mortality incidence at 22 years of age [41].

22.11.5 CLOVES Syndrome

The acronym CLOVES stands for congenital lipomatous overgrowth (CLO), vascular malformation (V), epidermal nevi (E) and scoliosis and spinal deformities (S) [42].

22.11.6 Characteristics of CLOVES (Fig. 22.8)

1. Various size lipomatous mass of the torso
2. Vascular malformations
3. Musculoskeletal deformities especially of hands and feet
4. Scoliosis and anomalies of the spine and chest
5. Neurologic involvement

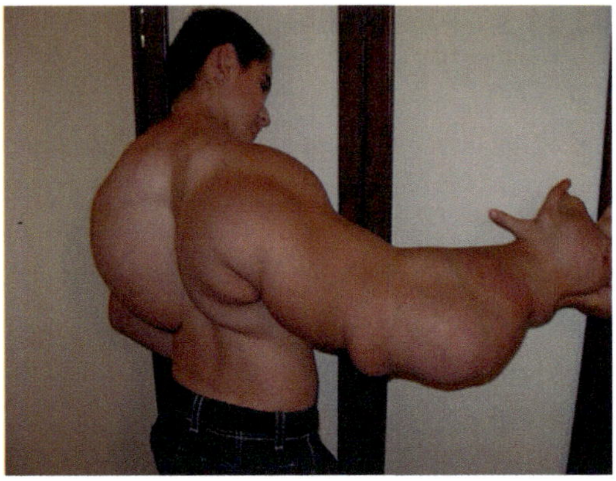

Fig. 22.8 CLOVES syndrome in a 9-year-old male

Unlike Proteus syndrome, CLOVES does not present with connective tissue nevi and consists of a lipomatous mass with an aggressive overgrowth and high rate of recurrence [42, 43].

This overgrowth leads to exhaustion due to the heavy weight of the overgrowing limb. When symptomatic treatment fails, surgical excision of the mass or amputation should be considered.

References

1. Lee BB, et al. Phlebology. 2007;22(6):283–6.
2. Marzella L. Indicazioni diagnostico terapeutiche per le Malformazioni vascolari dell'Arto superiore:valutazione dell'appropriatezza tra un gruppo di esperti e adozione di linee guida multidisciplinari. Chirurgia della Mano. 2016;53(3):77–87.
3. Belov S, Loose DA, Weber J. Vascular malformations. Reinbek: Einhorn Presse; 1989. p. 29.
4. Szilagyi DE, Smith RF, Elliott JP, et al. Congenital arteriovenous anomalies of the limbs. Arch Surg. 1976;111:423–9.
5. Gomes AS, Busuttil RW, et al. Congenital arteriovenous malformations. The role of transcatheter arterial embolization. Arch Surg. 1983;118:817–25.
6. Gomes MMR, Bernatz PE. Arteriovenous fistulas: a review and ten-year experience at the Mayo Clinic. Mayo Clin Proc. 1970;45:81–102.
7. Malan E, Pugliorisi A. Congenital angio-dysplasias of the extremities. I. Generalities and classification; venous dysplasias. J Cardiovasc Surg (Torino). 1964;5:87–130.
8. Malan E, Pugliorisi A. Congenital angiodysplasias of the extremities. II. Arterial, arterial and venous, and haemolymphatic dysplasias. J Cardiovasc Surg. 1965;6:255–345.
9. Wolfe SW, Pederson WC, Kozin SH, Cohen MS. Green's operative hand surgery, 2-volume. 6th ed. Philadelphia: Elsevier; 2011. p. 2236–9.
10. Angiome VR. Die Krankhaften Gerschwulste. Berlin: Hirschwald; 1863.
11. Mulliken J, Glowacky J. Hemangiomas and vascular malformations in infants and children: a classification based on endothelial characteristics. Plast Reconstr Surg. 1982;69:412–22.
12. Mattassi R. Hemangiomas and vascular malformation. Milan: Springer; 2009.
13. Konez O. Imaging in vascular anomalies. Medscape, October 2015
14. Cabbade EB. Xerography as an aid in planning resection of vascular malformation of the upper extremities. J Hand Surg Am. 1985;10:670–4.
15. Lee BB, Villavicencio L. Congenital vascular malformations: general considerations. In: Rutherford vascular surgery, vol. 68. Amsterdam: Elsevier; 2014.
16. Kennedy WP. Epidemiologic aspects of the problem of congenital malformations. In: Persaud TNV, editor. Problems of birth defects. Baltimore, MD: University Park Press; 1977. p. 35–52.
17. Stevenson AC, Johnston HA, Stewart MIP, Golding DR. Congenital malformations. A report of a study of series of consecutive births in 24 centres. Bull WHO. 1966;34(Suppl):9 and 100–102 (Extracts).
18. Myrianthopoulos NC, Chung CS. Congenital malformations in singletons. Epidemiologic survey. In: Bergsma D, editor. Birth defects original article series, vol. X, no II (Miami Symposia Specialists for the National Foundation-March of Dimes); 1974.
19. Kulungowski AM, Mulliken JB. Expression of androgen, estrogen, progesterone and growth hormone receptors in vascular malformations. Plast Reconstr Surg. 2012;129(6):919–24.
20. Luks VL, Kamitaki N, et al. Lymphatic and other vascular malformative/overgrowth disorders are caused by somatic mutations in PIK3CA. J Pediatr. 2015;166(4):1048–54.e1–5.
21. Ayturk UM, Couto JA. Somatic activating mutations in GNAQ and GNA11 are associated with congenital hemangioma. Am J Hum Genet. 2016;98(4):789–95.
22. Couto JA, Huang L. Endothelial cells from capillary malformations are enriched for somatic GNAQ mutations. Plast Reconstr Surg. 2016;137(1):77e–82e.
23. Couto JA, Huang L. Somatic MAP2K1 mutations are associated with extracranial arteriovenous malformation. Am J Hum Genet. 2017;100(3):546–54.
24. Belov S. Surgical treatment of congenital vascular defects. In: Chang JB, editor. Modern vascular surgery. New York: Springer; 1994. p. 383–97.
25. Hassanein HC, Mulliken JB. Evaluation of terminology for vascular anomalies in current literature. Plast Reconstr Surg. 2011;127(1):347–51.
26. Blei F. Basic science and clinical aspects of vascular anomalies. Curr Opin Pediatr. 2005;17(4):501–9.
27. Ek ET, Suh N. Vascular anomalies of hand and wrist. J Am Acad Orthop Surg. 2014;22:352–60.

28. Jacobs BJ, Anzarut A, Guerra S, Gordillo G, Imbriglia JE. Vascular anomalies of the upper extremity. J Hand Surg Am. 2010;35(10):1703–9.
29. Pearce WH, Rutherford RB, Whitehill TA, Davis K. Nuclear magnetic resonance imaging in patients with congenital vascular malformations of the limbs. J Vasc Surg. 1988;8:64–70.
30. Lee BB, Choe YH, Ahn JM, et al. The new role of MRI (magnetic resonance imaging) in the contemporary diagnosis of venous malformation: can it replace angiography? J Am Coll Surg. 2004;198: 549–58.
31. Coursley G, Ivins JC, Barker NW. Congenital arteriovenous fistulas in extremities. Angiology. 1956;7:201–17.
32. Park UJ, Do YS, Park KB, Park HS, Kim YW, Lee BB, Kim DL. Ann Vasc Surg. 2012;26(5):643–8.
33. Ahmad Khan RD. Glomus tumours: outcome based on tumour location in the hand. J Pak Med Assoc Nov. 2015;65(11 Suppl 3):S3–7.
34. Hill RA, Pho RW, Kumar VP. Resection of vascular malformations. J Hand Surg Br. 1993;18(1):17–21.
35. Upton J, Coombs CJ, Mulliken JB, Burrows PE, Pap S. Vascular malformations of the upper limb: a review of 270 patients. J Hand Surg Am. 1999;24(5):1019–35.
36. Di Giuseppe P. Surgical treatment of vascular malformation in the hand. In: Hemangiomas and vascular malformation. Milan: Springer; 2009. p. 287–92.
37. Amyere M, Dompmartin A. Common somatic alterations identified in Maffucci syndrome by molecular karyotyping. Mol Syndromol. 2014;5(6):259–67.
38. Kepler-Noreuil KM, et al. Am J Med Genet A. 2017;173(9):2359–65.
39. Ou M et al. Mol Clin Oncol. 2017;6(3):381–3.
40. Asillian A, et al. Adv Biomed Res. 2017;7:6–27.
41. Sapp JC, et al. Genet Med. 2017. https://doi.org/10.1038/gim.2017.65.
42. Bloom J, Upton J III. Cloves syndrome. J Hand Surg Am. 2013;38(12):2508–12.
43. Alomari AI. Characterization of a distinct syndrome that associates complex truncal overgrowth, vascular, and acral anomalies: a descriptive study of 18 cases of CLOVES syndrome. Clin Dysmorphol. 2009;18(1):1–7.

Macrodactilies

23

Scott N. Oishi, Marybeth Ezaki, Terri Beckwith, and Arena Sayavong

Abstract

Macrodactyly is the descriptive name for fingers or toes that are enlarged most often due to pathway mutations regulating growth, protein synthesis, and cellular proliferation. The enlargement in these patients is extremely variable and can affect the finger(s) only or the entire limb. These patients typically present for evaluation early in life as the enlarged digits/extremities are usually recognized at birth. It is critical to identify those children in which macrodactyly is extensive or progressive, as surgical and/or pharmacologic intervention may be warranted. Parental education and counseling about realistic expectations are imperative too.

Keywords

Macrodactyly · Overgrowth · PI3K-AKT · Fibroadipose hand · PROS

23.1 Introduction

As the name suggests, macrodactyly means abnormal enlargement of one or more digits of the hand or foot. Although associated with neurofibromatosis and Klippel-Trenaunay and Ollier syndromes, the most common etiology of this condition was only recently discovered using newly developed advanced sequencing techniques. A mutation in the PIK3CA (phosphatidylinositol-4,5-biphosphate 3-kinase) pathway was identified in affected tissues [1, 2]. This somatic mosaic gain-of-function mutation leads to dysregulation of growth through the mTOR pathway (Fig. 23.1) [2].

This pathway is involved with the regulation of growth, protein synthesis, and cellular proliferation and is also implicated in various adult malignancies. Other overgrowth conditions have been shown to be caused by mutations in this mTOR pathway, the so-called PIK3CA-related overgrowth spectrum (PROS) (Fig. 23.2).

The mutation occurs in the postzygotic embryonic period, thereby occurring in some cells and not in others. As a result, DNA sequencing of unaffected tissue will fail to show this upregulation in PIK3CA. Sanger sequencing is much less

S. N. Oishi (✉) · M. Ezaki · T. Beckwith · A. Sayavong
Charles E. Seay, Jr. Hand Center, Texas Scottish Rite Hospital for Children, Center for Excellence in Hand, Upper Extremity and Microvascular Surgery, Dallas, TX, USA
e-mail: Scott.Oishi@tsrh.org; Terri.Beckwith@tsrh.org; Arena.Sayavong@tsrh.org

G. Pajardi (ed.), *Pediatric Hand Surgery*, https://doi.org/10.1007/978-3-031-30984-7_23

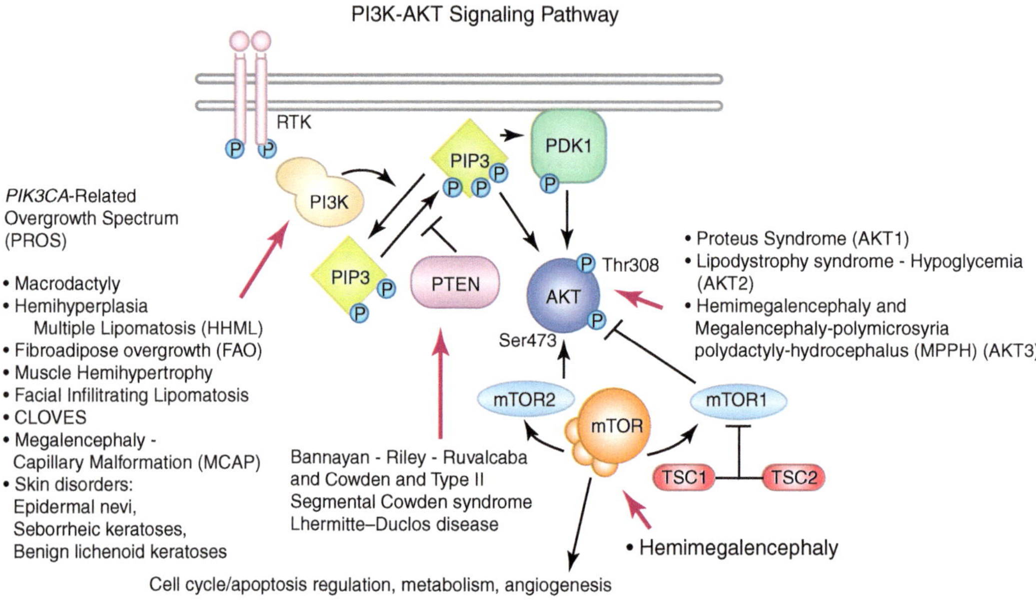

Fig. 23.1 Signaling pathway of PI3CA expression [2]

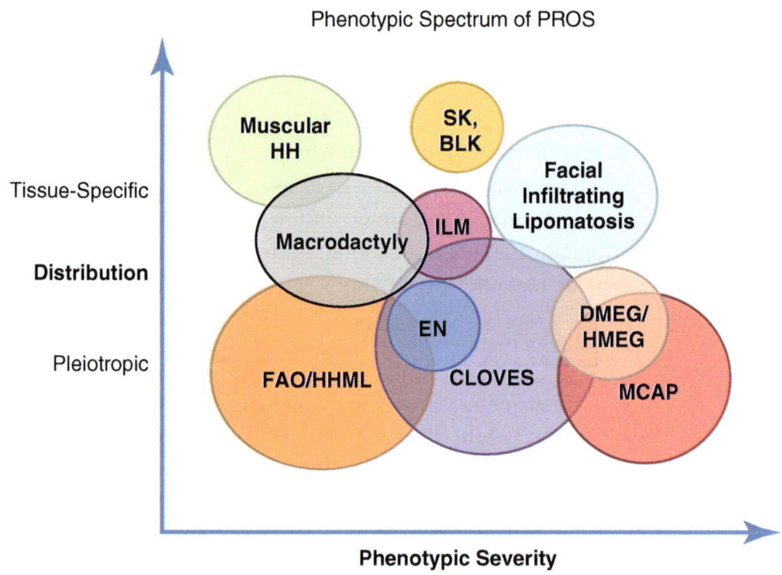

Fig. 23.2 Phenotypic variating related to the spectrum of PROS [2]

expensive than high-throughput but is slower and less sensitive and can have some false negatives because it has difficulty in distinguishing low-level mutations in the tissue. Next-generation sequencing (NGS) uses a technique of massively parallel sequencing and can pick up relatively low levels of mutation in the tissue. The burden of mutation in a cell population or the tissue is thought to be related to phenotype.

23.2 Clinical Presentation

The digits usually affected are in the median distribution of the hand, with the index finger being the most common (Fig. 23.3).

Occasionally, however, it can be isolated to the ulnar distribution of the hand (Fig. 23.4).

Macrodactyly was thought to be influenced by the associated nerve, which is grossly enlarged as

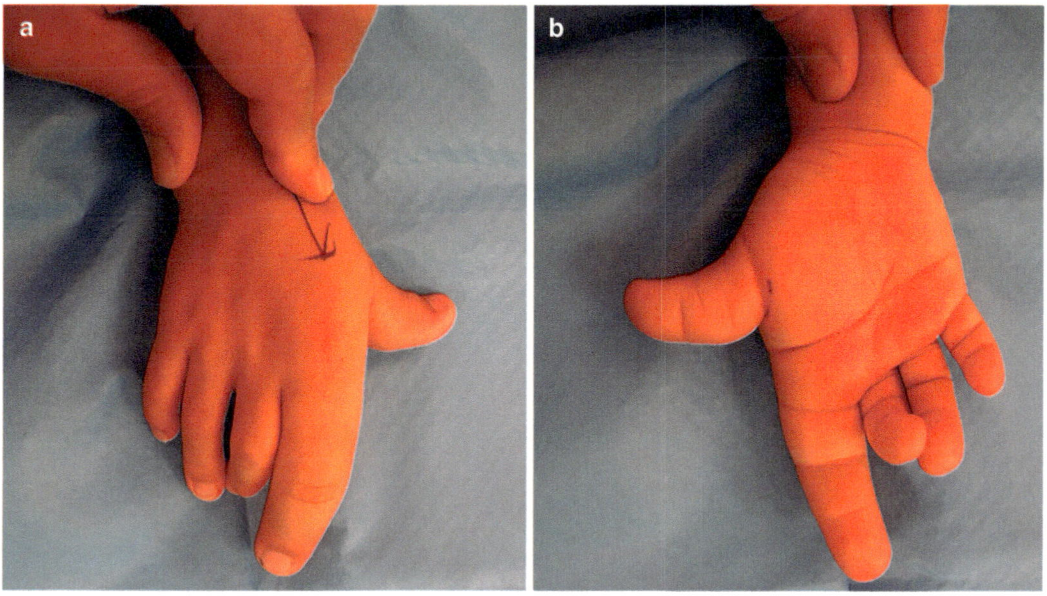

Fig. 23.3 (**a**, **b**) Macrodactyly involving the thumb and index fingers. Note the thumb hyperextension which is due to disproportionate palmar overgrowth

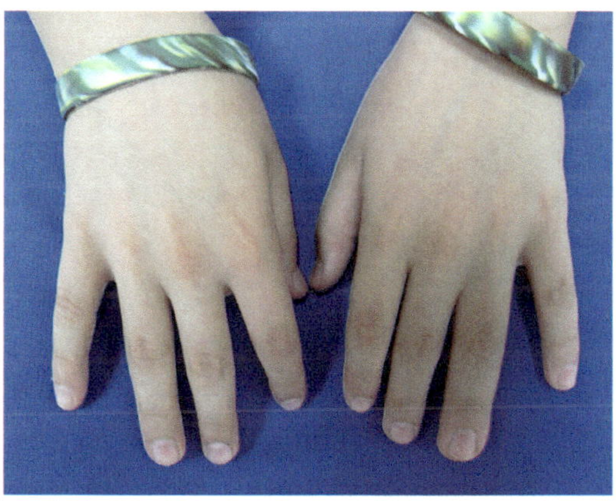

Fig. 23.4 Minimal enlargement of the ring finger with a normal thumb and index finger, defying the "nerve territory" concept

well. All soft and bony tissues of the digit are involved. The osseous structures enlarge and joints become stiff and hyperostotic. This enlargement needs not be limited to the digit, as proximal involvement of the hand and median nerve in the carpal tunnel is often seen. Nerve histology has been termed a lipofibromatous hamartoma, descriptive of fatty and fibrous enlargement, surrounding dispersed but otherwise functioning nerve fascicles. Enlargement of the nerve in the carpal canal may cause a compressive neuropathy (Fig. 23.5).

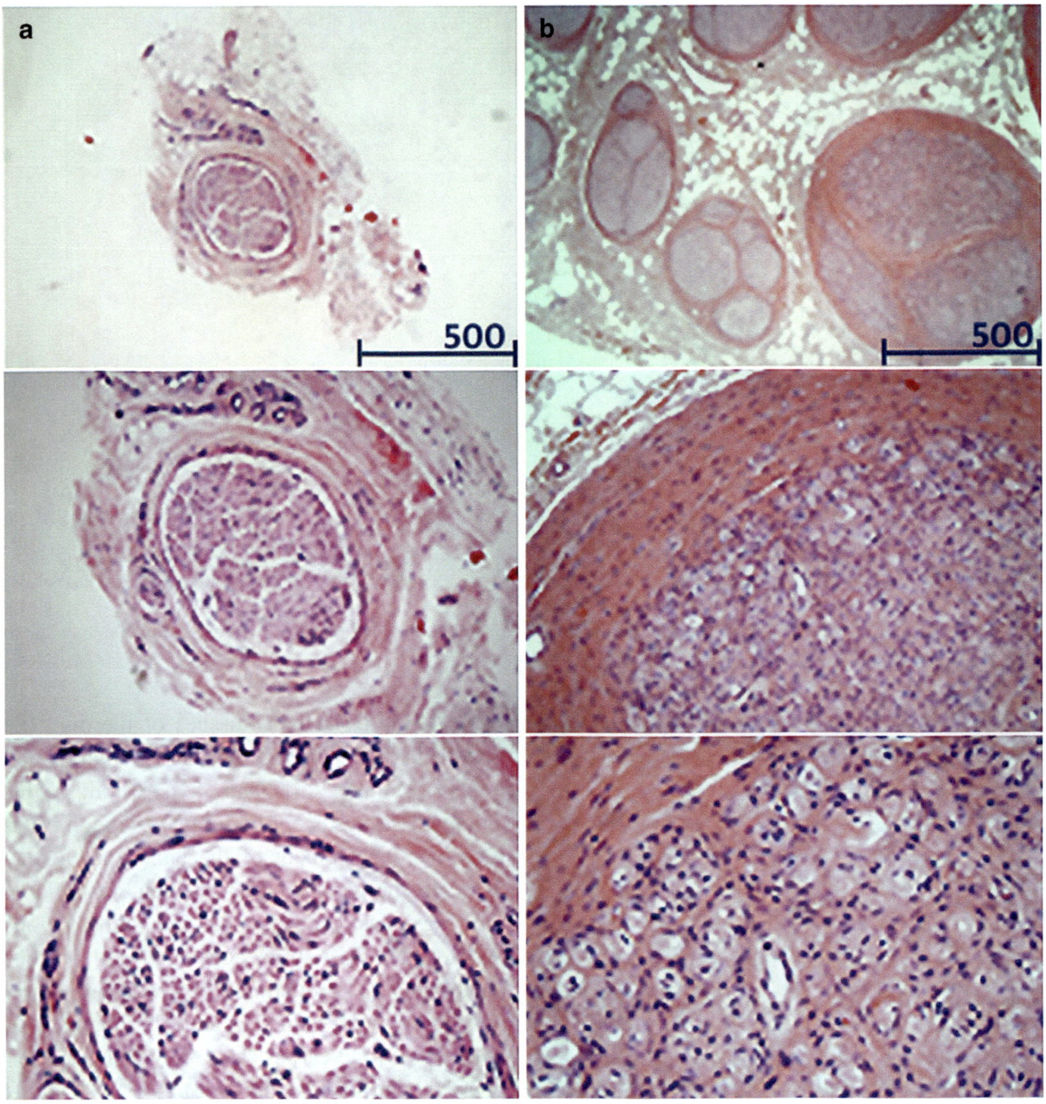

Fig. 23.5 Nerve histology in hematoxylin and eosin stain. (**a**) Normal nerve. (**b**) Macrodactyly nerve

23.3 Evaluation

Because of the disparity in digit/limb size, these patients are often seen at an early age [3, 4]. A thorough examination is mandatory to assess overall limb size as well as other findings possibly associated with PROS. It is especially important to identify those patients who have the macrodactyly associated with overall limb enlargement (macrodystrophic lipomatosis) (Fig. 23.6) as rapid growth may occur in the digits/limb and earlier surgical and/or medical intervention may be required. Macrodactyly can also be part of lymphatic overgrowth, so evaluation for vascular anomalies is also warranted. The macrodactylus digits are usually, and will be, stiff

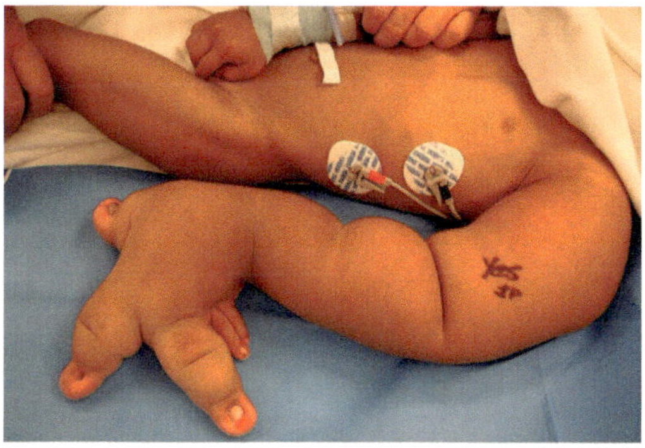

Fig. 23.6 Macrodystrophic lipomatosis. Note the entire limb enlargement with normal appearing ring and little fingers

and lacking full flexion. All physical findings should be pointed out to the parents to help inform their long-term expectations for the limb.

In patients who have growth proportionate to overall growth of the child, observation is warranted until the digits become the size of the parent of the same sex. Some digits may never need surgical intervention to slow growth (Fig. 23.7).

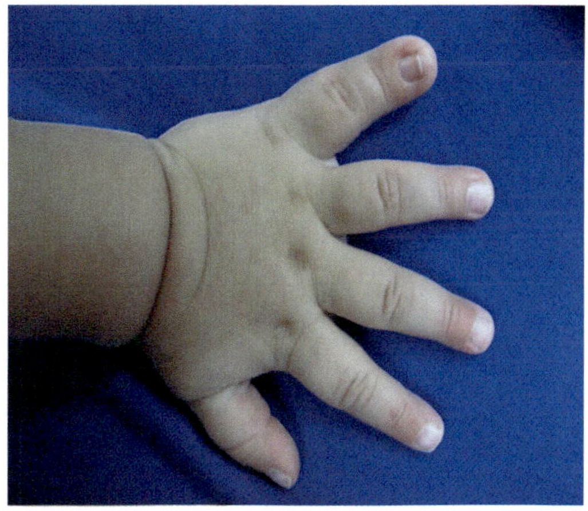

Fig. 23.7 Macrodactyly of the little finger that likely will never need surgical intervention to slow growth

Rapidly enlarging digits may develop angulation due to asymmetric growth plate involvement. In these instances, epiphysiodesis, corrective osteotomy, and debulking procedures are warranted (Fig. 23.8). A good algorithm for this strategy is outlined in a paper by Gluck and Ezaki (Fig. 23.9).

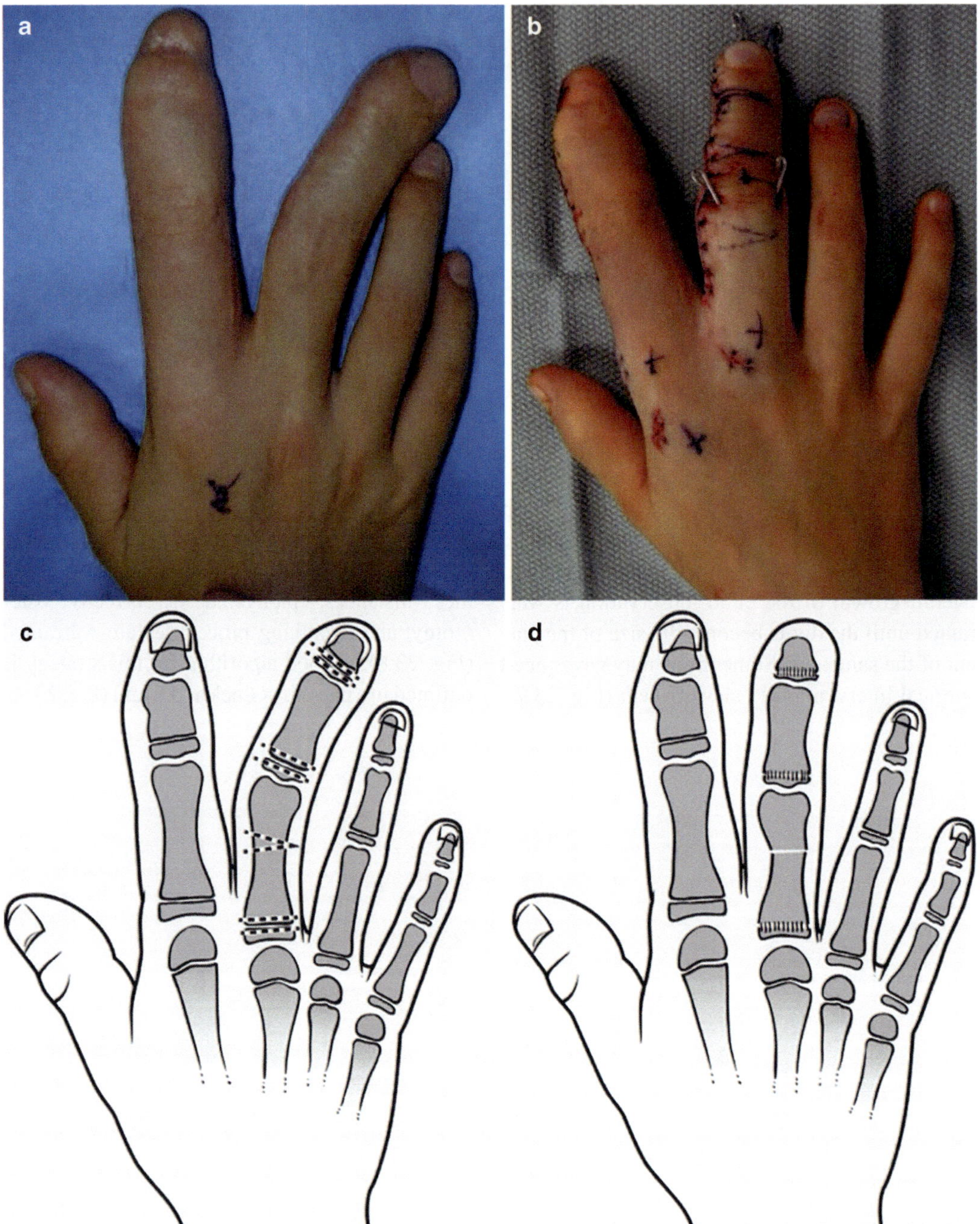

Fig. 23.8 Middle finger with angular deformity. (**a**, **b**) Before and after epiphysiodeses and shaft osteotomy. K-wires are used to maintain alignment until healing is complete. (**c**, **d**) The illustration portrays the cuts made at each level. "x" marks sites of planned epiphysiodeses [5]

23.4 Treatment

Treatment must be individualized to each patient. In patients who have rapidly enlarging digits or the macrodystrophic lipomatosis variety, referral to a hematologist may be warranted for possible institution of an mTOR blocker such as rapamycin [6]. Because of possible associated side effects and unknown long-term sequelae, routine use of rapamycin in all macrodactyly patients is not recommended.

Wound healing and scar formation are also affected by the mutated genetic pathway, and parents should be informed of possible problems before surgery. Meticulous wound care is especially important in these patients.

In most cases, surgery is undertaken when the child's digit reaches the size of the same sex parents. Surgery usually entails soft tissue debulking, physeal arrest, and osteotomy if significant angulation is present (Figs. 23.10 and 23.11). Digital vessels are typically thin, atretic, and often not well seen. Only one side of the finger should be debulked in this manner because of the risk of devascularizing the digit. A technical tip demonstrated in Fig. 23.10 is the placement of marker "darts" at the interphalangeal joint levels. This detail will help in aligning flaps during

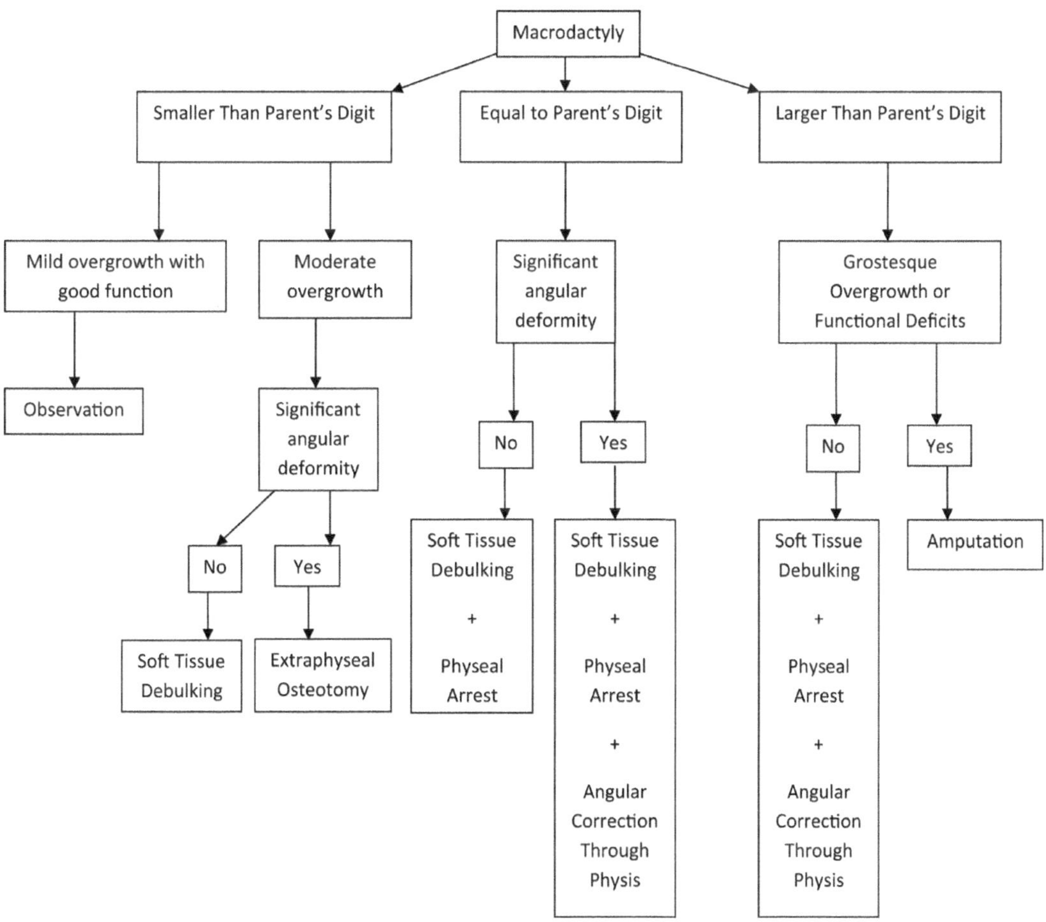

Fig. 23.9 Algorithm for intervention of macrodactyly [5]

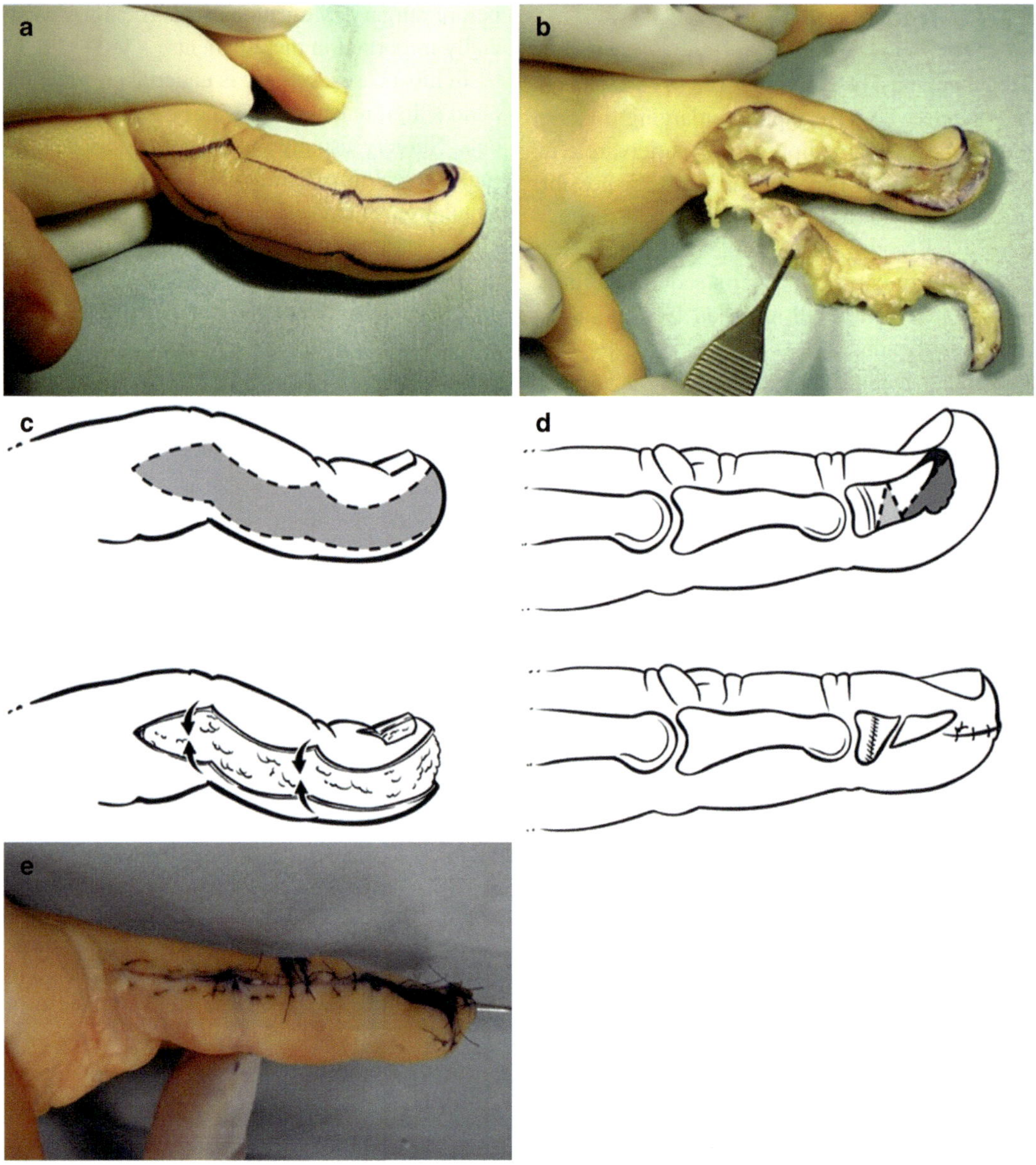

Fig. 23.10 (**a**) Planned soft tissue incision. (**b**) Soft tissue excised along with neurovascular bundle. (**c**) Illustration of how the soft tissue incision should come together. (**d**) Flexion osteotomy is used to correct hyperextension of the distal phalanx, and tuft excision narrows the dorso-palmar thickness of the fingertip. (**e**) End result of debulking and sagittal plan correction with K-wire in place [5]

wound closure and ensuring that the longitudinal scars remain dorsal to the mid-axial line. Excision of the distal portion of the nail plate and sterile matrix is also an option.

The parents should have clear understanding that these digits will never have the appearance of the unaffected contralateral digit, that they will be stiff, and that they may need multiple surgeries throughout life.

Figure 23.12 shows a typical patient with macrodactyly of the index and middle fingers. Note involvement of all the structures with significant angulation. As stated above, debulking on only one side of the finger is performed with

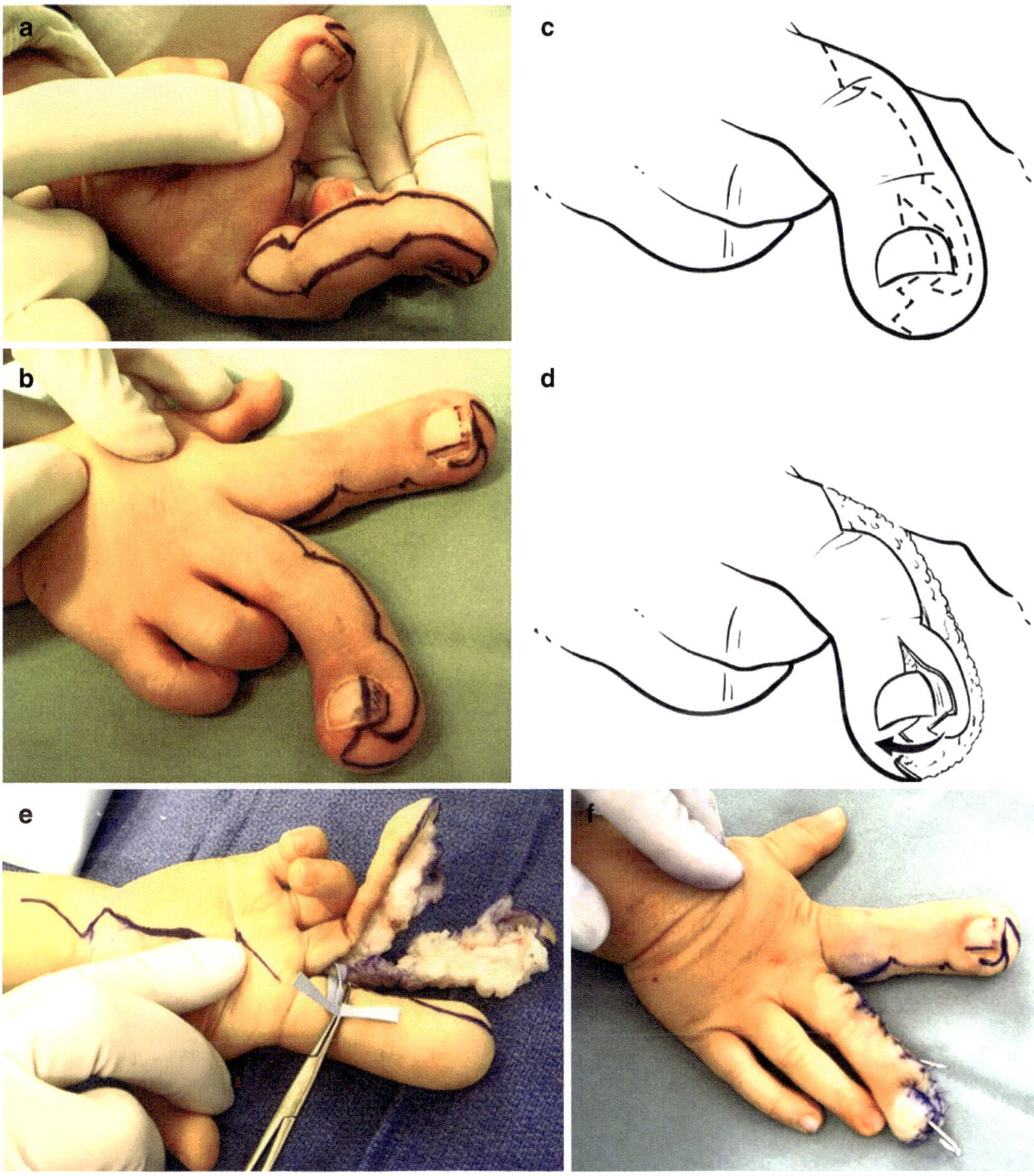

Fig. 23.11 (**a**, **b**) Incision planning for debulking and coronal plan correction of middle finger with planned incision illustration. (**c**) Nail plate to be excised. (**d**) Rotation of the soft tissue to create new perionychial fold. (**e**) Extensive debulking grossly overgrown digits. (**f**) Postoperative image after debulking and angular correction with pinning [5]

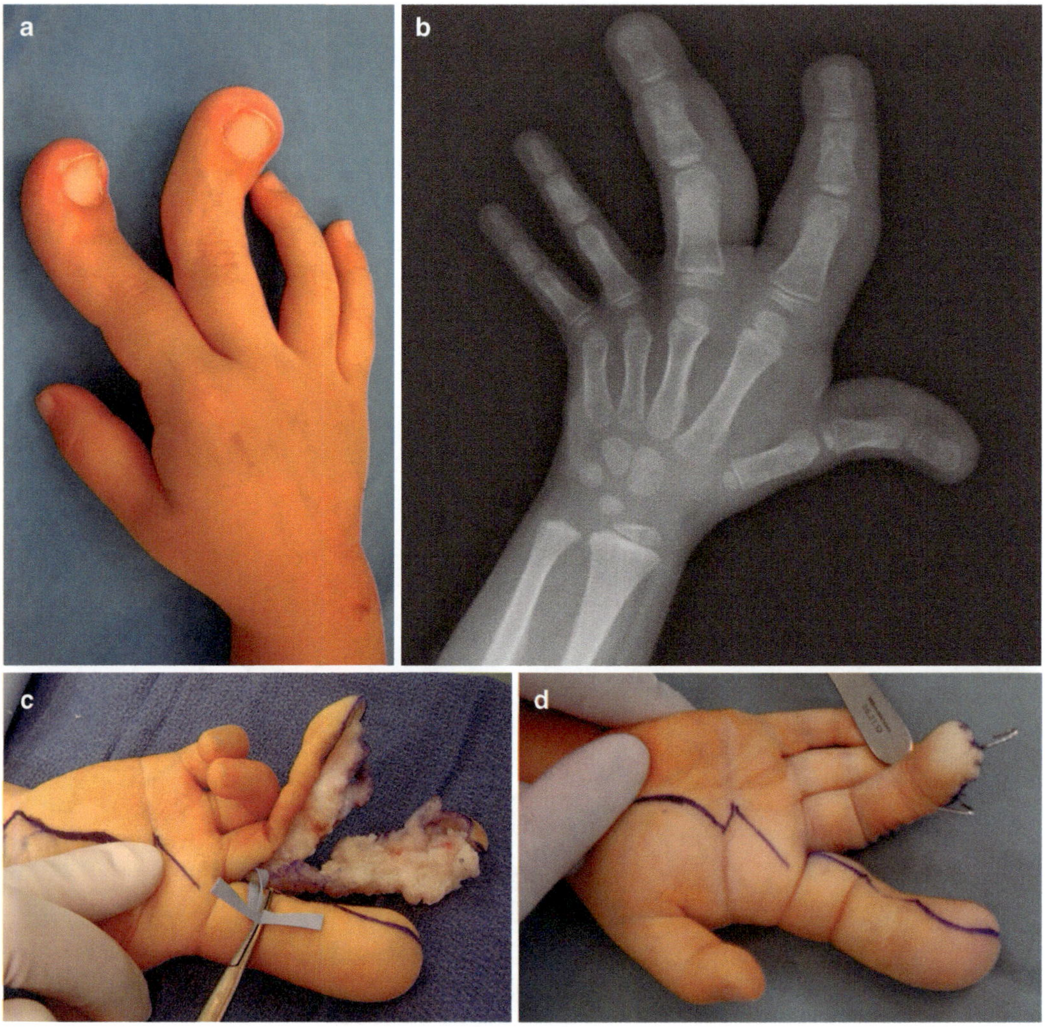

Fig. 23.12 (**a**, **b**) Clinical photograph and radiograph showing the large fingers with marked angulation. (**c**) The debulking procedure. Note the large digital nerve around the blue rubber band. (**d**) The appearance of the middle finger after debulking with markings for the debulking of the index finger. Note that the extension extends to the carpal tunnel to allow debulking in the hand and carpal tunnel release

excision of associated large digital nerve and the overlying skin supplied by that nerve. Despite removal of the nerve, these patients usually retain good sensation to the tip of the finger. Physeal closure was performed at the same setting as the fingers had achieved the length of the same sex parents. In addition, because of involvement of the hand and median nerve, the incision was extended proximally to the carpal tunnel to allow hand debulking and carpal tunnel release.

Because of the generalized overgrowth and stiffness present, amputation is a good option in some cases. This is especially true in situations where the large digits are syndactylized (Fig. 23.13).

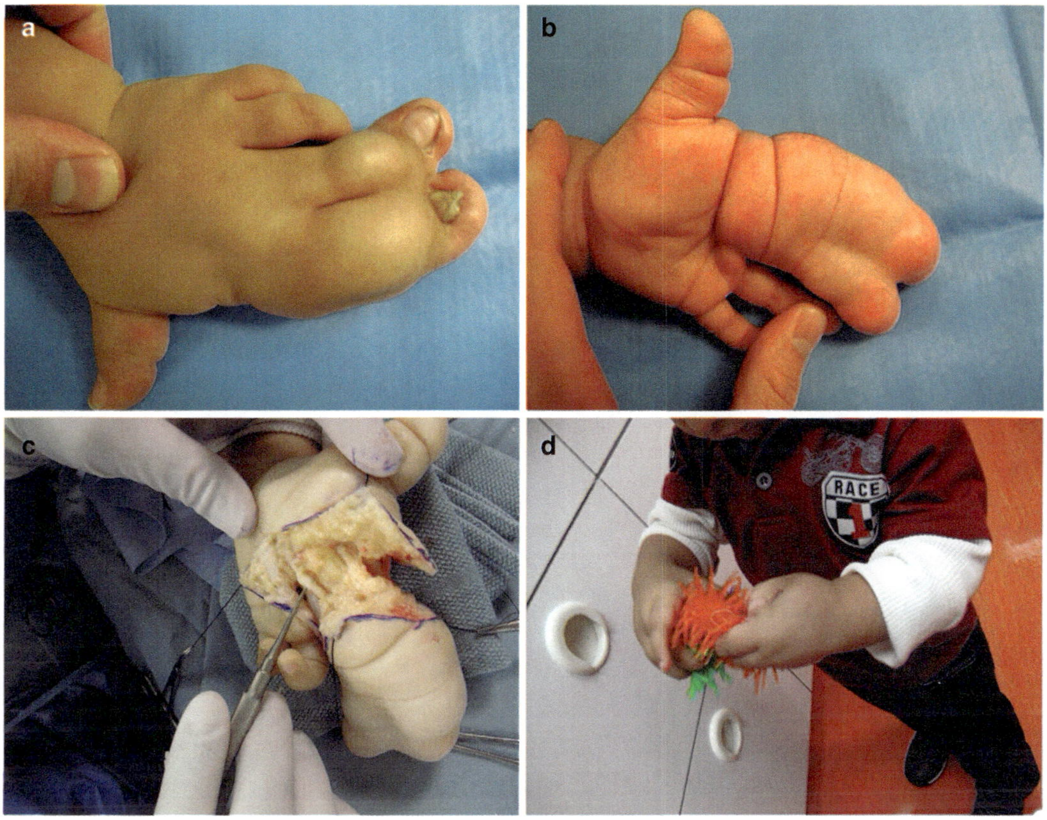

Fig. 23.13 (**a**, **b**) Syndactyly of macrodactylus digits. (**c**) Note the large digital nerves present in these digits. (**d**) Good function noted after primary ray amputation of the index and middle fingers

Even if successful syndactyly reconstruction is performed, patients will bypass the two stiff, large digits and grasp between the thumb and ring/little fingers. Long-term primary amputation is a much better option.

A patient may present with an index finger macrodactyly in which the finger is very stiff with very little motion or have a nonfunctional finger after attempted debulking, as shown in Fig. 23.14. Because the finger is very large and stiff, the child will bypass it. Ray amputation is an excellent option in these cases and can improve overall hand function.

In cases where the thumb is extremely large without much function, it would be tempting to perform a microvascular toe to thumb transfer. The issue has always been whether the transplanted digit would eventually be affected with the same overgrowth. Recently, there have been several isolated case reports describing successful transfer without enlargement, but certainly long-term follow-up is required before recommending this as standard treatment [7].

Macrodactyly patients need to be observed closely for carpal tunnel syndrome since a lipofibromatous hamartomas of the median nerve is frequently present (Fig. 23.15) [8].

Because this is present at a very young age, it is doubtful that complaints of paresthesias will be voiced and waiting until the presence of fingertip dryness or thenar wasting is not indicated.

Clinical manifestations may be frequent biting of the fingers or shaking the hands. Carpal tunnel release should be done through generous incisions that will provide coverage of the released nerve. Step-cutting of the transverse carpal liga-

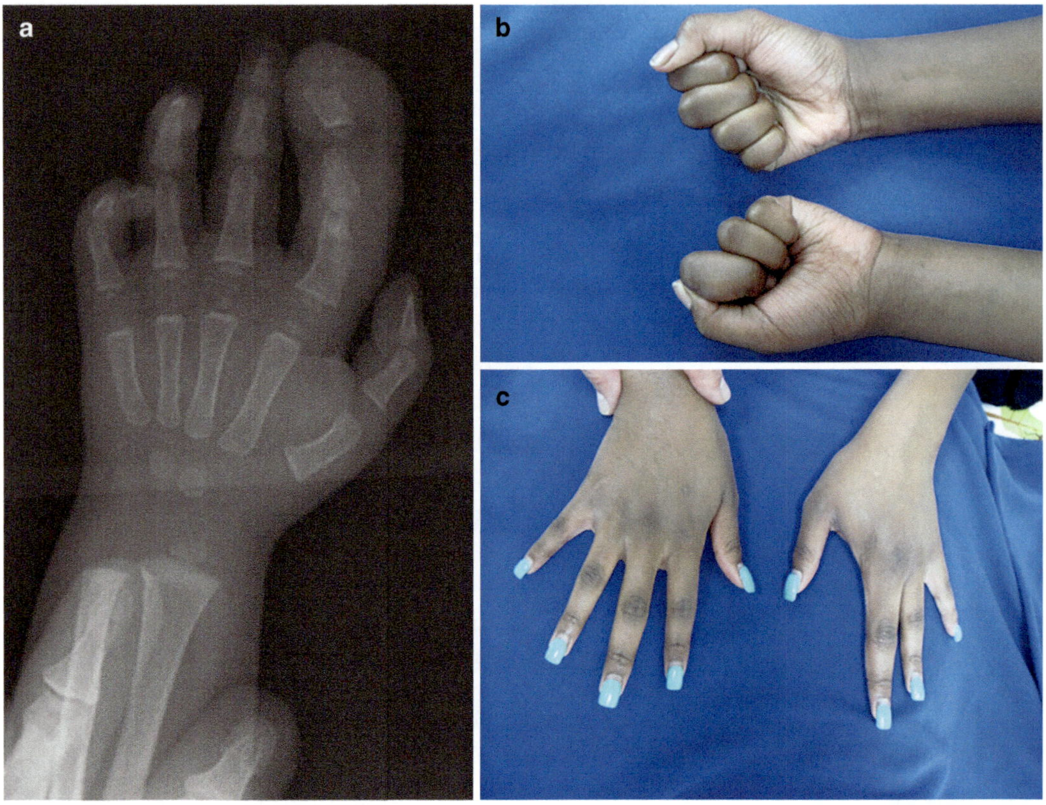

Fig. 23.14 (**a**) Large stiff macrodactylus index finger at 14 months of age. (**b**, **c**) Result after ray amputation of the index finger

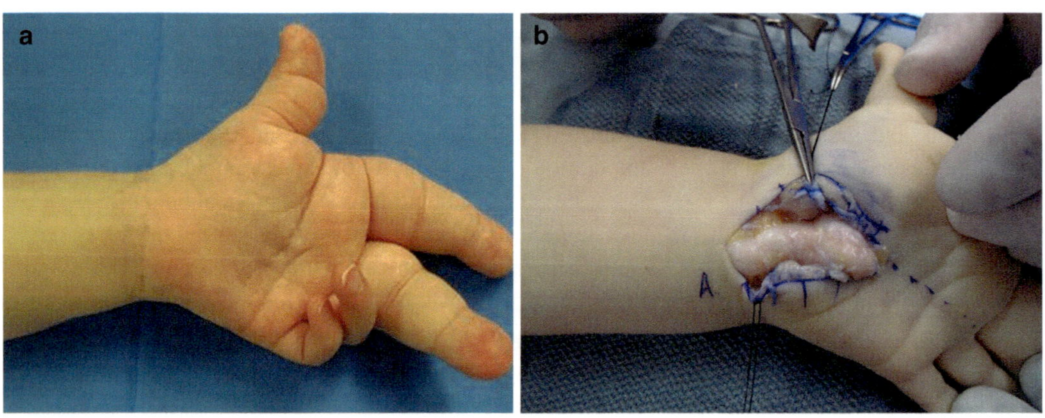

Fig. 23.15 (**a**, **b**) Patient with macrodactyly involving the median distribution of the hand. Note the large lipofibromatous hamartoma of the median nerve

ment to facilitate a loose repair will help prevent prolapse of the enlarge nerve. It is tempting to either debulk or shorten the nerve, but this should not be done, nor should a biopsy be taken, as these manipulations are not helpful and may result in difficult pain issues.

23.5 Conclusion

While macrodactyly can be associated with syndromes such as neurofibromatosis and Ollier and Klippel-Trenaunay syndromes, many cases are postzygotic mutations involving upregulation of PIK3CA and can be components of PROS. Close monitoring of these patients is warranted as rapid growth can be seen at an early age, with this subset of patients being candidates for mTOR inhibitor treatment. Surgical intervention is warranted in some patients, but stiff fingers will be expected despite aggressive debulking procedures. The goal for these patients is to achieve the most aesthetically pleasing finger(s) with minimal morbidity and good overall hand function. Parents must be counseled about realistic goals and expectations early on to assist them in making reasonable decisions for their child.

References

1. Rios JJ, Paria N, Burns DK, Israel BA, Cornelia R, Wise CA, et al. Somatic gain-of-function mutations in PIK3CA in patients with macrodactyly. Hum Mol Genet. 2013;22(3):444–51. Epub 2012/10/27.
2. Keppler-Noreuil KM, Rios JJ, Parker VE, Semple RK, Lindhurst MJ, Sapp JC, et al. PIK3CA-related overgrowth spectrum (PROS): diagnostic and testing eligibility criteria, differential diagnosis, and evaluation. Am J Med Genet A. 2015;167A(2):287–95. Epub 2015/01/06.
3. Ben-Bassat M, Casper J, Kaplan I, Laron Z. Congenital macrodactyly. A case report with a three-year follow-up. J Bone Joint Surg Br. 1966;48(2):359–64. Epub 1966/05/01.
4. Hardwicke J, Khan MA, Richards H, Warner RM, Lester R. Macrodactyly - options and outcomes. J Hand Surg Eur Vol. 2013;38(3):297–303. Epub 2012/06/28.
5. Gluck JS, Ezaki M. Surgical treatment of macrodactyly. J Hand Surg. 2015;40(7):1461–8. Epub 2015/06/08.
6. Li J, Kim SG, Blenis J. Rapamycin: one drug, many effects. Cell Metab. 2014;19(3):373–9. Epub 2014/02/11.
7. Cavadas PC, Thione A. Treatment of hand macrodactyly with resection and toe transfers. J Hand Surg. 2018;43(4):388.e1–6. Epub 2017/09/21.
8. Amadio PC, Reiman HM, Dobyns JH. Lipofibromatous hamartoma of nerve. J Hand Surg. 1988;13(1):67–75. Epub 1988/01/01.

Palliative Surgery in Obstetrical Brachial Plexus Palsy

24

Filippo M. Senes, Nunzio Catena, and Chiara Arrigoni

Abstract

The chance of recovering functional defects of obstetrical palsy through nerve surgical procedures has not reduced the role of palliative or secondary surgery, also called "functional surgery." Although nerve injury at birth is not a progressive lesion, growth changes of the upper limb and skeletal adaptations can significantly influence recovery, especially during adolescence, when body size changes and creates an imbalance that can impair already achieved functions. In particular, skeletal deformities can decrease joint range of motion as much as muscle imbalance due to nerve palsy. Secondary surgery would aim to achieve some essential functions of the upper limb (a satisfactory shoulder motion in external and internal rotation, a significant active flexion-extension of the elbow, good wrist control, and an opposable thumb with adequate hand grasp). Depending on patient's age, there are definite steps to perform surgery. In the article, indications to correct deformities induced by sequelae of obstetrical palsy of the upper arm are reported.

Keywords

Obstetrical brachial plexus palsy · Brachial plexus palsy sequelae · Shoulder motion limitation · Elbow motion limitation

24.1 Introduction

The chances of recovering from functional defects of obstetrical brachial plexus palsy (OBPP) through both early and late nerve repair have not reduced the importance of palliative or secondary surgery, also defined as functional surgery. It is well known that a severe functional impairment stems from the primary nerve lesion. Nerve palsy is consistently followed by muscular palsy and imbalance, both altering bone growth and triggering joint incongruence. Although nerve injury at birth is not a progressive lesion, growth changes of the upper limb and subsequent skeletal adaptations can significantly influence the recovery, especially during adolescence, when body size grows fast and creates an imbalance that impairs already achieved functions. In particular, skeletal deformities contribute to

F. M. Senes (✉)
Department of Hand Surgery and Rehabilitation, San Giuseppe Multimedica Hospital, Milan University, Milano, Italy
e-mail: filipposenes@fastwebnet.it

N. Catena
UOSD Microchirurgia Ricostruttiva e Chirurgia della Mano, IRCCS Istituto Giannina Gaslini, Genova, Italy

C. Arrigoni
Scuola di Specializzazione in Ortopedia e Traumatologia, Università degli Studi di Torino, Torino, Italy

G. Pajardi (ed.), *Pediatric Hand Surgery*, https://doi.org/10.1007/978-3-031-30984-7_24

decrease joint range of motion as much as the muscle imbalance due to nerve palsy [1].

A basic distinction between patients suffering from upper root involvement and those with partially recovered complete plexus involvement is mandatory: the weak muscle strength and reduced hand sensation indeed significantly impair the outcome of this latter group, even for shoulder function.

The success of palliative surgery depends on the extension of the palsy, which affects single segments of the upper arm. Multilevel malfunctioning of the upper arm, due to different root involvements, influences the outcome and worsens the motion of the upper arm. Indications for surgery mainly concern upper limb defects due to upper and intermediate lesions of the brachial plexus, whereas total involvement of the brachial plexus often discourages palliative surgery or reduces options for treatment.

Moreover, dealing with obstetrical brachial plexus palsy, we face a complex nerve lesion, totally different from peripheral nerve lesions in which there are sufficient muscular groups to compensate for defects. This is particularly true for upper arm distal defects, when the palsy involves several areas of the forearm and hand.

Secondary surgery should aim to achieve some basic functions, namely, a satisfactory shoulder motion in external and internal rotation, a significant active elbow function allowing flexion and extension movements, good wrist control, and an opposable thumb with adequate hand grasp. Nevertheless, hand motion recovery might be less predictable, because it is strongly influenced by the lack of sensation. Unfortunately, these conditions are difficult to achieve as a whole, particularly when hand involvement is so severe as to impair every surgical effort.

According to patients' age, there are definite steps to perform surgery.

Some surgical procedures in precise moments of growth are suitable for correcting deformities, whereas the same procedures performed in an inappropriate period might be ineffective or could even damage the child. Surgeons must be aware of this basic point and consider it before operating on patients.

Regarding surgical approaches, it is very important to avoid trying to reach an idealistic function of the limb, if this could determine a decrease of motion in others, particularly when advantages might be minimal.

From this standpoint, the therapeutic approach should aim to correct deformities and maximally increase the recovery. The final goal is not complete elimination of defects but the achievement of the highest degree of recovery.

24.2 Clinical Features and Therapeutic Options

Based on our experience and the literature, we would like to describe the chances of improving the upper arm motion through surgical procedures, keeping in mind the age of the child. Although some functional limitations are easily detected, multiple involvements of musculoskeletal areas have to be considered, especially because deformities influence each other.

Since the shoulder and elbow are more commonly involved by OBBP, we will describe in detail both districts that are more suitable for surgical procedures. However, some considerations about distal segments wil be reported at the end of the chapter.

24.2.1 Shoulder

In the natural history of neonatal brachial plexus palsy, the shoulder is constantly involved because of the injury of C5–C6 roots, which mainly results in a lack of abduction and external rotation. The characteristic aspect of the shoulder in the internal rotation is mainly due to muscular imbalance caused by nerve palsy; however, joint stiffness very often occurs in the first months after birth, futher impairing motion. Shoulder stiffness stems from subscapularis muscle contraction, which is very frequent, and from joint cuff and anterior soft tissue retraction; both conditions modify the shape of humeral epiphysis because of compressive forces and cause early loss of congruence of the humeral head that tends to flatten when in contact with the hypoplastic glenoid cavity [2]. Scapular winging is a typical feature due to the lack of congruence of the scapulothoracic girdle (Fig. 24.1). This deformity can be detected either for internal or external limitation of shoulder motion, often occurring in some planes of motion; it depends on flattening of the epiphyseal humeral head and misalignment of the glenoid cavity. Patients and their families often complain about the aberrant motion of the shoulder blade, rather than for limitation of motion [3].

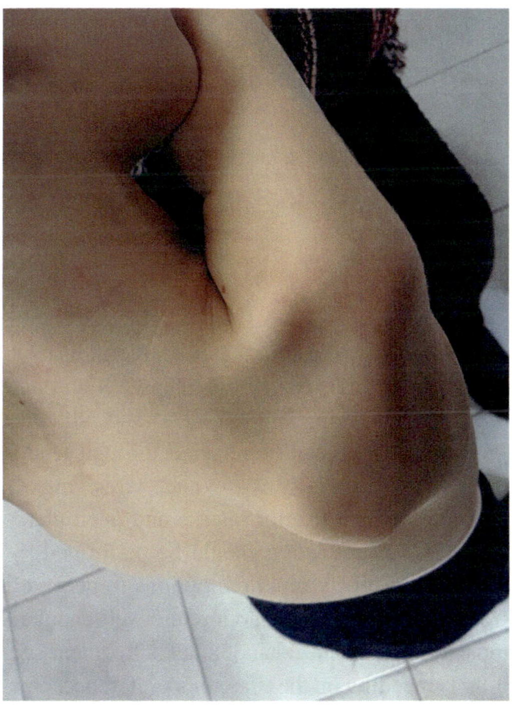

Fig. 24.1 Scapular winging: the scapular blade rotates along with the humeral head during the internal rotation and adduction of the arm showing an evident detachment of the scapula from the dorsi

An internally rotated shoulder with limited or no abduction, scapular winging, minimal or absent retroposition, and limited internal adduction toward the midline are constant features in children suffering from upper-intermediate OBPP sequelae. These patterns vary according to growth changes that occurre in some patients, namely, hypoplastic growth of the scapulohumeral girdle and upper arm involvement as a whole, particularly in the elbow.

In the early 1970s, Mallet assessed shoulder deformities by drawings of simple gestures scoring different degrees of disability (Fig. 24.2).

Later on, Gilbert and Raimondi described an improved classification through a detailed description of shoulder limitations, aiming at the detection of surgical indications. Over the years, other assessment methods have been presented with similar purposes [4, 5].

Indications for treatment might differ according to the severity of shoulder impairment that can address physical therapy alone or surgical procedures.

At anearly age, Physical therapy is the first therapeutic approach, particularly in shoulder motion recovery.

The aim of this chapter is not to discuss physical therapy in detail; however, some indications must be highlighted such as reduction of muscular imbalance, muscle strength renforcement, and joint motion increase.

Although physical therapy should be continued during growth, even including some sports, some clinical features of OBPP sequelae cannot be treated by physical therapy alone, and very often surgery is needed.

Swimming has been advocated for ages as the best solution, but in some conditions as posterior dislocation of the shoulder, it might worsen shoulder dislocation.

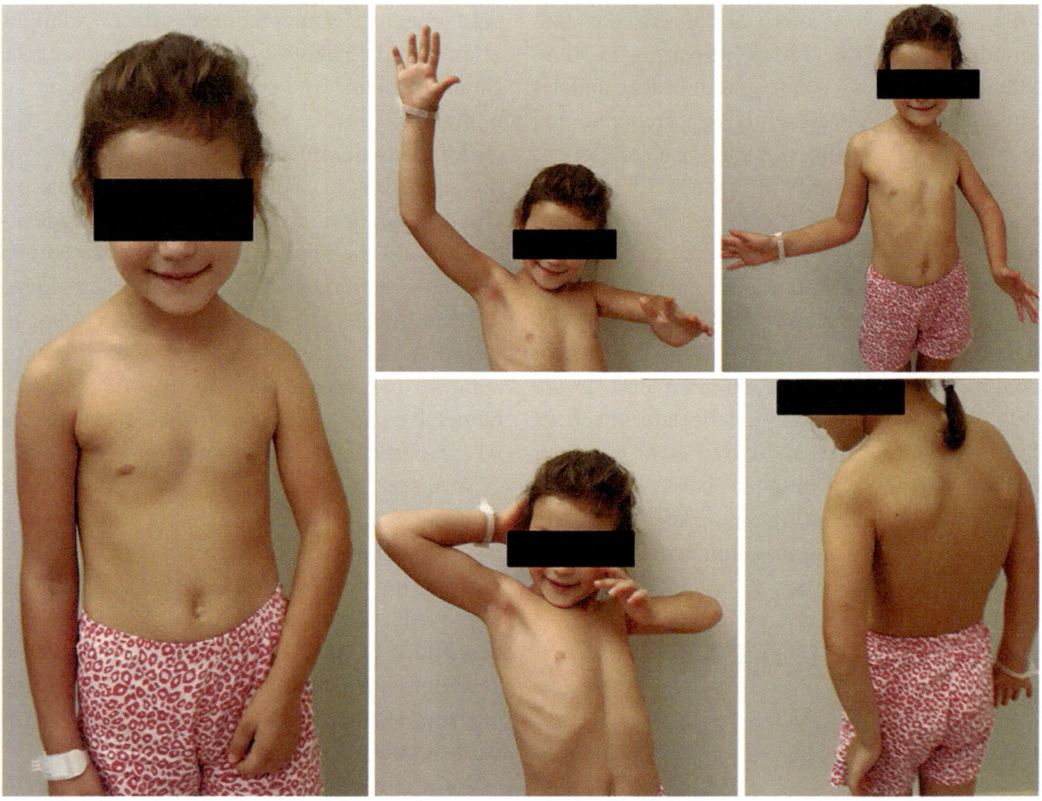

Fig. 24.2 According to Mallet's classification, clinical assessment of the shoulder can be explored with simple gestures to evaluate joint motion

24.2.1.1 Limited External Rotation

Apart from primary nerve surgery during the first months of life, which represents the best option for OBPP without prognostic signs of recovery, from one to two years of age, limitation of external rotation of the shoulder can be treated through nerve transfers. When there is a free passive shoulder motion regardless a complete lack of active external rotation, isolated transfer of accessory spinal nerve onto suprascapular nerve should be performed to reinnervate external rotator muscles. However, very often subscapularis muscle release or coracohumeral ligament section are needed to achieve a free passive motion of the humeral head [6].

Both the procedures act in decompressing the humeral head, favoring a balance among muscular groups to make up for palsied external rotator muscles function [7].

In the event of a lack of external rotation combined with soft tissue retraction and joint instability during the first years of life, many Authors state that a rebalancing of muscles and shoulder joint congruence can be attained through tendon transfers (latissimus dorsi and teres major). Additionally, an anterior release and open glenohumeral joint reduction should be performed [8–11]. As previously reported, options to achieve a free shoulder passive motion are subscapularis muscle release and coracohumeral ligament section. Depending on the surgeon's preference, anterior release of shoulder joint can be carried out by either an open or arthroscopic technique [12].

From two to four years of age, subscapularis muscle sliding or coracohumeral ligament release might be similarly performed to avoid asymmetrical forces acting on the mostly cartilaginous humeral head, preventing loss of head sphericity.

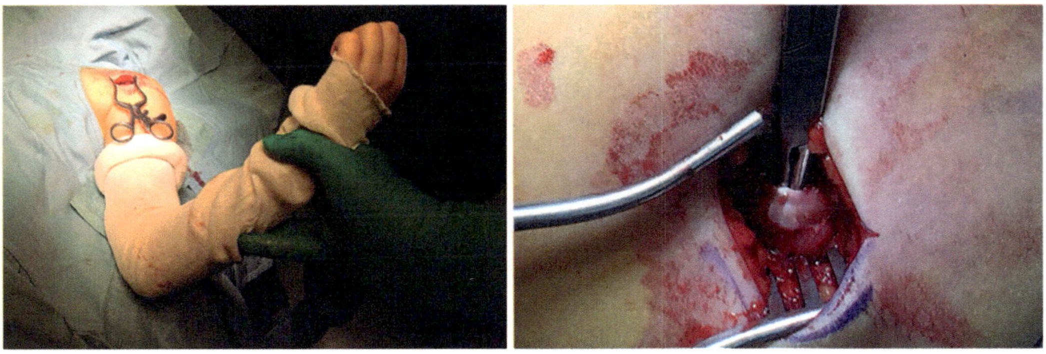

Fig. 24.3 Coracohumeral ligament is exposed before resection. Ligament resection allows the shoulder joint to achieve an increased external rotation

Unfortunately, subscapularis muscle release fails in about 50% of cases [13].

Although few reports have been published about a comparison of procedures, our impression is that coraco-humeral release seems to be more effective than subscapularis release. According to Gilbert's observations, the latter procedure seems to be inefficient after 4 years of age. In older children, subscapularis muscle release might represent one step of a multistage procedure, but we advise against using it as the first choice treatment at major age. On the other hand, the coraco-humeral release may be performed during the first years of life to obtain room for the motion of the humeral head that is expected to remodel during the residual growth (Fig. 24.3).

Preventive X-ray exploration to identify humeral head deformation is advisable, while at older ages, MRI (magnetic resonance imaging) and CT (computed tomography) scans are mandatory to confirm joint congruence.

Nerve transfer, as described above in very young children, might be a successful solution in addition to shoulder joint release. At any rate, whichever surgery might be used, a period of 3–6 weeks of immobilization in a brace or cast with the shoulder positioned in the abduction and external rotation is needed to allow the transfer (nervous or tendinous) to be stabilized.

From four to ten years of age, lack of active external rotation can be corrected by latissimus dorsi/teres major transfer to the rotatory cuff, as a first choice [8, 14].

In our experience, combined coracohumeral release and latissimus dorsi/teres major transfer can be effective, when residual stiffness of the shoulder is detected (Fig. 24.3).

When bone growth of proximal humeral physis is about to stop, approximately from ten years on, derotational osteotomy and plating at the upper third of humeral shaft in external rotation, performed above pectoralis major insertions, can be helpful to correct the internal rotational defect and compensate the anteposition of the shoulder girdle, additionally making up for cosmetic appearance [15, 16]. Muscle transfers, that is, latissimus dorsi muscle, can be added to reinforce motion (Fig. 24.4).

It is extremely important to perform a mild derotation of the bone stumps avoiding an extensive derotation over 25° to prevent from a loss of motion in internal rotation. Excessive derotation limits the capability to reach the median line of the body with the hand.

During growth, some patients who developed a severe defect of shoulder external rotation show a typical pattern with internal rotation of the shoulder and progressive flexion deformity of the elbow. After humeral derotation procedure, parents must be informed of the risk of losing some degrees of internal rotation because of the achievement of the same amount of degrees in external rotation.

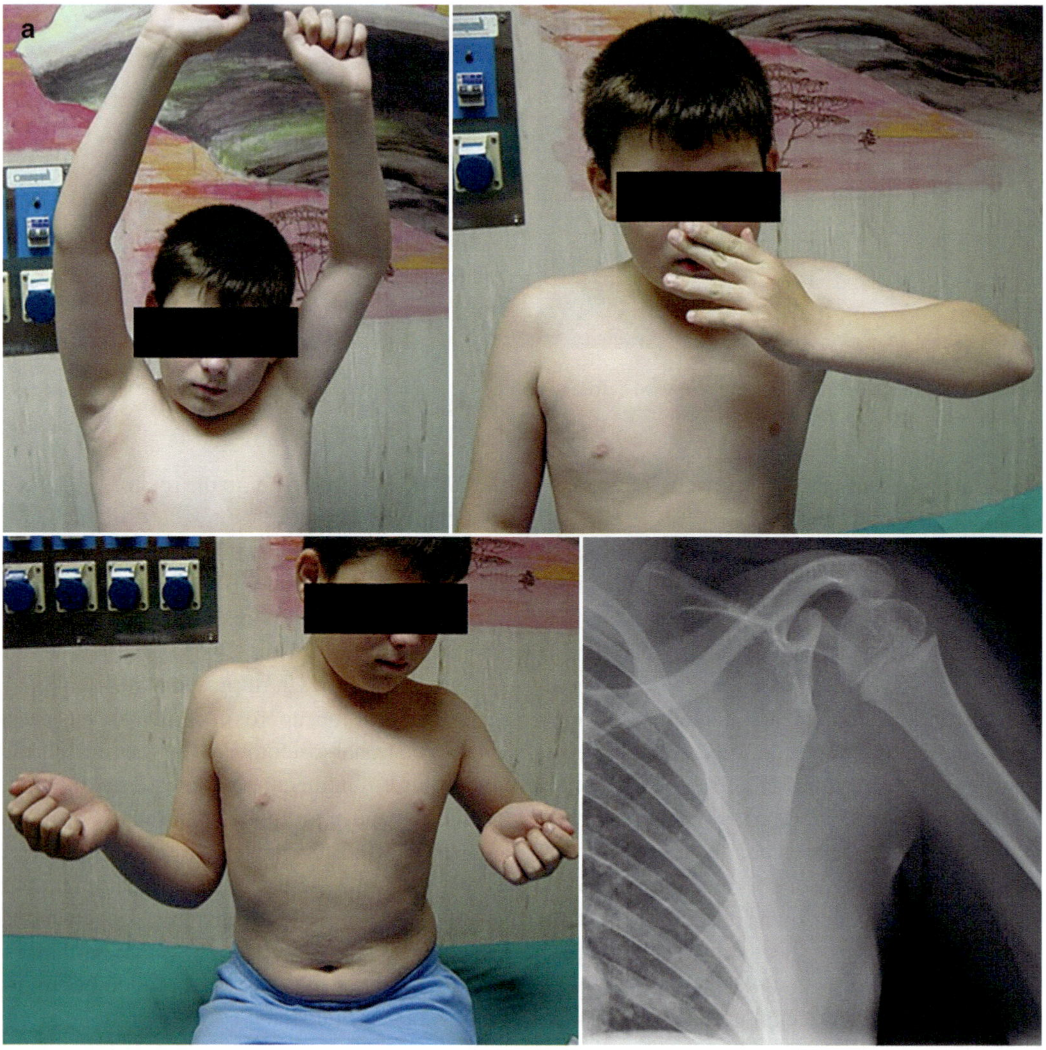

Fig. 24.4 (**a**, **b**) Derotational osteotomy of humeral proximal metaphysis provides a satisfactory improvement of external rotation motion of the shoulder, as is shown in preoperative (**a**) and postoperative images (**b**). X-ray images confirm the deformation of the humeral proximal epiphysis

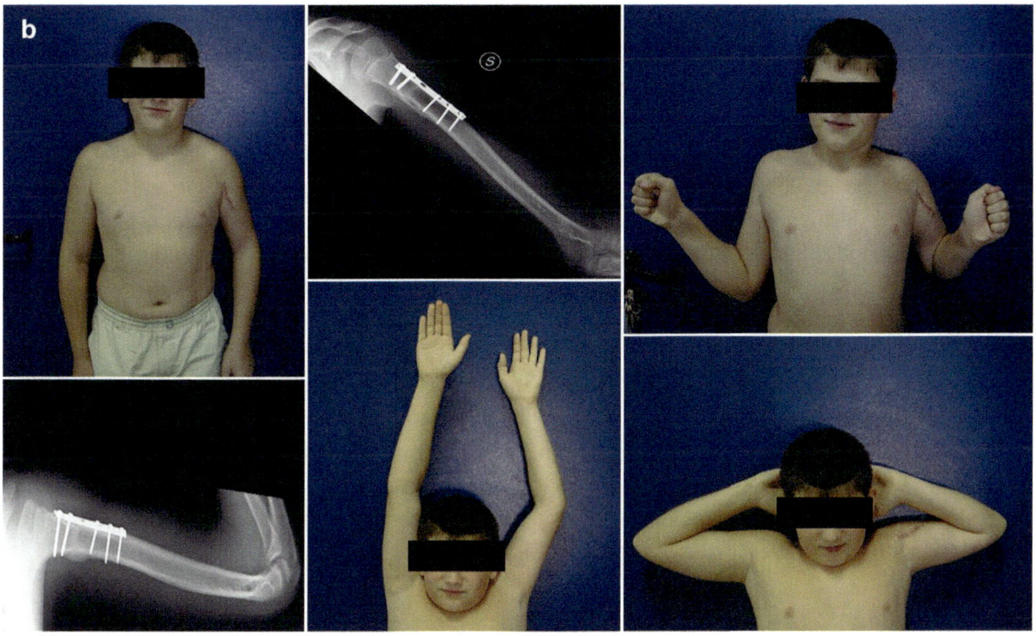

Fig. 24.4 (continued)

24.2.1.2 Limited Abduction

Limited abduction of the shoulder is one of the most common features of OBPP. There are different degrees of disability, so correction is required according to the severity of lesion.

Lack of abduction of the shoulder usually stems from different factors, above all insufficient deltoid muscle strength, but it can also be due to incongruence of the shoulder joint and unbalance of shoulder girdle muscles, particularly for the predominance of internal rotators.

During the first years of life, latissimus dorsi muscle transfer permits to attain a satisfactory external rotation along with a slight increasing of abduction. Inevitably, a loss of this minimal amount of abduction occurs during the following years, but this transfer is helpful for the development of the scapulo-humeral joint, favoring joint congruence and avoiding posterior dislocation of the humeral epiphysis.

Late nerve surgery through transfer of nerve branches of the long head of the triceps muscle to axillary muscle in very young children is a recent proposal which, however, is still debated on the risk of impair a relatively good triceps muscle [17].

In the event of severe lack of abduction, from six to ten years of age, trapezius muscle transferred onto the deltoid insertion can be a good solution, even though only a partial recovery of function is expected. In this procedure, a periosteal strip is elevated and sutured onto the deltoid insertion without skeletal anchorage to avoid progressive tightening of the transferred muscle during further growth. Excessive tension of transferred muscle results in abduction contracture with additional scapulohumeral stiffness. From 10 to 16 years of age, trapezius muscle transfer with olecranon graft fixed into humeral diaphysis is more appropriate.

Trapezius muscle transfer is effective for balancing a weak shoulder, particularly when combined with other muscle transfers, even though a limited amount of abduction is achieved [18–20].

In young adults, shoulder joint fusion is another option to better stabilize the scapulohumeral girdle.

24.2.1.3 Limited Internal Rotation

A typical feature of the defect is the incapability of reaching the median line of the body with the hand. This defect is far more limiting than the lack of external rotation because it has a severe impact on many basic daily functions. It is commonly observed during growth, but it becomes more limiting when other defects of motion are associated (Fig. 24.5).

Generally, the scapulohumeral girdle appears hypoplastic and placed in a forward position with a twisted clavicle. Scapular winging is always present, sometimes extremely evident.

Very often patients present with a lack of both external and internal rotations because of glenohumeral incongruence. Some patients show a paradoxical pattern in forced external rotation of the shoulder with no ability to internally rotate the upper arm.

Before ten years of age, coracoid process resection and subscapularis muscle release to reduce scapular winging might be helpful. Sometimes rhomboid muscle plication can reduce shoulder blade axis rotation.

From ten years of age on, internal derotational osteotomy of the humerus below pectoralis major insertion is a more advisable procedure that allows the patient to improve internal rotation and reach the anterior midline of the body with the hand. Similar to external derotational osteotomy, excessive internal derotation might be dangerous to the risk of losing the opposite function. Pectoralis muscle insertion laterally fixed onto the humeral shaft can help improve the internal rotation.

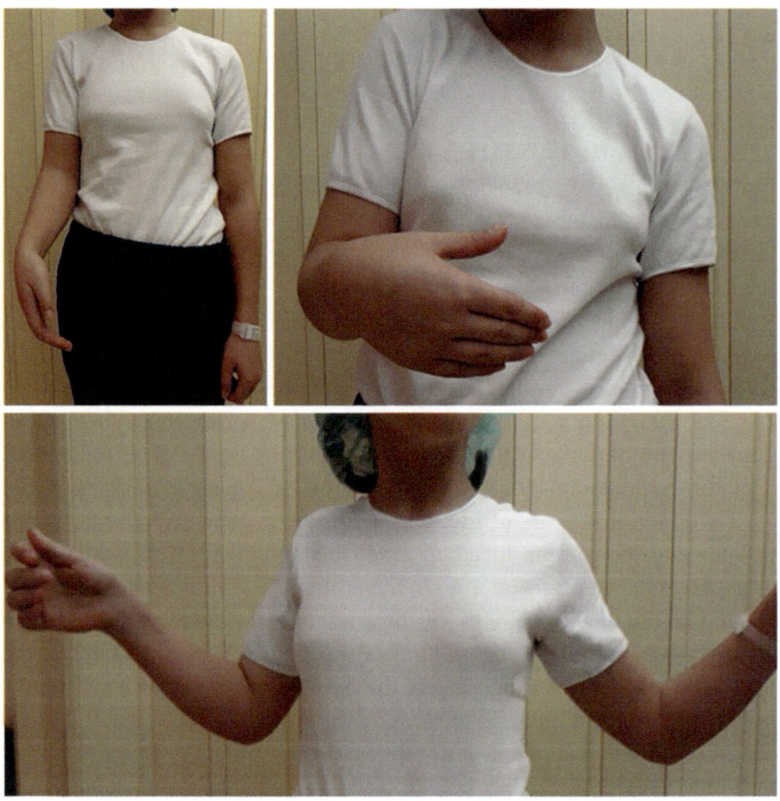

Fig. 24.5 During growth, this child developed a singular pattern in shoulder rotation. Despite a good external rotation, there is an evident lack of internal rotation that limits many basic daily functions

Retroposition is a complex combination of abduction and internal rotation of the shoulder. Retropositional defect is a constant feature of upper palsy that is usually treated through physical therapy, but rarely, it can be restored.

24.2.1.4 Posterior Subluxation

It usually occurs in adolescents with an internal rotational pattern, namely, hypoplastic development of the shoulder, modification of acromion, clavicle, coracoid process, and glenoid cavity [21] (Fig. 24.6).

The defect is due to incongruence between the anomalous shaped humeral head and the glenoid cavity. Hyperlaxity of the joint and muscle palsy trigger backward dislocation of the humeral head (Fig. 24.7).

Derotational osteotomy of the humeral shaft along with coracohumeral ligament release or coracoid resection and posterior capsuloplasty with or without glenoid osteotomy of re-orientation can help correct the instability [22].

These procedures are inconstantly rewarding because of the possible recurrence of deformity.

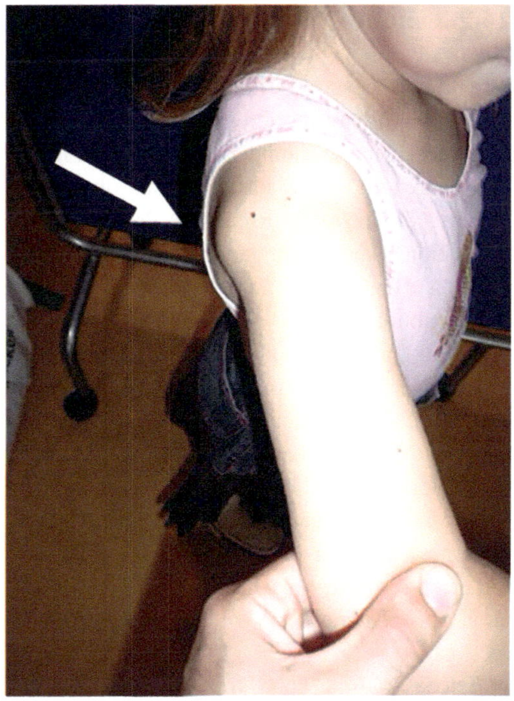

Fig. 24.7 Shoulder clinical evaluation demonstrates a severe posterior dislocation of the humeral head

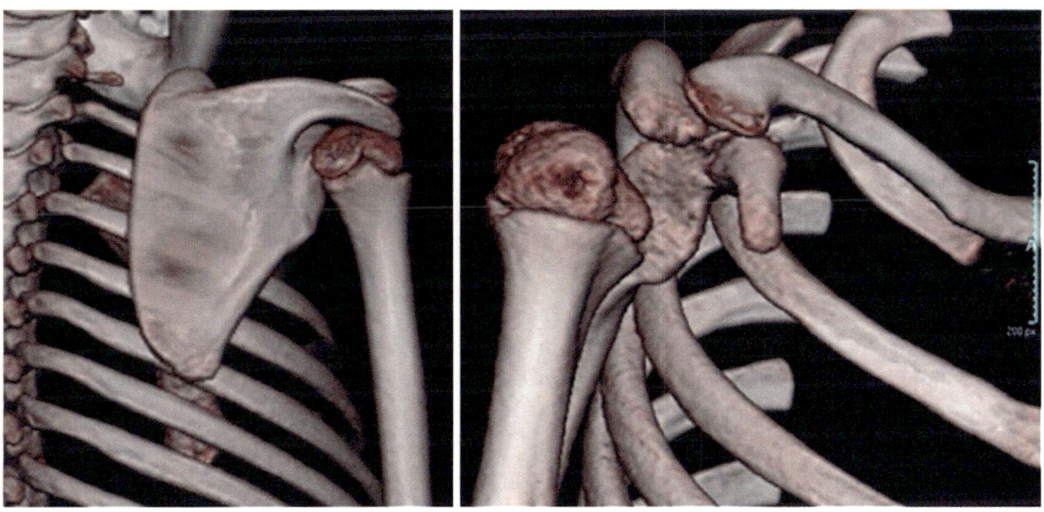

Fig. 24.6 During growth, a large group of patients present with severe skeletal deformities of the shoulder joint. Glenoid fossa dysplasia, coracoid process hypertrophy, and proximal humeral head dislocation significantly impair shoulder motion

24.2.2 Elbow

Impairment of elbow joint motion is another basic point that interferes with the outcome. Different from the shoulder which acts on multiple planes, the elbow has two axes of motion, namely, flexion and extension. Pronation and supination of the forearm are influenced by elbow position even though they do not take part in elbow motion.

Elbow joint morphology is altered by muscle imbalance, forced position of the elbow that causes the joint deformity, loss of perfect congruence, and growth changes due to physeal plate asymmetrical stimulation.

A weak elbow can present with two different patterns. The main important is due to palsy of the biceps muscle which stems from nerve palsy at birth, sometimes with partial strength recovery.

Triceps muscle palsy represents the opposit pattern but the predominance of the biceps muscle paradoxally causes a flexion deformity.

This flexion deformity posture is typical of upper-intermediate palsy in which internal rotation positioning of the shoulder and elbow flexion due to retraction of reinnervated biceps muscle results in a lack of elbow extension.

Elbow deformities are commonly assessed by the Raimondi and Gilbert's classification, which scores the severity of elbow limitation in degrees of flexion or extension.

24.2.2.1 Lack of Active Elbow Flexion

Lack of active elbow flexion is a typical feature in the majority of children presenting with OBPP in the first months of life, even though it tends to decrease during the first year of life. Its persistence is a typical feature of severe forms of neonatal palsy; currently, these patients are usually enrolled as candidates for early nerve surgery. However, older children lacking elbow flexion might be observed later in life, or they are exceptionally suffering sequela of unsuccessful brachial plexus surgery.

Palliative surgery can offer options for correcting the defect, but the number of procedures is limited.

Recent publications about nerve transfers in adults have shown the options to apply the same procedure to the child. Innervation of the biceps and/or brachialis muscle in the first years of life can be successful when proper indications are followed [23]. Active elbow flexion can be obtained through different nerve trunk transfers depending on the level of injury. In the event of a C5–C6 palsy, fascicles of the ulnar nerve assigned to the flexor carpi ulnaris can be transferred onto muscle cutaneous nerve or rather to biceps or brachialis muscle branches to achieve active elbow flexion. When there is C7 involvement or in the event of a partially recovered complete neonatal palsy, transfer of intercostal nerves connected to muscle cutaneous nerve trunk or its fascicles represents a better option to obtain elbow flexion [24].

In already grown children, elbow flexion can be achieved through pedicled muscle transfers (i.e., pectoralis major or minor, triceps, latissimus dorsi muscles) as well as using the classical Steindler procedure. However, very often local muscles are weak and unable to restore function [25].

Free muscle transfers (i.e., free vascularized gracilis muscle transfer) are another option, particularly in younger children when the lever arm of the elbow is favorable and body weight is limited [26, 27].

24.2.2.2 Lack of Elbow Extension

Although lack of elbow extension is a severe defect impairing upper limb function, lack of elbow active extension is thought to be partially compensated by gravitational forces (Fig. 24.8). Nevertheless, the involvement of the C7 root and posterior cord of the brachial plexus is not negligible. When posterior trunk involvement is seen in severely affected children, early nerve surgery is the correct indication. Conversely, indication for surgery might be more complicated when a

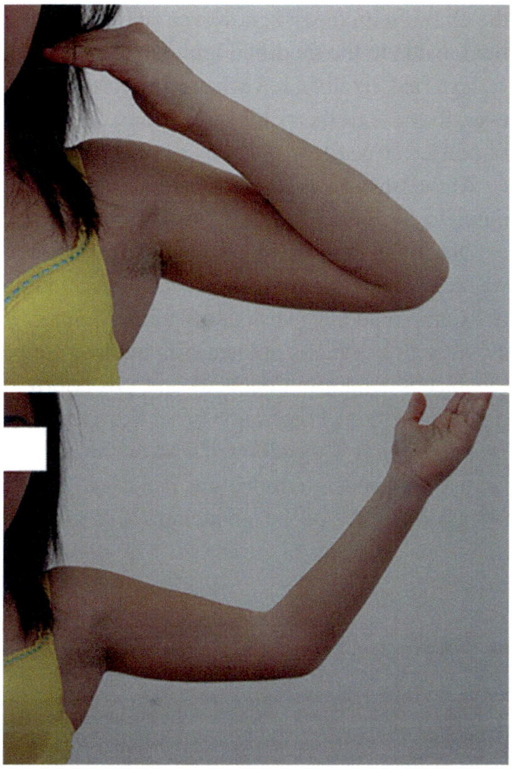

Fig. 24.8 Elbow extension limitation is constantly evident in the upper palsy. The deformity increases during growth impairing elbow motion and determining cosmetic problems in the patients

dissociated recovery of OBPP causes an isolated triceps muscle palsy or when the child is observed late.

In young children, nerve transfers can help restore triceps muscle activity, essential for contrasting biceps muscle flexion and avoiding progressive deformity of the joint, as described above. There is no general agreement about late nerve transfer and which nerve might be transferred.

Fascicles of the ulnar nerve assigned to the flexor carpi ulnaris can be transferred onto the radial nerve or rather on the branches of the long head of the triceps muscle to achieve active elbow extension. When there is C7 involvement or in the event of a partially recovered neonatal complete palsy, intercostal nerves connected to the radial nerve trunk or its fascicles can induce reinnervation of the triceps muscle. In already grown children, elbow extension can be obtained through pedicled muscles (latissimus dorsi muscle, deltoid muscle) [28].

24.2.2.3 Flexion Deformity for Limited Extension

A flexed attitude of the elbow with limitation of elbow extension is the commonest pattern, usually detected in the majority of patients presenting with OBPP sequelae. Flexion degree increases during growth, particularly during adolescence. Incidentally, patients particularly complain about this defect for functional and cosmetic reasons.

Progressive flexion degree of the elbow joint can reach >90°, particularly when a strong biceps muscle is not opposed by a weak triceps muscle. In this condition, elbow joint geometry is modified by muscle imbalance and loss of articular congruency. As a consequence, there is an alteration of the growing elbow, particularly the olecranon process that grows unhindered. These modifications result in a further decrease in motion due to the forced position of the elbow and physeal plate asymmetrical stimulation [29, 30].

Since the surgical correction of the defect is challenging, prevention is always attempted as the first step. Physical therapy can be effective in preventing worsening deformity. Repetition of exercises to increase the range of motion in flexion and extension along with prono-supination of the forearm permits to avoid increased flexed deformity of the elbow.

Static or dynamic nocturnal orthoses can be useful in keeping the elbow in extension, relaxing muscles and reducing joint stiffness. These devices are barely tolerated by toddlers. For this reason, progressive application of casts has been advised along with botulin toxin injections into the brachialis or internal rotator muscles of the shoulder to reduce the progression of flexion deformity [31].

At any rate, a correct approach to the shoulder represents in itself prevention against elbow progressive deformation.

Whenever elbow flexion appears severely limiting, surgery may be required for both functional and cosmetic purposes.

In the literature, biceps tendon lengthening, brachialis muscle release, and anterior open joint capsulotomy have been proposed during growth, even though recurrence of the deformity have been often reported. Furthermore, biceps muscle lengthening entails the risk of losing muscle strength that had undergone reinnervation during the first years of life [32].

A posterior wedged osteotomy in the distal humerus could obtain a satisfactory extension of the elbow, with the risk, however, of losing active flexion due to the modified joint angles.

External fixators have been proposed; however, they entail the risk of infections, stretching of palsied structures, stiffness, etc. [33].

At the time being, there are no definite procedures to completely correct the elbow.

Observing the pitfalls of the other techniques, we published an original procedure including both anteromedial incisions of elbow joint cuff along with brachialis aponeurosis incision (leaving biceps tendon untouched) and posteriorly a partial resection of olecranon tip so to increase the passive motion of the elbow. These two steps have been performed to remove mechanical obstacles on opposite sides of the elbow joint (Fig. 24.9).

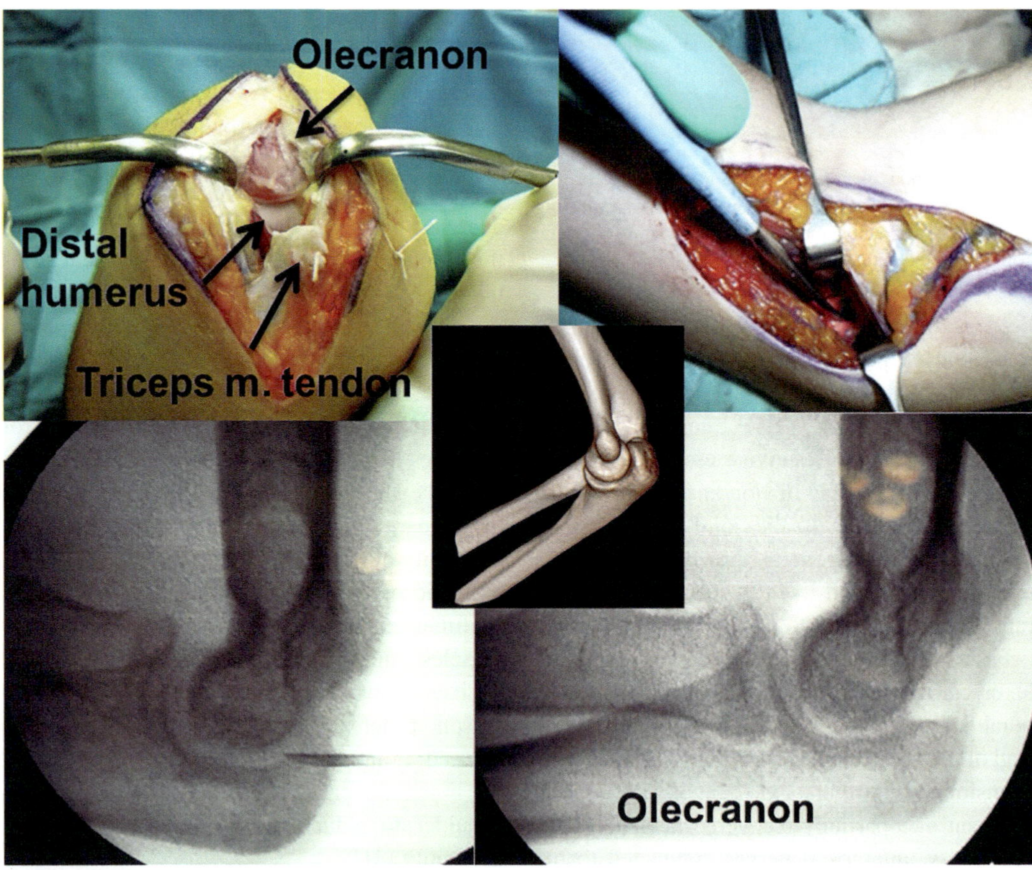

Fig. 24.9 Partial olecranon resection and anterior capsulotomy allow the flexed elbow to achieve a larger range of motion without losing flexion degrees. CT scan shows an increased length of the acromion, while X-ray pictures give details of the level of olecranon resection

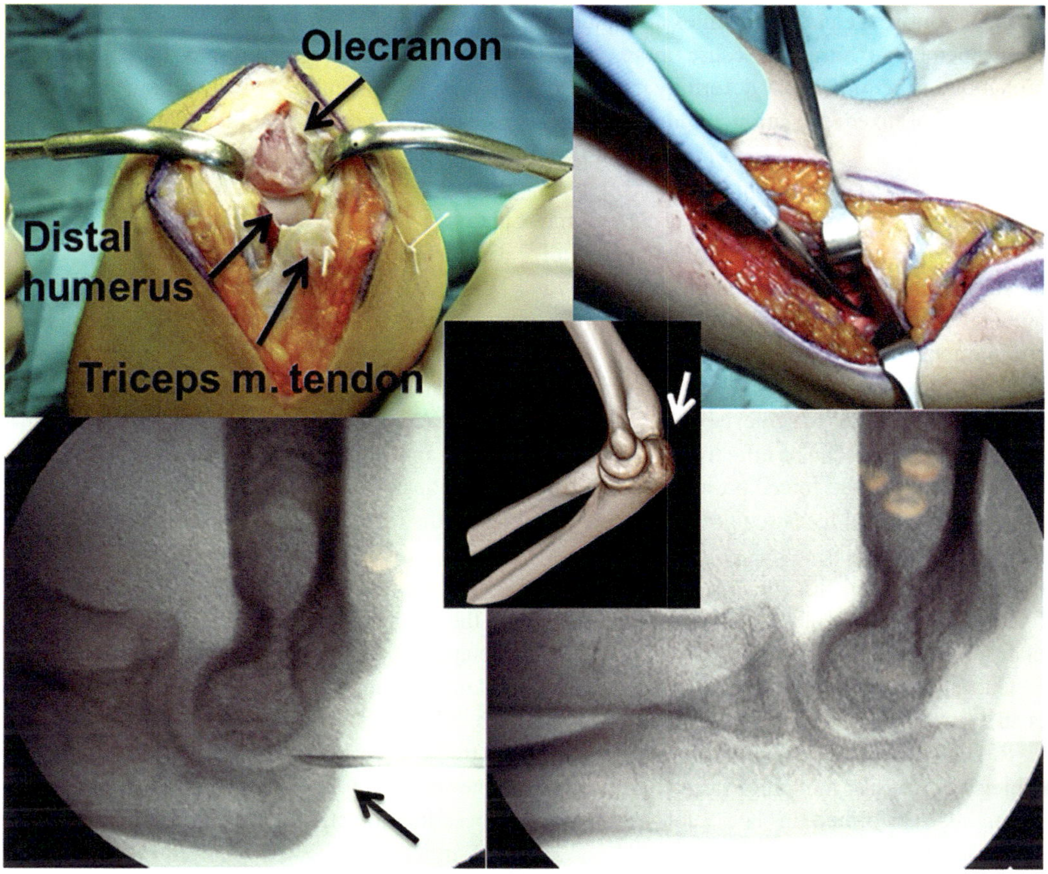

Fig. 24.9 (continued)

A mean increase of approximately 25° in elbow extension has been constantly reached. The results allow a good combination of functional and cosmetic advantages with the satisfaction of patients. The appropriate timing of the procedure is during adolescence when growth changes of the elbow joint do not lead to a recurrence of the deformity [34].

24.2.3 Forearm

The forearm is consistently involved in OBPP, both upper-intermediate and complete, showing different features according to palsy recovery.

Upper palsy presents with a pronation attitude, whereas severe intermediate and complete palsy usually shows a supinated posture.

24.2.3.1 Defect of Supination or Pronator Deformity

Pronator deformity is a typical upper trunk palsy sequela. The deformity stems from the imbalance of forearm pronator muscles which are active, whereas supinator muscles are palsied.

Apart from cases in which severe stiffness of the shoulder and elbow worsens forearm pronator deformity, a mild lack of supination is usually well tolerated. A good range of motion of the shoulder makes up adequately for the defect. Conversely, as the shoulder does not take part in forearm pronation movements, a lack of pronation cannot be compensated.

Physical therapy, taping, and orthosis in the intermediate position are conventional methods of treatment.

Inconstantly, skeletal deformities and interosseous membrane retraction cause more severe pronation of the forearm. A deformity exceeding two-thirds of fixed pronation requires surgical correction.

Uncommonly, subluxation of radial epiphysis in a backward position generally occurs in the oldest patients in whom uncontrolled growth of the radial epiphysis impinges on the distal part of humeral meta-epiphysis, further reducing forearm motion.

Some literature reports have proposed tendon releases and transfers to achieve better supination [35]. Some of them can be effective in the youngest patients; however, forced pronation in a much grown children and teens requires a derotational osteotomy. According to the age, Kirschner wire fixation and molded cast are adequate methods of fixation, whereas in older children, fixation by plate and screws is needed.

Currently, osteoclasis in very young children is an exceptional indication.

Radial head resection is appropriate for achieving a passive motion of the forearm and is commonly performed in late adolescence for severe limitation of pronation movement.

Although ten years of age has been identified as a hypothetical limit for performing soft tissue or skeletal procedures, in our opinion, timing of surgery should be established on a case-by-case basis.

24.2.3.2 Defect of Pronation or Supination Deformity

Supination deformity is a common feature of complete or intermediate palsy with severe impairment of the C7 root.

The typical appearance of the upper arm with a flexed elbow, supinated forearm, and hyperextended flail wrist springs from the dynamic imbalance among active supinator muscles, that is, biceps brachialis muscle and palsied pronator muscles. Since opposite forces are stemming from contracted muscles and gravitational forces of the elbow joint are not controlled by palsied muscles, further joint instability, namely radial head subluxation, consistently arises. Soft tissue defects, such as contracture and shortening of the interosseous membrane, biceps brachialis, supinator teres, and dorsal ligament of the distal radioulnar joint are worsened by skeletal deformities of bone and joints, namely, anterior subluxation of the proximal radial epiphysis and distal ulnar epiphysis subluxation.

Forearm fixed deformity, radial dislocation, and hand function empowering are the main indicators for surgery.

Surgical correction of forearm fixed supination is achieved using a tight interosseous membrane and joint capsule release to obtain a reduction of capital radial head subluxation. When the forearm can easily reach pronation, a Z lengthening of the biceps muscle insertional tendon at the radius is performed. The distal stump of the tendon is then rerouted around the radial metaphysis and sutured in adequate tension to obtain pronation motion when the elbow flexes [36, 37].

In the event of sufficient mobility of the two bones of the forearm, the first step can be skipped proceeding directly to biceps rerouting.

Surgical treatment is required in the event of progressive dislocation of the radial epiphysis at 4–6 years of age.

Hand impairment reduces chances for recovery, even though a correction of fixed supination provides chances for empowering some muscles of the wrist or the hand.

Many authors have proposed forearm osteotomy, reporting good cosmetically and functionally results in the oldest children [38–40].

When severe instability further impairs the chances of using the palsied forearm, radioulnar proximal fusion gives stability to the forearm, which, however, maintains poor function [41].

24.2.4 Wrist and Hand

Wrist and hand involvements are frequent in children suffering from OBPP sequelae, particularly in extensive paralysis.

Wrist extension is one of the goals of functional recovery of the upper arm. Lack of extension impairs hand function. Lack of wrist extension is one of the main indications for early nerve surgery. Therefore, any considerations about the outcome should be based on the expected result of the wrist.

Different patterns of wrist extension defects can be identified. First of all, wrist extension can stem from partial involvement of extensor carpi radialis tendons because of their prevalent innervation from C6 to C7 roots.

Along with physical therapy during the first years of life, nocturnal splints can be effective in balancing wrist muscles. In the event of a child over five years of age with persistent extension defect, despite good flexor muscles of the wrist and fingers, surgery might be appropriate. Flexor carpi ulnaris transfer onto extensor carpi radialis muscles is an effective procedure; however, loss of tension of transferred tendons or on the contrary excessive tension should be taken into account [42, 43].

When the posterior cord of the brachial plexus is severely injured with expectations of poor recovery, repair options considerably decrease.

Wrist flexion can be compensated by finger flexor transfers but tendon transfers are often ineffective or short lasting.

Different patterns of hand defects have been described so it is hard to standardize hand deformities. Raimondi and Gilbert's classification of palsied hand has grouped the majority of clinical aspects [44]. Different from single nerve palsy, in OBPP, frail muscles do not allow the hand to reach adequate strength. Lack of sensation in the hand should discourage any surgical procedure.

Thumb extension and opposition can be obtained using tendon transfer along with joint reinforcement or fusion. Other selected transfers are possible, but the outcome is constantly poor, particularly when transfers are performed too early in life. On the other hand, late transfers result to be constantly poor because the child neglects his affected hand.

24.3 Conclusions

To sum up, palliative surgery options allow patients to achieve satisfactory results, particularly those with a favorable prognosis of recovery but still missing functions.

The main factor determining a good outcome is the correct timing of surgery based on the age of the patients. Growth can undo even a satisfactory short term surgical result. Shoulder and elbow involvement can significantly improve through many surgical procedures that merge orthopedic techniques and nerve surgery. Surgical procedures for correcting distal segments are less effective because of the poor muscle recovery, particularly when a lack of sensation impairs the hand.

References

1. Gilbert A, editor. Brachial plexus injuries. London: Martin Dunitz Ltd; 2001.
2. Nixon M, Trail J. Management of shoulder problems following obstetric brachial plexus injury. Shoulder Elbow. 2014;6:12–7.
3. Waters PM. Comparison of the natural history, the outcome of microsurgical repair and the outcome of operative reconstruction in brachial plexus birth palsy. J Bone Joint Surg Am. 1999;81(5):649–59.
4. Mallet J. Paralysie obstétricale. Rev Chir Orthop Réparatrice Appar Mot. 1972;58(Suppl 1):166–8.
5. Haerle M, Gilbert A. Management of complete obstetric brachial plexus lesions. J Pediatr Orthop. 2004;24:194–200.
6. Sénès FM, Catena N, Sénès J. Nerve transfer in delayed obstetrical palsy repair. J Brachial Plex Peripher Nerve Inj. 2015;10(1):e2–e14.
7. Immermann I, Valencia H, Di Taranto P, Del Sole EM, Glait S, Price AE, Grossmann JA. Subscapular slide correction of the shoulder internal rotation contracture after brachial plexus birth injury: technique and outcomes. Tech Hand Up Extrem Surg. 2013;17(1):52–6.
8. Azburg JM, Kozin SH, Waters PM. Open glenohumeral joint reduction and latissimus dorsi and teres major tendon transfers for infants and children following brachial plexus birth palsy. Tech Hand Up Extrem Surg. 2017;21(2):30–6.
9. Breton A, Mainard L, De Gasperi M, Barbary S, Maurice E, Dautel G. Arthroscopic release of shoulder contracture secondary to obstetric brachial plexus palsy: retrospective study of children with an average

follow up of 4.5 years. Orthop Traumatol Surg Res. 2012;98:638–44.
10. Waters PM, Bae DS. Effect of tendon transfers and extraarticular soft tissue balancing on glenohumeral development in brachial plexus birth palsy. J Bone Joint Surg. 2005;87A(2):320–5.
11. Birch R. Late sequelae at the shoulder in obstetrical palsy in children. In: Randelli M, Karlsson J, editors. Surgical techniques in orthopaedics and traumatology: shoulder, vol. 3. Paris: Elsevier; 2001. 55-200-E-210.
12. Waters PM, Bae DS. The early effect of tendon transfers an open capsulorrhaphy on glenohumeral deformity in brachial plexus birth palsy. J Bone Joint Surg Am. 2008;90:2171–9.
13. Pagnotta A, Haerle M, Gilbert A. Long term results on abduction and external rotation after latissimus dorsi transfer for sequelae of obstetric palsy. Cain Orthop Relat Res. 2004;426:199–205.
14. Ozben H, Atalar AC, Bilsel K, Demirhan M. Transfer of latissimus dorsi and teres major tendons without subscapularis release for the treatment of obstetrical brachial plexus sequela. J Shoulder Elbow Surg. 2011;20(8):1265–74.
15. Chomiak J, Dungl P, Ostadal M, Frydychova M, Burian M. Muscle transfers in children and adults improve external rotation in cases of obstetrical brachial plexus paralysis: a comparative study. Int Orthop. 2014;38(4):803–10.
16. Abzug JM, Chafetz RS, Gaughan JP, Ashworth S, Kozin SH. Shoulder function after medial approach and derotational humeral osteotomy in patients with brachial plexus birth palsy. J Pediatr Orthop. 2010;30(5):469–74.
17. McRae MC, Borschel GH. Transfer of triceps motor branches of the radial nerve to axillary nerve with or without other nerve transfers provides antigravity shoulder abduction in pediatric brachial plexus injury. Hand (NY). 2012;7(2):186–90.
18. Aly A, Bahm J, Schuind F. Percutaneous humeral derotational osteotomy in obstetrical palsy: a new technique. J Hand Surg Eur. 2014;39(5):549–52.
19. Chen L, Gu YD, Hu SN. Applying transfer of and/or latissimus dorsi with teres major for reconstruction of abduction and external rotation of the shoulder in obstetrical brachial plexus palsy. J Reconstr Microsurg. 2002;18(4):275–80.
20. Gilbert A, Brockman R, Carlioz H. Surgical treatment of brachial plexus birth palsy. Clin Orthop. 1991;264:39–47.
21. Terzis JK, Kokkalis ZT. Primary and secondary shoulder reconstruction in obstetric brachial plexus palsy. Injury. 2008;39S:S5–S14.
22. Frich LH, Schmidt PH, Torfing T. Glenoid morphology in obstetrical brachial plexus lesion: a three dimensional computed tomography study. J Shoulder Elbow Surg. 2017;26(8):1374–82.
23. Di Mascio L, Chin FK, Fox M, Sinisi M. Glenoplasty for complex shoulder subluxation and dislocation in children with obstetric brachial plexus palsy. J Bone Joint Surg Br. 2011;93:102–7.
24. Murison J, Jehanno P, Fitoussi F. Nerve transfer to biceps to restore elbow flexion and supination in children with obstetrical brachial plexus palsy. J Child Orthop. 2017;11(6):455–9.
25. Kawabata H, Shibata T, Matsui Y, Yasui N. Use of intercostals nerves for neurotization of the musculocutaneous nerve in infants with birth related brachial plexus palsy. J Neurosurg. 2001;94(3):386–91.
26. Chwei Chin Chuang D, Hattori Y, Ma HS, Chen HC. The reconstruction strategy for improving elbow function in late obstetrical brachial plexus palsy. Plast Reconstr Surg. 2003;109(1):116–26.
27. El Gammal T, El Sayed A, Kobt MM, Saleh WR, Ragheb YF, Refai O, Morsy MM. Free functioning gracilis transplantation for reconstruction of elbow and hand function in late obstetrical brachial plexus palsy. Microsurgery. 2015;35(5):350–5.
28. Nath RK, Boutros SG, Somasundaram C. Eplasty. 2017:e34.
29. Senes FM, Catena N, Dapelo E, Senes J. Nerve transfer for elbow extension in obstetrical brachial plexus palsy. Ann Acad Med Singap. 2016;45(5):221–4.
30. Poyhia TH, Koivikko MP, Peltonen J, Kirjavainen MO, Lamminen AE, Mietosvaara AY. Muscle changes in brachial plexus birth injury with elbow flexion contracture: an MRI study. Pediatr Radiol. 2007;37:173–9.
31. Sheffler L, Lattanza L, Hagar Y, Bagley A, James MA. The prevalence, rate of progression and treatment of elbow flexion contracture in children with brachial plexus birth palsy. J Bone Joint Surg A. 2012;94:403–9.
32. Ho ES, Roy T, Stephens D, Clarke HM. Serial casting and splinting of elbow contracture in children with obstetrical brachial plexus palsy. J Hand Surg Am. 2010;35(1):84–91.
33. Garcia Lopez A, Sebastian P, Martinez LF. Anterior release of elbow flexion contractures in children with obstetrical brachial plexus lesions. J Hand Surg Am. 2012;37(8):1660–4.
34. Vekris MD, Pafilas D, Lykissas MG, Soucacos PN, Beris AE. Correction of elbow flexion contracture in late obstetrical brachial plexus palsy through arthrodiastasis of the elbow (Ioannina method). Tech Hand Up Extrem Surg. 2010;14(1):14–20.
35. Senes FM, Catena N, Dapelo E, Senes J. Correction of elbow flexion contracture by means of olecranon resection and anterior arthrolysis in obsttetrical brachial plexus sequelae. J Pediatr Orthop B. 2017;26(1):14–20.

36. Amrani A, Dendane MA, El Alami ZF. Pronator teres transfer to correct pronation deformity of the forearm after an obstetrical brachial plexus injury. J Bone Joint Surg Br. 2009;91(5):616–8.
37. Ruhmann O, Hierner R. Z plasty and rerouting of the biceps tendon with interosseous membrane release to restore pronation in paralytic supination posture and contracture of the forearm. Oper Orthop Traumatol. 2009;21(2):157–69.
38. Metsaars WP, Nagels J, Pijls BG, Langenhoff JM, Nelissen RG. Treatment of supination deformity for obstetric brachial plexus injury: a systematic review and meta-analysis. J Hand Surg Am. 2014;39(10):1948–58.
39. Gladstein AZ, Sachleben B, Ho ES, Anthony A, Clarke HM, Hopyan S. Forearm pronation osteotomy for supination contracture secondary to obstetrical brachial plexus palsy: a retrospective cohort study. J Pediatr Orthop. 2017;37(6):e357–63.
40. Van Kooten EO, Ishaque MA, Winters HA, Ritt MJ, Van der Sluijs HA. Pronating radius osteotomy for supination deformity in children with obstetric brachial plexus palsy. Tech Hand Up Extrem Surg. 2008;12(1):34–7.
41. Manfrini M, Valdiserri L. Proximal radio ulnar arthrosis in the treatment of supination deformity resulting from obstetrical paralysis. Ital J Orthop Traumatol. 1985;11(3):309–13.
42. Van Alphen NA, Van Doorn Loogman MH, Mass H, Van der Sluijs JA, Ritt MJ. Restoring wrist extension in obstetric palsy of the brachial plexus by transferring wrist flexors to wrist extensors. J Pediatr Rehabil Med. 2013;6(1):53–7.
43. Al Quattan MM. Tendon transfer to reconstruct wrist extension in children with obstetric brachial plexus palsy. J Hand Surg Br. 2003;28(2):153–7.
44. Raimondo PL. Evaluation of results in obstetrical brachial plexus palsy: the hand. In: Proceedings of international meeting of brachial plexus palsy, Helen, The Netherlands; 1993.

Nerve Injuries

25

Filippo M. Senes, Nunzio Catena, Luigi A. Nasto, and Chiara Arrigoni

Abstract

Commonly, peripheral nerve injuries (PNI) of the upper limb in children result from fractures or penetrating lesions. Patient's age significantly affects epidemiology and demographics of these lesions. In very young chidren, injuries of peripheral nerves can affect nerve maturations and impair distal joint motion and limb residual growth potential.

Nevertheless, child regeneration potential and neuronal plasticity allow for a better outcome than in adulthood injuries. Concerning the type and level of skeletal lesion, typical PNI patterns can be described. Cutting edges of fracture fragments can cause direct damage to nearby nerves, whereas joint dislocation often determines traction injuries. Early identification of nerve lesion is mandatory for planning the treatment that, depending on injury type and gap, consist of wait and see, direct suture, nerve grafting, and tubulization.

Keywords

Peripheral nerve · Upper limb · Children · Fractures · Penetrating lesions · Nerve graft

25.1 Introduction

Peripheral nerve injuries (PNI) of the upper limb after fractures and cutting lesions are a common occurrence in children, whereas canalicular (compression) syndrome is rare.

Although in the past, nerve injuries of the upper limbs were often grouped regardless of patient's age, researchers have focused on pediatric nerve injuries, particularly on nerve involvement following supracondylar humeral fractures.

Age significantly affects the occurrence of nerve lesions. Older children report a high rate of fracture-related PNI, probably because they are more commonly involved in road and sports accidents, while the youngest are usually under parental supervision [1].

Moreover, a basic approach to a pediatric nerve lesion should take into account that differences arise from the amount of myelinization of the nerve trunks, which is age- dependent.

F. M. Senes (✉)
Department oh Hand Surgery and Rehabilitation, San Giuseppe MultiMedica Hospital, Milan University, Milano, Italy
e-mail: filipposenes@fastwebnet.it

N. Catena
UOSD Microchirurgia Ricostruttiva e Chirurgia della Mano, IRCCS Istituto Giannina Gaslini, Genova, Italy

L. A. Nasto
UOC Ortopedia e Traumatologia, IRCCS Istituto Giannina Gaslini, Genova, Italy

C. Arrigoni
Scuola di Specializzazione in Ortopedia e Traumatologia, Università degli Studi di Torino, Torino, Italy

G. Pajardi (ed.), *Pediatric Hand Surgery*, https://doi.org/10.1007/978-3-031-30984-7_25

The absence of myelinated coating in peripheral nerve slows down nerve conduction velocity, which is about one-half compared with the ones detected in adults. A complete myelinated sheet in peripheral nerves develops at about 3 years of age.

Continue changes in the assessment of neurotrophins, neurotransmitters, and their receptors influence the maturation of the nervous system. In young children, any injury can affect the maturation process of the nerve, impairing motion, sensibility, and residual growth of the upper limb. Skeletal modifications of the upper limb, due to prolonged denervation, are exemplified by the shortening of the upper limb observed after a severe obstetrical brachial plexus palsy [2].

Apart from these potential issues, regeneration potential and neuronal plasticity in the child allow them to achieve a better outcome than in adulthood. Besides all, the risk of joint stiffness is very low, with exception of brachial plexus injuries.

In pediatric population, the age, growth, patterns of injuries and maturity level of peripheral nerve system will lead to peculiar tratment modalities.

25.2 Types and Sites of Nerve Lesions

In the upper limb, nerve injuries show typical features, depending on the single nerve and level of lesion. A basic distinction is the presence of a skin defect: open and closed injuries occur with different patterns at different upper arm levels.

Closed injuries are usually associated with fractures, which can trigger a direct nerve involvement by bone fragments; however, joint dislocation can cause nerve lesions by traction.

Considering nerve pathways, PNI are shown as follows:

- Axillary: shoulder dislocation and rarely proximal humeral fractures
- Radial: shaft humeral fractures
- Median, radial, and ulnar (isolated or in combination): supracondylar humeral fractures
- Median, ulnar, and elbow dislocation
- Posterior interosseous: acute or chronic anterior Monteggia lesions
- Median, ulnar; diaphyseal forearm fractures; median, distal radius fractures

Supracondylar humeral fracture is most commonly affected by PNI, because of two peculiar risk factors. Firstly, the close contact between nerves and bone at the elbow level is a major predisposing factor to nerve injury. Radial and ulnar nerves are often damaged because of their passage through definite osteofibrous tunnel and septa that prevent from their natural sliding. Secondly, the severe displacement of Gartland 3 supracondylar humeral fracture increases the chances of nerve kinking, entrapment, or laceration [3] (Fig. 25.1).

The pattern of nerve involvement is closely related to the type of fracture: the median nerve is commonly injured in the event of posterolateral Gartland 3 fractures whereas the radial nerve in posteromedial ones [4, 5].

Injuries of the ulnar nerve can be occasionally observed in rare flexion-type fractures, while sometimes iatrogenic lesions may happen after medial pinning.

Many authors have reported the radial nerve as the most commonly injured nerve; however, the recent literature has focused on the median nerve and particularly on its anterior interosseous branch (AIB).

In medical literature, anterior interosseous nerve involvement has been often neglected for two main reasons: on the one hand, median nerve trunk and related nerve branch injuries are usually difficult to differentiate each other, so medical reports group together these lesions as a whole; on the other hand, a sudden detection of anterior interosseous nerve involvement is hard to identify, especially in younger children who cannot adequately complain their discomfort [6].

Even though its incidence is underestimated, ABI palsy has to be probably considered the most

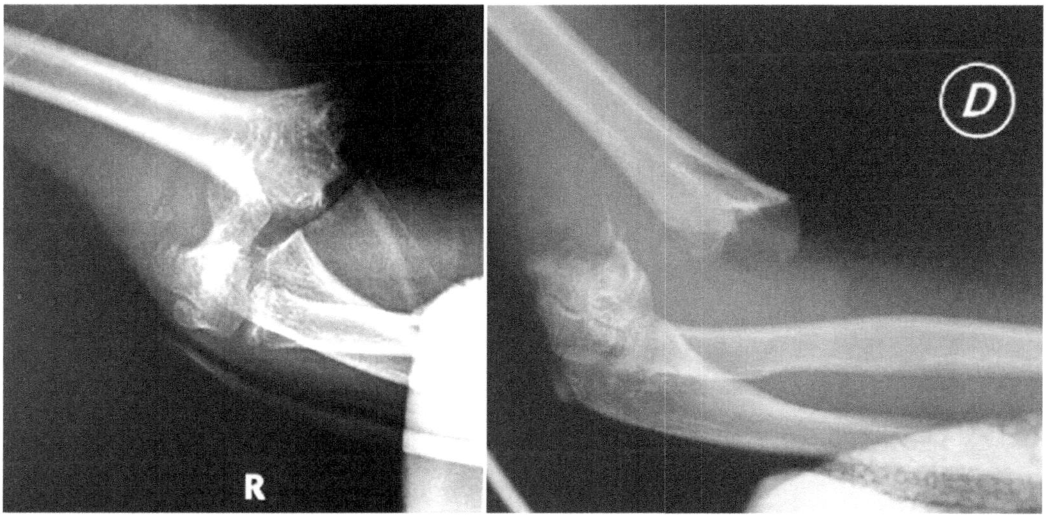

Fig. 25.1 Joint dislocation causing nerve traction and AIB injury

common nerve injury related to supracondylar fractures, even though its origin is far from the supracondylar region.

The peculiar anatomy of the median nerve may explain the prevalent involvement of AIB, which is due to two factors.

First of all, nerve fibers devoted to AIB are located in a posterior position in the main trunk of the median nerve, so that direct trauma triggered by the free edge of the proximal fragment of fracture might damage them before AIB (branch) detachment from the main nerve.

Moreover, after arising from the major trunk the AIB passes through the interosseous membrane in a deep position.

The narrow passage and angulation of the nerve trunk cause reduction of the natural sliding of the nerve and a predisposition to traction [7] (Fig. 25.2).

The radial nerve is commonly injured in fractures presenting with posteromedial dislocation. Notwithstanding the constant onset of the palsy, the recovery is usually spontaneous, as observed in the humeral shaft or Holstein–Lewis fractures [8, 9]. An unexpected radial nerve palsy that appears in the first weeks after trauma is possibly due to the compression or wrapping of the nerve by bone callus. As regards ulnar nerve injuries, there are minor chances of direct nerve injury in skeletal trauma, apart from rare fractures with flexion dislocation (2% of all supracondylar fractures).

Further causes of palsy might be a direct injury in the event of medial pinning for fracture fixation, which inconstantly causes nerve fascicle disruption or the arising of late palsy secondary to perineural fibrosis in the cubital tunnel.

Open injuries are commonly due to glass or sharp objects.

On the one hand, wounds of the upper arm are usually observed in older children because of their autonomy, which exposes them to the risk of cutting with penetrating glass fragments, metal plates, knives, or cutting blades. On the other hand, little children are easily injured by the same sharp objects but more commonly are suffering from crush injuries, without significant impairment of nerve trunks.

The wrist, palmar surface of the hand, and fingers are the most common sites of injury. Very often, multiple cuttings are detected, interesting both the vessels, tendons and muscles, and nerves as well.

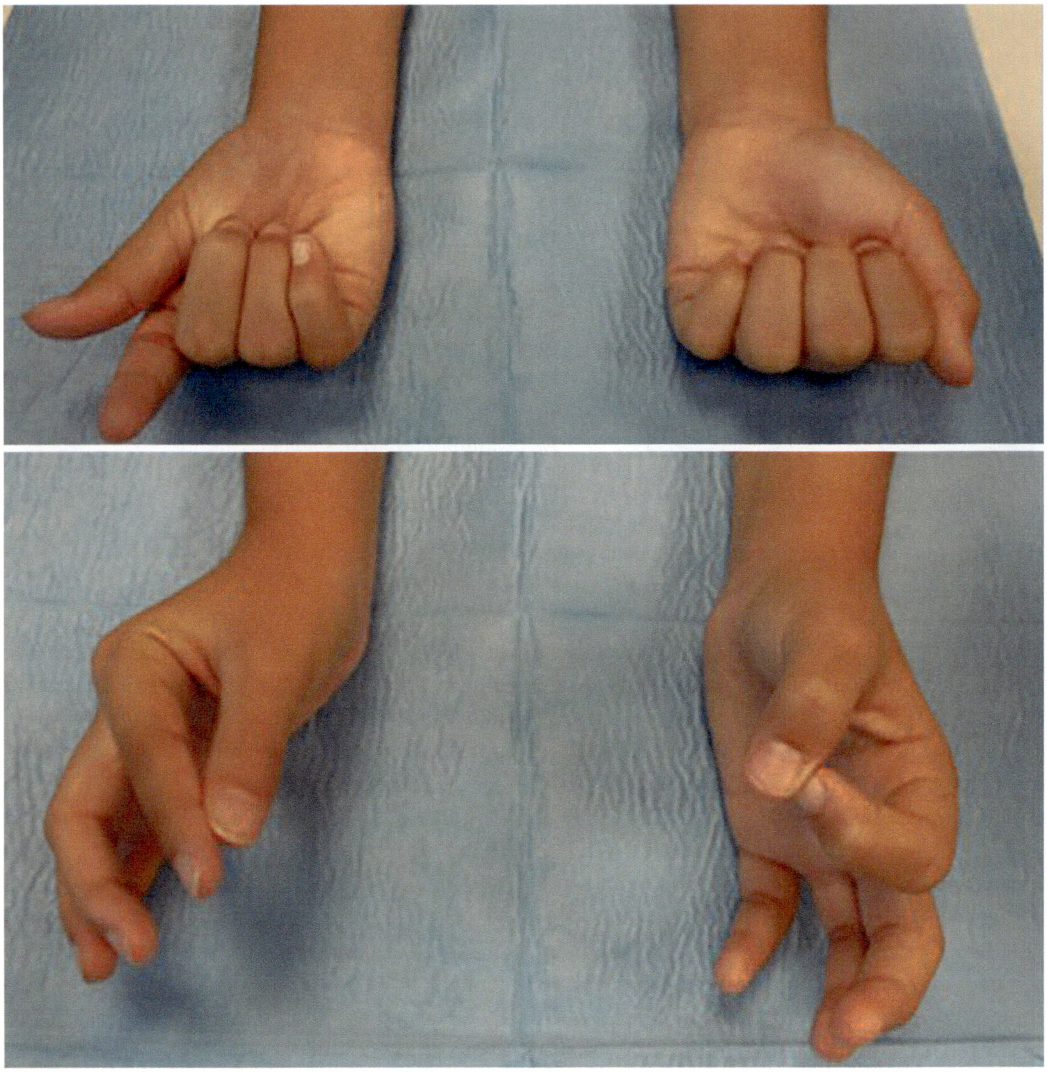

Fig. 25.2 Kiloh–Nevin syndrome: impossibility to distal phalanx flexion of the thumb and index finger after AIB injury

Physicians must be aware of thoroughly exploring any minimal glass wounds because a skin laceration might be expression of deep structures damaging.

Although a clinical examination might be difficult in the child, especially in the youngest, vessels, tendons, and nerve interruption should be detected in the first exploration [10] (Fig. 25.3).

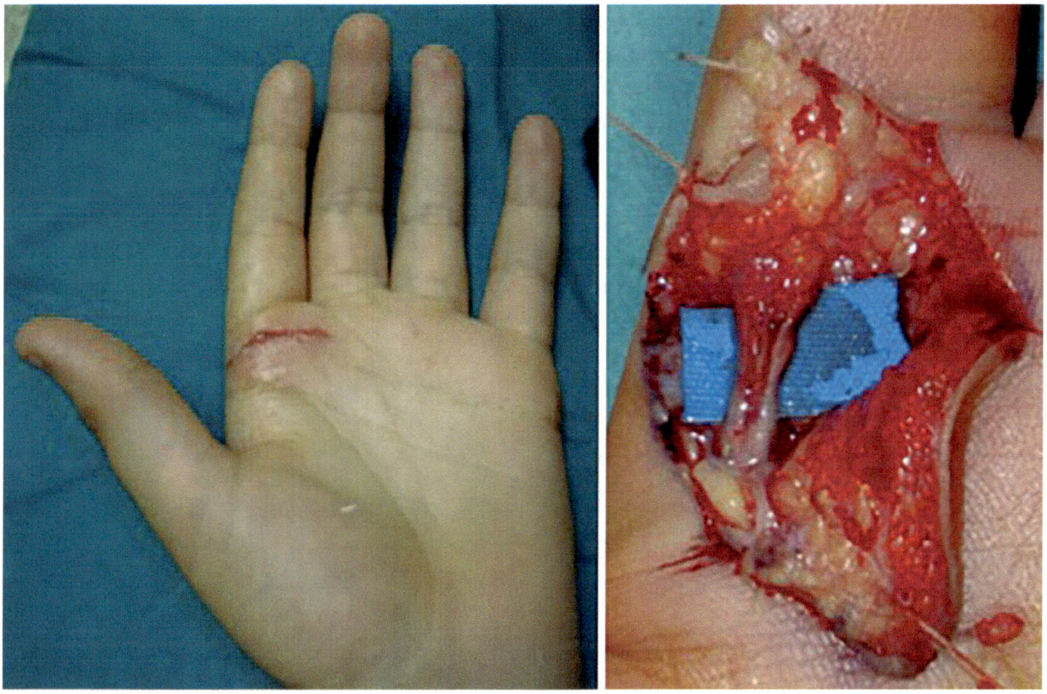

Fig. 25.3 Small wound in the palmar region with a lesion of the collateral radial nerve for the index finger

25.3 Diagnosis

Early identification of nerve palsy is basic either for the treatment or forensic aspect. Medical reports should clearly show if the paralysis were already present at the admission of the patient to the emergency room. Although detection of nerve palsy might be independent of the treatment, very often reports lack this information, so in case of legal disagreement, it might be hard to explain a nerve lesion that occurred at the trauma [11]. Clinical examination should be accurately carried out to give the right information and decide on strategies for treatment.

Nevertheless, the examination might be challenging, especially in the youngest child presenting with bone fractures. Usually, they are uncooperative because of their age, anxiety, pain, and swelling. For those reasons, assessment methods commonly applied to test active motion and sensibility cannot be used, because of the risk of underestimating the palsy.

To solve the problem, some authors have proposed to assess the sensibility of uncooperative children by submerging the hand in water, soaking or wet cloth, and then observing the capability to wrinkle [12]. Immediate sign of nerve involvement is neuropraxia; however, during the first weeks after trauma, it does not need to carry out any early diagnostic examination. Closed nerve injury of the upper limb has a high chance of spontaneous recovery. On the contrary, in the event of a palsy not showing any sign of recovery from 4–6 months after the trauma, it is advisable to study the nerve through ultrasound and neurophysiological exams. Similarly, early surgery should be performed in the event of persistent palsy with a Tinel's sign remaining at the fracture site, which might be the expression of nerve entrapment in the bone regeneration callus.

The key point is to detect whether the nerve is in-continuity or not and about perilesional tissues [13].

Neurophysiological exams are still considered the gold standard to study nerve palsy, although they are not always reliable, especially in the acute phase of the palsy or in uncooperative patients [14]. Sonography, giving more information on the morphology, continuity, and motility of the nerve, can easily identify nerve damage that requires early surgical treatment.

Being not influenced by tissue changes following the trauma or by the presence of metallic devices, this examination can be carried out during the first weeks after the injury.

It is usually well tolerated by the child, allowing it to be repeated to assess the recovery [15].

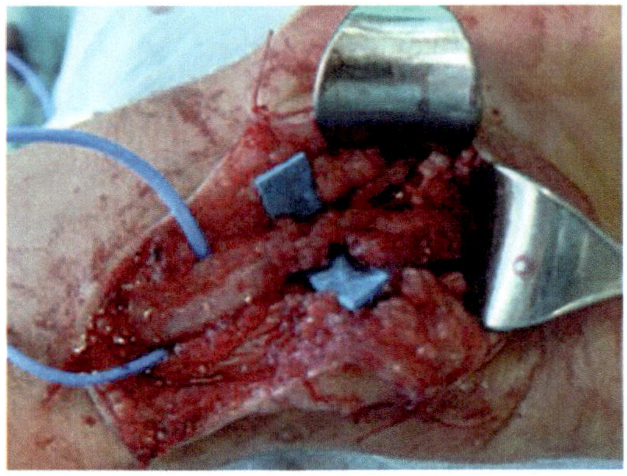

Fig. 25.4 Ulnar nerve lesion treated with direct suture

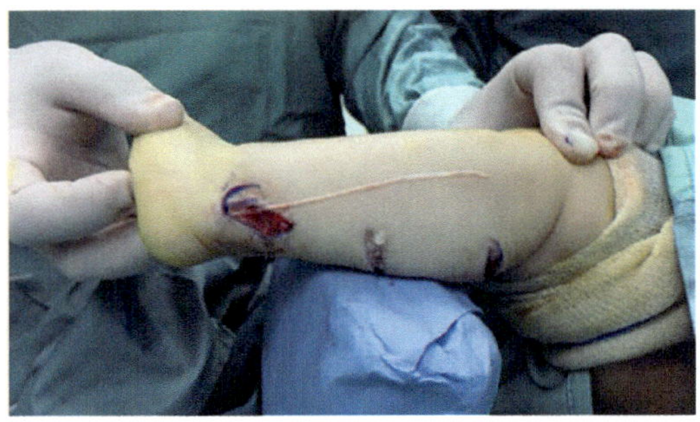

Fig. 25.5 Sural nerve graft for nerve reconstruction

25.4 Treatment

The approach to PNI differs from the type of injury, namely, open or closed, and the presence of a nerve gap.

The treatment of open injuries should be theoretically carried out as soon as possible to avoid the formation of scar tissue which might hinder nerve regeneration.

However, a new opinion has arisen about delayed reconstruction within 3 weeks after the trauma, especially in the event of extended or complicated multiple tissue lesions.

Moreover, this option of delayed treatment could be useful for surgeons who do not usually deal with nerve surgery, allowing them to address the injured child at a hub center where nerve surgery is commonly carried out.

According to nerve damage, nerve reconstruction can be performed through different techniques: direct suture (Fig. 25.4), nerve graft (Fig. 25.5), and tubulization are the options (Fig. 25.6).

Neurorrhaphy is the best procedure because it can provide the right orientation of the axons. However, in open injuries, a nerve gap is often shown so to impose substitution of the gap through nerve grafts or conduits.

To fill the gap, nerve grafts are the best solution. Schwann cells of interposed nerve graft contribute to nerve regeneration, both for mixed and sensitive nerves.

The conduits represent an alternative to bridge the gap, but some concerns still remain. Although many types of tubes have been proposed to improve nerve regeneration (i.e., *biological* or *synthetic*), at the time being there are still contrasting results apart from some good outcome in sensitive nerves.

On the contrary, regarding mixed nerves its application remains controversial [16].

Notwithstanding, considering the overall good recovery of nerve injury in children, the use of nerve conduits in repairing nerve defects of the upper limb may be considered even for mixed nerves [17].

Another matter that is widely debated is the approach to a closed nerve injury, especially for those associated with supracondylar humeral fractures.

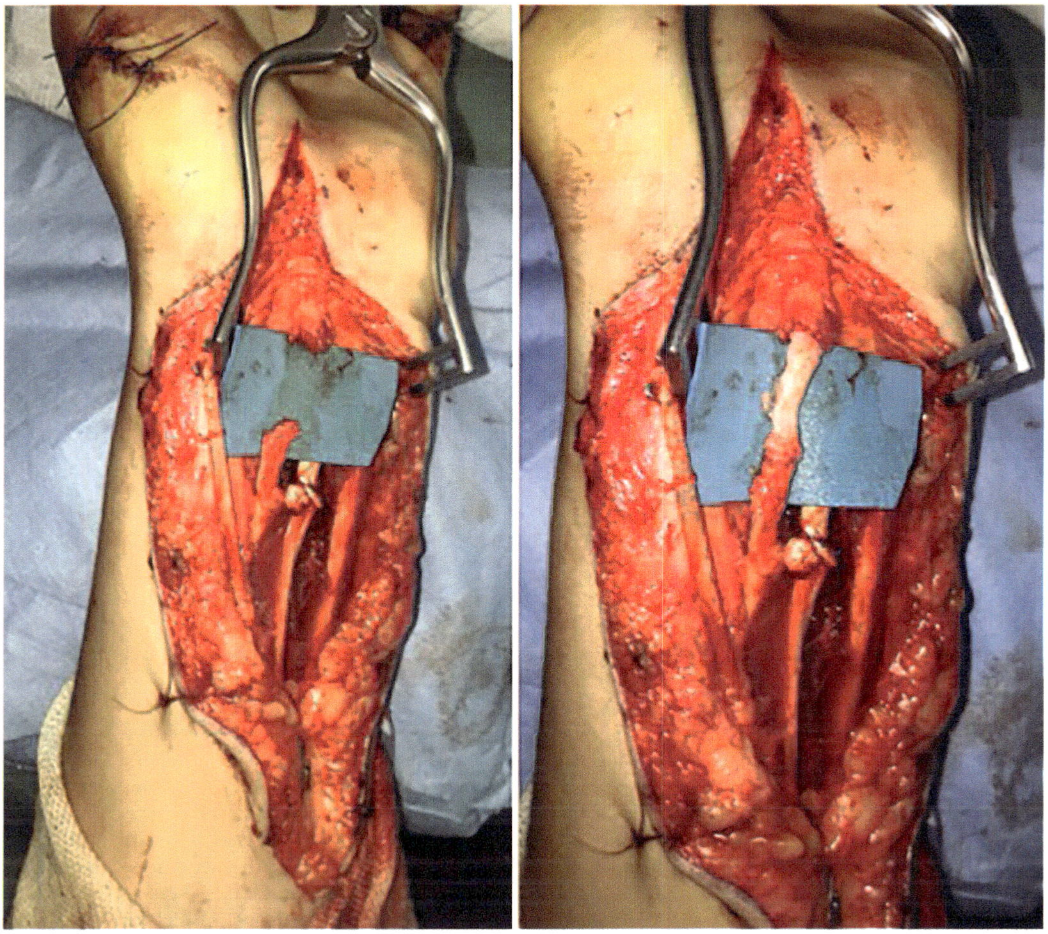

Fig. 25.6 Median nerve reconstruction with saphenous vein tubulization

On the one hand, the majority of these lesions tend to a complete recovery: a waiting attitude should be considered, postponing any treatment before 6 months from the trauma [18, 19].

If nerve palsy does not shortly appear after the trauma but is detected in the following weeks, a nerve entrapment into bone callus formation should be suspected.

Radial and median nerves are commonly involved, although the first one has a major risk because of its close location to the bone.

In the event of late paralysis, sonography can show the nerve morphology and surrounding bone callus formation.

If compression is confirmed, early exploration can establish whether the nerve might be freed or repaired through autografts.

In the event of neglected nerve injuries in adults, tendon transfers are commonly performed to restore function. On the contrary, tendon transfers in children should not be considered as a first option, because of their nerve spontaneous repair or recovery achievement through delayed nerve reconstruction.

25.5 Conclusion

To sum up, PNI are common occurrences in pediatric traumatology, particularly in upper limbs than in the lower ones.

Although open lesions are not negligible, the majority of lesions are closed injuries. Unlike adulthood, closed injuries require a waiting attitude without surgery because of a spontaneous recovery that might happen within a few months, whereas open lesions are in need of immediate treatment as in adults.

Even though the outcome is generally good, a small percentage of failure has to be taken into consideration, particularly those related to open or closed ulnar nerve injuries.

References

1. Missios S, Bekelis K, Spinner RJ. Traumatic peripheral nerve injuries in children: epidemiology and socioeconomics. J Neurosurg Pediatr. 2014;10:1–7.
2. Birch R, Achan P. Peripheral nerve repairs and their results in children. Hand Clin. 2000;16(4):579–95.
3. Waters PM, Bae DS. Distal humerus fracture. In: Pediatric hand and upper limb surgery. A practical guide. Philadelphia: Lippincott Williams and Wilkins; 2012. p. 287–315.
4. McGraw JJ, Akbarnia BA, Hanel DP. Neurological complications resulting from supracondylar fractures of the humerus in children. J Pediatr Orthop. 1986;6:647–50.
5. Iqbal M, Habib R. Nerve injuries associated with supracondylar fracture of the humerus in children. J Pak Med Assoc. 1994;44:148–9.
6. Babal JC, Mehlman CT, Klein G. Nerve injuries associated with pediatric supracondylar humeral fractures: a meta-analysis. J Pediatr Orthop. 2010;30(3):253–63.
7. Vincelet Y, Journeau P, Popkov D, Haumont T, Lascombes P. The anatomical basis for anterior interosseous nerve palsy secondary to supracondylar fractures in children. Orthop Traumatol Surg Res. 2013;99:543–7.
8. Holstein A, Lewis GM. Fractures of the humerus with radial nerve palsy. J Bone Joint Surg. 1963;45:1382–8.
9. Rocchi M, Tarallo L, Mugnai R, Adani R. Humeral shaft fractures complicated by radial nerve palsy: is surgical exploration necessary? Musculoskelet Surg. 2016;100(Suppl 1):S53–60.
10. Waters PM, Bae DS. Traumatic peripheral nerve injuries. In: Pediatric hand and upper limb surgery. A practical guide. Philadelphia: Lippincott Williams and Wilkins; 2012. p. 462–77.
11. Lyons JP, Ashley E, Hoffer MM. Ulnar nerve palsies after percutaneous cross pinning of supracondylar fractures in children's elbow. J Pediatr Orthop. 1998;18:43–5.
12. Tindall A, Dawood R, Povlsen B. Case of the month: the skin wrinkle test a simple nerve injury test for pediatric and uncooperative patients. Emerg Med J. 2006;23(11):883–6.
13. Barisic N, Perovic D, Mitrovic Z, Jurenic D, Zagar M. Assessment of war and accidental nerve injuries in children. Pediatr Neurol. 1999;21(1):450–5.
14. Carter GT, Robinson LR, Chang VH, Kraft GH. Electrodiagnostic evaluation of traumatic nerve injuries. Hand Clin. 2000;16:1–12.
15. Lee J, Bidwell T, Metcalfe R. Ultrasound in pediatric peripheral nerve injuries: can this affect our surgical decision making? A preliminary report. J Pediatr Orthop. 2013;33(2):152–8.
16. Yang M, Rawson JL, Zhang EW, Arnold PB, Lineaweaver W, Zhang F. Comparison of outcomes from repair of median and ulnar nerve defect with nerve graft and tubulization: a meta-analysis. J Reconstr Microsurg. 2011;27:451–60.
17. Senes FM, Catena N, Senes J. Use of tubulization (nerve conduits) in repairing nerve defects in children. Indian J Orthop. 2015;49(5):554–60.
18. Senes FM, Campus R, Becchetti F, Catena N. Upper limb nerve injuries in developmental age. Microsurgery. 2009;29(7):529–35.
19. Shore BJ, Gillespie BT, Miller PE, Bae DS, Waters PM. Recovery of motor nerve injuries associated with displaced, extension-type pediatric supracondylar humerus fractures. J Pediatr Orthop. 2017;39(9):e652–6.

26 Flexor Tendon Lesions in Children: Diagnosis, Treatment, and Early Active Motion Rehabilitation

Chiara Parolo, Greta Culicchia, Rossella Pagliaro, and Giorgio Pajardi

Abstract

Flexor tendon injuries in children represent a diagnostic and therapeutic challenge for surgeons. These injuries can go unnoticed and rehabilitation is difficult, but good results are achieved after treatment. In the recent years, with the evolution of repair techniques of flexor tendons, in adult patients, an early active motion regime was introduced. In pediatric age, there is not still common consensus for surgical technique and for postoperative rehabilitation. In children aged between 3 and 7 years, we prefer the pullout technique while in children aged between 8 and 12 years the four-strand suture associated with the peripheral epitendinous suture. Partial early active motion protocol is started no later than 7 days after the repair. Between April and December 2018, four children were treated. There were no complications such as rupture, inflammation, infection, or contractures of the proximal interphalangeal joint at the final follow-up. No patient needs tenolysis. Good and excellent results were registered in all four digits, respectively, with the TAM score and the Strickland method. We do believe that early active motion by promoting tendon gliding immediately avoids the exclusion of the hand and the loss of the motor pattern and favors the return to play activities.

Keywords

Flexor tendons · Rehabilitation · Mobilization Injuries

Flexor tendon injuries in children represent a diagnostic and therapeutic challenge for surgeons. These injuries can go unnoticed and rehabilitation is difficult, but good results are achieved after treatment.

The incidence of these lesions in children has been estimated at 3.6/100,000 children per year [1]. Flexor zones II and V are the most commonly affected, and it is very strange to see these lesions in children younger than 2 years old, although they have been described in newborns occurring during emergency cesarean deliveries [2]. "Buds" or higher incidence peaks have also been observed in holiday times, in which children tend to manipulate sharp instruments [2].

The most common trauma mechanism is caused by cutting glass, followed by sharp object injuries (knives). Associated neurological injuries are commonly found in flexor zones III and V, and

C. Parolo (✉) · G. Culicchia · R. Pagliaro
Milan, Italy
e-mail: chiara.parolo@multimedica.it; grata.culicchia@multimedica.it; rossella.pagliaro@multimedica.it

G. Pajardi
Department of Hand Surgery and Rehabilitation, S. Giuseppe Hospital IRCCS MultiMedica, Milan University, Milan, Italy
e-mail: gpajardi@centrostudimano.it

G. Pajardi (ed.), *Pediatric Hand Surgery*, https://doi.org/10.1007/978-3-031-30984-7_26

they are not frequently associated with finger fractures or extensor tendon injuries [1]. These injuries are more common in men than in women and most commonly affect the right hand [1, 3].

In the recent years, with the evolution of repair techniques of flexor tendons, in adult patients, an early active motion regime was introduced. There are several articles that support this concept seeing as it improves the gliding of tendons and the strength of tensile and reduces the adhesion formation and complications. In pediatric age, there is not still common consensus for surgical technique and for postoperative rehabilitation. In fact, rehabilitation program after flexor tendon repair is highly controversial. Some authors prefer immobilization while others support different rehabilitation protocols. Postoperative rehabilitation programs are strictly influenced by the patient's age. In literature, preschoolers (less than 5 years old) are immobilized while for children between 5 and 10 years old recommend an early motion program under the supervision of the hand therapist. In this study, we reported the cases of children between 3 and 12 years old with flexor tendon injury in zones I, II, and III repaired with four-strand suture associated with epitendinous suture and with pullout technique. After surgery, they performed the early active motion protocol.

In children aged between 3 and 7 years, we prefer the pullout technique while in children aged between 8 and 12 years the four-strand suture associated with the peripheral epitendinous suture. The pullout technique, described for the first time by Bunnel in 1940, is used for the repair of the profundus flexor tendon in zone I with the aim of transferring the tendon suture to the button placed on the digital apex (Fig. 26.1). This technique allows the two tendon stumps to be brought together, eliminating tension during muscle contraction. In recent decades, a four-strand repair associated with a peripheral epitendinous suture has been the main repair technique for flexor tendons. This promotes greater resistance and sealing force and less gapping at the repair site and allows for inherent healing by limiting adhesion formation. The associated peripheral epitendinous suture has the purpose of leveling and reducing the repair thickness ensuring greater sliding. When the tendon is too small, we use a smaller suture than adults in order to permit a four-strand technique.

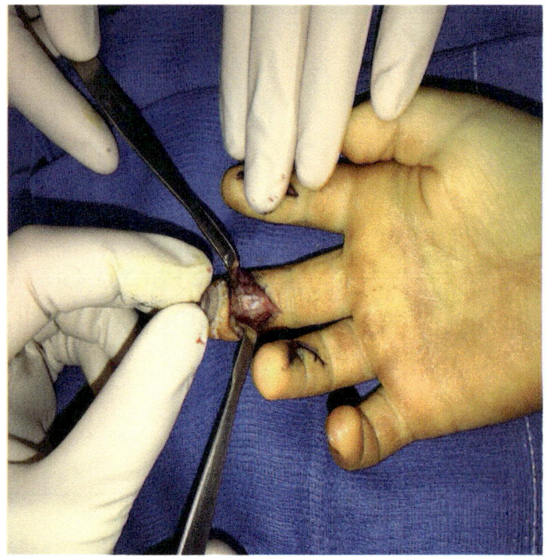

Fig. 26.1 Pull-out technique

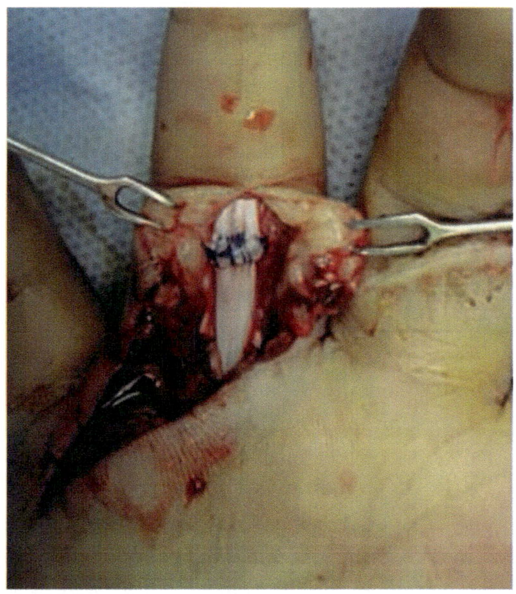

Fig. 26.2 Double 4 strand in flexor tendon repair

After surgery, a dorsal thermoplastic splint was applied at the end of surgery to protect the tendon suture, and this is usually worn for 6 weeks. The splint keeps the wrist at 0–30° of extension, the metacarpophalangeal joints at 30° of flexion, and the interphalangeal joints fully extended. Prior to initiating an active motion regime, maximal passive digital flexion should be restored (Fig. 26.2). This will assist in reducing the work of flexion on the repaired tendon and preventing joint stiffness. Edema also plays a significant role in the limitation of motion, especially in the early phase following surgery. For this reason, active mobilization regime begins on the third to fifth days in line with current thinking on the subsidence of postoperative edema. Active flexion exercises were initiated from the distal interphalangeal (dip) joint, and motion should be confined to the outer range or first third of flexion. In fact, resistance to digital flexion increases over the first two-thirds of flexion increasing five- to tenfold in the final third. The degrees of digital active flexion will be increased after 1 week until reaching the complete active flexion in the fourth week. Active IP (interphalangeal) joint extension exercises are very important and should be performed regularly to prevent the loss of extension at the IP joints, which is a common complication in this type of injury. Patients did not move the wrist until the third week and performed passive and active digital exercises with the wrist immobilized inside the splint. From the third to the sixth weeks, the patient removed the splint only to perform the exercise (Table 26.1). With the pullout technique, the risk of tendon rupture is lower. For this reason, the active mobilization regime of the fingers and wrist begins immediately without any limit in the degrees of movement. The splint was worn only at night and in dangerous activities. The pullout is removed at 6 weeks after a surgical check (Table 26.2).

The study was conducted from 2017 to 2018 in the Hand Surgery and Rehabilitation department

Table 26.1 Rehabilitation regime for flexor tendon repair with a four-strand suture

- Begin the motion at 3–5 days postoperative
- Protective dorsal splint applied to be worn for 6 weeks
- Prioritize restoration of full passive digital flexion
- Start early active motion from the DIP joint
- Encourage active digital extension exercise
- Move the wrist at 3 weeks
- Begin the complete active flexion of fingers at 4 weeks
- At 6 weeks, remove splint during the day but worn it for the night
- At 6 weeks, commence stretching and splinting of residual flexion deformity
- Return to normal activity between 10 and 12 weeks

Table 26.2 Rehabilitation regime for flexor tendon repair with pullout technique

- Begin the motion at 3–5 days postoperative
- Protective dorsal splint worn at night and in dangerous activities for 6 weeks
- Prioritize restoration of full passive digital flexion
- Start active movement of the fingers in all degrees of flexion
- Encourage active digital extension exercise
- Stimulate to use the fingers in activity of the day
- At 6 weeks, remove the pullout
- At 6 weeks, commence stretching and splinting of residual flexion deformity
- Return to normal activity between 10 and 12 weeks

at the IRCCS (Scientific Institute of Recovery and Care) Multimedica group of Lombardy. Small patients aged 3–12 years with lesions of the flexor tendons in areas 1, 2, and 3 operated from 2017 to 2018 were included. The inclusion criteria were lesion of the flexor digitorum profundus tendon, of the flexor digitorum superficialis, a combination of the FDP (flexor digitorum profundus) and FDS (flexor digitorum superficialis) tendon, and of the flexor pollicis longus; injury zones I, II, and III; concomitant neurovascular injury; surgical repair with a four-strand suture associated with epitendinous suture or with pullout technique; and start of the partial early active motion protocol no later than 7 days after repair. The exclusion criteria were associated injuries such as fractures, volar plate, and pulley injury. In children aged 8–12 years, the flexor tendons were repaired with a four-strand associated with epitendinous suture using the Prolene 3.0 for the central suture and Prolene 5.0 for the peripheral suture. The pullout technique was used for children aged 3–7 years. After the surgical repair, a dorsal thermoplastic splint (photo) was applied and the patients were started the rehabilitation regimen based on the partial early active motion protocol. The exercises were performed several times a day at home under parental supervision and with the hand therapist three times a week. The evaluation scales used were AROM (active range of motion), TAM (total active motion), % TAM, Strickland, Buck-Gramcko, and Scala Vas.

Active flexion and extension at the proximal and distal interphalangeal joints of the injured fingers were measured by a hand therapist using a goniometer. Postoperative outcome for joint function was assessed using the total active of motion (TAM) scoring system suggested by the American Society for Surgery of the Hand. The results were also established using Buck-Gramcko score and the Strickland and Glogovac Grading System with excellent (85–100%), good (70–84%), fair (50–69%), and poor (<50%) postoperative function.

Between April and December 2018, four children were treated. Of them, two were males and two were females. The mean age was 6 years (range 3–9 years). In total, four digits were affected: thumb $n = 1$, middle finger $n = 2$, and small finger $n = 1$. The flexor digitorum profundus (FDP) tendon was affected in two fingers, the flexor pollicis longus (FLP) tendon in one finger and the combination of the flexor digitorum profundus (FDP) and the flexor digitorum superficialis (FDS) tendons in one finger. The number of tendon laceration in zone I was two and in zone II was two. Concomitant neurovascular transection was diagnosed in two patients. The patients were subdivided by age into two groups: 3–7 years (two digits) whose tendons were repaired with pullout technique and 8–12 years (two digits) whose tendons were repaired with a four-strand suture associated with the epitendinous suture. There were no complications such as rupture, inflammation, infection, and contractures of the proximal interphalangeal joint at the final follow-up. No patient needs tenolysis. Good and excellent results were registered in all four digits, respectively, with the TAM score and the Strickland Method. According to the Buck-Gramcko evaluation system, all digits showed excellent functional results. Mean Vas score was 1 only given to the 8–12 years' group and the final mean was 1. All parents were happy with the final results.

In adults, early active motion is the principle of flexor tendon rehabilitation. The need for a stronger central suture to resist the early active movement regimen has been underlined for several years in adults. Several studies have shown excellent results with the four-strand technique associated with the epitendinous suture. The suture technique is a critical factor in children compared to adults. Although it is possible to place more than one core suture in an adult-size tendon, this might not always be possible in the smaller pediatric-size tendon. In this study, we have not wanted to compare different suturing techniques, but the suture technique and the post-operative rehabilitation program are greatly influenced by the age group and by the cooperation of child. In literature, many different forms of early mobilization programs have been used. Preschoolers are frequently immobilized in a cast for 3–4 weeks, while for children between 5 and 10 years of age, most of the recent articles recommends a modified early mobilization program under the supervision of a hand therapist but the fingers are immobilized between physiotherapy sessions [4]. In our experience, the children aged 0–2 years are frequently immobilized with splint for 3–4 weeks [5] in children between 3 and 7 years of age with flexor tendon injury in zone I, we use the pullout repair technique and the active motion regime start immediately without any limitation of the movements at the level of the fingers and wrist. This is because the pullout technique is safer and the possibility of tendon rupture is lower. So it is used in younger children where the use of splint is difficult to manage and rehabilitation does not require complex exercises. For patients between 8 and 12 years, we use an early active motion regimen after the tendon reparation with a four-strand suture associated with the epitendinous suture, as for adult injuries. In this case, our postoperative rehabilitation protocol involves an early but partial active movement of the fingers for the first 3 postoperative weeks because resistance to digital flexion increases over the first two-thirds of flexion increasing five- to tenfold in the final third week. The wrist is immobilized inside the splint until 3 weeks, and only after this period it is possible to move it. There was not any difference in the post-operative outcomes between groups of age in this study. In fact, using the Strickland criteria and Buck-Gramcko evaluation, all children qualified for an excellent outcome in all four fingers. Comparing our data with the Nietosvaara and

Al-Qattan's studies who promote immediate active mobilization, we obtained 50% of the excellent results before a year according to the Strickland criteria. Moreover, in our study, there were not cases of tendon rupture and of contractures of the proximal interphalangeal joint and tenolysis. The VAS scale was administered only to the 8–12 years' group by reason of poor compliance and understanding of children under 7 years old, and we had a very low score at the end of the treatment.

We did not evaluate the grip strength and the DASH (Disabilities of the Arm, Shoulder, and Hand) questionnaire because it was developed and validated for adults. However, the results obtained with early active motion after flexor tendon repair are encouraging considering the tendency to reduce complication rates and early recovery of finger movement and functionality. In addition, we believe that early active motion by promoting tendon gliding immediately avoids the exclusion of the hand and the loss of the motor pattern and favors the return to play activities. We have shown that it can easily be applied to children and is well tolerated by them and their families.

References

1. Nietosvaara Y, Lindfors NC, Palmu S, Rautakorpi S, Ristaniemi N. Flexor tendon injuries in pediatric patients. J Hand Surg Am. 2007;32(10):1549–57.
2. Al-Qattan MM. Flexor tendon injuries in the child. J Hand Surg Eur. 2013;39(1):46–53.
3. Sikora S, Lai M, Arneja JS. Flexor tendon injuries pediatric: a 10-year outcome analysis. Can J Plast Surg. 2013;21(3):181–5.
4. Moehrlen U, Mazzone L, Bieli C, Weber DM. Early mobilization after flexor tendon repair in children. Eur J Pediatr Surg. 2009;19(2):83–6.
5. Kato H, Minami A, Suenaga N, Iwasaki N, Kimura T. Long term results after primary repairs of zone 2 flexor tendon lacerations in children younger than age 6 years. J Pediatr Orthop. 2002;22(6):732–5.

27 Pediatric Hand Fractures

Filippo M. Senes, Luigi A. Nasto,
Nunzio Catena, and Chiara Arrigoni

Abstract

Pediatric hand fractures can be anatomically classified as fractures or dislocations of the wrist, carpus, metacarpals, and phalanxes. Wrist fractures (i.e., distal metaphyseal radius and/or ulna fractures) represent 20% of all fractures in growing children. These injuries can be classed as simple fractures with no displacement, greenstick fractures, and complete fractures with dislocation and overlapping of the fracture fragments. However, in almost 90% of cases they require conservative treatment. Pediatric carpal fractures are rare, commonly observed in adolescents rather than in children because of the cartilaginous matrix of carpal bones. Metacarpal and phalanxes show typical fracture patterns: metacarpal fractures are most commonly metaphyseal compression fractures or Salter-Harris (SH) type II physeal fractures and are frequently observed in the I and V rays; phalangeal fractures are the most common hand fractures in children and the distal phalanx is the most injured. Dislocation of metacarpophalangeal (MP) and interphalangeal (IP) joints is not frequently reported in children. Minor fingertip injuries are very common instead. Sometimes simple wound care will be enough in achieving complete healing, but in cases of larger skin loss with exposed fractures, advancement flap or, more rarely, regional flaps or skin grafts could be required.

Keywords

Pediatric · Children · Hand · Fractures · Dislocations · Wound

F. M. Senes (✉)
Department of Hand Surgery and Rehabilitation, S. Giuseppe MultiMedica Hospital, Milan University, Milano, Italy
e-mail: filipposenes@fastwebnet.it

L. A. Nasto
UOC Ortopedia e Traumatologia, IRCCS Istituto Giannina Gaslini, Genova, Italy

N. Catena
UOSD Microchirurgia Ricostruttiva e Chirurgia della Mano, IRCCS Giannina Gaslini, Genova, Italy

C. Arrigoni
Scuola di Specializzazione in Ortopedia e Traumatologia, Università degli Studi di Torino, Torino, Italy

27.1 Introduction

Pediatric hand fractures can be classified anatomically as fractures and dislocations of the wrist region, carpus, metacarpals, and phalanxes [1].

27.1.1 Wrist Region Fractures

Wrist fractures (i.e., distal metaphyseal radius and/or ulna fractures) represent 20% of all frac-

G. Pajardi (ed.), *Pediatric Hand Surgery*, https://doi.org/10.1007/978-3-031-30984-7_27

tures in growing children. These injuries can be classified as simple fractures with no displacement, greenstick fractures (i.e., monocortical fractures), and complete fractures with dislocation and overlapping of the fracture fragments [2]. Finally, epiphyseal fractures of the distal radius are also very common and can be associated with a fracture of the distal ulna.

Pain, tenderness, and local swelling are the three most common findings in wrist fractures. In displaced fractures, there is an obvious clinical deformity of the wrist, typically a bayonet deformity with dorsal displacement of the distal fragment. X-ray imaging helps in establishing a correct diagnosis, although it can be negative in cases of SH type I of the distal radius.

Not displaced fractures, greenstick fractures, and complete fractures can be treated with cast immobilization. If some significant displacement or angulation is present, this can be usually reduced in the casting room after a brief procedural analgesia. This allows conservative treatment for almost 90% of fractures in the distal radius and ulna region. However, displaced fractures with significant overlapping of the fracture fragments will require reduction under anesthesia. If the reduction is unstable, temporary pinning of the fracture is advised. The upper limb is immobilized in a well-molded cast after the procedure, with flexion of the wrist if needed. X-ray imaging is obtained 1 week after reduction to exclude any loss of correction, and the cast is removed at 5 weeks.

Displaced SH type I or II distal radius fractures are very easy to diagnose, and an X-ray shows the direction of the displacement. The complete reduction can be achieved at this level by closed means and short procedural anesthesia. The wrist is immobilized in a closed well-molded cast for 4 weeks. X-ray imaging is always obtained 1 week after reduction to rule out any loss of correction.

Fractures and epiphyseal injuries of the wrist show very good healing with almost complete restoration of the anatomy even in cases of moderate displacement. This is due to the great growth and repair potential of this anatomical region in growing children and pediatric patients.

27.1.2 Carpal Bone Fractures

Pediatric carpal bone fractures are rare and usually observed in adolescents [3]. Carpal bones are largely cartilaginous in children, thus less prone to fractures. Higher-energy trauma normally causes multiple fractures of the carpal bones with associated metacarpal fractures [4].

The scaphoid is the most commonly injured carpal bone. The scaphoid fracture can be observed either in isolation or with a distal radius fracture. This fracture is exceedingly rare before the age of seven [4, 5]. In more than 50% of cases, a distal pole fracture is observed, while fractures of the body or proximal pole are less common [6, 7].

Clinically, focal tenderness is observed at the anatomical snuffbox and along the axis of the first ray. A scaphoid fracture can be easily missed on X-rays, especially if only a small angulation is present or a limited interruption of the cortex. However, if focal tenderness can be elicited at the anatomical snuffbox in presence of negative X-ray, a short period of immobilization (2 weeks) with a cast is advised. X-ray is then repeated at the end of the immobilization period to confirm the presence of a fracture. In children, treatment is nonoperative. Cast immobilization is maintained for 4 weeks in incomplete fractures, while complete fractures are splinted for 4–8 weeks. In cases of belated diagnosis or delayed healing, cast immobilization can be extended up to 8–16 weeks until complete healing is achieved.

Ossification of the scaphoid bone proceeds in a distal to proximal direction. This is followed by rapid vascularization, which explains why complications typical of adult patients (i.e., nonunion, bone necrosis) are usually absent in children. At the end of the ossification period, vascularization of the bone decreases and becomes more similar to the adult pattern. Avascular necrosis is very rare in children [6–8]. Similarly, nonunion is very rare in pediatric patients [9–12] (Fig. 27.1).

Interestingly, the lack of ossification or complete bone bridging on the X-ray is not necessarily a demonstration of nonunion in pediatric patients. Often, a fibrous tissue bridge develops between the fracture fragments. Nevertheless,

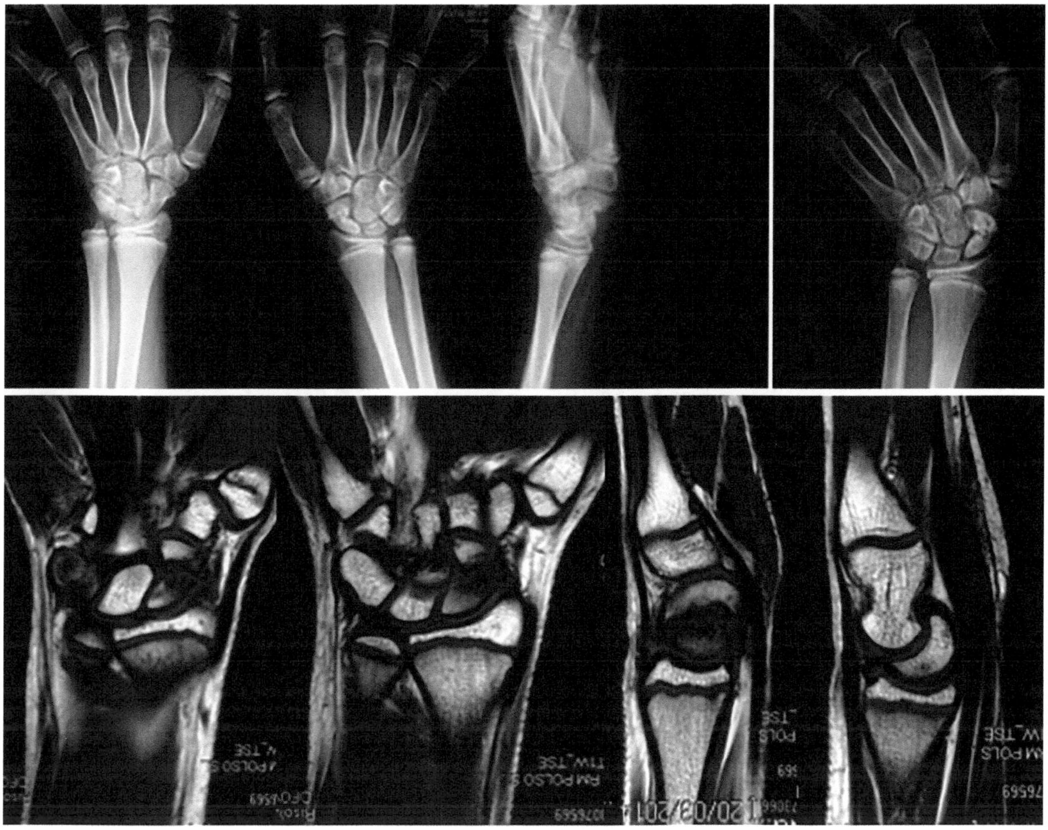

Fig. 27.1 Shaft scaphoid fracture hesitated in nonunion

prolonged immobilization allows complete healing of the fracture. The rare cases of pediatric scaphoid bone nonunion have been successfully treated with bone grafting through a volar approach to the fracture site [13, 14] (Fig. 27.2).

Very rare fractures of other carpal bones (Fig. 27.3).

27.1.3 Metacarpal Fractures and Dislocations

Metacarpals and phalanxes show typical fracture patterns. The presence of a single growth plate explains the typical fracture patterns seen in these bones.

Metacarpal fractures are most commonly observed in I and V rays. These injuries are generally metaphyseal compression or SH type II physeal fractures. The epiphysis of the I metacarpal is located at the base of the bone, while in the remaining metacarpals, the epiphysis is located distally, at the head of the bone.

Diaphyseal fractures of metacarpals are unusual. Oblique or spiral fracture pattern and modest displacement occur, as adult fractures. These are most commonly observed in the II and III metacarpal. Isolated or multiple diaphyseal fractures can be immobilized in a cast with MCP joints flexed and PIP and DIP joints extended. If bone fragments are severely displaced, closed reduction should be attempted and followed by 4 weeks cast splinting. Sometimes, Kirshner wire pinning is needed to maintain reduction; rarely, plate and screw fixation are required (Fig. 27.4).

Fractures of the distal third of II, III, and IV metacarpals are rare in children and adolescents [15, 16]. In distal metaphyseal fractures, the metacarpal heads are always tilted on the

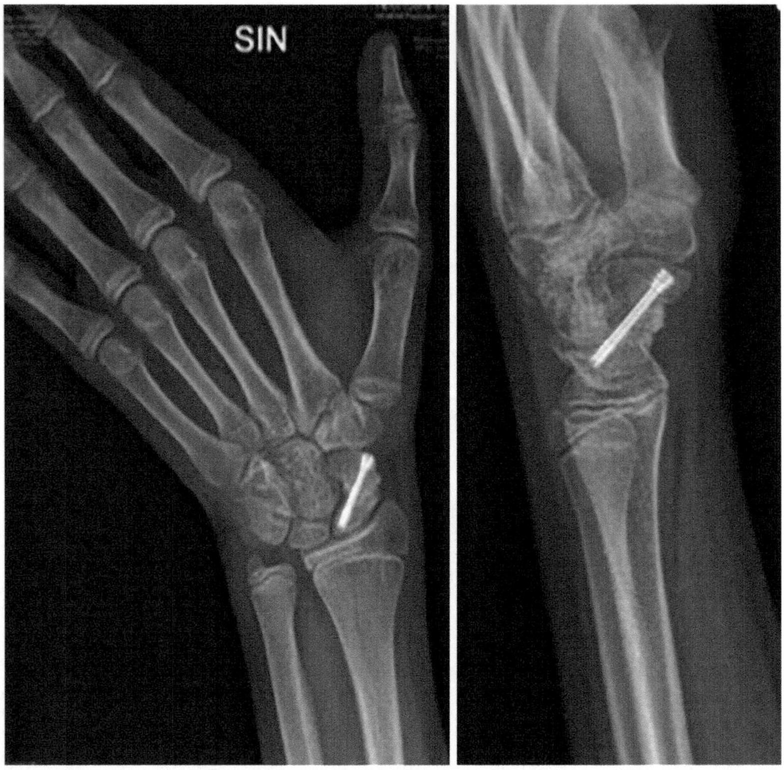

Fig. 27.2 Scaphoid nonunion treated with allograft from the distal radius

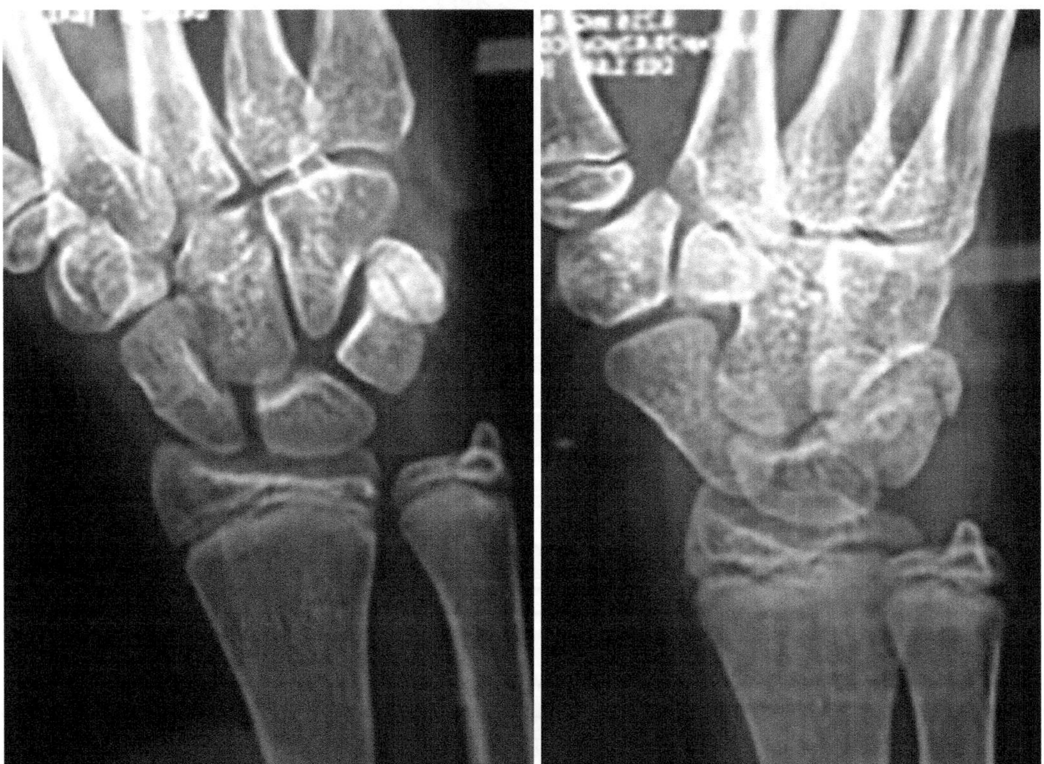

Fig. 27.3 Triquetral fracture

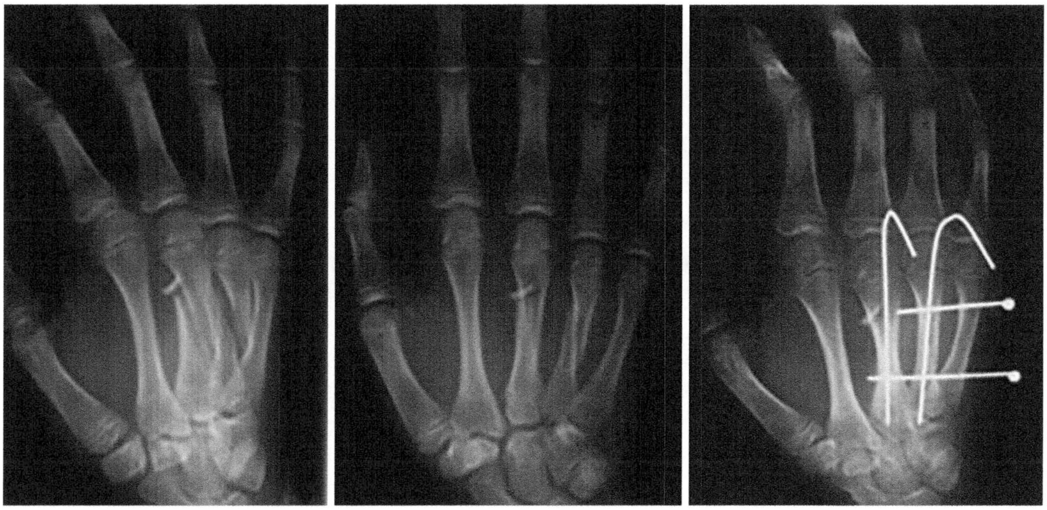

Fig. 27.4 Spiral diaphyseal displaced fractures of III and IV metacarpals treated with closed reduction and Kirshner wire pinning

volar side because of the strong action of flexor tendons. Often, ulnar angulation is also observed.

Greenstick metaphyseal or SH type II epiphyseal fractures are most commonly observed at the level of the V and IV rays. These fractures are typically due to direct trauma (punch injury) and are displaced into flexion. Acceptable angular deformities and indications for reduction have been discussed elsewhere [17–19].

In adolescents, when growth plates are about to close, the loss of physiological prominence of metacarpals and the decreased growth potential of metacarpals require an almost anatomical reduction. Closed reduction of the angular deviation and cast immobilization are usually performed. Unstable and irriducible fractures are treated through percutaneous Kirshner wires pinning. Odgen advises against the use of endomedullary Kirshner wires in metacarpals to avoid growth retardation and prevent from growth plate damage. In our opinion, growth plate injury is due to repeated attempts at cannulating the metacarpal rather than physis transfixion by a single wire.

The incomplete correction or reduction determine a metacarpal shortening. This can be due to epiphyseal healing in a flexed position, or to posttraumatic epiphysiodesis as a result of growth plate injury. The latter mechanism is more common in SH type III and IV fractures than in type II injuries [20, 21].

Fractures of the first metacarpal are tipically located at the base/proximal third of the bone as a SH type II injury. Open growth plate differs these fractures from Bennet and Rolando's fractures observed in adult patients [22, 23]. The displacement pattern is determined by the strong intercapsular volar oblique ligament, which spans from the trapezium to the base of the I metacarpal (Fig. 27.5).

There is huge variability in terms of clinical presentation, radiographic findings, and amount of displacement of the metaphyseal fragment [24–26]. Generally, metacarpal diaphysis is dorsally and proximally displaced. Furthermore, diaphyseal shaft is also twisted in supination by the abductor pollicis longus muscle, and radially displaced by the adductor pollicis muscle. The abundant and thick periosteum limits a marked fracture fragments displacement while it provides stability to closed reduction.

Although minimal displacement can be treated with cast immobilization, an anatomical reduction

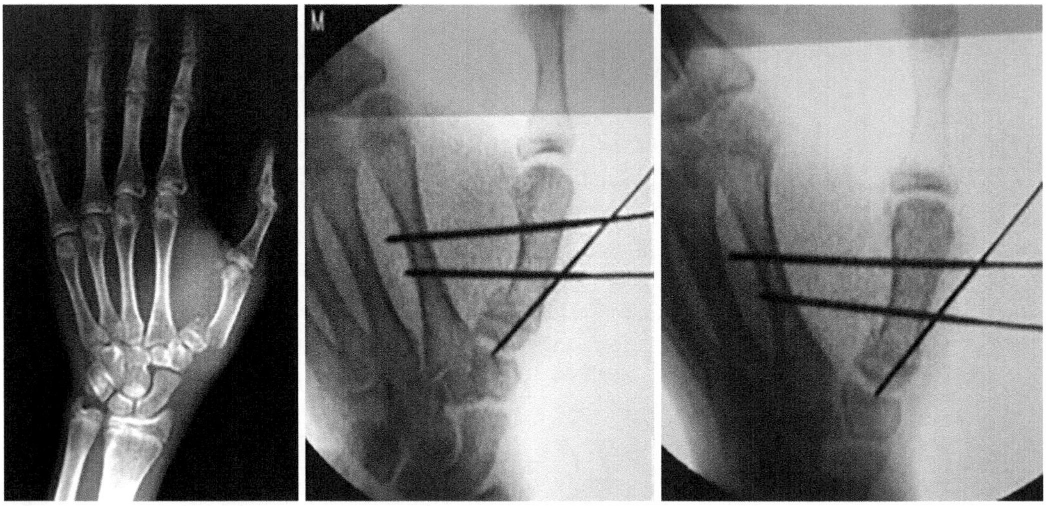

Fig. 27.5 First metacarpal base displaced fracture treated with closed reduction and Kirshner wire pinning

is always advisable. In any case, displacement >30° must be always corrected and reduced.

Reduction is achieved with longitudinal traction on the extremity of the thumb, along with abduction, extension, and pronation of the metacarpal. Hyperextension of the metacarpal should be avoided. The maneuver is completed by pushing at the base of the first finger while applying an opposing force on the head of the first metacarpal.

Less commonly, a fracture with complete dislocation of the metaphysis through a buttonhole of the periosteum can be observed. This can prevent closed reduction and makes open reduction necessary. In these cases, ulnar deviation of the base of the metacarpal is most often noted.

Non-displaced diaphyseal metacarpal fractures are conservatively treated, while displaced fractures are reduced following the metacarpal longitudinal axis. As with other metacarpals, immobilization is maintained for 4 weeks and can be extended for an extra 2–4 weeks if bone healing is insufficient.

27.1.4 Phalangeal Fractures and Dislocations

Phalangeal fractures are the most common hand fractures in children. Although all three phalanxes can be interested from bone damage, the distal phalanx is the most frequently injured. Fractures of phalanxes can be classified as fractures of proximal part of the bone (physeal injuries), fractures of the diaphysis (extraphyseal injuries), and fractures of distal part of the bone (extraphyseal injuries) (Fig. 27.6).

Most commonly, only a small cortical defect is identified on the X-rays. These injuries can be treated with a short period of immobilization, achieving a complete resolution of the symptoms.

Fractures of the proximal phalanx of the thumb are commonly physeal injuries and are clinically equivalent to adult ligamentous injuries interesting the metacarpophalangeal joint. All types of physeal injuries can be seen at this level; however, while SH type III and IV fractures usu-

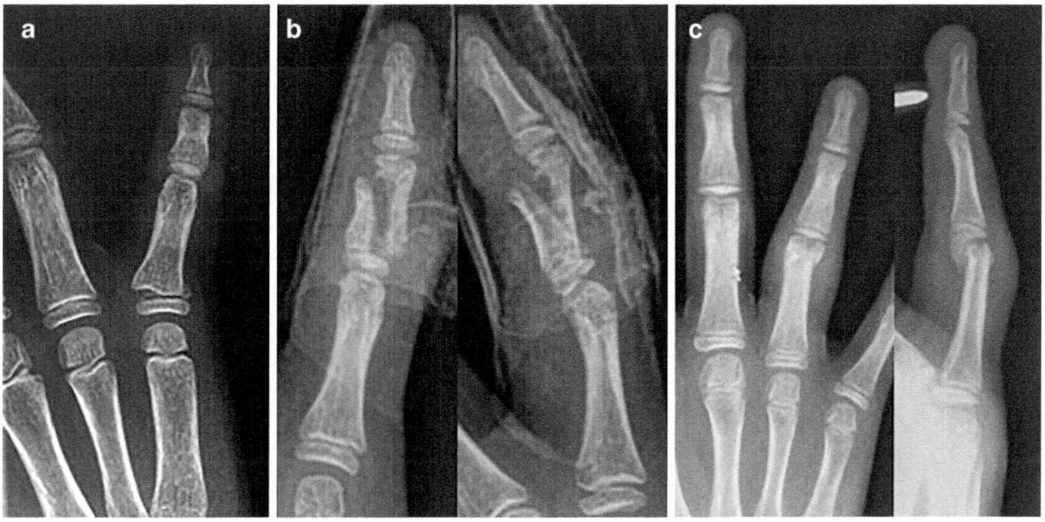

Fig. 27.6 Phalangeal fractures can be classified as proximal physeal fractures (**a**), diaphyseal fractures (**b**), and distal extraphyseal fractures (**c**)

ally require open reduction and internal fixation, SH types I and II can be treated conservatively by spinting the thumb into adduction to prevent later displacement. Similarly, neck (subcapital) fractures of proximal phalanx of the thumb must be adequately immobilized because they can easily displace and undergo malunion.

Tubercle fractures of the distal phalanx usually result from a crush injury and are typical in younger children. On the other hand, epiphyseal fractures of the distal phalanx are less common and are seen in older children after a crush injury. These fractures are at risk of infection, growth plate damage, and secondary epiphysiodesis. Furthermore, volar insertion of the FDP tendon leads to secondary flexion displacement of the distal fragment, while dorsal insertion of the extensor tendon leads to extension displacement of the proximal (physeal) fragment. Counteraction of these forces can be obtained with Kirshner wire fixation, especially in SH type III and IV injuries.

Basal proximal phalanx fractures of the long fingers are usually SH type II injuries with large metaphyseal fragment (Thurstan-Holland fragment). In older children, these are less commonly SH type III and IV injuries. SH type V fractures are exceedingly rare and treatment depends on the amount of displacement. These fractures are at risk of growth arrest. In proximal phalanxes, compression fractures of the proximal third of the bone are volarly angulated because of flexion and extension deforming forces of either intrinsic hand muscles or extensor tendons. On the X-rays, the fracture looks like a greenstick fracture, usually by the ulnar side of the cortex. Closed reduction and spinting are generally successful in obtaining realignment of the fracture. Sometimes, a full control of the proximal fragment can be difficult to attain. In these cases, a finger spacer (e.g., a pencil) can be used to displace radially the distal fragment (Fig. 27.7). Alternatively, MCP joints can be flexed to >90° and fracture reduced by re-tensioning collateral ligaments and pushing volarly the distal fragment.

In greenstick fractures, a complete breakage of contralateral cortex is sometimes needed to allow reduction of the fracture. However, preserving some continuity of the bone and periosteum allows preservation of some stability and prevents hypercorrection.

Treatment of non-displaced epiphyseal fractures requires 15–20 days of immobilization with a tongue blade and elastic bandage. When the alignment is not acceptable, closed reduction is needed. After reduction, the finger is

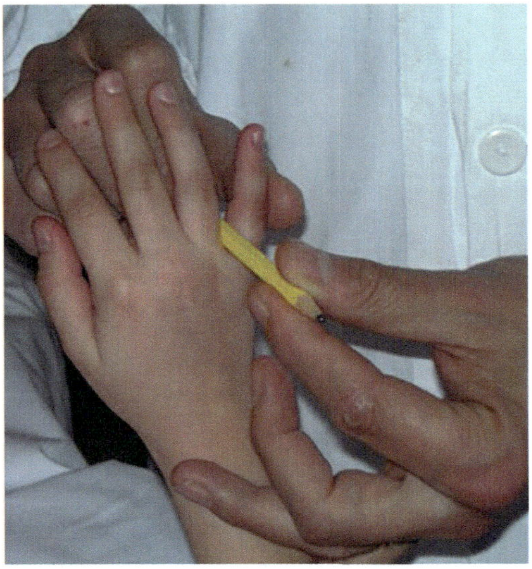

Fig. 27.7 Finger spacer technique for closed reduction

splinted along with the adjacent finger (i.e., buddy taping) for 3 weeks. The involved fingers are immobilized with MCP joints flexed at 60° and PIP joints flexed at 15°, making sure that fingers are kept parallel. While in adolescents and older children, elastic bandages are preferable, cast immobilization is advisable in younger children. The inclusion of the V metacarpal for ulnar side fingers, or thenar eminence for radial side fingers and thumb, allows for a safe and effective restriction from the activity and better stability. Open reduction and Kirshner wire fixation are preferred methods when closed reduction is failed, residual rotatory deformity, or a small epiphyseal fragment is impeding the reduction [27]. Usually, close reduction and kirshner wire percutaneous pinning are successful. In case of severe palmar displacement of distal fracture fragment, open reduction is needed [26].

At the level of proximal phalanxes, up to 10° of coronal displacement can be tolerated because of the compensatory action of the adjacent MCP joint. However, middle and distal phalanxes show a minimal adaptation to coronal displacement. Shaft fractures of the proximal and middle phalanxes follow similar patterns and treatment strategies. More than 75% of phalanx fractures are treated conservatively with a brief period of immobilization. Only 15% of fractures require a closed reduction, while roughly 10% will require open procedures. According to Leonard and Dubravcik, in 40% of cases surgically treated fractures are located in the metaphyseal area, while 26% are diaphyseal [27, 28].

Non-displaced diaphyseal fractures of the phalanxes are conservatively treated by 3 weeks of immobilization. In cases of displaced or unstable fracture patterns (e.g., oblique or spiral fractures), an open reduction is indicated with Kirshner wire fixation followed by 6 weeks of immobilization. Surgical approach should be cautious in diaphyseal fractures because of the poor vascularity of the distal fragment. Delayed angulation can be prevented by immobilizing MCP and interphalangeal joints into flexion. Loss of correction and malunion leads to loss of digital cascade during flexion with overlapping of the fingers.

As long as axial and transverse plane alignment is preserved, pediatric patients can make up for malalignment of phalanx fractures. Rotatory defects are the main complication of diaphyseal finger fractures and must be prevented through a careful clinical examination. There are three main causes of rotatory defects: a missed rotatory displacement at the time of the fracture, incomplete reduction of the fracture, and inappropriate immobilization. A thorough X-ray examination of the fracture through lateral and oblique views allows early recognition of a rotatory defect. In cases of a delayed diagnosis, a rotational osteotomy is the only viable option of treatment. In well-aligned fractures involving only one cortex and presenting with minimal metaphyseal angulation, a 15–20 days of casting or splinting period is sufficient.

Neck (subcapital) fractures of the phalanxes are equally common. They usually present with a dorsal displacement of the distal fragment. Furthermore, rotatory malalignment is often present due to the action of the volar plate on the condylar fragment, which can be incarcerated in the capsule and the collateral ligament. The presence of rotatory malalignment must be ruled out on X-ray lateral views, before and after a closed reduction. Percutaneous fixation with Kirshner wires is advised, whether an open or closed reduction is performed. Healing of these fractures happens as early as 3 weeks, and malalignment at this level leads to a reduction of the range of motion of the adjacent joints. Furthermore, the risk of malunion or nonunion is increased [29].

A frequent fracture of fifth digit proximal phalanx is the "extra-octave" fracture, which involves the base of the proximal phalanx with extreme ulnar deviation of the distal fragment. It is a type II epiphyseal fracture that can be easily reduced with closed manipulation. Reduction is achieved by placing a pencil in the web space and pushing the fifth digit radially. The reduced finger is splinted to the adjacent, uninjured finger. Immobilization is maintained for 3 weeks. Rarely, open reduction with pinning is required to maintain reduction until complete fracture healing.

Small epiphyseal fractures of the phalanxes can be observed at the insertion of the collateral ligaments. These are almost always pure cartilaginous fractures and do not affect bone growth. In cases of bigger fractures, articular involvement should be ruled out as this may lead to loss of articular congruence.

Fractures of the distal phalanx with mallet finger deformity are similar to adult lesions, although there are some anatomical differences between the two age groups. In small children, SH type I or II fractures are typical, while in adolescents SH type III and IV lesions are more common. Extensor tendon detachment at the distal phalanx is rare in children. Furthermore, ossification of the epiphyseal portion of the phalanx lately occurs, making diagnosis and treatment more difficult. Epiphyseal fractures require DIP joint casting into hyperextension for 3 weeks, while 4–6 weeks immobilization is advised in cases of isolated tendon injuries. If closed anatomical reduction cannot be obtained, surgery is indicated, and an open reduction is performed with Kirshner wire fixation (Fig. 27.8).

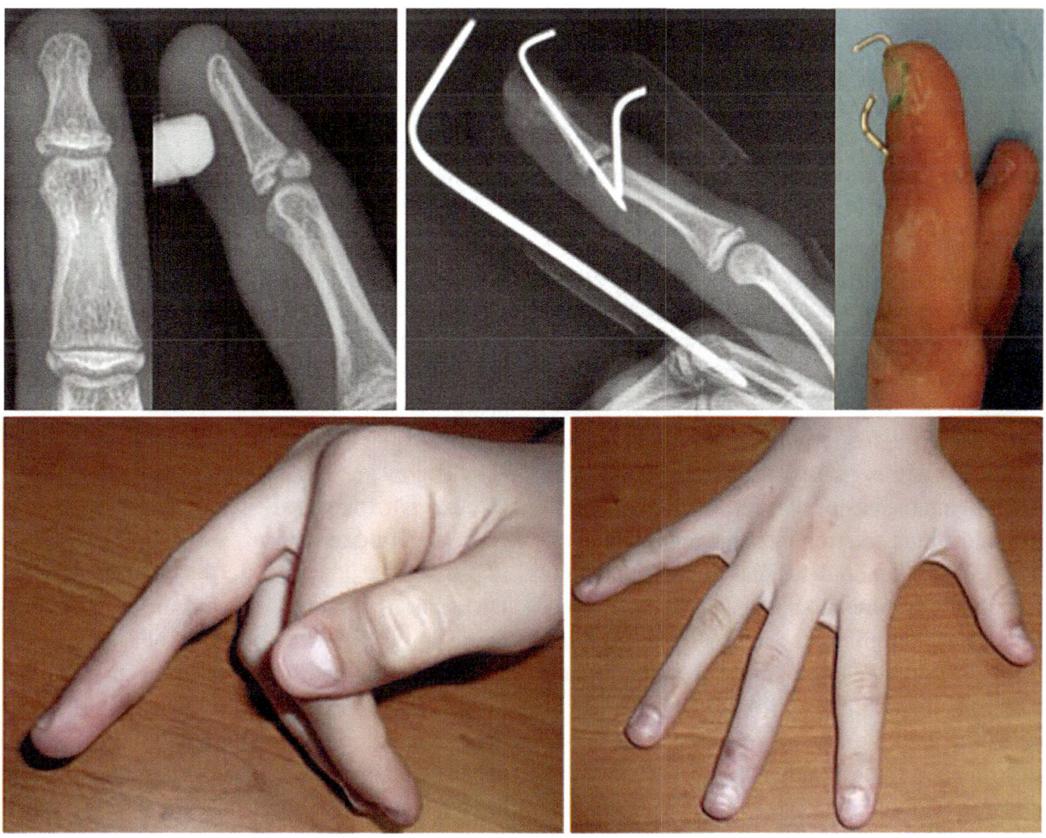

Fig. 27.8 Mallet finger injury treated with Kirshner wire pinning through closed reduction (Ishiguro technique)

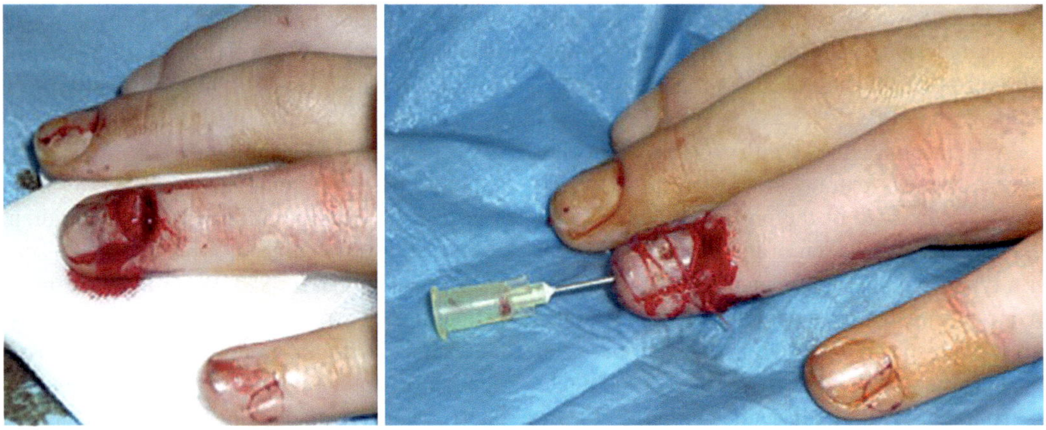

Fig. 27.9 Open fractures with nail avulsion

Open reduction and fixation are also indicated in doubtful cases with rupture of the extensor tendon. A similar technique can be used in rare lesions of the volar portion of the distal phalanx with displacement due to FDP insertion [30, 31].

Open fractures with mallet finger deformity in distal phalanxes can be seen after crush injuries. These fractures are in high-stakes of infection. Debridement of the nail bed at the fracture site (Seymour fracture), repair of the nail bed, and repositioning of the nail with immobilization are usually performed.

Fractures of the tubercle or meta-epiphyseal region of the distal phalanx are associated with nail laminal or germinal matrix injuries. As open fractures, bacterial contamination and infection are typical complications [32]. Severe diastasis of the fracture fragments is uncommon because of the presence of fibrous septa. Treatment consists of nail repositioning into its bed and suture fixation to allow regrowth of the nail. Stitches should be placed atraumatically (with 5–6/0 sutures) to allow a rapid reconstruction and minimize residual deformities (Fig. 27.9) [33]. A wound soft bandage acts like fracture fixation until complete healing is obtained.

Minor fingertip injuries are very common in children and young adolescents. Simple wound care is sufficient in achieving complete healing of the wound and preserving the length and neurological function of the finger. In cases of larger skin loss with tubercle exposure, a simple advancement flap can be used for coverage. Less commonly, regional flaps (e.g., cross-finger flap, thenar eminence flap) or a skin graft from the wrist or forearm can be used. The choice of the graft/coverage strategy depends on the amount of skin loss, age of the patient, surgeon's experience, and parents' expectations. If apical skin loss is minimal, a local V-Y skin flap can be used with very good results (Fig. 27.10).

In cases of subamputation with a thin skin pedicle, a simple wound margin apposition with stitching can be attempted. Most of the time, satisfactory healing can be obtained. Nevertheless, it is of utmost importance to carefully and regularly check the repair process until complete healing is obtained.

27.1.5 Metacarpal-Phalangeal Dislocations

Dislocations of the MCP joints are a quite common in children, although not frequently reported. The I and II rays are typically involved [34]. A forceful hyperextension of the II finger due to a fall on the floor with open hand is the usual injury mechanism. The volar plate is broken at the level of the metacarpal head. Dorsal displacement of the phalanx leads to the intra-articular dislocation of the volar plate

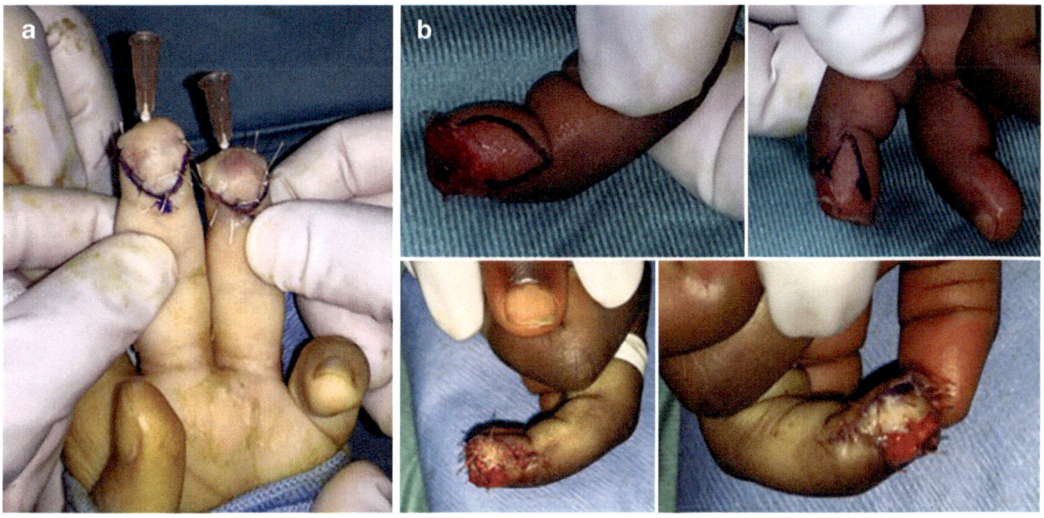

Fig. 27.10 Local flaps in skin loss: V-Y (**a**) and bilateral Kutler (**b**)

(complex dislocation). The resulting ulnarization of the flexor tendons and radialization of the lumbricals locks trigger the volar dislocation of the metacarpal head, which loses its natural fibrocartilaginous stabilizers. The metacarpal head also penetrates through the metacarpal transverse ligament and superficial palmar fascia, further obstructing the reduction.

Closed reduction can be difficult and sometimes impossible because of the intra-articular dislocation of the volar plate (Fig. 27.11).

It is preferable to avoid repeated attempts at closed reduction and proceed with an open procedure. The surgical approach consists of a volar exposure of the ray through a Brunner-type incision with a complete A1 pulley opening. A small longitudinal incision of the volar plate is performed to reduce the tension of the collateral ligament and allow atraumatic reduction of the metacarpal head. In cases of delayed diagnosis and treatment (usually after 3–4 weeks), an additional dorsal surgical approach is needed to cut and release ulnar collateral ligament [34]. After surgery, cast immobilization is applied to avoid hyperextension of the joint and keep MCP joints in flexion.

MCP joint dislocation at the thumb determines a volar dislocation of the metacarpal head through the thenar muscles (i.e., flexor pollicis brevis) and the articular capsule. The buttonhole through the joint capsule locks the metacarpal head impeding reduction. Closed reduction is attained by flexing the proximal phalanx to release intrinsic musculature and applying longitudinal traction. When closed reduction is unsuccessful, an open reduction is indicated.

27.1.6 Collateral Ligament of the Thumb

Isolated lesions of the ulnar collateral ligament of the thumb (i.e., Stener lesion) are rare in children. These injuries are usually due to an SH type III fracture of proximal phalanx epiphysis, while they are inconstly associated with a metacarpal basal fracture [35]. Surgery is often required to reconstruct the articular surface and avoid instability at the base of the thumb.

27.1.7 Interphalangeal Dislocations

Interphalangeal dislocations are rare pediatric injuries that typically occur in adolescents. They are due to direct trauma and common it found in the PIP joint. Diagnosis is easy and clear from clinical presentation. Sometimes, an associated epiphyseal fracture can be observed. This is due to the strong insertion of

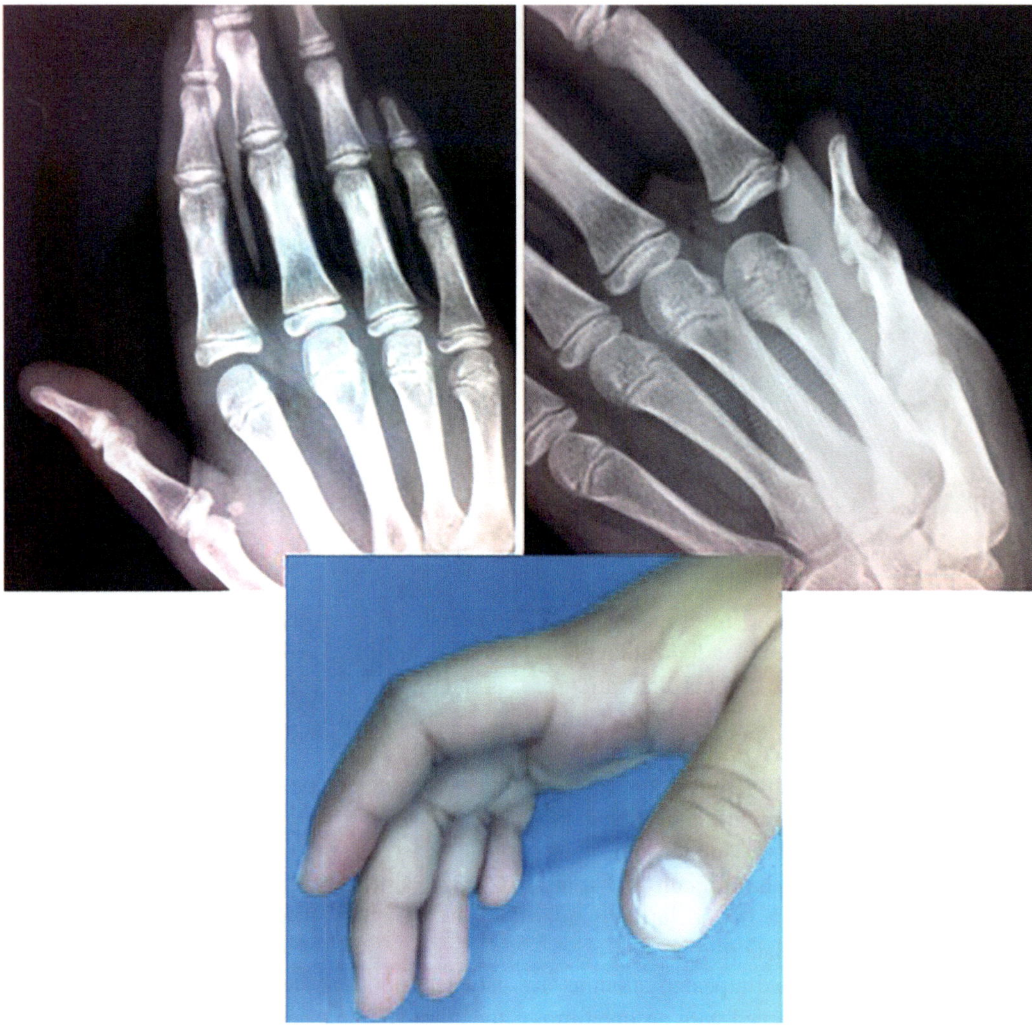

Fig. 27.11 Suspected intra-articular dislocation of the volar plate in the metacarpophalangeal joint

the collateral ligaments around the joint [36]. Malalignment of an untreated epiphyseal fracture can be permanent; therefore, this must be always ruled out before and after reduction. Reduction of interphalangeal joint dislocations is obtained by hyperextending the joint and then distally and volarly pushing the distal fragment. In cases of unsuccessful closed reduction interposition of the volar plate or epiphyseal fracture fragment should be take into consideration. After reduction, the stability of collateral ligaments and joint range of motion should be checked by comparison to the contralateral side. Post-reduction splinting (15 days) will be followed by active mobilization. In older children, buddy taping can be used instead of rigid immobilization.

References

1. Beatty E, Light TR, Belsole RJ, Ogden JA. Wrist and hand skeletal injuries in children. Hand Clin. 1990;6:723–38.
2. Herring J. Tachdjian's pediatric orthopaedics. Philadelphia: Saunders; 2013.
3. Goddard N. Carpal fractures in children. Clin Orthop Relat Res. 2005;(432):73–6.

4. Smida M, Nigrou K, Soohun T, Sallem R, Jalel C, Ben Ghachem M. Combined fracture of the distal radius and scaphoid in children. Report of 2 cases. Acta Orthop Belg. 2003;69(1):79–81.
5. Greene MH, Hadied AM, LaMont RL. Scaphoid fractures in children. J Hand Surg Am. 1984;9:536–41.
6. Larson B, Light TR, Ogden JA. Fracture and ischemic necrosis of the immature scaphoid. J Hand Surg Am. 1987;12:122–7.
7. Mussbichler H. Injuries of the carpal scaphoid in children. Acta Radiol. 1961;56:361–8.
8. Vahvanen V, Westerlund M. Fracture of the carpal scaphoid in children. A clinical and roentgenological study of 108 cases. Acta Orthop Scand. 1980;51:909–13.
9. Onuba O, Ireland J. Two cases of non-union of fractures of the scaphoid in children. Injury. 1983;15:109–12.
10. Southcott R, Rosman MA. Non-union of carpal scaphoid fractures in children. J Bone Joint Surg Br. 1977;59:20–3.
11. Maxted MJ, Owen R. Two cases of non-union of carpal scaphoid fractures in children. Injury. 1982;13:441–3.
12. Pick RY, Segal D. Carpal scaphoid fracture and non-union in an eight-year-old child. Report of a case. J Bone Joint Surg Am. 1983;65:1188–9.
13. Wilson-MacDonald J. Delayed union of the distal scaphoid in a child. J Hand Surg Am. 1987;12: 520–2.
14. García-Mata S. Carpal scaphoid fracture nonunion in children. J Pediatr Orthop. 2002;22(4):448–51.
15. Light TR, Ogden JA. Metacarpal epiphyseal fractures. J Hand Surg Am. 1987;12:460–4.
16. Steinert V, Knorr P. [Metacarpal and finger fractures in childhood]. Zentralbl Chir. 1971;96:113–24.
17. Almquist EE. Hand injuries in children. Pediatr Clin North Am. 1986;33:1511–22.
18. Valencia J, Leyva F, Gomez-Bajo GJ. Pediatric hand trauma. Clin Orthop Relat Res. 2005;(432):77–86.
19. Kelsch G, Ulrich C. Intramedullary k-wire fixation of metacarpal fractures. Arch Orthop Trauma Surg. 2004;124:523–6.
20. Rajesh A, Basu AK, Vaidhyanath R, Finlay D. Hand fractures: a study of their site and type in childhood. Clin Radiol. 2001;56:667–9.
21. Brown JE. Epiphyseal growth arrest in a fractured metacarpal. J Bone Joint Surg Am. 1959;41-A:494–6.
22. Hastings H, Simmons BP. Hand fractures in children. A statistical analysis. Clin Orthop Relat Res. 1984;(188):120–30.
23. Breen TF, Gelberman RH, Jupiter JB. Intra-articular fractures of the basilar joint of the thumb. Hand Clin. 1988;4:491–501.
24. Cannon SR, Dowd GS, Williams DH, Scott JM. A long-term study following Bennett's fracture. J Hand Surg Br. 1986;11:426–31.
25. Griffiths JC. Bennett's fracture in childhood. Br J Clin Pract. 1966;20:582–3.
26. Pellegrini VD. Fractures at the base of the thumb. Hand Clin. 1988;4:87–102.
27. Leonard MH, Dubravcik P. Management of fractured fingers in the child. Clin Orthop Relat Res. 1970;73:160–8.
28. Barton NJ. Fractures of the phalanges of the hand in children. Hand. 1979;11:134–43.
29. Simmons BP, Peters TT. Subcondylar fossa reconstruction for malunion of fractures of the proximal phalanx in children. J Hand Surg Am. 1987;12:1079–82.
30. McFarlane RM, Hampole MK. Treatment of extensor tendon injuries of the hand. Can J Surg. 1973;16:366–75.
31. Niechajev IA. Conservative and operative treatment of mallet finger. Plast Reconstr Surg. 1985;76:580–5.
32. Engber WD, Clancy WG. Traumatic avulsion of the fingernail associated with injury to the phalangeal epiphyseal plate. J Bone Joint Surg Am. 1978;60:713–4.
33. Ashbell TS, Kleinert HE, Putcha SM, Kutz JE. The deformed fingernail, a frequent result of failure to repair nail bed injuries. J Trauma. 1967;7:177–90.
34. Whipple TL, Evans JP, Urbaniak JR. Irreducible dislocation of a finger joint in a child. A case report. J Bone Joint Surg Am. 1980;62:832–3.
35. Stener B. Skeletal injuries associated with rupture of the ulnar collateral ligament of the metacarpophalangeal joint of the thumb. A clinical and anatomical study. Acta Chir Scand. 1963;125:583–6.
36. Ogden JA. Skeletal injury in the child. New York: Springer; 2000.

Replantation

28

Mona I. Winge and Magne Røkkum

Abstract

Most replantations are indicated in children due to their advantageous nerve regeneration, greater healing potential and functional outcome. A replanted limb has better functional results than a prosthesis. The proper care of the amputated extremity is essential during an expedient transfer to a replantation centre. The ischaemia time of an amputated part with musculature should not exceed 6 h, and a vascular shunt must be considered if possible. Vasospasms are more often encountered in children and must be recognised promptly and treated as early as possible considering the small vessel size. The outcomes depend on the type of injury, level of injury, the child`s weight, the ischaemia time and microsurgical competence of the surgical team. Increased survival rates are present when two veins are repaired. The follow-up is multidisciplinary and long term.

Keywords

Amputation · Children · Digit · Hand injuries Lower limb · Microsurgery · Paediatric Replantation · Revascularisation · Upper extremity

28.1 Background

The operating microscope was first used in 1921 for a middle ear operation with an introduction to ophthalmology in 1946 [1]. The first reported microvascular anastomosis using an operating microscope was performed by Jacobsen and Suarez in 1960 [2]. In 1962, Malt and McKhann successfully replanted a completely amputated upper extremity in a 12-year-old boy [3]. Kleinert and Kasdan performed the first successful anastomosis of a digital artery and revascularised a subtotally amputated thumb in 1962 [4]. Komatsu and Tamai replanted a completely amputated thumb in 1965 [5]. The refinement of suture materials and delicate microsurgical instruments made possible the development of microvascular surgical techniques [1]. In addition to replantations, microsurgical advances led to the introduction of free vascularised autotransplantations of the skin, bone, joints and toes [6, 7]. The first free vascularised composite allotransplantation of the upper extremity using modern immunosuppression was performed in an adult in 1998 and in an eight-year-old child in 2017 [8–10].

M. I. Winge (✉)
Division of Orthopaedic Surgery, Oslo University Hospital, Oslo, Norway
e-mail: mwinge@ous-hf.no

M. Røkkum
Oslo, Norway
e-mail: mrokkum@ous-hf.no

G. Pajardi (ed.), *Pediatric Hand Surgery*, https://doi.org/10.1007/978-3-031-30984-7_28

Replantation centres with a 24 h service exist today all over the world. These should include a team of several microvascular surgeons, an anaesthesiologist, theatre and ward nurses specialised in microvascular surgery and units for intensive and pre- operative/post-operative care, physiotherapy and occupational therapy [11]. Countries around the world organise differently their replantation centres. In the USA, a declining volume in the number of replantations has resulted in a reduction in microsurgical experience and success rate. A decline in success rates has been observed in the USA since 2000 from 80–90% to 48–57% [12]. This decline in replantations is associated with fewer industrial accidents and narrower indications for digital replantations. According to Squitieri, 52% of paediatric digit replantations were performed in centres with an annual volume of 1–2 such operations per year [13]. The outcome after surgery is dependent on microsurgical competence and frequency of replantations per surgeon per year. The creation of regional replant centres has been suggested as a solution to better the situation [12]. Sabapathy highlights the need for education and training of health professionals [14].

28.2 Terminology

Replantation is defined as the reattachment of an amputated part that was completely severed from the body. Revascularisation implies vascular insufficiency and an incomplete amputation of a part still attached to the body by the skin, nerve, tendon or bone (Fig. 28.1a–c). In both cases, vascular repair with reestablishment of the circulation is needed [11, 15–17].

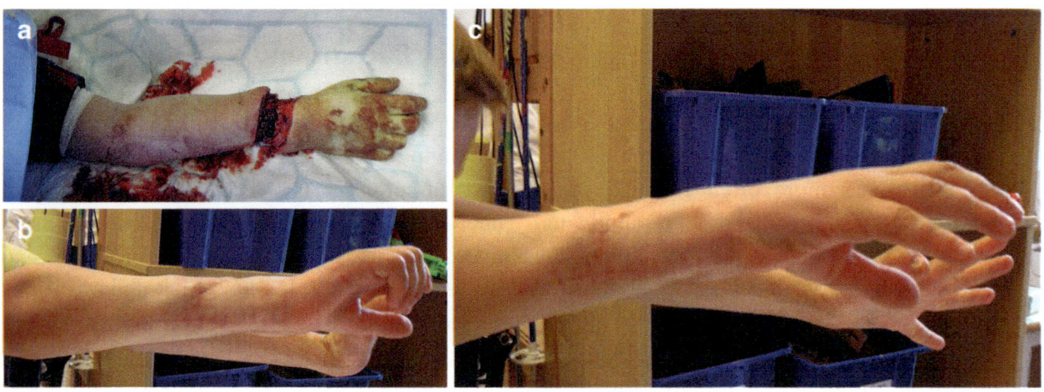

Fig. 28.1 (**a**) Wood splitter accident in an 8-year-old boy resulting in a partial amputation at distal radius level right side. (**b**, **c**) Functional result 3 years later

28.3 Epidemiology

The incidence rate of upper extremity amputations in children <18 years of age is relatively low and seems to vary considerably between the countries. The estimated incidence of serious amputations in the upper extremity (thumb, more than two fingers and proximal injuries) ages 0–19 years in Sweden in 1979 was 0.15 per 100,000 person years [18]. The incidence for total amputations ages 0–16 years in Southern Finland was 0.18 per 100,000 person years [19] whereas in Greece ages 0–14 years the incidence was 19.7 per 100,000 person years [20].

Injuries in the upper extremity needing a replantation or revascularisation in children 0–14 years of age have an incidence of 0.9 per 100,000 person years in an epidemiological study done in Southern Sweden [21]. The annual replantation incidence for adults and children was estimated to be 0.5–0.7 per 100,000 persons in Denmark [22], 1.9 per 100,000 person years in Sweden [21] and 1.9–3.4 per 100,000 in Finland (0.2–0.6 per 100,000 persons for serious amputations) [23].

In the USA, Taras reported that 9% of replantation patients were younger than 10 years of age and 20% between 11 and 20 years [24]. Squitieri found that amputations occurred more commonly in the white male population with an average age of 10 [13]. Jaeger however found two ages of peak incidence of amputation, at 5 and 15 years of age [25]. The youngest children are most inquisitive and injure themselves after placing their fingers in inappropriate places. The older children start participating more in activities outside the home which can end in very serious injuries [26, 27]. Replantation rates vary depending on the type of injury but also on the type of health-care system in each country. The rate of attempted finger replantation in children in the USA was 40% from 2000 to 2006. Blacks (odds ratio 0.47), Hispanics (odds ratio 0.37) and uninsured children (odds ratio 0.38) were significantly less likely to undergo replantation than Whites and children with health care [13].

Our upper extremity and microsurgical unit has, since 1994, been the Norwegian National Unit for Replantation Surgery for all injured limbs with compromised vascular supply needing replantation or revascularisation. We receive patients from the whole of Norway including the islands of Svalbard in the Arctic Ocean. The population of Norway was 5.3 million with a paediatric population below the age of 18 of 1.1 million in 2018. We perform replantations of digits, hands, more proximal upper extremities, lower extremities and other amputated body parts on approximately 50–70 patients per year with an incidence of 0.35 per 100.000 person years for children (0–18 years) and 1.4–1.7 per 100.000 person years for adults.

28.4 Mechanisms, Classifications and Causes of Injury

The mechanisms of upper limb amputations are guillotine, crush and avulsion or a combination most frequently of crush and avulsion injuries. Guillotine injuries are sharp with minimal soft tissue damage beyond the injury (Fig. 28.2a, b). Crush amputations are the most common causing blunt soft tissue damage to the close surrounding area (Fig. 28.3a–d). Depending on the external forces at the time of injury, the crush injury will be classified as either mild or major, for example, caused by a fine-toothed blade from a table saw or a wider saw blade like the circular saws or wood splitters. Avulsions can extend the damage to a varying distance. The avulsive injuries have the poorest outcomes as they tear and disrupt the tissue at different levels. The vessels commonly tear away from the amputate whereas the nerves usually avulse from more proximally. The arteries are stronger and more elastic than the veins. They stretch and rupture at their weakest point often distal to the level of amputation, in the area of smaller calibre. Intima lesions may occur a distance from the amputation. The veins are weak and will rupture easily at the level of injury without affecting the rest of the vessel.

Several classification systems exist for distal amputations at different digital levels. Foucher and Sebastin and Chung have classified amputations distal to the insertion of flexor digito-

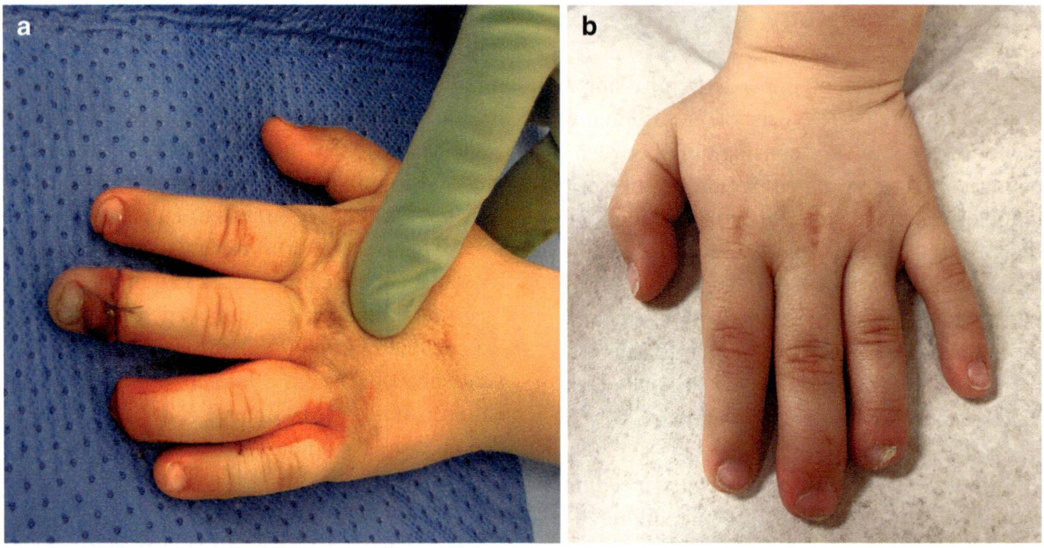

Fig. 28.2 (**a**) Axe injury in a 4-year-old boy resulting in a partial amputation of third finger and total amputation of fourth finger left side. (**b**) End result after revascularisation of third finger and composite grafting of fourth finger

rum superficialis (FDS) [28]. Ishikawa and Tamai classify amputations from the distal interphalangeal joint (DIP) joint whereas Hirase's is distal to the flexor digitorum profundus (FDP) insertion [29, 30]. Classification systems by Wei, Vilkki and del Piñal for major hand injuries follow a severity scale and give guidelines as to their management [31, 32]. De Piñal divides the amputations into radial, ulnar, metacarpal, carpal and forearm amputations. The levels of amputation determine the functional outcome of a limb. More favourable levels are distal amputations at finger/mid-hand level at the palmar arch and proximal to radiocarpal joint whereas less favourable is proximal forearm where the innervation to the musculature can be affected [33].

Micro replantations are defined as the reattachments at digit, hand and wrist level. The replantations more proximal to the wrist are classified as macro replantations. Children can in rare cases sustain a major segment amputation, often due to traction injuries in a domestic-agricultural environment [34–36].

The most common causes of paediatric amputations vary from country to country. The guillotine injury was the most frequent mechanism in children <13 years of age in Thailand [37] whereas in the West different types of mild and major crush injuries were most often seen, due to saws, axes, machinery, power tools and lawn mowers [13, 20, 38]. The causes of injury in the USA are mild crush (18%), machinery (16%), lawn mowers (12%), motor vehicle collisions (8%), gunshot wound (6%) and off-road transport (6%). The motor vehicle collisions were the main cause of all adolescent amputations (19%) which increases with age to 55% in driving-age patients between the ages 16 and 17 [27]. Hostetler's overview of products associated with amputations includes tools (9%) of which power saws account for 18% [26]. The most common causes of fingertip injury are 93% crush, followed by 4% sharp laceration [39]. Stationary exercise bicycles cause avulsion-type injuries ranging in severity from lacerations and fractures to amputations [40, 41].

From 1984 to 1999, our unit treated 47 children (8 girls/39 boys) with a total of 66 digital amputations (30 partial and 36 complete). The mean age was eight years (20 months–15 years) with two age peaks at 1–5 and 10–15 years of

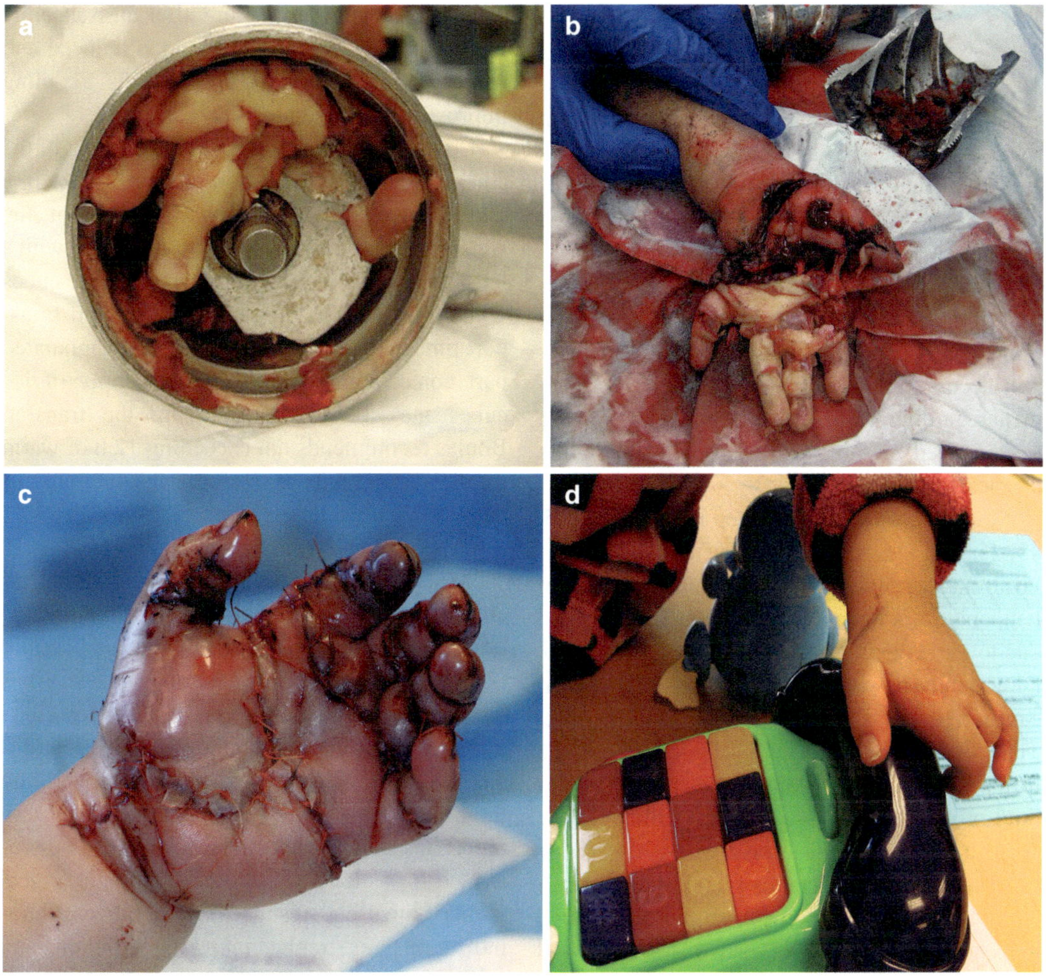

Fig. 28.3 (**a**) Mincing machine accident in a 2-year-old girl left hand. (**b**) Left hand removed from the mincing machine. Mangled hand and multi-level injury. No sign of circulation in second, third and fourth fingers. (**c**) End result after revascularisation. (**d**) Third and fourth finger left hand did not survive. End result 7 months later

age. The four most common causes of digital amputation were wood splitter (32%), crush injury (21%), guillotine injuries (13%) and circular saw (11%).

The mutilating hand injuries in the child can be put in three categories, either accidental, non-accidental (abuse) or self-mutilating. Lesch-Nyhan disease is a very rare inherited disorder associated with abnormal motor development, mental retardation, hyperuricemia and self-injurious behaviour which includes chewing off digits [42, 43]. The treatment of the self-mutilation should be limited to controlling infections and revisions without any reconstructive surgery.

28.5 Care for and Transportation of Amputated Parts

Optimal care of the amputate and an expedient transfer to a microvascular replantation centre is essential. Many inappropriate methods of transporting an amputated part have been used throughout the years of which placement of an amputated digit in the mouth is one and in formalin another. The amputated part should not be immersed in saline or water for many hours as it will become macerated. There is general agreement regarding wrapping of an amputated limb in a moistened sterile gauze, alternatively in the cleanest cloth available [44].

Suggestions for the next step have varied [15, 43, 45–47]. Our unit has experienced better survival rates of replanted digits preserved at room temperature compared to cooling. This may be due to unrecognised frostbite in the latter group. Direct contact with ice, snow or ice packs will cause frostbite and permanent tissue damage. This is caused by direct cellular injury due to the formation of ice crystals and denaturation of lipid-protein complexes. Indirect cellular injury is more severe and ensues as a result of thawing and microvascular thrombosis continuing the cell injury and death [48]. Some frostbitten amputated parts will thaw during the end of transport and replantation might be attempted. The success rate after such attempts is low. Hence, for amputated parts without muscle and a transportation time within 6–8 h, we recommend storage at room temperature.

Whereas fingers and limbs without musculature have a higher tolerance for prolonged ischaemia, this is not the case for limbs with musculature. Several experimental models have shown that warm ischaemia can be tolerated by muscle tissue up to 4 hours before myocyte death begins [39, 40]. Prolonged ischaemia will lead to muscle tissue necrosis or the "no-reflow" phenomenon which is described as flow through the arterial anastomosis but not through to the capillaries, thus not revascularising the tissue, resulting in arterial thrombosis [41, 42]. A rat study has demonstrated that even small reductions of the ambient temperature can have a substantial protective effect on musculature after an ischaemic period [49]. The oxygen demand is reduced and metabolic activity diminished as cooling improves the ischaemic tolerance.

Cooling can be performed by placement of the amputated part in a saline-moistened gauze in a closed waterproof bag and placement of the waterproof bag in another bag or box filled with a lot of water and a minimum amount of ice cubes with an ideal temperature of 10–12 °C. If transport time is expected to be long or the amputated part contains muscle, additional supply of ice cubes may be provided during the transfer. Boulas recommends not exceeding 12 h of warm ischaemia for digits or 6 h for limbs with musculature which can be extended to 24 h and 10–12 h, respectively, if kept at a temperature of 4–10 °C [45]. Li however found no statistical difference in survival rates of digits between preservation at room temperature and low temperature (2–6 °C) [50]. Prolonged warm ischaemia has been proposed as more than 10–12 h for digits and 6 h for amputated limbs with muscles [51, 52]. Broad agreement exists around the world on the 6 h limit for limbs with musculature. A case report has shown that cold ischaemia can be prolonged for as long as 94 h for amputated fingers with positive end results [53]. Relative contraindications for replantation for children and adults are prolonged warm ischaemia and inadvertently frozen amputated parts.

A partially amputated limb should be placed in a near anatomic alignment, covered by sterile-moistened gauze and pressure dressing and stabilised by a splint. Direct pressure on the area(s) of bleeding, elevation and the application of cold packs on proximal injuries will most often control the situation. In most cases, bleeding will stop if the vessels are completely transected due to vasoconstriction and haemostasis. A partial arterial lesion can cause continuous bleeding because the intact portion of the vessel wall does not retract and prevents closure.

There is no need for a tourniquet after injury or during transport of the patients. A tourniquet can cause pressure injuries on the soft tissue and vessels resulting in an ischaemic environment in the whole extremity, affecting its survival and limiting also the tourniquet time during surgery [43]. After a while, the tourniquet will not be able to limit the arterial pressure and gradual venous congestion will develop. Shock from a venous haemorrhage and hypovolemia can happen at the removal of the tourniquet. No clamping or haemostat should be placed on the vessels as this will often injure the neurovascular bundle [46].

28.6 Indications for Replantation in Children

The decision to replant is not always an easy one. Broader general indications exist for replantation in children than in adults. Unless the amputated part is severely damaged, most replantations are indicated in children. They have superb healing capacity and recover and adapt more quickly to traumatic events or surgical procedures [51, 54, 55]. The difficulty of the procedure and rate of success are dependent on the type of injury and patient's body weight rather than age [56, 57]. Baker's review of 33 children under 34 months and 41 digits found that body weight greater than 11 kg will have the most influence on vein availability and thereby digit survival [56]. Children have the advantage of faster nerve regeneration which can often result in normal nerve function due to the short distance to the target. This is probably the most important explanation of the favourable results after replantation in children. If successful, good function and healthy bone growth are seen.

The indications for replantation are the same in children as in adults: thumb, multiple digits and proximal amputations distal to the glenohumeral joint. In addition, the replantation of single digits is indicated in children. If the patient has no other life-threatening injuries, a major replantation of the upper [34, 58, 59] or lower limb [60–64] can be performed with greater success in the child than in the adult. One of the main concerns in replantation surgery of the lower limb is nerve regeneration and sensibility of the sole. The second is the length of limb which is a lesser concern in children due to compensatory growth.

28.7 Contra-indications to Surgery

Treatment of the concomitant life-threatening injuries must take priority. Amputation and severe mutilations have a very dramatic primary appearance which can sometimes mask other more serious proximal or general injuries. The small size of the vessels in children is no contra-indication to replantation. No significant morbidity or mortality has been associated with microsurgery done in the paediatric population [47].

A "thumb test" can be done on larger replants to test for prolonged ischaemia diagnosing established rigor mortis if rigid and immobile, when passively moving the thumb in the amputated part [43]. Prolonged warm ischaemia and severe muscle injury are expected to result in poor muscle function and strength with the occurrence of contractures. Metabolic and infectious complications with subsequent vascular thrombosis are seen [65]. Replantation should not be done if revascularisation of the limb is not possible within 6 h of warm ischaemia from time of injury, due to the expected extent of muscle necrosis. Serious and even life-threatening infections can develop resulting in sepsis or gas gangrene.

The following injuries are possible contra-indications to replantation for children: concomitant life-threatening injury, avulsed brachial plexus in proximal amputations, multilevel or segmental injuries, severe crush, mangling, burning or degloving injuries. Each case must be thoroughly discussed within the replantation team as no two cases are alike. The "red line sign" (also known as "Chinese streaks") on the lateral borders of the digit is a sign which suggests complete avulsion of all digital arterial side branches resulting in the leakage of blood from the avulsed vessels and the appearance of reddish lines along the sides of the digit. A resection of a considerable length of vessel past the first side branch is necessary if replantation is to be attempted as the intima injury usually stops at this level. Biemer suggested using vein grafts in 1977 to bridge a vessel defect, avoid excessive shortening of a replanted finger, lessen the risk of thrombosis and increase survival [66].

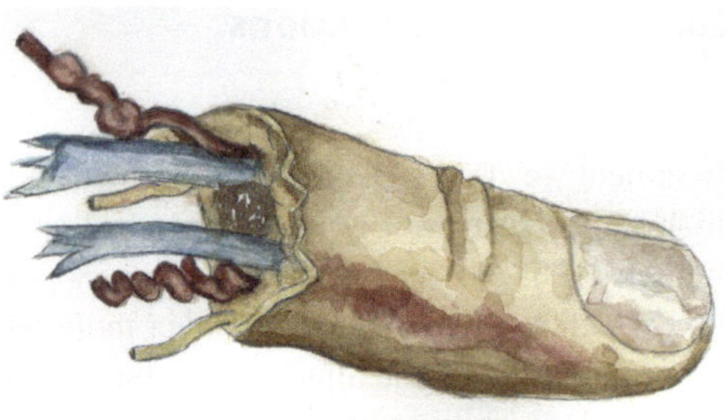

Fig. 28.4 "Red line sign" and "Ribbon sign" (Ill.: Roald Sivertsen)

Another sign present after severe avulsion injuries is the "ribbon sign" characterised by marked tortuosity of the digital arteries indicating stretched and injured vessels 0.5–1 cm from the site of transection (Fig. 28.4). A resection of the injured section of vessel combined with vein grafting is essential [67].

Children are generally healthy patients without adult medical conditions (hypertension, vascular disease), drug, alcohol or tobacco use and economic factors (i.e. early return to work) which adults can struggle with [24, 43, 45].

28.8 Initial Evaluation

The child and parents being sent from another hospital must not be promised that a replantation will be done or that it will be successful. They should be told that they are being transferred to be evaluated for replantation. It is the ultimate decision of the microsurgical centre treating the child if there is indication for replantation or not. The paediatric patient should be evaluated by the replantation team at their arrival in the emergency department. When communicating with child and parents, it is important to use tact and be calm, reassuring but firm. Information about the different treatment options should be given to the parents and child, if possible, with receipt of consent, pre-surgery [43].

28.9 Pre-operative Preparation

Advanced trauma life support and paediatric resuscitation are prioritised first. Major upper limb amputation patients have often lost significant amounts of blood and should be volume resuscitated. Attention is then turned to the extremity where direct compressive dressings have been applied. Removal of the dressing in the emergency department can prevent it from maintaining haemostasis. Determining the vascularity of the limb will identify the patients needing direct transport to the operating room to limit ischaemia time. A speedy transfer is necessary from the emergency room to the operating theatre. The initial assessment of the youngest children and full limb assessment must be done by the replantation team in the operating theatre under a general anaesthetic [59].

X-rays of the amputated part, the injured extremity and the healthy arm for comparison can be taken on the way to surgery or alternatively with fluoroscopy in the operating theatre. These will show the epiphyseal plates but not the unossified osseous structures. Comminution or segmental bone injury on X-rays will give a first assessment of the severity of the injury and probable extent of soft tissue damage.

An optimal pre-operative preparation of the child is important either in the emergency room or directly in the operation theatre. Painkillers, tetanus and antibiotic prophylaxis are given. In many countries, first-generation cephalosporins (cefalotin 30 mg/kg) are chosen for prophylaxis and in other countries second-generation cephalosporins. Metronidazole (20–30 mg/kg) prophylaxis is added for farm machinery-related injuries, lawn mower injuries or heavily soiled wounds. Farm machinery is associated with environmental contamination such as animal excreta. Ciprofloxacin 20 mg/kg is therefore recommended to be included due to the presence of Gram-negative microbes. Harkness recommends taking wound swabs intra-operatively. As soon as the culture results are ready, the empirical regimen should be modified. If the cultures are negative, the child is well and showing no signs of infection at time of wound inspection; the empirical therapy can be stopped [68].

Blood chemistry analysis, complete blood count (red blood cells, white blood cells, platelets, haemoglobin, haematocrit), coagulation status (fibrinogen, APTT, INR), liver function analysis and blood typing with cross-matching are ordered. IV cannulas, central venous catheter and brachial plexus block with catheter are placed [24]. The indwelling catheter with sympathetic blockade is recommended for the procedure with a continuous infusion post-operatively [69–71]. Ropivacaine 2 mg/ml is the drug of choice in our hospital as it is less cardiotoxic than bupivacaine [72]. This will help minimise pain and anxiety, decrease vasospasm and increase surface temperature. Children can experience vasospasms more easily than adults which is an important factor to recognise and treat should it occur [73]. The placement of a plexus block must not delay surgery. An indwelling urethral catheter is inserted.

28.10 Operative Technique

Microvascular replantation surgery should be managed by a replantation team (minimum two competent microsurgeons, anaesthesiologist, theatre and ward nurse staff specialised in microsurgery) available around the clock everyday [51]. Sophisticated knowledge of the physiology and anatomy of microcirculation is essential and will help surgeons achieve higher patency rates when anastomosing ≤1 mm vessels.

Children are usually given a general anaesthesia, although surgery is possible with an intra-operative regional anaesthesia. Appropriate loupe magnification to 3.5–4.5 times and an operating microscope (diploscope) under magnification of 20–30 times with a foot control are essential for paediatric microsurgery. Microsurgical instruments and 10-0 or 11-0 non-absorbable nylon sutures are needed. Choose the right size tourniquet for the child in question, and inflation pressure, 200–220 mmHg, is often adequate. Note the time when the tourniquet is applied. It should not exceed the maximum of 2 h. Much of the surgery can be done without a tourniquet and repeated applications should be avoided.

While the child is being prepared for surgery, one part of the replantation team can start preparing the amputated part under magnification. Meticulous debridement is of great importance as well as locating vessels and nerves. The vessels are flushed through with heparinised saline and tagged with micro-vessel clamps, the nerves with 9-0 sutures. Based on Saba and Zinberg's findings, we are using 20 U/ml of heparinised saline in our clinic. This gives an ideal patency rate without the complications of excessive bleeding that higher concentrations can experience. It also takes into account the neutralising effect of heparin on prostacyclin and increased risk of thrombosis at lower concentrations [74–76]. The distal tendon stump is retrieved and prepared and a suture is inserted. Loose bone splints can be removed at this point. The proximal stump is prepared as soon as the child is anaesthetised. The tourniquet should only be applied after the proximal flow of the vessels has been checked and pulsatile arterial spurt obtained.

Some authors prioritise bone shortening to minimise tension on arteries, veins and nerves. We have experienced that an exact reduction of the amputated part without shortening will often improve alignment and stability. Cheng concurs stating that children's vessels are more elastic than adults' [56, 77]. Autogenous venous grafts can be needed to repair the arterial injury. The veins are more easily mobilised and can generally be sutured directly. Efforts should be made to avoid compromising the epiphyseal plates in children, choosing smooth pins [46, 47]. Bony fixation in the hand and fingers is managed with K-wires (0.7, 0.89 mm), sometimes with additional interosseous cerclage wires. Plates may be used on the humerus or forearm [47, 51]. A rapid osteosynthesis with K-wires (0.89, 1.0 mm) can sometimes be chosen before vascular anastomosis to save time. Microsurgical suture of vessels can only start when a stable osteosynthesis has been obtained.

The surgical sequence during replantation is bony fixation first for both distal and proximal amputations, avoiding digital rotation. In digital replantations, the next steps are the repair of the flexor tendons, digital nerves and arteries followed by the extensor tendons and veins. In major limb replantations, it is essential to reestablish vascular continuity as early as possible after osteosynthesis.

Before any arterial anastomosis is attempted, the proximal flow must be checked. Flushing of the artery, complete resection of injured sections of artery and removal of thrombotic clots are essential till a pulsatile spurting flow is obtained. Only then can one continue with the anastomosis, after having prepared proximal and distal arterial ends, relieving tension, resected intima and overhanging adventitia. No tension must be put on the anastomosis and vein grafting will be needed in some cases. They must be reversed after their harvest from the forearm so as to respect the direction of flow past the venous valves.

We aim to repair one digital artery and two veins in both adults and children. An increase in survival has been shown when repairing ≥2 veins compared to only 1 anastomosed vein, which has been corroborated by Lee for replanted digits in zone II with the equal or higher number of veins repaired to arteries repaired [78, 79]. Vein grafts might be needed and can be taken from the volar aspect of the forearm. The calibre of the digital vessels is small, but both artery and vein repair are feasible in children with an expected diameter of 0.2–0.8 mm from the distal phalanx to the proximal phalanx [80].

The risk of vasospasm is a well-known complication which is also our experience [73]. Others though do not experience this complication during elective microsurgery [81] and hypothesise that a relative lack of the muscularis layer is insufficient to produce vasospasms in paediatric vessels [82]. Many microsurgeons use topical vasodilators intra-operatively to combat vasospasms, most often papaverine 40 mg/ml or lidocaine 100 mg/ml [83–85]

No consensus exists as to the intra-operative administration of IV heparin during replantation surgery. The survival of free flaps in animals and humans did not improve with systemic heparin [86]. A review by Conrad however supports using intra-operative heparin as a bolus agent and topical irrigant [87]. Some authors administer systemic heparin right before starting on the anastomosis at a dose of 1000 units for younger children and 3000 units for those closer to adult weight. Serial doses of heparin at 500–1000 units/hour have been recommended if the procedure is lengthy [24]. Our standard routine is a bolus dose of IV heparin 2500 units to adults and approximately 1000 units to younger children of 20 kg (50–100 IE/kg) one minute before clamps are removed.

In major limb amputations, some authors recommend a perfusion washout of stagnant blood and its haemolytic products from the intravascular tree with University of Wisconsin fluid for pre-operative management before transfer (1 L UW solution at a temperature of 10 °C). This provides also rapid cooling of the entire limb [88]. A vascular shunt should be considered for major limb amputations if time from amputation to arrival in the operation theatre is expected to be longer than 4–6 h with the advantage of shortening the ischaemia time [17, 51, 59, 89]. This must however be weighed up against the disadvantage of working around a shunt, in a bloody field, the blood loss and the swelling of the extremity. Daigle used a shunt in 2/15 (13%) patients where ischaemia time was prolonged (11 and 15.5 h). One of two limbs survived [59]. Perfusion or at least flushing of the amputation with heparinised saline should be started as soon as possible at arrival at the replant centre, clearing out blood and microthrombi, eliminating metabolite breakdown products from prolonged ischaemia and assuring vascular patency. Continuous cooling of a major limb can extend ischaemia time by slowing down the cellular metabolic processes. A surgical glove filled with cold water can be placed along or under the amputate during the surgical procedure. Radical debridement of devitalised parts is essential to reduce possible post-operative complications such as myonecrosis and infections, leaving only well-vascularised tissue and avoiding dead space susceptible to infection [90].

In forearm surgery, we recommend repairing both ulnar and radial arteries. Arterial dominance is difficult to predict in any given situation, creating an uncertain situation if only one artery is repaired [43]. Limb engorgement is a problem in upper limb replantation. Suture as many veins as possible before clamps are removed. If necessary venous grafts from the leg should be harvested to avoid vascular sutures under tension with subsequent risk of thrombus formation. It is mandatory to restore the arterial inflow before venous repair in major limb replantations permitting further washout of toxic metabolites in the amputated part. Sabapathy recommends guidelines dependent on the time from injury to arrival at the hospital and level of injury. Should the ischaemia time permit it, arterial repair is done after debridement and bony fixation. If the ischaemia time is prolonged and the level of injury is more proximal, a preliminary shunt placement with later arterial repair is suggested. Intermittent perfusion of the limb can be done for 5–10 min by releasing the arterial clamp before and during the repair of the remaining structures [91]. Fasciotomy of the injured muscular compartments is routinely performed. The area can be covered immediately by a mesh skin graft. In major limb replantation, a return to the operating theatre should be planned within 48 h for exploration and supplementary debridement. Several debridements might be necessary.

Adequate haemostasis should be achieved intra-operatively to minimise post-operative bleeding. The skin is loosely approximated with interrupted nylon non-absorbable or synthetic absorbable 4/0 to 5/0 sutures. The vessels should be covered by vital soft tissue, alternatively a vascularised flap. Full- or split-thickness grafts can cover smaller areas of exposed vessel if the wounds are difficult to approximate due to oedema. The other wounds can be left open to allow decompression of the digital vessels.

The wounds are covered with non-adherent, loosely wrapped dressing to avoid constriction and pressure, and a big bulky supportive bandage is applied. Some authors apply a splint or a cast over the elbow in the youngest children which is not a standard routine for our paediatric patients [92]. Fingertips should remain exposed for later frequent observations and temperature monitoring.

28.11 Post-operative Medical Therapy and Monitoring

The post-operative care is essential to obtain good results [15]. In paediatric microvascular surgery, one must be aware that technical difficulties will occur, and perfect anastomoses will not always be achievable [77]. The small vessel sizes will make the child prone to post-operative arterial and venous spasms as well as thrombosis. Minimising possible vasospasms by controlling pain and room temperature is the main goal for the post-operative treatment. Continuing the intra-operative regional anaesthesia in the post-operative phase can adequately control pain as well as narcotic and non-narcotic drugs. The hand is placed in a big bandage and the extremity is kept elevated with complete bedrest for the first five days in an ambient room (23–24 °C). Individual blankets can be used to keep the operated extremity warm.

No standardised anticoagulation therapy exists for replantation surgery, even though a combination of heparin (which counteracts the effects of thrombin on platelets and fibrinogen), aspirin (which decreases platelet function) and dextran (which increases blood flow or decreases blood viscosity) was suggested as early as 1978 [93–95]. Some surgeons give no prophylaxis and others only aspirin.

The dose of oral acetylsalicylate given varies between 3 mg/kg/day [96], 4 mg/kg [95] and 6 mg/kg/d for six weeks [37]. Some recommend avoiding it [43]. Masotti demonstrated on healthy volunteers that aspirin is dose-related and acts differently on platelets than on the vessel wall requiring an average dose of 3.5 mg/kg for inhibitory effect on platelet aggregation [97]. Our regimen is 3–5 mg/kg/day which is approximately 75 mg/day for a younger child of 20 kg. This dose of 75 mg/day should not be exceeded in the older child.

Some authors give heparin at a dose of 100 units/kg to children and adjusted to maintain the activated partial thromboplastin time at 1.5 times normal. Others choose to give an IV infusion of heparin (3U/kg body weight/h) for the first 12–24 h and then reduced gradually [43]. A retrospective study comparing acetylsalicylic acid (ASA) + IV heparin treatment with ASA and ASA+ SC heparin showed that continuous IV heparin post-operatively gives more complications with no more favourable anti-thrombotic effects [98]. We deem the IV heparin anticoagulation treatment given at time of anastomosis repair and clamp removal sufficient. Betancourt has shown that the highest risk of critical thrombosis following a finger replantation is during the first three post-operative days [99].

Previous anticoagulation treatments have included Dextran 40 given at time of vessel anastomosis and continued for 3–5 days post-operatively [87, 93, 100]. As a volume expander with an antiplatelet effect, it needs the monitoring of other IV fluids given to avoid overload. IV Promiten prophylaxis is given against anaphylaxis before the infusion of Dextran. Other rare complications are volume overload, pulmonary oedema, cerebral oedema, platelet dysfunction and acute renal failure [101].

Some suggest giving chlorpromazine (thorazine) to reduce anxiety, as a sedative and peripheral vasodilator in children at a dose of 0.3 mg/kg body weight three times a day for five days [17, 102]. Chlorpromazine has not been part of our regimen for many years. This has had no resulting negative consequences.

Pressors have a peripheral vasoconstrictive effect and have no place in post-operative care. Some suggest high doses of vitamins A and E to combat venous insufficiency. Ferrous sulphate or ferrous fumarate, at a dose of 5 mg/kg/day divided twice a day and to be continued for 2–3 months after haemoglobin has normalised, is recommended to prevent iron deficiency anaemia.

Our post-operative follow-up of an extremity is done by recording clinical appearance (colour, pulp turgor, capillary refill of the fingertip and nail bed) and skin temperature with a non-injured finger as reference. The monitoring of surface skin temperature is a reliable indicator of digital viability though not widely used [103, 104]. Through the years, different methods have been tested such as pulse oximetry, Doppler probes, thermometer with wired probe and later wireless infrared thermometer [105]. Jones recommends the differential pulse oximetry as a superior post-operative method of monitoring paediatric toe-to-hand transfers [106].

Authors have different routines as to the intervals between observations. Most recommend hourly observations the first 24 h with reduction to every other hour for the second 24 h, if the surgery seems to have been a success [15, 19]. The protocol from Nancy, France, only lasts for five days with a gradual reduction of intervals as long as favourable observations of the amputated part are noted [92]. Monitoring needs to be done by competent adequate staff. In our unit, the extremity is monitored every hour until the observations are stable with a subsequent gradual reduction of intervals until day 10.

The child must not get cold and observations are to be maintained at once per hour if the replanted part is stable. One must refrain from being noisy and keep the child warm, calm, unstressed and pain-free. Some centres used warming lamps post-operatively in earlier years and have discontinued whereas others still continue [92, 107, 108]. Other centres keep the entire upper extremity warm by wrapping it in a Bair Hugger [109]. Our theatre nurses make a warm hat out of a stocking and padding bandages to cover the whole extremity (Fig. 28.5). With comprehensive care including repeated observations with both clinical and objective evaluations, it is expected that arterial or venous insufficiencies can be detected early [108].

A reoperation should be considered if the temperature has fallen below 32 °C or if the clinical appearance of the finger indicates a vascular insufficiency [19]. Thirkannad finds a drop of temperature of 3 °C significant compared to a non-injured finger [43]. We consider a fall in temperature of 2 °C combined with a change in colour or capillary refill warning factors deter-

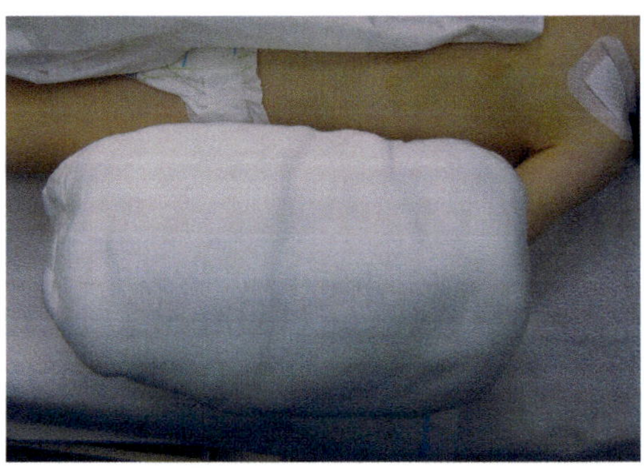

Fig. 28.5 Warm hat made by our theatre nurses out of a stocking and padding bandages covering the whole extremity in a child

mining the need for a reoperation, the latter two being the most important.

Some suggest nil per os the first 24 h just in case, which is not the case in our unit. Chocolate, caffeine and nicotine are strictly prohibited as they can induce vasospasm.

Some give IV antibiotic prophylaxis for 5–8 days or until the digit has survived [15, 92] and continue orally till the wounds have healed [37]. We administer IV antibiotic prophylaxis the first 24 h and continue orally till there is no sign of oozing from the wounds. The dressing is cautiously changed at signs of excessive bleeding to avoid development of a cold environment and the risk of a tight bandage.

28.12 Complications

Despite the experience of skilled microsurgeons and favourable conditions of the injured hand, failures due to vascular thrombosis do happen, most often during the first three days postoperatively [99]. Either arterial or venous problems can occur. Pallor and slow or no capillary refill will indicate an arterial inflow problem whereas signs of congestion with bluish colours and a rapid capillary refill will indicate a venous outflow problem. The elevation of the extremity will in some cases increase venous return and make apparent capillary refill. In both cases, the temperature will fall gradually, more abruptly in arterial failure. If the clinical appearance is difficult to assess, a needle prick of the finger pulp with an 18-gauge needle (green) can be done. Dark blood indicates a venous insufficiency whereas an absence of blood suggests an arterial insufficiency.

It is important to check that the bandage is not too tight and constrictive. An elevation or depression of the hand may increase outflow/inflow to the hand/digit. Check that the regional block is effective since correct pain relief might release a vasospasm. A patient must be kept warm and adequately hydrated with a haemoglobin >9 g/dl and haematocrit 24–30%. The child must be returned immediately to the operating theatre for exploration of the patency of the vessels if simple procedures on the ward do not help. If thrombosis has occurred in a venous or arterial anastomosis, resection of the anastomosis is done, and a new repair with or without vein graft is performed.

Post-operative external bleeding in the dressing should raise questions of its source from the wound edges, potential thrombosis and decreased blood flow through the anastomosis.

A venous anastomosis is not always possible in distal replantations. An incision is therefore made in the pulp tip to relieve the venous congestion. Bloodletting is then part of the primary treatment. It is secondary in other situations when venous insufficiency is observed. We use a transverse pulp incision directly under the nail to prevent unacceptable secondary scarring in the area of grip (Fig. 28.6a–c). Another manner of treating venous congestion is rubbing a sponge/gauze soaked in heparin over a scratched surface on the digit [92]. Shi recommends a transverse or oblique fish mouth incision at the pulp tip, limiting the incision to the dermis layer to ensure oozing, finding deeper incisions unnecessary [30]. Regular observations of the colour of the replant will determine the frequency of the follow-up and scratching of the digit. According to Shi, it takes 4–6 days for a replanted paediatric digit to reestablish a venous circulation. Han suggests taking into account the soft tissue trauma of the replanted digit and waiting until the fifth day before the first attempt at stopping the bleeding [107]. Other methods to treat venous congestion have been a para-ungual stab incision [107], nail removal and scraping of the nail matrix with heparin soaks, creating an arteriovenous or venocutaneous fistula [110, 111] or delayed venous anastomosis [112]. Puhaindran suggests dermal pocketing as an alternative method, especially for social cultures where leeches are not easily accepted, after a distal finger replantation when no veins are found. Osteosynthesis and arterial anastomosis are performed followed by de-epithelisation on the amputate and on a suitable site on the palm for venous drainage [113].

A salvage procedure to treat venous outflow is bloodletting using medicinal leeches, *Hirudo medicinalis* (Fig. 28.7). In a recent review, the success rate of digital replant salvage was 62.3%

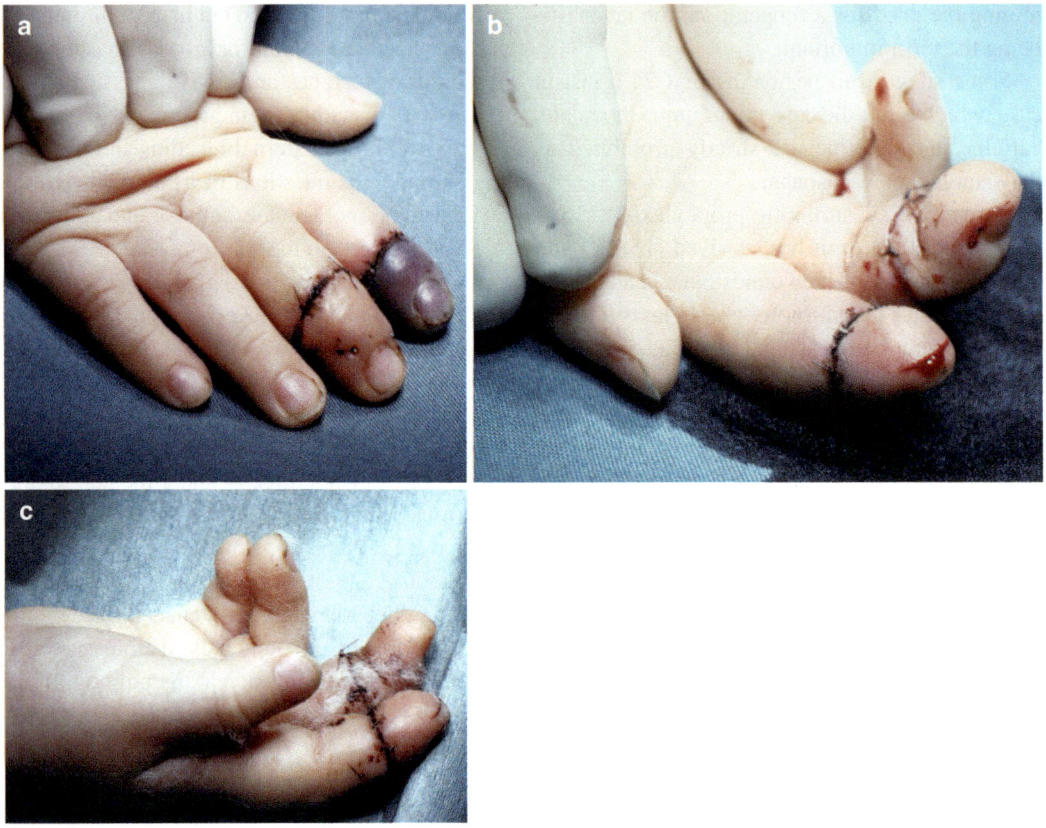

Fig. 28.6 (**a**) Venous insufficiency in right second digit in 2-year-old boy. (**b**) Status after reanastomosis of vein and transverse fish-mouth pulp incision. (**c**) End result after 10 days

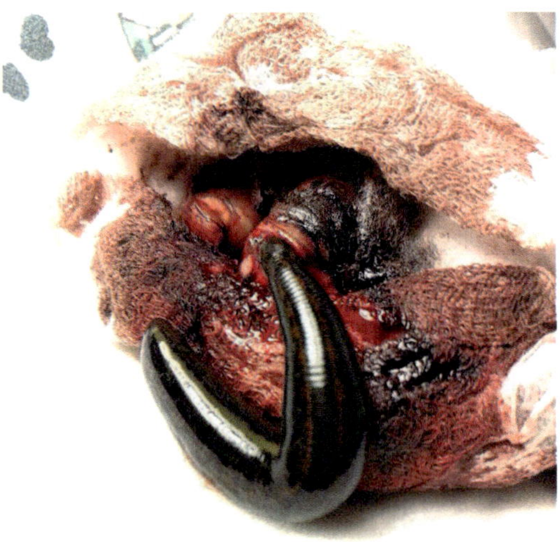

Fig. 28.7 Leech therapy in 4-year-old boy

[114]. The mechanisms of leeches are to remove a volume of blood (about 5 ml) at each feed and to secrete a local anticoagulant, hirudin, through saliva as a potent heparin analogue. This allows decompression of the incised digit and prolonged bleeding for 8–12 h, thereby preventing congestion. A new leech is applied when the bleeding stops. Antibiotic prophylaxis with third-generation cephalosporin or ciprofloxacin has been recommended during leech therapy because of the bacteria *Aeromonas hydrophila* present in their intestinal tract and the water they live in [115]. Our Welsh leech provider confirms that *Aeromonas hydrophila* is part of the normal intestinal flora and helps to suppress other bacteria. Our post-operative routine comprises a change of antibiotics to ciprofloxacin at the start of leech treatment. Wound swabs should be taken if signs of infection develop during leech therapy and then *Aeromonas* should be specified as a possible bacterial agent. One must be very aware of the probable need for transfusions during bleeding, and strict monitoring of the patient's haemoglobin and haematocrit is mandatory.

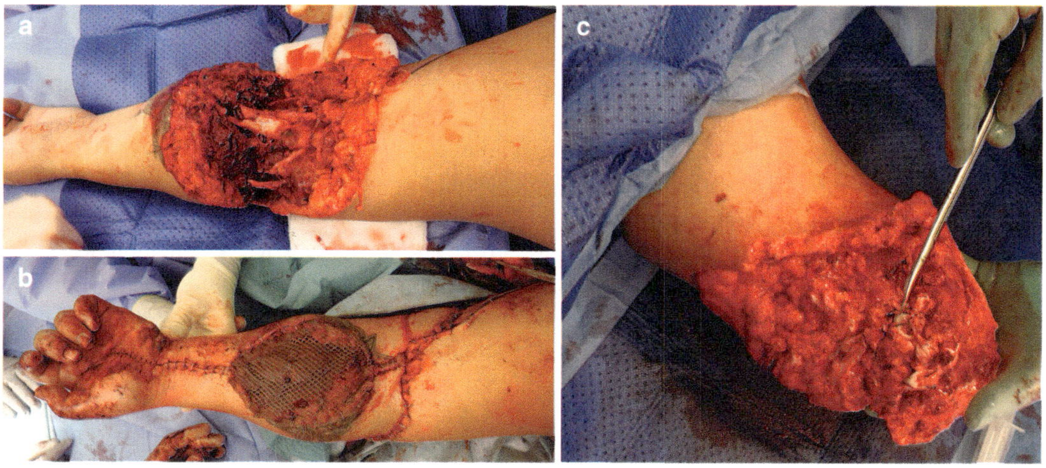

Fig. 28.8 (**a**) Partial amputation of left upper extremity at proximal forearm level in a 17-year-old girl injured in a car accident. (**b**) Revascularisation done within 5 h after time of injury. (**c**) Numerous attempts at revisions and revascularisations because of recurrent signs of arterial insufficiency. Reperfusion injury and sepsis developed resulting in the need for the amputation of the left arm

Reperfusion injury is a complication specific to proximal limb replantations with major muscle mass and warm ischaemia time greater than 4 hours as a risk factor (Fig. 28.8a–c). Skeletal muscle is especially prone to reperfusion injury. It can cause more tissue damage than the ischaemia alone, and the amount of re-perfused devitalised tissue will determine morbidity. The severely injured tissue generates inflammatory mediators which cause local and systemic effects. The local inflammatory response includes the release of reactive oxygen species and other inflammatory breakdown products of injured ischaemic cells. This will lead to oedema in the 4–6 h after reperfusion. The most active area for the inflammatory response is seen between the damaged and dead muscle tissues. The inflammatory mediators are released through several mechanisms, one being the coagulation system, which activates clotting. This can aggravate endothelial damage, causing arterial vasoconstriction, microvascular thrombosis and the propagation of the no-reflow phenomenon. The systemic response depends on the muscle mass involved in the ischaemic process. The resulting inflammatory reaction will cause either a local response alone or a local and a systemic response. Hypotension, hyperkalaemia, acidosis, myoglobinuria, disseminated intravascular coagulation and end-organ failure can be seen. In the severe ischaemia, the systemic inflammatory response will lead to a diffuse vascular permeability problem not localised to any organ and to third space fluid loss. If left untreated, hypovolemia and hypoperfusion of the kidneys with acute renal failure will occur. If the third space is recognised and overtreated, it can lead to pulmonary oedema. The reperfusion injury can become severe and threaten limb, and life, resulting in the need for intensive care treatment and re-amputation as the only surgical option [89, 116, 117]. Extracorporeal perfusion might be able to prolong limb preservation according to animal studies [118].

If a complete failure of circulation in a replanted finger has occurred, there is no need to remove the digit straight away. The digit can be left to demarcate as occasionally only partial failure is seen and the amputation level might be more distal than the primary injury.

Once confirmation of healed bone is seen on X-rays, one can plan for the removal of K-wires. Most wounds heal spontaneously but some will need secondary revision and/or secondary coverage. Non-unions are rarely seen in children. Tenolysis and/or arthrolysis might be needed at a later stage.

28.13 Physical Therapy

A regular supervised post-operative follow-up after limb amputation and replantation surgery by physiotherapists and occupational therapists is essential. Without this, a good functional result cannot be expected [119]. Physiotherapy starts as early as possible with careful manual stretching and active movement when stable osteosynthesis and tendon sutures are in place. Splints are used to stabilise the extremity and to continue manual stretching when signs of healing are present. The hand therapy given to the children needs to be age assessed. The treatment is anticipated to be long, a minimum of 1–2 years, all depending on the severity of the injury.

28.14 Outcomes

The paediatric patient is generally healthy without comorbidity, with greater healing, less scar formation, better nerve regeneration, enhanced tendon gliding, easier joint mobilisation and regenerative and adaptation potential [25, 120]. Individual assessments focusing on function as the main goal must be made when considering indications for replantation. Long-term follow-up studies show good functional outcomes in children [108]. We recommend that future studies include age-adapted patient-reported outcome measures when possible. The sensory recovery after nerve suture can be excellent in a guillotine injury due to the proximity to the end organ in digits and the high regeneration power in children [80]. Results can be surprisingly good post-neurotisation in replantation cases where nerve repair was not possible distal to the nerve trifurcation [121]. The digital replantation distal to DIP joint is still technically difficult in children, and thus the success rate will be lower than in adults [30]. The most challenging procedures are the amputation with degloving involving a vascular injury over a long segment of the artery. The survival rate was higher in children younger than nine years of age than children 9–16 years old, with no relationship found to the type of injury. The child's body weight over 11 kg has the most influence on vein availability and thereby digit survival [56]. In Baker's four patients under 11 kg, no suitable veins were found. There was no relationship between the survival of the part and the sex of the patient, the level of the injury, the injured digit, the pre-operative duration of ischaemia, the number of arteries or veins that had been anastomosed and the use of venous grafts [16]. The outcome after replantation will vary depending on the level of injury [122]. Digits tolerate longer ischaemia times; even cold ischaemia up to 96 h have had little consequence [53]. The situation is very different in more proximal amputations when muscle is involved. The success of a proximal limb replantation is dependent on reestablishing circulation within as short period of time as possible [34].

The success rate was significantly higher after revascularisation (88%) than after replantation (63%) [16]. The success rate is higher after primary surgery than after revision surgery. A salvage rate of 50% has been described, arterial problems being more amendable than venous ones. The success rate in children is lower than in adults due to the extremely small vessel size and nature of the injury (crush and avulsion). The survival rate of 60 replanted parts in 41 children was 94% after guillotine injury and 80% and 74%, respectively, for crush and avulsion injuries [25]. The mechanism of injury did not however affect survival in a study done on single finger replantations [79].

A retrospective thumb avulsion study on 27 patients, mean age 33 years (range 2–78), presented survival rates of 83% at or proximal to the MP joint and 38% distal to the MP joint [123]. This variation in survival was related to the difference in vessel size. The overall success rates for digital replantation in children are 63–97% [16, 24, 25, 37, 50, 56, 80, 102, 124]. A review of paediatric major limb replantations found success rates from 42% to 88% with very few long clinical series and many heterogenous groups [59]. Daigle and Raimondi report an overall major limb survival rate of 87% and 100%, respectively [34, 59]. The functional results were dependent on the level of amputation. A study on 59 patients, mean age 22.7 years (10 weeks to 53 years), of which 20 patients were <16 years of age, showed that a reconstruction distal to the flexor digitorum superficialis (FDS) insertion gave a mean joint motion of 82°, compared with a reconstruction proximal to the insertion resulting in mean joint motion of 35° [79].

Cold intolerance was experienced by 53% of the patients but was seasonal and could be reduced by wearing protective garments [59].

28.15 Paediatric Fingertip Composite Grafts

A distally amputated paediatric digit will have a better chance of survival if replantable vasculature is present on the amputate [56]. Shi replanted 12 digits in children, 4–10 years of age, with only 1 failure distal to or at the nail bed [30]. When an amputation of a fingertip happens distal to the trifurcation of the digital arteries, a replantation is challenging or impossible. The average survival rate of a paediatric composite graft is 24%, which can increase with the cooling of the amputated part [43]. Murphy presents 96 patients treated with a non-vascularised "replantation" of fingertips, 11-year follow-up, median age 2.4 years (range 0–16) where there was no graft take in 32% of cases, 52% partial graft take and 16% complete graft take [39]. The morbidity is low. Composite grafting has a better success rate in the amputations distal to the DIP joint and in children younger than three years of age [125] (Fig. 28.9a–d).

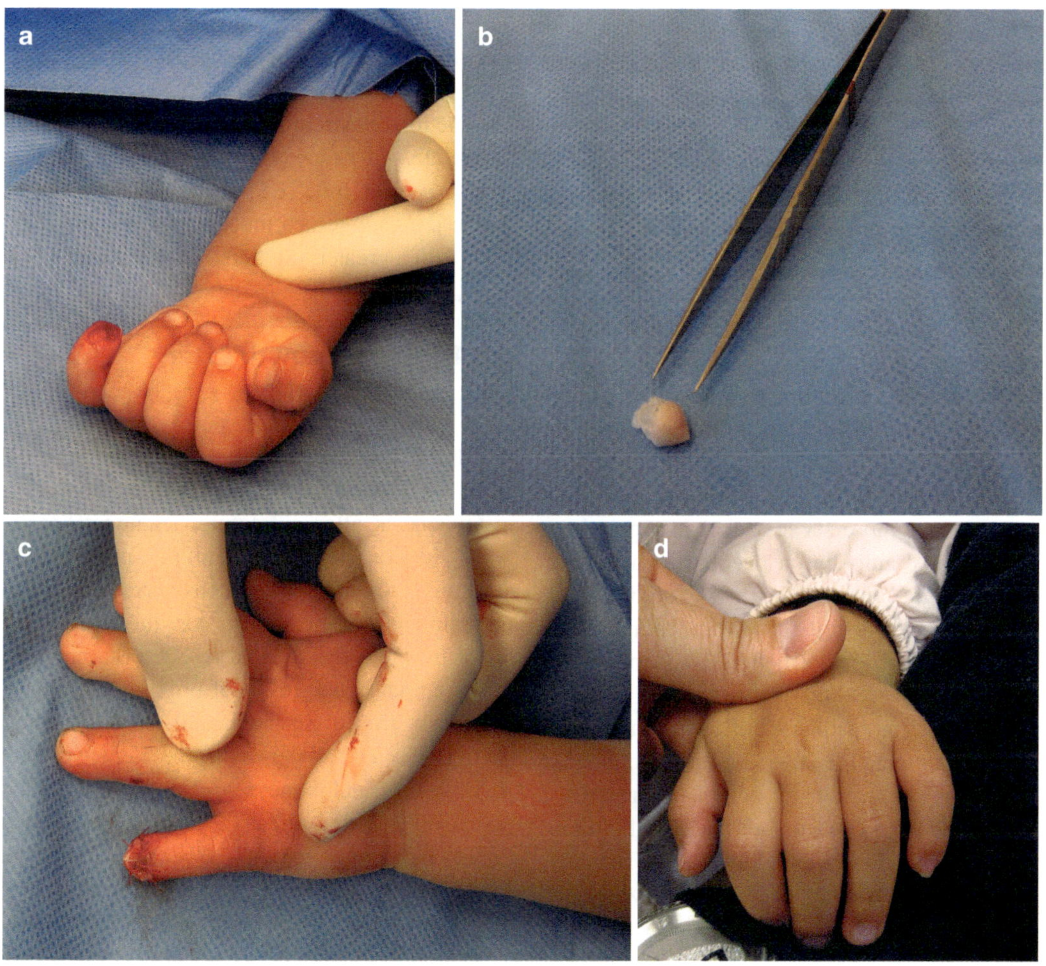

Fig. 28.9 (**a**) Amputation of fingertip in a door distal to replantable vasculature in a 2-year-old girl. (**b**) Amputated fingertip. (**c**) Composite grafting of fingertip. (**d**) End result 2 months later

28.16 Psychological Aspects

The parent(s) or any sibling/adult involved in a paediatric amputation injury will feel enormous guilt [43]. Professional counselling will be of great support for everybody and will thus ensure a better follow-up of the child's treatment. This counselling should continue during the patient's rehabilitation when necessary [126]. The parents are key to any rehabilitation, and a good relationship with health-care professionals is essential for best results [127]. One can expect that a successful replantation will be a great relief for a family. Children show a high degree of cooperation with health-care professionals [54]. Grob gives recommendations for promoting a positive outcome after a severe hand injury [128]. A biopsychosocial perspective towards treatment and management should be adopted by the multidisciplinary team giving a positive influence on immediate and long-term outcomes. Good functional results are expected in the paediatric patient and optimal treatment, and care must be given to ensure that potential psychological issues will not impede their outcome [129].

28.17 Prosthetic Usage in Children

A first priority at the time of injury is to consider if the replanted limb will be of use to the patient or if a revision could be the better solution. The functional result of a replanted major segment was more successful than a prosthetic in a bilateral amputation paediatric case report [130]. Daigle confirms that 93% of studied cases <18 years of age felt that their replanted arm functioned and looked better than a prosthesis [59, 131].

A long-term paediatric follow-up in a multidisciplinary team (orthopaedic surgeon, physical therapist, occupational therapist, prosthetist, social worker) is needed after the loss of multiple fingers or limb loss at a proximal level. This team can help ascertain the child's need or wish for a prosthesis. If the injury occurred at a very young age, many patients will cope surprisingly well, similar to children with a congenital limb deficiency. Some rehabilitate very well and can often choose not to use a prosthesis. Children have a greater regenerative potential and adapt much better than adults after injury. The professionals assisting the patients and families must be familiar with the available prostheses and mechanical aids [54]. The prostheses for below-elbow amputations are much better than for above-elbow amputations since restoring the elbow flexion is a very complex function [122]. Less than 50% of the above-elbow amputees will use their prostheses whereas the below-elbow amputees will more probably use theirs [132]. One obvious reason for patients not using their prosthesis is the lack of sensation, which remains a significant challenge. The osseointegrated prostheses can be possible alternatives in certain situations, especially for proximal humeral amputations in the skeletally mature patient.

The lower extremity prostheses function well, especially in below-knee amputations and in young people [59]. The presence of a knee or an ankle joint suggests a much easier prosthetic fitting with a greater functional outcome [133].

28.18 Bone Growth After Replantation

Paediatric bones are different from those of adults with thick periosteum and induction of intense osteogenesis after a fracture, leading to faster consolidation and infrequent non-unions [54]. The level of amputation is considered to be a significant prognostic factor for the epiphyseal growth of the replanted part. An assessment of longitudinal bone growth of proximal and distal segments after digital replantations with a long-term follow-up has shown that the average growth in the proximal bone segment was 94.5% of expected growth whereas the distal replanted part had an average growth of 92.7% of normal [134]. Cheng found that the bone growth in replanted digits with and without joint involvement had a mean relative length of 88% and 93%, respectively, compared to normal digits [80]. The injury to the epiphyseal plate during a traumatic amputation is an important factor influencing its normal growth. With an affected epiphysis, the bone growth of replanted digits was reduced from 93% to 86% of the contra-lateral non-injured side [135]. The distal radius and ulna growth plates account for about 80% of longitudinal forearm growth and 80% of humeral growth takes place at the proximal end. Some authors noticed an "all-or-none" growth phenomenon after replantation where no growth, overgrowth and normal growth were found in their group of patients [25]. In major limb replantations, multiple causes explain the problem of growth: direct lesion of the growth plate, excessive shortening of the bone, iatrogenic damage of the growth plate during osteosynthesis and possibly a decreased oxygen rate after replantation due to reduced blood flow.

28.19 Reconstruction Surgery

The free flap coverage of injured limbs is an acceptable procedure in children as it is in adults after trauma [73]. The thenar flap to cover major pulp loss and the heterodigital flap for salvage of degloved digits have been recommended [136, 137]. Al-Qattan suggests that the pedicled groin and abdominal flaps should be considered as options for hand and finger coverage especially in the younger children [138]. Song describes two cases, a 44- and 23-year-olds, follow-up of 10 and 9 years, where devitalised bone was preserved in necrotic fingers after crush injuries and covered with free tissue transfer with good short- and long-term results [139]. An index finger pollicisation is an option for the hand injuries with a severely mutilated first ray [140]. If digital salvage is impossible, a reconstruction with toe transfers should be considered in the paediatric population, especially in the metacarpal hand [32, 141, 142]. The toe-to-antebrachial stump transplantation as described by Vilkki for amputations at wrist level is an alternative to a prosthesis and is designed to create a pincer grip [143].

28.20 Prevention

Many amputation injuries are preventable with awareness-raising campaigns and active safety counselling [20]. Paediatric injuries caused by doors, home exercise bicycles, lawn mowers and farms can be prevented through design changes and education [40, 41, 144–147]. Davis recommends several steps to prevent farming injuries including formal education especially of older children on the operation of farming equipment and the application of nonremovable automatic safety devices on farming equipment by manufacturers [148]. In the USA, Borne recommends preventative measures for adolescents who are more prone to motor vehicle and firearm injuries due to their driving inexperience, their increased risk taking behaviour, overestimation of skills and the influence of peer pressure [27]. A high cost is associated with upper extremity injuries, both emotionally and economically; thus aggressive efforts towards prevention should be a main aim.

References

1. O'Brien BM. Replantation and reconstructive microvascular surgery. Part I. Ann R Coll Surg Engl. 1976;58(2):87–103.
2. Jacobsen JH, Suarez EL. Microsurgery in anastomosis of small vessels. Surg Forum. 1960;11:243.
3. Malt RA, McKhann C. Replantation of severed arms. JAMA. 1964;189:716–22.
4. Kleinert HE, Kasdan ML. Anastomosis of digital vessels. J Ky Med Assoc. 1965;63:106–8.
5. Komatsu S, Tamai S. Successful replantation of a completely cut-off thumb. Plast Reconstr Surg. 1968;42(4):374–7. https://doi.org/10.1097/00006534-196810000-00021.
6. Tamai S. History of microsurgery–from the beginning until the end of the 1970s. Microsurgery. 1993;14(1):6–13.
7. Baudet J, Martin D, Bakhach J, Demiri E. Microvascular surgery in Europe: the early achievements and development. Microsurgery. 1993;14(4):234–40.
8. Gurnaney HG, Fiadjoe JE, Levin LS, Chang B, Delvalle H, Galvez J, et al. Anesthetic management of the first pediatric bilateral hand transplant. Can J Anaesth. 2016;63(6):731–6. https://doi.org/10.1007/s12630-016-0625-y.

9. Cetrulo CL Jr, Kovach SJ. Procurement of hand and arm allografts. Tech Hand Up Extrem Surg. 2013;17(4):232–8. https://doi.org/10.1097/bth.0000000000000031.
10. Dubernard JM, Owen E, Herzberg G, Lanzetta M, Martin X, Kapila H, et al. Human hand allograft: report on first 6 months. Lancet. 1999;353(9161):1315–20. https://doi.org/10.1016/s0140-6736(99)02062-0.
11. Biemer E. Definitions and classifications in replantation surgery. Br J Plast Surg. 1980;33(2):164–8.
12. Hadley SR, Capo JT. Digit replantation the first 50 years. Bull Hosp Jt Dis. 2015;73(2):148–55.
13. Squitieri L, Reichert H, Kim HM, Steggerda J, Chung KC. Patterns of surgical care and health disparities of treating pediatric finger amputation injuries in the United States. J Am Coll Surg. 2011;213(4):475–85. https://doi.org/10.1016/j.jamcollsurg.2011.07.017.
14. Raja SS. Management of complex tissue injuries and replantation across the world. Injury. 2006;37(11):1057–60. https://doi.org/10.1016/j.injury.2006.07.026.
15. Michalko KB, Bentz ML. Digital replantation in children. Crit Care Med. 2002;30(11):S444–7.
16. Saies AD, Urbaniak JR, Nunley JA, Taras JS, Goldner RD, Fitch RD. Results after replantation and revascularization in the upper extremity in children. J Bone Joint Surg Am. 1994;76(12):1766–76.
17. Urbaniak JR. Replantation in children. In: Serafin D, Georgiade N, editors. Pediatric plastic surgery. St. Louis: C.V. Mosby; 1984. p. 1168–85.
18. Nylander G, Vilkki S, Ostrup L. The need for replantation surgery after traumatic amputations of the upper extremity–an estimate based upon the epidemiology of Sweden. J Hand Surg (Br). 1984;9(3):257–60.
19. Lindfors N, Marttila I. Replantation or revascularisation injuries in children: incidence, epidemiology, and outcome. J Plast Surg Hand Surg. 2012;46(5):359–63. https://doi.org/10.3109/2000656x.2012.700012.
20. Panagopoulou P, Antonopoulos CN, Iakovakis I, Dessypris N, Gkiokas A, Pasparakis D, et al. Traumatic hand amputations among children in Greece: epidemiology and prevention potential. Inj Prev. 2012;18(5):309–14. https://doi.org/10.1136/injuryprev-2011-040121.
21. Atroshi I, Rosberg HE. Epidemiology of amputations and severe injuries of the hand. Hand Clin. 2001;17(3):343–50. vii
22. Kiil J. The epidemiology of replantation cases. Scand J Plast Reconstr Surg Suppl. 1982;19:78–80.
23. Vilkki SK, Goransson H. Traumatic amputations and the need for a replantation service in Finland. Ann Chir Gynaecol. 1982;71(1):2–7.
24. Taras JS, Nunley JA, Urbaniak JR, Goldner RD, Fitch RD. Replantation in children. Microsurgery. 1991;12(3):216–20.
25. Jaeger SH, Tsai TM, Kleinert HE. Upper extremity replantation in children. Orthop Clin North Am. 1981;12(4):897–907.
26. Hostetler SG, Schwartz L, Shields BJ, Xiang H, Smith GA. Characteristics of pediatric traumatic amputations treated in hospital emergency departments: United States, 1990-2002. Pediatrics. 2005;116(5):e667–74. https://doi.org/10.1542/peds.2004-2143.
27. Borne A, Porter A, Recicar J, Maxson T, Montgomery C. Pediatric traumatic amputations in the United States: a 5-year review. J Pediatr Orthop. 2017;37(2):e104–e7. https://doi.org/10.1097/bpo.0000000000000693.
28. Foucher G. Distal digital replantation. One of the best indications for microsurgery. International. J Microsurg. 1981;3:263–70.
29. Jazayeri L, Klausner JQ, Chang J. Distal digital replantation. Plast Reconstr Surg. 2013;132(5):1207–17. https://doi.org/10.1097/PRS.0b013e3182a3c0e7.
30. Shi D, Qi J, Li D, Zhu L, Jin W, Cai D. Fingertip replantation at or beyond the nail base in children. Microsurgery. 2010;30(5):380–5. https://doi.org/10.1002/micr.20743.
31. del Pinal F. Severe mutilating injuries to the hand: guidelines for organizing the chaos. J Plast Reconstr Aesthet Surg. 2007;60(7):816–27. https://doi.org/10.1016/j.bjps.2007.02.019.
32. Kotkansalo T, Vilkki SK, Elo P. The functional results of post-traumatic metacarpal hand reconstruction with microvascular toe transfers. J Hand Surg Eur. 2009;34(6):730–42. https://doi.org/10.1177/1753193409337958.
33. Tamai S. Twenty years' experience of limb replantation–review of 293 upper extremity replants. J Hand Surg Am. 1982;7(6):549–56.
34. Raimondi PL, Petrolati M, Delaria G. Replantation of large segments in children. Hand Clin. 2000;16(4):547–61.
35. McClure SK, Shaughnessy WJ. Farm-related limb amputations in children. J Pediatr Orthop. 2005;25(2):133–7.
36. Koul AR, Cyriac A, Khaleel VM, Vinodan K. Bilateral high upper limb replantation in a child. Plast Reconstr Surg. 2004;113(6):1734–8; discussion 9-41.
37. Waikakul S, Sakkarnkosol S, Vanadurongwan V, Un-nanuntana A. Results of 1018 digital replantations in 552 patients. Injury. 2000;31(1):33–40.
38. Conner KA, McKenzie LB, Xiang H, Smith GA. Pediatric traumatic amputations and hospital resource utilization in the United States, 2003. J Trauma. 2010;68(1):131–7. https://doi.org/10.1097/TA.0b013e3181a5f2ec.
39. Murphy AD, Keating CP, Penington A, McCombe D, Coombs CJ. Paediatric fingertip composite grafts: do they all go black? J Plast Reconstr Aesthet Surg. 2017;70(2):173–7. https://doi.org/10.1016/j.bjps.2016.11.002.

40. Benson LS, Waters PM, Meier SW, Visotsky JL, Williams CS. Pediatric hand injuries due to home exercycles. J Pediatr Orthop. 2000;20(1):34–9.
41. Lehrer MS, Bozentka DJ, Partington MT, Lee B, Osterman AL. Pediatric hand injuries due to exercise bicycles. J Trauma. 1997;43(1):100–2.
42. McCarthy GT, Green EM, Ogunbona O, Simmonds HA, Fairbanks L, Pountney T, et al. A population study of Lesch-Nyhan disease in the UK. Dev Med Child Neurol. 2011;53(1):34–9. https://doi.org/10.1111/j.1469-8749.2010.03786.x.
43. Thirkannad SM. Mutilating hand injuries in children. Hand Clin. 2016;32(4):477–89. https://doi.org/10.1016/j.hcl.2016.07.007.
44. VanGiesen PJ, Seaber AV, Urbaniak JR. Storage of amputated parts prior to replantation–an experimental study with rabbit ears. J Hand Surg Am. 1983;8(1):60–5.
45. Boulas HJ. Amputations of the fingers and hand: indications for replantation. J Am Acad Orthop Surg. 1998;6(2):100–5.
46. Abzug JM, Kozin SH. Pediatric replantation. J Hand Surg Am. 2014;39(1):143–5. https://doi.org/10.1016/j.jhsa.2013.09.002.
47. Kim JY, Brown RJ, Jones NF. Pediatric upper extremity replantation. Clin Plast Surg. 2005;32(1):1–10. https://doi.org/10.1016/j.cps.2004.09.003.
48. Handford C, Thomas O, Imray CHE. Frostbite. Emerg Med Clin North Am. 2017;35(2):281–99. https://doi.org/10.1016/j.emc.2016.12.006.
49. Skjeldal S, Grogaard B, Nordsletten L, Reikeras O, Svindland A, Torvik A. Protective effect of low-grade hypothermia in experimental skeletal muscle ischemia. Eur Surg Res. 1992;24(4):197–203.
50. Li J, Guo Z, Zhu Q, Lei W, Han Y, Li M, et al. Fingertip replantation: determinants of survival. Plast Reconstr Surg. 2008;122(3):833–9. https://doi.org/10.1097/PRS.0b013e318180ed61.
51. Goldner R, Urbaniak J. Replantation. In: Green D, Hotchkiss R, Pederson W, Wolfe S, editors. Green's operative hand surgery. 5th ed. Philadelphia: Elsevier; 2005. p. 1569–86.
52. Kuri M, Watt A, Buncke G. Replantation at the level of the radiocarpal joint. In: Salyapongse AN, Poore SO, Afifi AM, Bentz ML, editors. Extremity replantation: a comprehensive clinical guide. New York: Springer; 2015. p. 67–81.
53. Wei FC, Chang YL, Chen HC, Chuang CC. Three successful digital replantations in a patient after 84, 86, and 94 hours of cold ischemia time. Plast Reconstr Surg. 1988;82(2):346–50.
54. Valencia J, Leyva F, Gomez-Bajo GJ. Pediatric hand trauma. Clin Orthop Relat Res. 2005;432:77–86.
55. Shenaq SM, Dinh TA. Pediatric microsurgery. Replantation, revascularization, and obstetric brachial plexus palsy. Clin Plast Surg. 1990;17(1):77–83.
56. Baker GL, Kleinert JM. Digit replantation in infants and young children: determinants of survival. Plast Reconstr Surg. 1994;94(1):139–45.
57. Mohan R, Panthaki Z, Armstrong MB. Replantation in the pediatric hand. J Craniofac Surg. 2009;20(4):996–8. https://doi.org/10.1097/SCS.0b013e3181ae21e5.
58. Zuker RM, Stevenson JH. Proximal upper limb replantation in children. J Trauma. 1988;28(4):544–7.
59. Daigle JP, Kleinert JM. Major limb replantation in children. Microsurgery. 1991;12(3):221–31.
60. Hierner R, Betz AM, Comtet JJ, Berger AC. Decision making and results in subtotal and total lower leg amputations: reconstruction versus amputation. Microsurgery. 1995;16(12):830–9.
61. Durban CM, Lee SY, Lim HC. Above-the-knee replantation in a child: a case report with a 24-year follow-up. Strat Trauma Limb Reconstr. 2015;10(3):189–93. https://doi.org/10.1007/s11751-015-0230-6.
62. Jones NF, Shin EK, Mostofi A, Oppenheim WL. Successful replantation of the leg in a pre-ambulatory infant. J Reconstr Microsurg. 2005;21(6):359–64. https://doi.org/10.1055/s-2005-915202.
63. Park EH, Mackay DR, Manders EK, Segal LS. Replantation of the midfoot in a child–six-year follow-up with pedobarographic analysis. J Reconstr Microsurg. 1999;15(5):337–41. https://doi.org/10.1055/s-2007-1000112.
64. Datiashvili RO. Simultaneous replantation of both lower legs in a child: 23 years later. J Reconstr Microsurg. 2009;25(5):323–9. https://doi.org/10.1055/s-0029-1215528.
65. Goldner RD, Urbaniak JR. Indications for replantation in the adult upper extremity. Occup Med. 1989;4(3):525–38.
66. Biemer D. Vein grafts in microvascular surgery. Br J Plast Surg. 1977;30(3):197–9.
67. Van Beek AL, Kutz JE, Zook EG. Importance of the ribbon sign, indicating unsuitability of the vessel, in replanting a finger. Plast Reconstr Surg. 1978;61(1):32–5.
68. Harkness B, Andresen D, Kesson A, Isaacs D. Infections following lawnmower and farm machinery-related injuries in children. J Paediatr Child Health. 2009;45(9):525–8. https://doi.org/10.1111/j.1440-1754.2009.01552.x.
69. Kurt E, Ozturk S, Isik S, Zor F. Continuous brachial plexus blockade for digital replantations and toe-to-hand transfers. Ann Plast Surg. 2005;54(1):24–7.
70. Su HH, Lui PW, Yu CL, Liew CS, Lin CH, Lin YT, et al. The effects of continuous axillary brachial plexus block with ropivacaine infusion on skin temperature and survival of crushed fingers after microsurgical replantation. Chang Gung Med J. 2005;28(8):567–74.
71. Phelps DB, Rutherford RB, Boswick JA Jr. Control of vasospasm following trauma and microvascular surgery. J Hand Surg Am. 1979;4(2):109–17.
72. Graf BM, Abraham I, Eberbach N, Kunst G, Stowe DF, Martin E. Differences in cardiotoxicity of bupivacaine and ropivacaine are the result

of physicochemical and stereoselective properties. Anesthesiology. 2002;96(6):1427–34.
73. Duteille F, Lim A, Dautel G. Free flap coverage of upper and lower limb tissue defects in children: a series of 22 patients. Ann Plast Surg. 2003;50(4):344–9. https://doi.org/10.1097/01.sap.0000044143.36516.32.
74. Cox GW, Runnels S, Hsu HS, Das SK. A comparison of heparinised saline irrigation solutions in a model of microvascular thrombosis. Br J Plast Surg. 1992;45(5):345–8.
75. Saba HI, Saba SR, Blackburn CA, Hartmann RC, Mason RG. Heparin neutralization of PGI2: effects upon platelets. Science. 1979;205(4405):499–501.
76. Zinberg EM, Choo DI, Zotter LA. Effect of heparinized irrigating solutions on patency of experimental microvascular anastomoses. Microsurgery. 1989;10(2):103–7; discussion 8-9.
77. Cheng GL, Pan DD, Yang ZX, Fang GR, Gong XS. Digital replantation in children. Ann Plast Surg. 1985;15(4):325–31.
78. Lee BI, Chung HY, Kim WK, Kim SW, Dhong ES. The effects of the number and ratio of repaired arteries and veins on the survival rate in digital replantation. Ann Plast Surg. 2000;44(3):288–94.
79. Urbaniak JR, Roth JH, Nunley JA, Goldner RD, Koman LA. The results of replantation after amputation of a single finger. J Bone Joint Surg Am. 1985;67(4):611–9.
80. Cheng GL, Pan DD, Zhang NP, Fang GR. Digital replantation in children: a long-term follow-up study. J Hand Surg Am. 1998;23(4):635–46. https://doi.org/10.1016/s0363-5023(98)80049-x.
81. Devaraj VS, Kay SP, Batchelor AG, Yates A. Microvascular surgery in children. Br J Plast Surg. 1991;44(4):276–80.
82. Parry SW, Toth BA, Elliott LF. Microvascular free-tissue transfer in children. Plast Reconstr Surg. 1988;81(6):838–40.
83. Gherardini G, Gurlek A, Cromeens D, Joly GA, Wang BG, Evans GR. Drug-induced vasodilation: in vitro and in vivo study on the effects of lidocaine and papaverine on rabbit carotid artery. Microsurgery. 1998;18(2):90–6.
84. Johns RA, DiFazio CA, Longnecker DE. Lidocaine constricts or dilates rat arterioles in a dose-dependent manner. Anesthesiology. 1985;62(2):141–4.
85. Vargas CR, Iorio ML, Lee BT. A systematic review of topical vasodilators for the treatment of intraoperative vasospasm in reconstructive microsurgery. Plast Reconstr Surg. 2015;136(2):411–22. https://doi.org/10.1097/prs.0000000000001431.
86. Couteau C, Rem K, Guillier D, Moris V, Revol M, Cristofari S. Improving free-flap survival using intra-operative heparin: ritualistic practice or evidence-base medicine? A systematic review. Ann Chir Plast Esthet. 2017;63:1–5. https://doi.org/10.1016/j.anplas.2017.06.010.
87. Conrad MH, Adams WP Jr. Pharmacologic optimization of microsurgery in the new millennium. Plast Reconstr Surg. 2001;108(7):2088–96; quiz 97.
88. Lloyd MS, Teo TC, Pickford MA, Arnstein PM. Preoperative management of the amputated limb. EMJ. 2005;22(7):478–80. https://doi.org/10.1136/emj.2003.008797.
89. Waters M, Harley B. Replantation of the forearm or arm. In: Salyapongse AN, Poore SO, Afifi AM, Bentz ML, editors. Extremity replantation : a comprehensive clinical guide. New York: Springer; 2015. p. 83–102.
90. Godina M. Early microsurgical reconstruction of complex trauma of the extremities. Plast Reconstr Surg. 1986;78(3):285–92.
91. Sabapathy SR, Venkatramani H, Bharathi RR, Bhardwaj P. Replantation surgery. J Hand Surg Am. 2011;36(6):1104–10. https://doi.org/10.1016/j.jhsa.2011.03.039.
92. Barbary S, Dautel G. Digital replantation in children. Chir Main. 2012;31(5):221–6. https://doi.org/10.1016/j.main.2012.08.001.
93. Ketchum LD. Pharmacological alterations in the clotting mechanism: use in microvascular surgery. J Hand Surg Am. 1978;3(5):407–15.
94. Davies DM. A world survey of anticoagulation practice in clinical microvascular surgery. Br J Plast Surg. 1982;35(1):96–9.
95. Askari M, Fisher C, Weniger FG, Bidic S, Lee WP. Anticoagulation therapy in microsurgery: a review. J Hand Surg Am. 2006;31(5):836–46. https://doi.org/10.1016/j.jhsa.2006.02.023.
96. Chang WH, Petry JJ. Platelets, prostaglandins, and patency in microvascular surgery. J Microsurg. 1980;2(1):27–35.
97. Masotti G, Galanti G, Poggesi L, Abbate R, Neri Serneri GG. Differential inhibition of prostacyclin production and platelet aggregation by aspirin. Lancet. 1979;2(8154):1213–7.
98. Nikolis A, Tahiri Y, St-Supery V, Harris PG, Landes G, Lessard L, et al. Intravenous heparin use in digital replantation and revascularization: the Quebec provincial replantation program experience. Microsurgery. 2011;31(6):421–7. https://doi.org/10.1002/micr.20900.
99. Betancourt FM, Mah ET, McCabe SJ. Timing of critical thrombosis after replantation surgery of the digits. J Reconstr Microsurg. 1998;14(5):313–6. https://doi.org/10.1055/s-2007-1000183.
100. Buntic RF, Brooks D, Buncke HJ, Buncke GM. Dextran-related complications in head and neck microsurgery: do the benefits outweigh the risks? Plast Reconstr Surg. 2004;114(4):1008; author reply-9.
101. Disa JJ, Polvora VP, Pusic AL, Singh B, Cordeiro PG. Dextran-related complications in head and neck microsurgery: do the benefits outweigh the risks? A prospective randomized analysis. Plast

Reconstr Surg. 2003;112(6):1534–9. https://doi.org/10.1097/01.prs.0000083378.58757.54.
102. Beris AE, Soucacos PN, Malizos KN. Microsurgery in children. Clin Orthop Relat Res. 1995;314:112–21.
103. Khouri RK, Shaw WW. Monitoring of free flaps with surface-temperature recordings: is it reliable? Plast Reconstr Surg. 1992;89(3):495–9; discussion 500-2.
104. Reagan DS, Grundberg AB, George MJ. Clinical evaluation and temperature monitoring in predicting viability in replantations. J Reconstr Microsurg. 1994;10(1):1–6. https://doi.org/10.1055/s-2007-1006563.
105. Ruopsa N, Kujala S, Kaarela O, Ohtonen P, Ryhanen J. Wireless infrared thermometer in the follow-up of finger temperatures. J Hand Surg Eur. 2009;34(4):526–9. https://doi.org/10.1177/1753193409102456.
106. Jones NF, Gupta R. Postoperative monitoring of pediatric toe-to-hand transfers with differential pulse oximetry. J Hand Surg Am. 2001;26(3):525–9. https://doi.org/10.1053/jhsu.2001.24132.
107. Han SK, Lee BI, Kim WK. Topical and systemic anticoagulation in the treatment of absent or compromised venous outflow in replanted fingertips. J Hand Surg Am. 2000;25(4):659–67. https://doi.org/10.1053/jhsu.2000.6920.
108. Goldner RD. Postoperative management. Hand Clin. 1985;1(2):205–15.
109. Pereira C, Azari K. Replantation of the digits. In: Salyapongse A, Poore S, Afifi A, Bentz M, editors. Extremity replantation: a comprehensive clinical guide. New York: Springer; 2015. p. 49–65.
110. Kamei K, Sinokawa Y, Kishibe M. The venocutaneous fistula: a new technique for reducing venous congestion in replanted fingertips. Plast Reconstr Surg. 1997;99(6):1771–4.
111. Sakamoto A, Yoshida T, Matsumoto Y, Kozuma M, Iwamoto Y. Revascularization of complete and incomplete distal finger amputations in children below 2 years of age: a report of three cases. J Hand Surg Eur. 2011;36(8):677–81. https://doi.org/10.1177/1753193411409839.
112. Mihara M, Nakanishi M, Nakashima M, Narushima M, Gonda K, Koshima I. Distal phalanx replantation using the delayed venous method: a high success rate in 21 cases without specialised technique. JPRAS. 2008;61(1):88–93. https://doi.org/10.1016/j.bjps.2007.02.004.
113. Puhaindran ME, Paavilainen P, Tan DM, Peng YP, Lim AY. Dermal pocketing following distal finger replantation. JPRAS. 2010;63(8):1318–22. https://doi.org/10.1016/j.bjps.2009.06.039.
114. Whitaker IS, Oboumarzouk O, Rozen WM, Naderi N, Balasubramanian SP, Azzopardi EA, et al. The efficacy of medicinal leeches in plastic and reconstructive surgery: a systematic review of 277 reported clinical cases. Microsurgery. 2012;32(3):240–50. https://doi.org/10.1002/micr.20971.
115. Mumcuoglu KY. Recommendations for the use of leeches in reconstructive plastic surgery. eCAM. 2014;2014:205929. https://doi.org/10.1155/2014/205929.
116. Beyersdorf F. Protection of the ischemic skeletal muscle. Thorac Cardiovasc Surg. 1991;39(1):19–28. https://doi.org/10.1055/s-2007-1013924.
117. Blaisdell FW. The pathophysiology of skeletal muscle ischemia and the reperfusion syndrome: a review. Cardiovasc Surg. 2002;10(6):620–30.
118. Kueckelhaus M, Fischer S, Sisk G, Kiwanuka H, Bueno EM, Dermietzel A, et al. A mobile extracorporeal extremity salvage system for replantation and transplantation. Ann Plast Surg. 2016;76(3):355–60. https://doi.org/10.1097/sap.0000000000000681.
119. Wang SH, Young KF, Wei JN. Replantation of severed limbs–clinical analysis of 91 cases. J Hand Surg Am. 1981;6(4):311–8.
120. Van Beek AL, Wavak PW, Zook EG. Microvascular surgery in young children. Plast Reconstr Surg. 1979;63(4):457–62.
121. Faivre S, Lim A, Dautel G, Duteille F, Merle M. Adjacent and spontaneous neurotization after distal digital replantation in children. Plast Reconstr Surg. 2003;111(1):159–65; discussion 66. https://doi.org/10.1097/01.prs.0000037758.54135.4b.
122. Wei F-C, Mardini S. Bilateral high upper limb replantation in a child. Plast Reconstr Surg. 2004;113(6):1734–8.
123. Aziz W, Noojin F, Arakaki A, Kutz JE. Avulsion injuries of the thumb: survival factors and functional results of replantation. Orthopedics. 1998;21(10):1113–7.
124. Ikeda K, Yamauchi S, Hashimoto F, Tomita K, Yoshimura M. Digital replantation in children: a long-term follow-up study. Microsurgery. 1990;11(4):261–4.
125. Heistein JB, Cook PA. Factors affecting composite graft survival in digital tip amputations. Ann Plast Surg. 2003;50(3):299–303.
126. Ezerins S, Harm C, Kempton C, Salyapongse A. Rehabilitation following replantation in the upper extremity. In: Salyapongse AN, Poore SO, Afifi AM, Bentz ML, editors. Extremity replantation : a comprehensive clinical guide. New York: Springer; 2015. p. 191–206.
127. Buncke GM, Buntic RF, Romeo O. Pediatric mutilating hand injuries. Hand Clin. 2003;19(1):121–31.
128. Grob M, Papadopulos NA, Zimmermann A, Biemer E, Kovacs L. The psychological impact of severe hand injury. J Hand Surg Eur. 2008;33(3):358–62. https://doi.org/10.1177/1753193407087026.
129. Meyer TM. Psychological aspects of mutilating hand injuries. Hand Clin. 2003;19(1):41–9.
130. Peacock K, Tsai TM. Comparison of functional results of replantation versus prosthesis in a patient with bilateral arm amputation. Clin Orthop Relat Res. 1987;214:153–9.

131. Graham B, Adkins P, Tsai TM, Firrell J, Breidenbach WC. Major replantation versus revision amputation and prosthetic fitting in the upper extremity: a late functional outcomes study. J Hand Surg Am. 1998;23(5):783–91.
132. Wright TW, Hagen AD, Wood MB. Prosthetic usage in major upper extremity amputations. J Hand Surg Am. 1995;20(4):619–22. https://doi.org/10.1016/s0363-5023(05)80278-3.
133. Le JT, Scott-Wyard PR. Pediatric limb differences and amputations. Phys Med Rehabil Clin N Am. 2015;26(1):95–108. https://doi.org/10.1016/j.pmr.2014.09.006.
134. Demiri E, Bakhach J, Tsakoniatis N, Martin D, Baudet J. Bone growth after replantation in children. J Reconstr Microsurg. 1995;11(2):113–22; discussion 22-3. https://doi.org/10.1055/s-2007-1006518.
135. Beyermann K, Hahn P, Mutsch Y, Lanz U. Bone growth after finger replantation in childhood. Handchir Mikrochir Plast Chir. 2000;32(2):88–92. https://doi.org/10.1055/s-2000-19254.
136. Fitoussi F, Ghorbani A, Jehanno P, Frajman JM, Pennecot GF. Thenar flap for severe finger tip injuries in children. J Hand Surg (Br). 2004;29(2):108–12. https://doi.org/10.1016/j.jhsb.2003.10.006.
137. Hashem AM. Salvage of degloved digits with heterodigital flaps and full thickness skin grafts. Ann Plast Surg. 2010;64(2):155–8. https://doi.org/10.1097/SAP.0b013e3181a2c602.
138. Al-Qattan MM, Al-Qattan AM. Defining the indications of pedicled groin and abdominal flaps in hand reconstruction in the current microsurgery era. J Hand Surg Am. 2016;41(9):917–27. https://doi.org/10.1016/j.jhsa.2016.06.006.
139. Song F, Pan Y, Zhao Z, Deng J, Sun C. Preservation of devitalized bone in necrotic digits following crush injury with free tissue transfer. J Hand Surg Am. 2017;42(9):755. https://doi.org/10.1016/j.jhsa.2017.03.019.
140. Yu G, Xu HY, Lei HY, Guo S, Huang JH, Li DB. Combined index finger pollicization with an anterolateral thigh flap for thumb reconstruction. Chin J Traumatol. 2014;17(6):354–7.
141. Herrera FA, Lee CK, Brooks D, Buntic R, Buncke GM. Simultaneous double second toe transplantation for reconstruction of multiple digit loss in traumatic hand injuries. J Reconstr Microsurg. 2009;25(6):369–76. https://doi.org/10.1055/s-0029-1215527.
142. Kotkansalo T, Vilkki S, Elo P. Long-term results of finger reconstruction with microvascular toe transfers after trauma. J Plast Reconstr Aesthet Surg. 2011;64(10):1291–9. https://doi.org/10.1016/j.bjps.2011.04.036.
143. Vilkki SK, Kotkansalo T. Present technique and long-term results of toe-to-antebrachial stump transplantation. JPRAS. 2007;60(7):835–48. https://doi.org/10.1016/j.bjps.2007.02.018.
144. Smith GA. Technical report: lawn mower-related injuries to children. Pediatrics. 2001;107(6):E106.
145. Rathje C, Venegas A, Helmer SD, Drake RM, Ward JG, Haan JM. Pediatric farm injuries: morbidity and mortality. Kans J Med. 2017;10(4):1–12.
146. Yorlets RR, Busa K, Eberlin KR, Raisolsadat MA, Bae DS, Waters PM, et al. Fingertip injuries in children: epidemiology, financial burden, and implications for prevention. Hand. 2017;12(4):342–7. https://doi.org/10.1177/1558944716670139.
147. Loder RT. Demographics of traumatic amputations in children. Implications for prevention strategies. J Bone Joint Surg Am. 2004;86(5):923–8.
148. Davis JB Jr, Howell CG, Parrish RA. Childhood farm injury: the role of the physician in prevention. Am Surg. 1988;54(4):192–4.

Hand Transplantation in Children

29

Shaun D. Mendenhall, Todd J. Levy, Sandra Amaral, Benjamin Chang, and L. Scott Levin

Abstract

Pediatric hand transplantation is a recent addition to the field of vascularized composite allotransplantation. After careful patient selection, thorough preoperative planning, and repeated rehearsals by a large multidisciplinary team, we recently completed the world's first bilateral distal forearm level hand transplant in an eight-year-old child who was already on immunosuppression following a living donor kidney transplant. Short-term outcomes at 30 months have been promising including return of hand intrinsic motor function, return of sensibility of the hands, and ability to perform self-care and age-appropriate play. The sequelae of long-term systemic immunosuppression and incomplete nerve recovery will continue to be a limiting factor in pediatric hand transplantation, but with careful patient selection, planning, and modern medical and surgical care, hand transplantation is now an option for children with upper limb loss.

Keywords

Hand transplantation · Hand transplant · Vascularized composite allotransplantation · Upper extremity transplant · Heterologous hand transplant · Pediatric hand surgery · Hand amputation · Prosthetics

29.1 Introduction

Vascularized composite allotransplantation (VCA) refers to the transplantation of multiple tissue types together as a single functional unit such as an upper extremity or face, which contain bone, muscle, fat, vessels, nerves, and skin [1]. Beginning in 1998 with the first successful hand transplant in an adult [2], the modern era of VCA has been a worldwide effort with transplants and research taking place on nearly every continent

S. D. Mendenhall · L. S. Levin (✉)
Division of Plastic, Reconstructive, and Oral Surgery, Division of Orthopaedic Surgery, Children's Hospital of Philadelphia, Perelman School of Medicine at the University of Pennsylvania, Philadelphia, PA, USA
e-mail: mendenhals@chop.edu; Scott.levin@pennmedicine.upenn.edu

T. J. Levy
Center for Rehabilitation, The Children's Hospital of Philadelphia, Philadelphia, PA, USA
e-mail: levyt@chop.edu

S. Amaral
Division of Nephrology, Children's Hospital of Philadelphia, Perelman School of Medicine at the University of Pennsylvania, Philadelphia, PA, USA
e-mail: amarals@chop.edu

B. Chang
Division of Plastic, Reconstructive, and Oral Surgery, Division of Orthopaedic Surgery, Children's Hospital of Philadelphia, Perelman School of Medicine at the University of Pennsylvania, Philadelphia, PA, USA

Division of Plastic Surgery, Department of Orthopaedic Surgery, Perelman School of Medicine at the University of Pennsylvania, Philadelphia, PA, USA
e-mail: benjamin.chang@pennmedicine.upenn.edu

G. Pajardi (ed.), *Pediatric Hand Surgery*, https://doi.org/10.1007/978-3-031-30984-7_29

of the world [3]. Since then, many major milestones have been reached in this growing field including the world's first bilateral hand transplantation in a child performed by our team at the Children's Hospital of Philadelphia in 2015 [4–8]. This chapter will present the historical, ethical, psychosocial, donor, surgical, immunological, and rehabilitation considerations of this case as well as the outcomes at 30 months.

29.1.1 Hand and Upper Extremity Transplantation

With approximately 150 transplants in over 100 patients worldwide, transplantation of the hand and upper extremity has become by far the most widely performed VCA to date [3]. The first modern-era hand transplant occurred in Lyon, France, when Jean-Michel Dubernard led a team of international surgeons in a unilateral dominant hand transplant in 1998 [2]. Patient noncompliance with immunosuppression led to rejection of this allograft and the subsequent need for transplant removal, but long-term success was found in the second modern-era hand transplant four months after the first [9]. Dr. Warren Breidenbach and his team led this transplant in Louisville, which would become the longest VCA transplant in the world currently at nearly 25 years posttransplant. Since then, many bilateral transplants and even above-elbow transplants have been performed worldwide which have demonstrated technical success and excellent functional outcomes in select patients. Patient survival has been good with only one patient death from isolated upper extremity transplantation in the worldwide experience [10]. The five-year allograft survival rate for upper extremity transplants approaches 90% [3, 11], which is better than that of other deceased donor solid organ transplants, with the best outcomes reported for heart transplants at a 75% five-year survival rate [12, 13].

Functional outcomes of hand transplantation have been promising. Nearly all hand transplant patients recover protective sensation of the hand and 84% recover discriminative touch [14]. Motor function is more dependent on the level of the transplant with wrist-level transplants generally obtaining the best functional outcomes. Nevertheless, even above-elbow transplants can regain meaningful function [15]. Outcomes data from the International Registry on Hand and Composite Tissue Allotransplantation (www.handregistry.com) and others demonstrate an overall trend toward continued functional improvement over the life of the allograft [14, 16]. Of note, starting just one year after transplant, the Disability of the Arm, Shoulder, and Hand (DASH) scores are on average better for transplants than for prosthetic users [14, 16, 17].

As with solid organ transplantation, VCA outcomes have been tempered by the sequelae of lifelong immunosuppression including opportunistic bacterial, fungal, and viral infections, metabolic complications, and malignancies [18, 19]. Since these transplants are not lifesaving but quality of life enhancing, the benefits of improved function and appearance must be carefully weighed with the complications of immunosuppression.

29.1.2 Upper Extremity Transplantation in Children

Transplantation of the upper extremity in children is a very recent and limited addition to the field of vascularized composite allotransplantation. The first upper extremity transplant in a child was performed in Malaysia between two identical twins in 2000 by Pathmanathan [20, 21]. This case consisted of an above-elbow arm transplant for congenital absence of the hand in one twin from the other who had a fatal meningoencephalocele. Although under reported, the child went on to have excellent function of the transplanted arm as of the report on her eight-year follow-up [20]. Because the donor was her twin sister, no immunosuppression was needed. The second attempt at a pediatric arm transplant, and the first allotransplant requiring immunosuppression, took place in Mexico City ten years later. A 17-year-old female underwent bilateral proximal arm transplantation 3 years after a high-voltage electrical injury. Unfortunately, this patient had massive intraoperative blood loss and resuscitation and died in the early perioperative

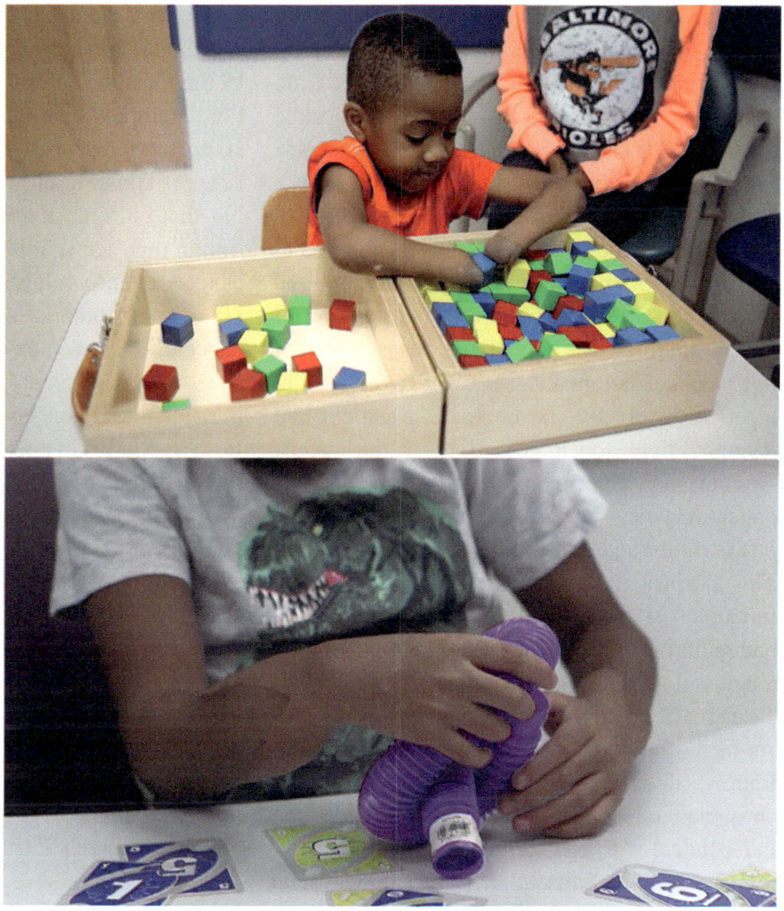

Fig. 29.1 Preoperative photo of the world's first bilateral hand transplant recipient (top) and at 25 months posttransplant (bottom). Photos courtesy of the Children's Hospital of Philadelphia

period of a cardiopulmonary event attributed to a severe cytokine release syndrome associated with thymoglobulin [10]. In 2015, our team performed a bilateral hand transplant on an eight-year-old quadrimembral amputee at the Children's Hospital of Philadelphia in the United States (Fig. 29.1) [4–7]. This child had lost all four limbs and his kidneys due to staphylococcal sepsis at the age of two and had previously undergone living-related donor kidney transplantation from his mother at the age of four. The patient continues to do well 8 years posttransplant and has gained remarkable function of the hands. A review of his case follows that demonstrates the importance of careful patient selection, thorough preoperative planning, intraoperative technical expertise, and postoperative medical and rehabilitation care by a large multidisciplinary team.

29.2 Case Report of the First Pediatric Bilateral Hand Transplant

Complete details of the first bilateral hand transplantation performed on a child were previously reported [4]. Briefly, after two years of evaluation and planning by a large multidisciplinary team including orthopedic, plastic, and transplant surgeons, transplant immunologists, occupational and physical therapists, social workers, pediatric psychologists, pediatric pharmacists, and ethicists, the decision was made to proceed with transplant. The risks of slightly increased immunosuppression over the patient's current kidney transplant regimen were deemed worth the benefits of having arms. The Institutional Review Board viewed the transplant as novel clinical care and considered the procedure exempt from full review. Multiple preoperative rehearsals took place in preparation for the surgery. After a little over two months on the waitlist, an appropriate donor was found and the transplant was performed in a 10 h and 40 min operation with a large surgical team. In the early postoperative period, one of the hands became ischemic due to thrombosis of the ulnar artery which required immediate take back to the OR and revision of the anastomosis. The patient was hospitalized for five weeks as an inpatient and for two weeks in inpatient rehab. By six months, the patient had regained light touch sensation of the hands. Around an eight-month posttransplant, the patient had clear intrinsic muscle function return in the right hand and by ten months in the left. This intrinsic function was also confirmed by functional MRI. During the first year the patient had multiple bouts of acute rejection treated with a bolus of steroids and topical agents along with an increase in maintenance immunosuppression. As of 30-month follow-up, he has continued to improve in sensation, motor function, and psychosocial integration of the hands and is more independent with self-care such as eating, toileting, and clothing himself. He is also able to write and to play sports such as baseball and football. Serial functional brain imaging studies including diffusion tensor imaging MRI and magnetoencephalography have demonstrated that the massive cortical reorganization associated with amputation is reversible back to similar patterns to the pre-amputation state after transplantation of new hands [22].

29.2.1 Ethical Considerations

Vascularized composite allotransplantation has had significant ethical implications since its inception [23–25]. Traditionally, VCA transplants have been considered nonlifesaving but quality of life-enhancing procedures. Therefore, one of the biggest ethical dilemmas for VCA is weighing the risks of lifelong immunosuppression (IS) with the benefits of improved function, appearance, and independence that transplantation offers. With children, this is obviously a bigger dilemma, since with longer exposure to IS the risks of untoward side effects are greater. For example, the incidence of nonmelanoma skin cancer in the solid organ transplant patient is approximately 50% at 20 years, demonstrating that children undergoing hand transplantation in their teens are at substantial risk for skin cancers in early adulthood [26–28]. In addition, other nonmelanoma skin cancers and nonskin cancers, such as non-Hodgkin lymphoma, are also more prevalent in pediatric solid organ transplant recipients over time (Yanik, Francis). In one study of pediatric kidney transplant recipients, nearly 17% experienced a posttransplant cancer over a median follow-up of 13 years (Francis). The risk of renal failure from calcineurin inhibitors is another important consideration and is both dose and time dependent [29]. Children and their caregivers should understand that there is a possibility of needing a kidney transplant before they reach middle age. The advantage of our patient was that he was already on IS for a renal transplant which made the decision easier to proceed with bilateral arm transplantation.

Some authors have recently argued that VCA transplants are actually lifesaving, thus tipping the risk benefit ratio [30]. In this view, the concept of "social death" is introduced which includes ostracism, social isolation and loneliness, and loss of personhood and a worthwhile life [30]. People suffering from social death have higher mortality rates, suicidal ideation, and attempts. Those with severe disfigurement including amputations (especially quadrimembral amputees and facial disfigurement) are at high risk for social death and therefore can have a lifesaving benefit from VCA. The concept of social death should be considered with screening children for hand transplantation and other VCAs.

Another ethical consideration for pediatric transplantation is the likelihood of experiencing chronic rejection leading to graft loss at some point in the future. We are now starting to appreciate chronic rejection in vascularized composite allotransplantation since the first of these transplants is now nearing 25 years of follow-up. Although the first US hand transplant patient Matthew Scott is still doing very well and has an excellent appearance and function of his hand, there have been reports in other patients of changes consistent with chronic rejection including graft fibrosis, thinning of the skin, loss of fingernails and adnexal structures, accelerated aging, and even graft vessel thrombosis from intimal hyperplasia leading to removal of the allograft [31–33]. This means children receiving VCAs will face the real threat of having to deal with loss of the allografts in early middle age and potentially the possibility of re-transplantation. These possibilities should be discussed with caregivers and included in the informed consent process for pediatric VCA. There are many other ethical considerations for pediatric VCA that are beyond the scope of this chapter [23–25, 34–37].

29.2.2 Psychosocial Considerations

Psychosocial considerations are extremely important for successful VCA transplantation in adults and children. The worldwide experience in adult hand transplantation has demonstrated that one of the biggest risk factors for allograft failure is patient noncompliance [3, 38, 39]. Experience with pediatric solid organ transplantation has demonstrated significant problems with patient noncompliance with IS therapy, especially in the adolescent patient [34, 40, 41]. Strong parental and family support is associated with better pediatric compliance and should be an important factor in the screening process for hand transplantation in children [42, 43]. In addition to compliance with IS, children who are being considered for hand VCA should also have a certain amount of maturity and determination that will allow them to cope with the potentially long hospital stay (seven weeks in our patient) and the vigorous hand therapy regimen following transplantation. A psychosocial subcommittee including social workers, psychologists, and psychiatrists should be involved in the screening process to help determine if a candidate has the psychological stability and resilience needed to cope with the vigorous demands of postoperative therapy, medical treatment, and close follow-up. The team should be prepared to provide the pediatric recipient with increased support as he/she transitions to adolescence and adulthood.

29.2.3 Donor Considerations

One of the biggest challenges in pediatric VCA is finding a suitable donor. We analyzed the United Network on Organ Sharing (UNOS) database and found that in the United States only about 8% of all organ donors are pediatric (ages 0–17) and that only about 15 children per year in the entire country would be a match for our recipient based on blood type, age ±2 years, and ethnicity [44]. Another issue is the sensitive nature of obtaining authorization from family members once an appropriate donor is found. We conclude that pediatric VCA donors are rare and may require longer travel times for procurement. This will be a limiting factor for pediatric VCA moving forward. In our particular case, despite the odds, an appropriate donor was found in just over two months after listing our patient. We did travel a considerable distance for procurement but were able to limit the cold ischemia time to approximately 6 h. We utilized three-dimensional printed hand models for size comparison between our recipient and the donor (Fig. 29.2) [8].

29.2.4 Surgical Considerations

29.2.4.1 Surgical Team

There are a number of important surgical considerations in pediatric hand transplantation. It is important to develop a surgical team familiar with pediatric hand surgery and pediatric microsurgery. The team must dedicate themselves to the significant time commitment required for preoperative planning, surgical rehearsals, the lengthy transplant operations, and as in our case the potential for vascular compromise and urgent

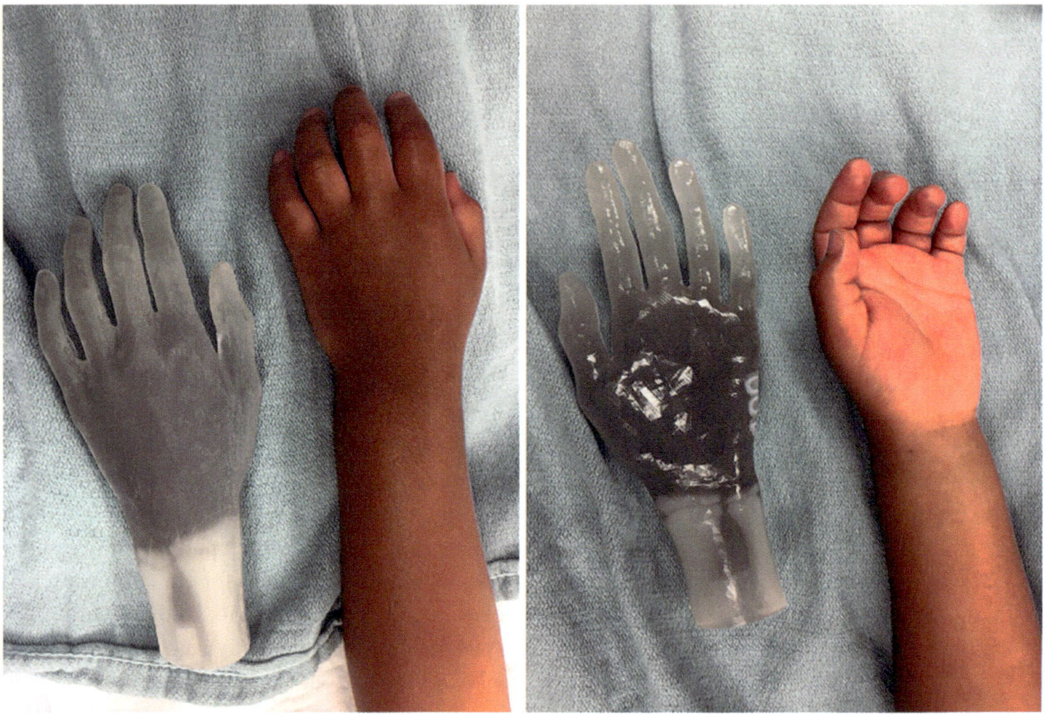

Fig. 29.2 Photos of three-dimensional printed hand next to donor hand for size comparison prior to procurement

reexploration in the OR. The team must be willing to be available at all times and to expeditiously return home if travelling for the moment when an appropriate donor is found.

29.2.4.2 Procedure

The donor limbs were procured and perfused with Belzer UW cold storage solution. Cold ischemia time was 6 h. Operating room preparation of the recipient included bilateral upper extremity indwelling axillary nerve block catheters, large bore lines for vascular access, and thymoglobulin and intravenous methylprednisolone induction. Four teams worked simultaneously on the donor and recipient limbs, identifying and attaching sterile labels to major peripheral nerves, tendons, and vessels to facilitate repair following bony fixation (Fig. 29.3). Osteosynthesis was done with Materialise (Leuven, Belgium) custom cutting guides applied to the donor and recipient radius and ulna, based on preoperative CT planning and three-dimensional printing, saving approximately 1 h of ischemia time (Fig. 29.3) [6]. Following rigid osteosynthesis with plates and screws, microsurgical repair of the radial and ulnar arteries was followed by multiple vein repairs and reperfusion (Fig. 29.4). Tenorrhaphy

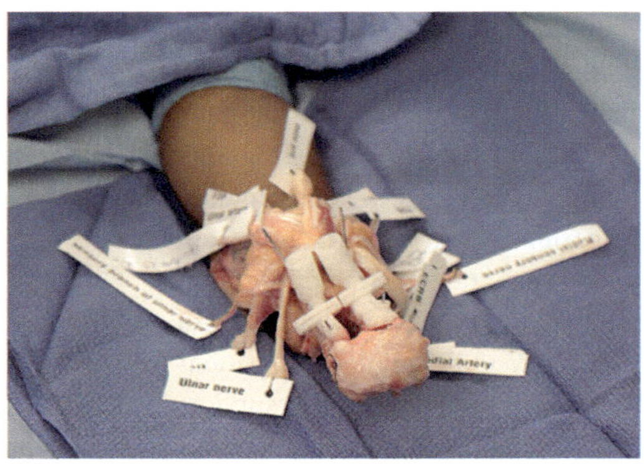

Fig. 29.3 Intraoperative view of the recipient limb being prepared for transplant by identifying and tagging all key structures. Used with permission from Amaral S, Levin LS. Pediatric and congenital hand transplantation. Current opinion in organ transplantation. 2017;22(5):477-83

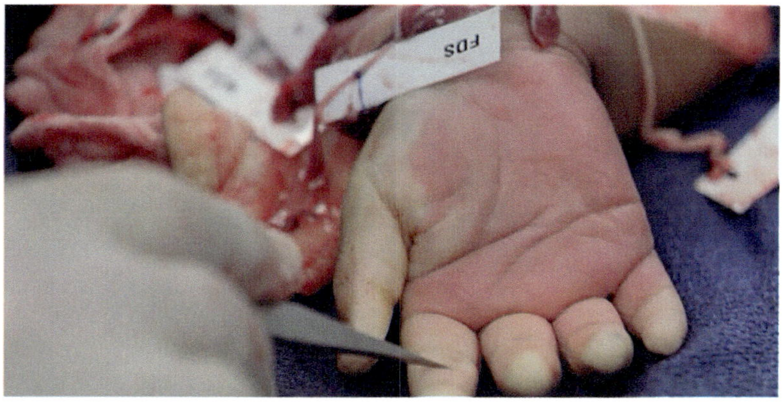

Fig. 29.4 Right hand transplant immediately after reperfusion

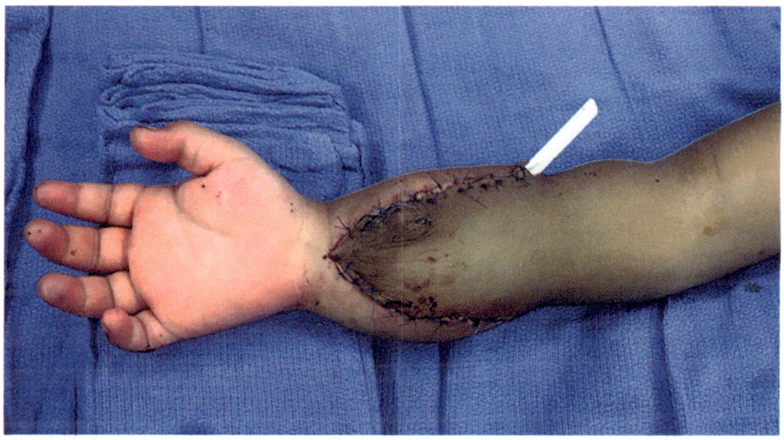

Fig. 29.5 Right hand immediately after transplantation surgery

of the flexor and extensor tendons of the wrist, thumb, and digits was then performed while keeping the wrist in 30° of extension and the hand in a fist. This was followed by repair of the median, superficial radial, and ulnar nerves. Interdigitating skin flaps were closed with excess donor skin included for accommodation of swelling and subsequent biopsies (Fig. 29.5).

Despite anticoagulation with heparin infusion, 2 h after the operation, the right hand was noted to be poorly perfused (Fig. 29.6) likely due to postoperative edema and redundancy of the ulnar artery repair that led to kinking. This was recognized immediately, and the patient was returned to the operating room for vascular revision, which included shortening the ulnar artery repair and performing an additional venous anastomosis of a vena comitans of the ulnar artery using an arterial interpositional graft that was banked from the donor. There were no further vascular events.

29.2.4.3 Early Postoperative Monitoring

Posttransplantation surveillance included daily physical examination of the limbs as well as continuous pulse oximetry to monitor tissue perfusion. Weekly skin biopsies were done and graded by the 2008 Banff criteria [45]. The patient received standard antimicrobial prophylaxis with valganciclovir and trimethoprim–sulfamethoxazole. He transitioned from heparin to aspirin by day 3 after the operation.

29.2.5 Immunological Considerations

Postoperatively, the patient received thymoglobulin induction with intravenous methylprednisolone (10 mg/kg), mycophenolate mofetil (600 mg/m^2 per dose), and tacrolimus. Goals trough

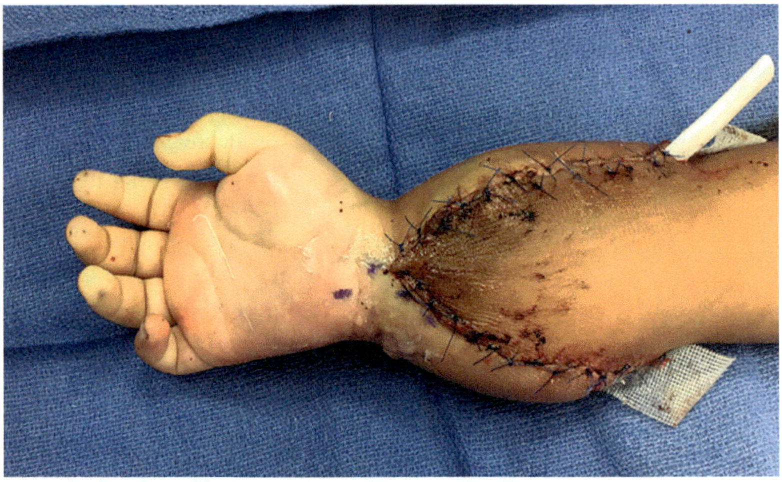

Fig. 29.6 Right hand 2 h after completion of transplantation surgery, now pale with evidence of arterial thrombosis and poor perfusion. The patient was immediately taken back to the OR for exploration and revision

tacrolimus concentrations of 10–12 ng/mL were difficult to achieve. In this setting, at week 3, the child experienced his first rejection episode, grades I–II bilaterally, which improved with intravenous methylprednisolone and topical betamethasone dipropionate (0.05% ointment) with topical tacrolimus (0.03%). Fluconazole (3 mg/kg once a day) was added to boost systemic tacrolimus concentrations. When tacrolimus concentrations increased to 12–15 ng/mL, the rejection resolved. One month later, bilateral grade I rejection recurred but responded to topical betamethasone. Concomitantly, the serum creatinine concentration increased from 0.5 g/dL to 0.7 g/dL. The creatinine increase was presumed to be secondary to tacrolimus toxic effects. In response, at three months after transplantation, sirolimus was added to the treatment regimen to enable reduction in tacrolimus.

Serious rejection episodes occurred in month 4 (grade III) and month 7 (grade II–III), presenting as erythematous rash with edema of both hands. Both episodes were successfully treated with topical betamethasone, topical tacrolimus, and intravenous methylprednisolone for three days. Oral prednisone was tapered gradually over 2–4 weeks depending on the timing of the resolution of the rejection episode. After month 8, several episodes of grade I rejection occurred but cleared with topical treatment and adjustments to tacrolimus or sirolimus doses. All rejection episodes have been T cell mediated, with no evidence of B cell or antibody mediated rejection. As of December 2017, 30 months after transplantation, he was stable on mycophenolate mofetil (200 mg BID), sirolimus (target trough 50–80 ng/mL), tacrolimus (target trough 7–8 ng/mL), and prednisone (5 mg daily) with a serum creatinine of 1.0 mg/dL.

Adverse events in the first year included a urinary tract infection, rhinovirus, two episodes of acute kidney injury associated with dehydration, and neutropenia responsive to granulocyte colony-stimulating factor. Related to the sirolimus, the patient experienced mouth ulcers, responsive to triamcinolone paste, and hyperlipidemia, treated with a statin. There was no proteinuria or hypertension. Viral studies for cytomegalovirus and EpsteinBarr virus have been persistently negative.

29.2.6 Posttransplant Rehabilitation

The initial therapy schedule for our patient was arduous and tailored to the attention span, occupations, and emotions of a child. Therapy was initiated six days postsurgery and provided daily for five weeks in acute care and then two weeks in inpatient rehabilitation, followed by ongoing outpatient and school therapy [4]. The team must secure appropriate resources prior to transplantation, both for the hand transplantation center and continued therapy in the patient's hometown. Four occupational therapists (OTs) worked with this patient during hospitalization, often in teams, and were on-call at all times. He spent most of each day in therapy with time allotted for naps, patient-caregiver bonding, and child life activities. The quality of therapy closely resembled outpatient hand therapy. The OTs sent a daily progress report to the surgical team with pictures/videos and attended morning rounds to collaborate and ensure dressings accommodated his orthoses and functional rehabilitation.

Considering the patient's developed motor strategies without the use of hands from two to eight years of age, an intense therapy program was implemented to restore active hand movements. This included motor imagery, biofeedback, and psychosocial interventions to facilitate acceptance of the hands, new habits, and cortical reorganization. Rote exercises, functional exercises, and splinting interventions were tailored to the patient's age. With intense therapy, he transitioned from using the allografts passively (e.g., pressing them together against objects for carrying, using proximal movements to push and pull objects) to using active prehensile patterns. Physical therapists addressed balance and mobility.

Our patient transitioned to a Day Hospital program in his community where he received therapy and schooling five days per week and then outpatient OT. Therapy is ongoing at 30 months postsurgery. Therapists from the transplantation center continue to follow him and collaborate with the medical team to target therapies. Our therapists suggest continuing therapy and minimizing compensatory motor strategies for two years following plateau of sensorimotor function and cortical plasticity. Collaboration between transplant center therapists and local therapists is especially important given the pediatric subspecialty care required.

29.2.7 Follow-Up and Outcomes

At 30 months of follow-up, our patient continues to progress in motor function, sensibility, and integration of the hands as his own. He has remarkably improved in his ability to provide self-care and to experience play in a manner similar to his peers. The box and block (Fig. 29.7) and nine-hole peg tests (Fig. 29.8) elucidate progress at the functional activity level, particularly efficiency of upper extremity gross motor skills compared to baseline [46, 47]. Tests of simulated functional activities such as the

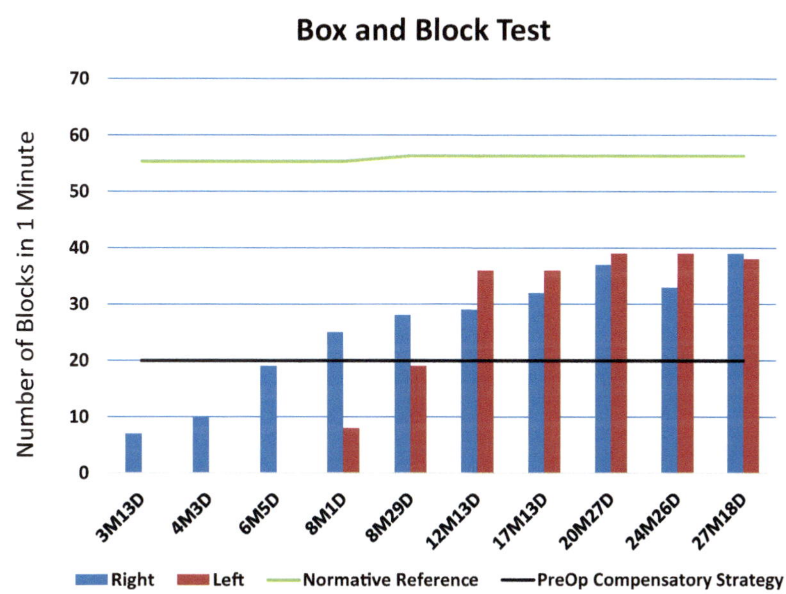

Fig. 29.7 Results of repeated box and block test measurements up until 27 months postoperative showing improvement in hand function. The black line shows the patient's preoperative state, and the green line shows aged-matched normal controls. Of note, the 27-month assessment may be slightly skewed by the fact that the patient had lidocaine injections for skin biopsies 2 h before the assessment and had some residual numbness of the fingers

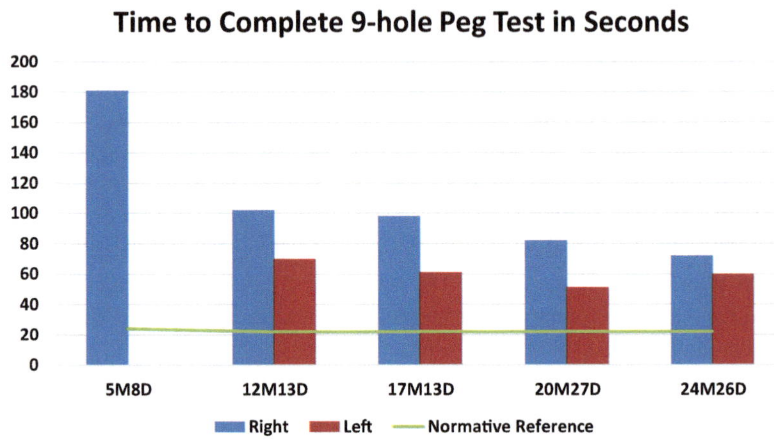

Fig. 29.8 Results of repeated nine-hole peg test measurements up until 25 months postoperative showing improvement in hand function. The green line shows aged-matched normal controls

Sollerman Hand Function Test [48] and the Carroll Quantitative Test of Upper Extremity Function [49] are less appropriate for children. He has obvious function of the intrinsic muscles of the hands and has no evidence of clawing. His sensation and specific finger localization continues to improve. His Semmes-Weinstein monofilament testing currently puts him in the "emerging normal sensation" range with most of the finger pulps. His left hand, which was a slightly more distal level of amputation than the right, has always done better than his right; however, he has always preferred this hand and is successful using this as the lead hand for most daily activities. His growth plates have all remained open and his ossification centers have expanded since transplant, although his hand is measuring small for his age (Fig. 29.9).

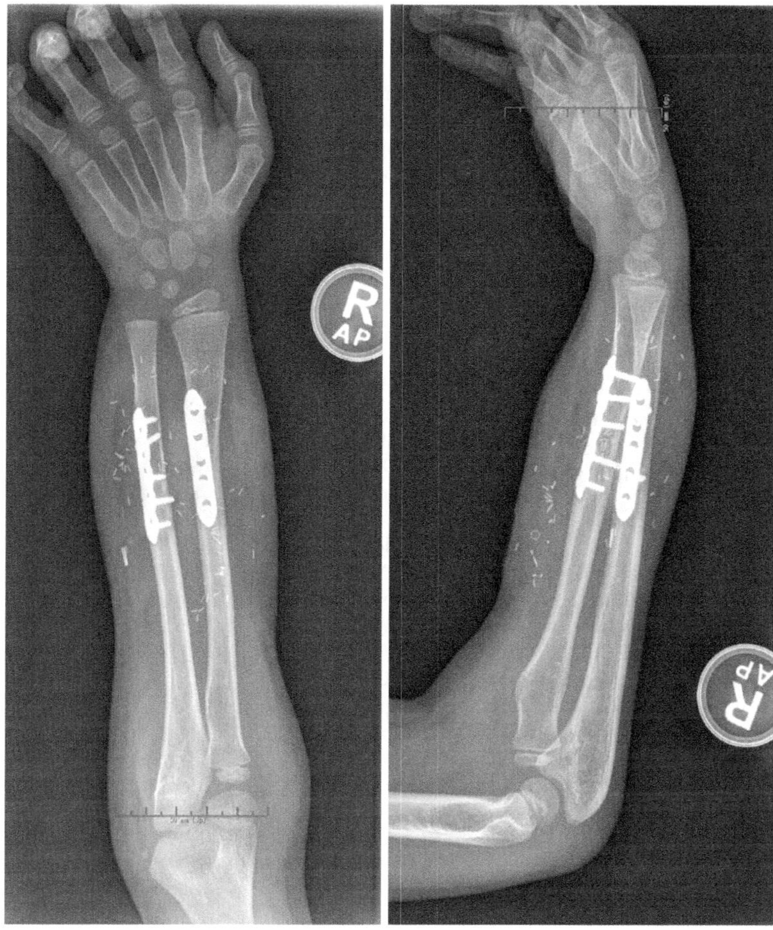

Fig. 29.9 AP and lateral X-rays of the transplant right hand at 25-month follow-up showing good bone healing at the osteosynthesis and open growth plates

29.3 Future of Hand/Arm Transplantation in Children

The future of hand transplantation in children is still unknown. We have shown good short-term success in the world's first pediatric bilateral hand transplant, but there is much yet to be learned in this emerging field of VCA. We remain cautiously optimistic. The two factors that will continue to limit the widespread applicability of both pediatric and adult hand transplantations are the needs for systemic immunosuppression with its side effects and the long distance needed for nerve regeneration. As the science behind these two issues improves, more widespread application of vascularized composite allotransplantation will follow. In the meantime, careful patient selection, thorough preoperative planning, intraoperative technical expertise, and postoperative medical and rehabilitation care by a large multidisciplinary team remain paramount for success in this new treatment option for children with upper limb loss.

References

1. Tintle SM, Potter BK, Elliott RM, Levin LS. Hand transplantation. JBJS Rev. 2014;2(1):e3.
2. Dubernard JM, Owen E, Herzberg G, Lanzetta M, Martin X, Kapila H, et al. Human hand allograft: report on first 6 months. Lancet. 1999;353(9161):1315–20.
3. Shores JT, Brandacher G, Lee WP. Hand and upper extremity transplantation: an update of outcomes in the worldwide experience. Plast Reconstr Surg. 2015;135(2):351–60.
4. Amaral S, Kessler SK, Levy TJ, Gaetz W, McAndrew C, Chang B, et al. 18-month outcomes of heterologous bilateral hand transplantation in a child: a case report. Lancet Child Adoles Health. 2017;1(1):35–44.

5. Amaral S, Levin LS. Pediatric and congenital hand transplantation. Curr Opin Organ Transplant. 2017;22(5):477–83.
6. Galvez JA, Gralewski K, McAndrew C, Rehman MA, Chang B, Levin LS. Assessment and planning for a pediatric bilateral hand transplant using 3-dimensional modeling: case report. J Hand Surg Am. 2016;41(3):341–3.
7. Gurnaney HG, Fiadjoe JE, Levin LS, Chang B, Delvalle H, Galvez J, et al. Anesthetic management of the first pediatric bilateral hand transplant. Can J Anaesth. 2016;63(6):731–6.
8. Momeni A, Chang B, Levin LS. Technology and vascularized composite allotransplantation (VCA)-lessons learned from the first bilateral pediatric hand transplant. J Mater Sci Mater Med. 2016;27(11):161.
9. Jones JW, Gruber SA, Barker JH, Breidenbach WC. Successful hand transplantation. One-year follow-up. Louisville Hand Transplant Team. N Engl J Med. 2000;343(7):468–73.
10. Iglesias M, Leal P, Butron P, Santander-Flores S, Ricano-Enciso D, Gonzalez-Chavez MA, et al. Severe complications after bilateral upper extremity transplantation: a case report. Transplantation. 2014;98(3):16–7.
11. Shores JT, Malek V, Lee WP, Brandacher G. Outcomes after hand and upper extremity transplantation. J Mater Sci Mater Med. 2017;28(5):72.
12. Scientific Registry of Transplant Recipients (SRTR) 2012 annual data report 2012. Available https://srtr.transplant.hrsa.gov/annual_reports/2012/Default.aspx.
13. Mendenhall SD, Schmucker RW, De la Garza M, Lutfy J, Levin LS, Neumeister MW. Osteosynthesis in forearm transplantation using a novel ulnar-shortening osteotomy system for simultaneous both bone fixation. Vascul Compos Allotranspl. 2015;2(3):53–9.
14. Petruzzo P, Lanzetta M, Dubernard JM, Landin L, Cavadas P, Margreiter R, et al. The international registry on hand and composite tissue transplantation. Transplantation. 2010;90(12):1590–4.
15. Cavadas PC, Ibanez J, Thione A, Alfaro L. Bilateral trans-humeral arm transplantation: result at 2 years. Am J Transplant. 2011;11(5):1085–90.
16. Landin L, Bonastre J, Casado-Sanchez C, Diez J, Ninkovic M, Lanzetta M, et al. Outcomes with respect to disabilities of the upper limb after hand allograft transplantation: a systematic review. Transpl Int. 2012;25(4):424–32.
17. General DoVAOoI. Healthcare inspection prosthetic limb care in VA facilities 2012. Available http://www.va.gov/oig/pubs/VAOIG-11-02138-116.pdf.
18. Pomahac B, Gobble RM, Schneeberger S. Facial and hand allotransplantation. Cold Spring Harb Perspect Med. 2014;4(3):a015651.
19. Khalifian S, Brazio PS, Mohan R, Shaffer C, Brandacher G, Barth RN, et al. Facial transplantation: the first 9 years. Lancet. 2014;384(9960):2153–63.
20. Pathmanathan V. Arm transplantation for congenital absence of the hand: the 8 year outcome. EUROHAND 2008, XIIIth congress of the federation of European Societies for Surgery of the hand, Lausanne, Switzerland, 2008.
21. Mukesh N, Bramstedt KA. Perspectives of US and Australian hand therapists about pediatric hand transplantation. Prog Transplant. 2017;27(1):73–8.
22. Gaetz W, Kessler SK, Roberts TPL, Berman JI, Levy TJ, Hsia M, et al. Massive cortical reorganization is reversible following bilateral transplants of the hands: evidence from the first successful bilateral pediatric hand transplant patient. Ann Clin Transl Neurol. 2017;5(1):92–7.
23. Simmons PD. Ethical considerations in composite tissue allotransplantation. Microsurgery. 2000;20(8):458–65.
24. Rohrich RJ, Longaker MT, Cunningham B. On the ethics of composite tissue allotransplantation (facial transplantation). Plast Reconstr Surg. 2006;117(6):2071–3.
25. Barker JH, Brown CS, Cunningham M, Wiggins O, Furr A, Maldonado C, et al. Ethical considerations in human facial tissue allotransplantation. Ann Plast Surg. 2008;60(1):103–9.
26. Francis A, Johnson DW, Craig JC, Wong G. Incidence and predictors of cancer following kidney transplantation in childhood. Am J Transplant. 2017;17(10):2650–8.
27. Yanik EL, Shiels MS, Smith JM, Clarke CA, Lynch CF, Kahn AR, et al. Contribution of solid organ transplant recipients to the pediatric non-hodgkin lymphoma burden in the United States. Cancer. 2017;123(23):4663–71.
28. Yanik EL, Smith JM, Shiels MS, Clarke CA, Lynch CF, Kahn AR, et al. Cancer risk after pediatric solid organ transplantation. Pediatrics. 2017;139(5):e20163893.
29. Naesens M, Kuypers DRJ, Sarwal M. Calcineurin inhibitor nephrotoxicity. Clin J Am Soc Nephrol. 2009;4(2):481–508.
30. Katrina AB. A Lifesaving view of vascularized composite allotransplantation: patient experience of social death before and after face, hand, and larynx transplant. J Patient Exp. 2017;2017:2374373517730556.
31. Kaufman CL, Ouseph R, Blair B, Kutz JE, Tsai TM, Scheker LR, et al. Graft vasculopathy in clinical hand transplantation. Am J Transplant. 2012;12(4):1004–16.
32. Krezdorn N, Pomahac B. Chronic allograft deterioration: a clinical reality in vascularized composite allotransplantation. Am J Transplant. 2017;17(7):1703–4.
33. Morelon E, Petruzzo P, Kanitakis J, Dakpe S, Thaunat O, Dubois V, et al. Face transplantation: partial graft loss of the first case 10 years later. Am J Transplant. 2017;17(7):1935–40.
34. Colen DL, Bank J, McAndrew C, Levin LS. Reconstruction for all: the case for pediatric hand transplantation. Vascul Compos Allotranspl. 2015;2(3):47–52.
35. Benghiac AG, Garrett JR, Carter BS. Ethical issues in pediatric face transplantation. Pediatr Transplant. 2017;21:7.

36. Bartlett SP, Chang B, Levin LS. Discussion: ethical issues in pediatric face transplantation: should we perform face transplantation in children? Plast Reconstr Surg. 2016;138(2):455–7.
37. Marchac A, Kuschner T, Paris J, Picard A, Vazquez MP, Lantieri L. Ethical issues in pediatric face transplantation: should we perform face transplantation in children? Plast Reconstr Surg. 2016;138(2):449–54.
38. Kumnig M, Jowsey SG, Moreno E, Brandacher G, Azari K, Rumpold G. An overview of psychosocial assessment procedures in reconstructive hand transplantation. Transpl Int. 2014;27(5):417–27.
39. Kumnig M, DiMartini AF, DiMartini AF. Psychological aspects of hand transplantation. Curr Opin Organ Transplant. 2014;19(2):188–95.
40. Lefkowitz DS, Fitzgerald CJ, Zelikovsky N, Barlow K, Wray J. Best practices in the pediatric pretransplant psychosocial evaluation. Pediatr Transplant. 2014;18(4):327–35.
41. Nevins TE, Nickerson PW, Dew MA. Understanding medication nonadherence after kidney transplant. J Am Soc Nephrol. 2017;28(8):2290–301.
42. Burra P, Ferrarese A, Feltrin G. Quality of life and adherence in liver transplant recipients. Minerva Gastroenterol Dietol. 2017;64(2):180–6.
43. Burra P, Germani G, Gnoato F, Lazzaro S, Russo FP, Cillo U, et al. Adherence in liver transplant recipients. Liver Transpl. 2011;17(7):760–70.
44. Mendenhall SD, Sawyer JD, West BL, Neumeister MW, Levin LS. Pediatric vascularized composite allotransplantation—what's the landscape for obtaining appropriate donors in the United States? Pediatr Transplant. 2019;23(5):e13466.
45. Schneider M, Cardones AR, Selim MA, Cendales LC. Vascularized composite allotransplantation: a closer look at the banff working classification. Transpl Int. 2016;29(6):663–71.
46. Jongbloed-Pereboom M, Nijhuis-van der Sanden MW, Steenbergen B. Norm scores of the box and block test for children ages 3-10 years. Am J Occup Ther. 2013;67(3):312–8.
47. Wang YC, Bohannon RW, Kapellusch J, Garg A, Gershon RC. Dexterity as measured with the 9-Hole Peg Test (9-HPT) across the age span. J Hand Ther. 2015;28(1):53–9.
48. Sollerman C, Ejeskär A. Sollerman hand function test: a standardised method and its use in tetraplegic patients. Scand J Plast Reconstr Surg Hand Surg. 1995;29(2):167–76.
49. Carroll D. A quantitative test of upper extremity function. J Chronic Dis. 1965;18(5):479–91.

Rehabilitation in Pediatric Hand Trauma

30

Rossella Pagliaro, Luigi Bartolomeo, Silvia Minoia, and Elena Marta Mancon

Abstract

A trauma can be for an adult a sudden change of status, the patient is immediately more helpful from caregivers, and the same is for children. Everyday life can change temporarily or definitively, and the child needs help and attention to accept this new status of his/her upper limb.

The trauma often modifies our motor image, and the little patient needs to adapt to this new functional or aesthetic situation, and this can be hard for the child and his family.

One of the first health workers that the family has to deal with is the hand surgeon, for a decision plan of therapy.

A good relationship with the health workers can increase the satisfaction of the patient and of caregivers, and this can be useful and positive also for the psychological aspect of acceptance of the new situation; this also helps to increase the compliance of the patient and of the family.

When it is necessary, a request of a psychological support is given to the child and family, together or separately.

During the physical therapy, it is very important for the patient to have a high compliance, because it plays an important role in it. Rehabilitation can be very difficult for pediatric patients, much more than with adults, especially for very traumatic accidents.

The younger is the child, the easier is for him/her to adapt to new situations; the same works with neuroplasticity.

Keywords

Hand · Traumas · Children · Motor image Functional limitation

A trauma can be for an adult a sudden change of status and the same is for children. Everyday life can change temporarily or definitively, and the child needs help and attention to accept this new status of his/her upper limb.

The trauma often modifies our motor image, and the little patient needs to adapt to this new functional or aesthetic situation and this can be hard for the child and his/her family. Sometimes children focus on their difference or limitation so

R. Pagliar (✉) · L. Bartolomeo · S. Minoia
E. M. Mancon
Hand Surgery and Rehabilitation Department, San Giuseppe Hospital IRCCS MultiMedica, Milan University, Milan, Italy

Milan, Italy
e-mail: rossella.pagliaro@multimedica.it; luigi.bartolomeo@multimedica.it; silvia.minoia@multimedica.it; elenamarta.mancon@multimedica.it

G. Pajardi (ed.), *Pediatric Hand Surgery*, https://doi.org/10.1007/978-3-031-30984-7_30

much that this aspect becomes the most important feature of their bodies.

Emotionally children are ashamed and desire to hide the hand, they try to put the hand in the pockets, sometimes they do not want to wear T-shirts, or they avoid public situation like school and playground.

One of the first health workers that the family has to deal with is the hand surgeon, for a decision plan of therapy.

A good relationship with the health workers can increase the satisfaction of the patient and of caregivers, and this can be useful and positive also for the psychological aspect of acceptance of the new situation; this also helps to increase the compliance of the patient and of the family.

When it is necessary, or a request of a psychological support is given to the child and family, together or separately; this can help both to express the expectations and realize the real possibilities and abilities that the child will have at the end of the surgical treatment and rehabilitation.

After the surgery, the limb of the little patient is protected by a bandage, often the dressing covers also some healthy segments, and this can contribute to an inappropriate and miraculous image of the hand. However, this is necessary to protect properly the limb after the surgical approach.

The postsurgery is a lapse of time in which the little patient and family have the chance to deal with anxiety and loss of the total control of the usual status of heath we all have in everyday life. This is the time of rehabilitation; the patient starts to get used to: be touched by the therapist's hands, to see the injured segment and the whole hand or arm. During the physical therapy, it is very important for the patient to have a high compliance, because it plays an important role in it. The aim of the therapist is to rehabilitate the whole limb through games and playing with children. Rehabilitation can be very difficult for pediatric patients, much more than with adults, especially for very traumatic accidents.

It can be very hard to obtain a high level of compliance for the whole section of physical therapy; in fact children can be shy or worried or even terrified sometimes; this is why the therapist needs to be patient, especially if some particular movements are required for the situation. Often a good observation of the child, respecting the motor milestones and the cognitive growth, can be the key for a good rehabilitation and also change often games and toys, choosing something appropriate for the aim of the physiotherapy, but fun in the meantime is essential.

The younger is the child, the easier is for him/her to adapt to new situations; the same works with neuroplasticity: with a good rehabilitative plan and a good relationship between the little patient and the therapist, the child will be able to regain dexterity and good motor skills, and this means good functionality and quality of life.

30.1 Fractures

Over 25% of traumas in pediatrics are fractures: in particular in the early stages of age, crushing traumas often occur in adolescents who often injure themselves while they are playing or doing sports.

In crushing traumas, distal phalanges and external rays of the hand are often involved. Interphalangeal joint traumas and volar plate lesions are also quite common.

All muscular-skeletal injuries have a different evolution in children compared to the same injury on an adult; in fact the elasticity of the different tissues and the presence of the growth plate needs a different therapeutic approach.

Particularly surgeon will pay attention on the possibility of interfering with the correct growth of the limb or segment or having distal problems on nerves or lately with secondary arthritis, stiffness, or chronic pain.

Bones in children can change quite quickly in shape, rotation, and alignment, if it they are subjected to stress.

Many fractures of the hand and wrist in children can be treated in a conservative way, with a cast or splint, and do not need surgery.

30.1.1 Conservative Treatment

Immobilization needs to be done immediately after the reduction of the fracture, particularly if the little patient is under anesthesia. A cast is probably the better choice for children; casts in fact are very resistant. Often the immobilization is wider than it should be for adults, for example, in a very young patient with a fracture of a phalange, it can be necessary to include the wrist too. If the cast is small or light, the risk is that the child can be able to remove it or damage while he/she plays or sleeps.

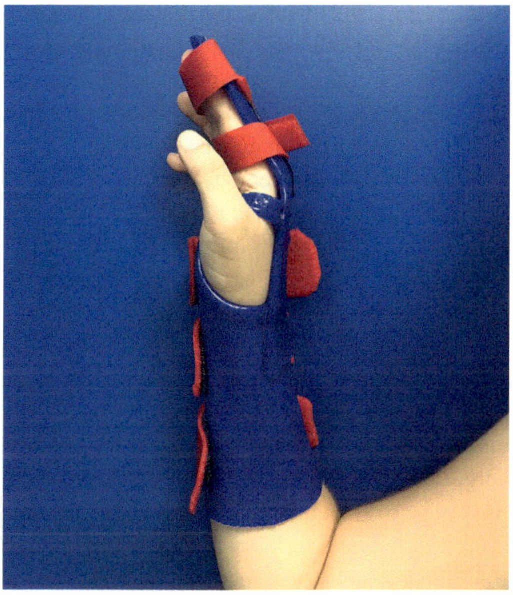

Fig. 30.1 Removal splint made by therapist after cast immobilization in the hand fractures

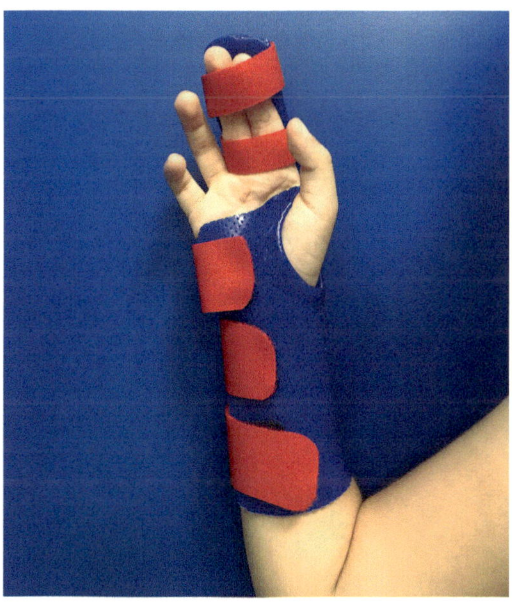

Fig. 30.2 Removal splint with wrist and fingers included to start mobilization after hand fractures

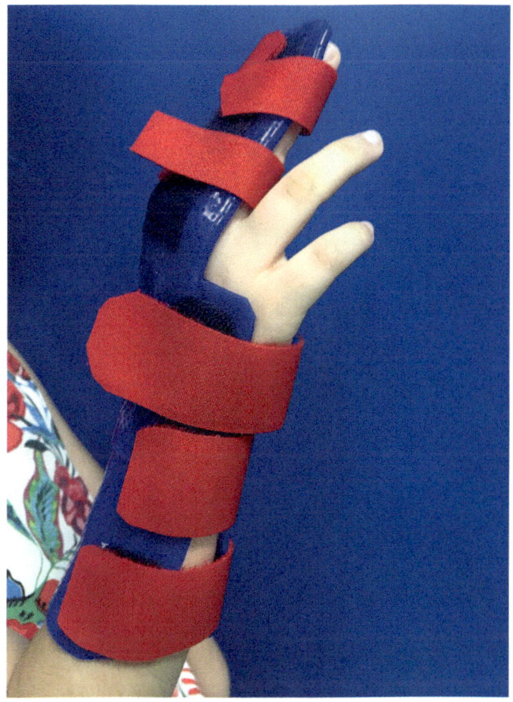

Fig. 30.3 Removal splint with wrist and fingers included to start mobilization after hand fractures

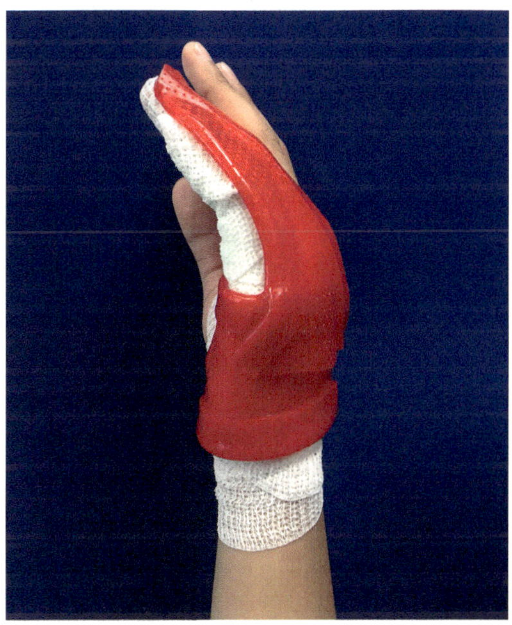

Fig. 30.4 Cast for fingers fractures

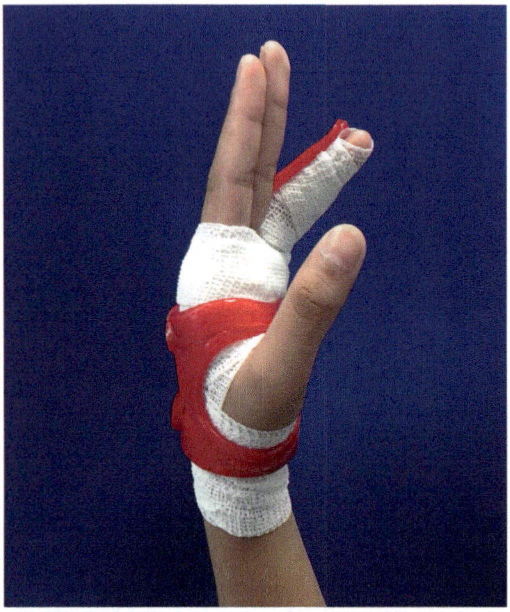

Fig. 30.5 Cast for fingers fractures

In compound fractures, normally the treatment is cast immobilization for three/four weeks and then a visit after an X-ray; when the cast is taken off, a removal splint is made by the therapists (Figs. 30.1, 30.2, 30.3, 30.4, and 30.5). During the following days, a specific rehabilitative with a hand therapist begins.

30.1.2 Surgical Treatment

Surgery in pediatrics is very different from surgery in adults: the periosteum is thick; growth plates are delicate, so the surgeon has to pay attention during the whole surgical approach.

30.1.3 Apical Traumas: Rehabilitative Part

In pediatrics, distal phalangeal traumas are quite common; crushing traumas represent the most of apical traumas but also hyperflexion or hyperextension.

Crushing can generate lesions of the nail or sub-nail hematoma or more complex trauma like complete lesion of the nail bed, fracture of the distal phalanx, or a lesion of the flexure or extension tendon.

In case of surgical flap suture also with microfractures after four weeks with a fixed digital splint (Fig. 30.6), the patient can start the active mobilization with a selective recruitment of the flexor digitorum profundus and exercises for the recruitment of extensor tendons. When the wound will be completely healed, the therapist can begin the treatment of the scar with a hydrating cream and with the use of a silicone elastomer during the night (Fig. 30.7), associated with a CoBan bandage to give the finger the correct compression for a proper skin remodeling.

The therapist will teach the parents how to do exercises for sensibility in order to manage the alteration of sensibility that is completely normal in this situation; this can help a quicker recovery and a quicker corticalization.

A digital and removable splint will be used during the night and in risky situation like schools and playgrounds until eight weeks from the surgery.

In case of subamputation of the distal phalanx, the postoperative period will be of immobilization with a digital splint in protection of the amputation stump (Fig. 30.6).

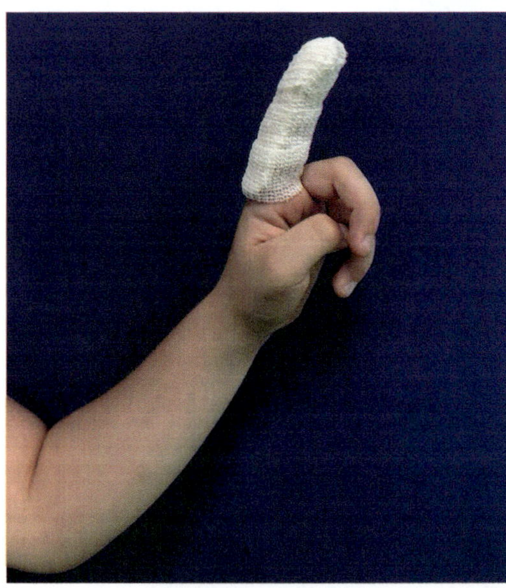

Fig. 30.6 Digital fix splint for fractures' fingers

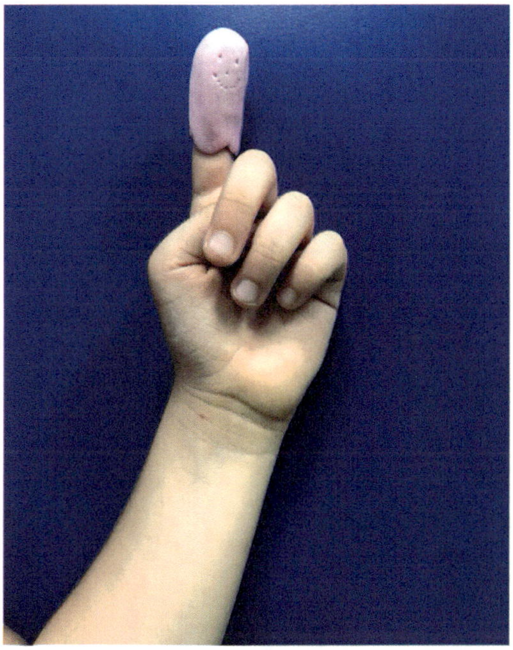

Fig. 30.7 The silicone elastomer used in the night time to treat the scar

When all the wounds will be completely healed, the hand therapist will make a removable splint in order to protect the stump, the parents will learn how to massage the scars, and the use of silicon sheets will be suggested for the night. Also in this case, sensibility has to be stimulated through different tissues. It is very important that the little patient at the end of the therapy is able to use the fingers involved in the trauma for all the activities of daily living (Fig. 30.8).

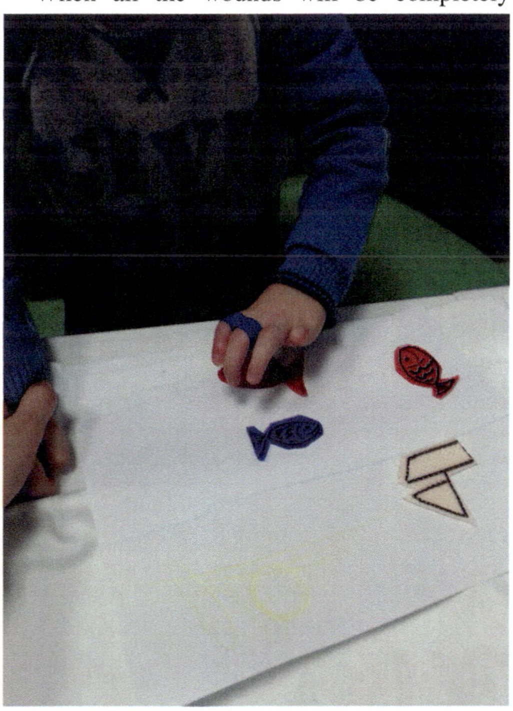

Fig. 30.8 A kind of exercise to stimulate hand using in manual play and daily living activity

30.2 Tendon Lesions in Pediatrics

Tendon lesions in children have a high incidence because they explore the world outside with their little hands often without paying attention. If these lesions are not treated properly, they can cause important functional deficits and deficits of growth; the child in fact can learn daily activities with the complete exclusion of the segment or of the whole hand.

However, it is very difficult to treat children with this kind of lesions because sometimes they have a very low compliance and little hands and little fingers which are very difficult to treat and to splint.

The major difference between the treatment of an adult and a child in this field is that treating a child means a bigger immobilization and bigger splints that can include also digit and joint that are not directly involved in the trauma, with the aim of giving more stability and to be safer (Fig. 30.9a–c).

The time of immobilization is on average longer than in adults, for example, in the lesion of flexor tendons, we begin to physiotherapy at the end of the fourth week keeping the splint that will be made removable, with the wrist extended 0–20°, metacarpal-phalangeal joint at about 30°, and interphalangeal joint extended (Fig. 30.10a). Disposition is chosen in order to avoid intrinsic muscle retraction.

Sometimes the surgeon chooses the pullout technique (Fig. 30.11); this can allow the immediate mobilization. The little patient will have of course a limit in the maximum open extension. The splint is going to be removable from the very beginning and will be made in the same position

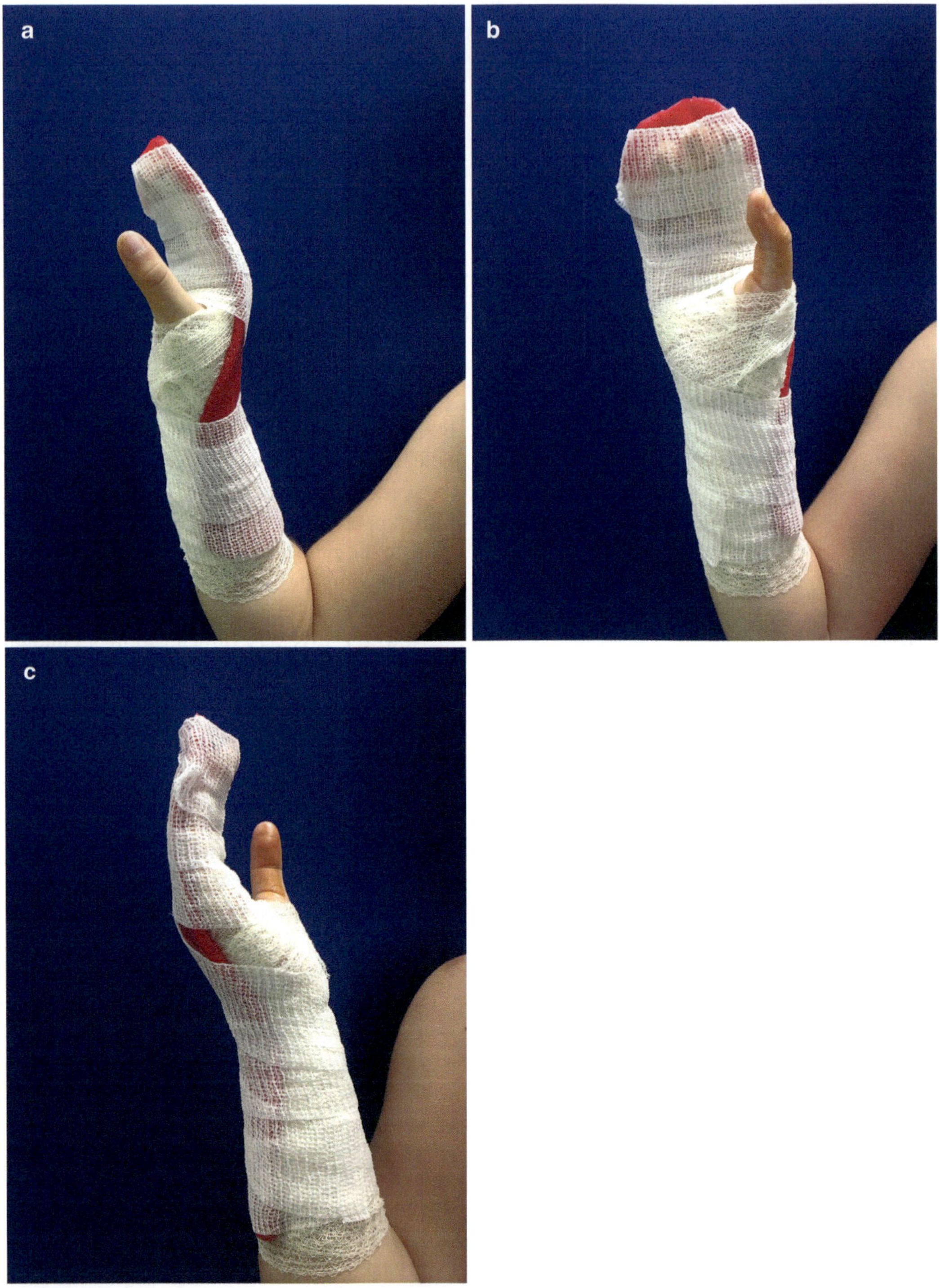

Fig. 30.9 Immobilization splint in pediatric hand tendon lesion

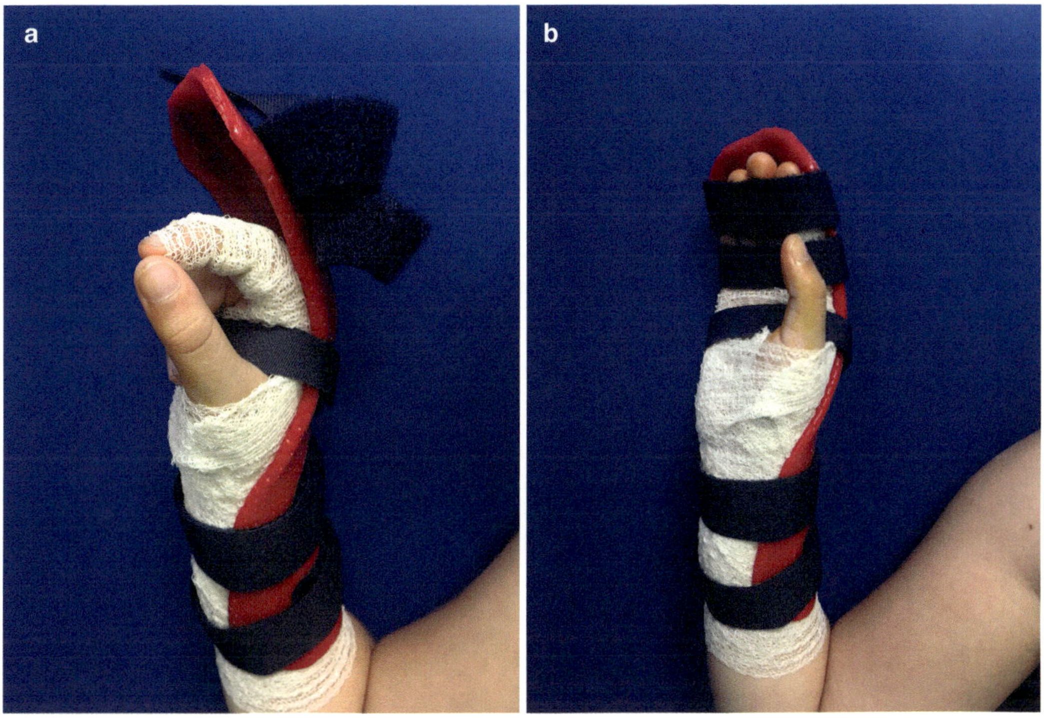

Fig. 30.10 Flexor tendons removable splint to start physiotherapy

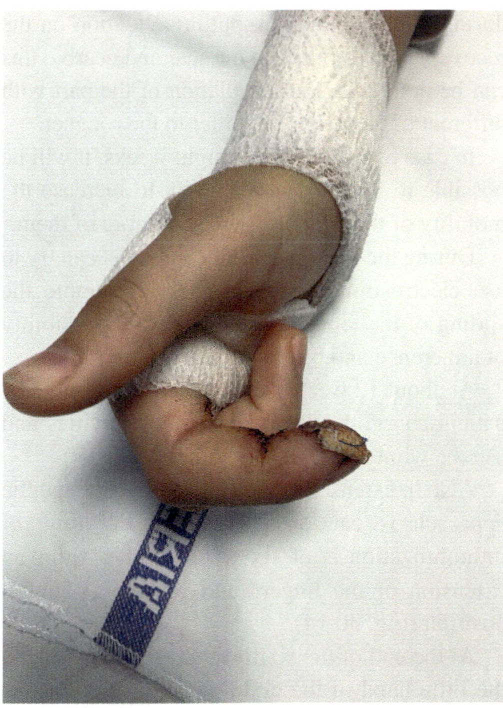

Fig. 30.11 Start rehabilitation with flexor tendon pull out technique repair

that we explain before in order to protect the suture of the tendon.

The wearing of the splint will take a little bit longer for your patients, especially during the night and in risky situation.

The recovery will be placed basically on playing; the therapist will choose with the little patient games and toys that can be appropriate for the situation and the age (Fig. 30.12a).

Fortunately in children, the elasticity of the tissues helps to reduce the post-immobilization stiffness (Fig. 30.13).

The massage of the scar will be extremely important and has to be done more than four times a day, not very long but very often during the day. The technique of the massage is to do it slowly with pressure in order to avoid a thickening of the scar and to limit the establishment of adherence in the deep tissues.

Another tool that needs to be associated with the massage is the use of silicon sheets, to wear during the night, which means for at least 8 hours per night. It is very important to spend some time

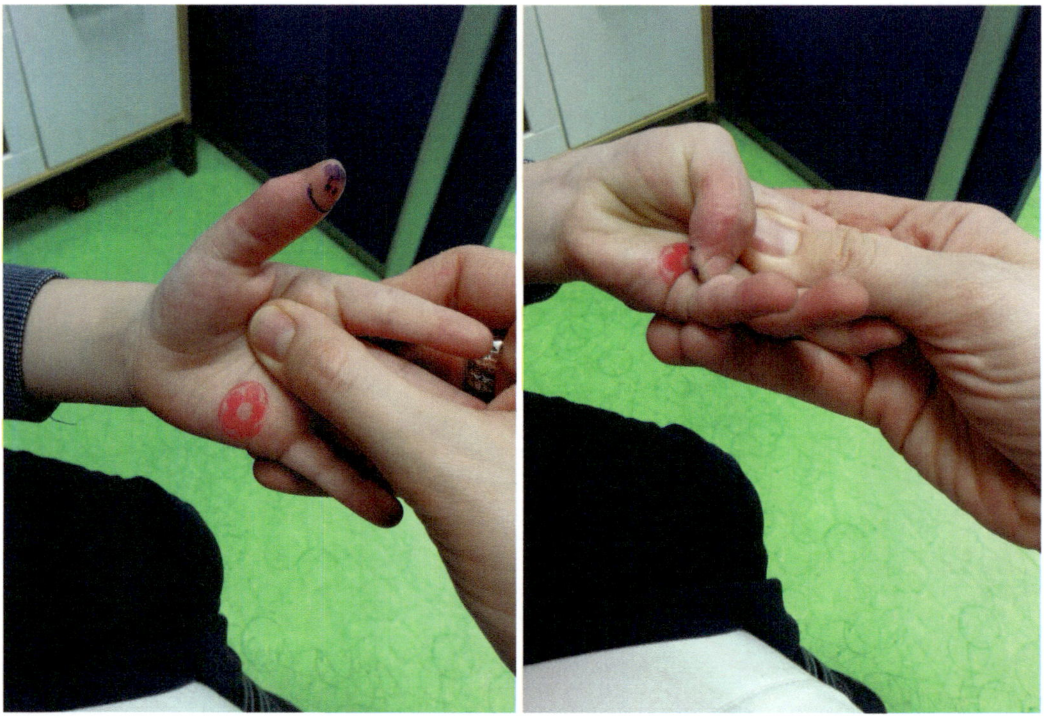

Fig. 30.12 Example of exercise in rehabilitation in flexor tendon lesion

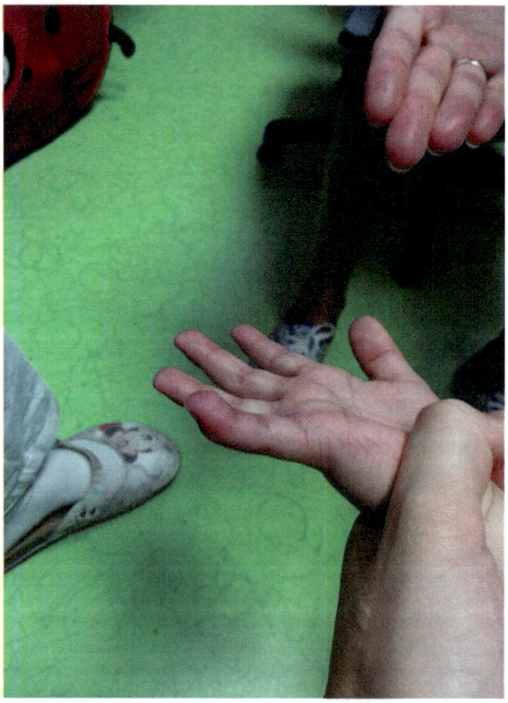

Fig. 30.13 Result of flexor tendon lesion

during the rehabilitation, putting attention on the recovery of sensibility on the scar and nearby; this can be done with the stimulation of the part with different tissues from the softer to the rougher.

In case of stiffness after eight weeks, it will be possible to make dynamic splint to increase the mobility of the single finger or of more of them.

During the tenth week. The therapist can try to use electrostimulation in order to promote the sliding of the tendons and reduce the possibility of adherence and bio-feedback.

At about 12 weeks, if there are no deficits, the patient can go back to the normal activities and use the whole limb like the other.

Also in extensor tendon lesion, the therapeutic approach is cautious. Normally, the time of immobilization is of six weeks with a splint in extension of the fingers and wrist in a neutral position (Fig. 30.14).

At the end of the sixth week, we start to move the little hand of the child, making a removable splint. The therapist will teach the little patient

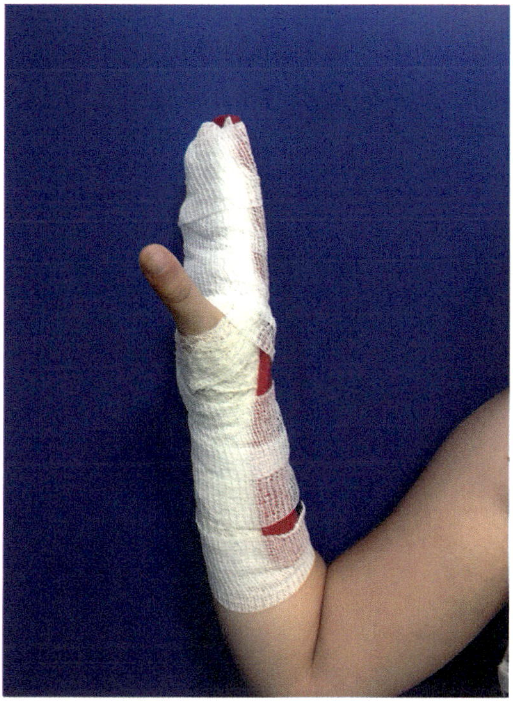

Fig. 30.14 Example of cast immobilization for extensor tendon lesion

and parents some exercises for the fingers like the "hook" and the "roof," so gradually as the flexion improves, the patient will be able to do a complete fist. To help the patient to understand how to close the hand, the therapist will provide some targets, like cylinders from bigger ones to smaller ones. During the rehabilitative session, different kinds of grips will be offered to the child in order to recorticalize the correct gesture of the single hand and of both in bimanual grips.

For sure also in this case, the treatment of this scar when healed will be very important and will follow the rules that we have explained before such as multiple massages during the day and the use of silicon sheets during the night. The extensor tendons slide immediately under the skin; this means that normally a scar has more possibility to do adherence with the next tissues and this can limit the range of motion. For this reason the parents need to learn from the therapist how to do dynamic sliding in schools; this means that they fix the skin in one way and they asked the child to extend or flex which has a double effect on the scar, and this can be very useful. Also in this case during the week, if there is stiffness, the therapist can make dynamic splint in flexion to increase the range of motion.

At about 12 weeks like for flexor tendons, the rehabilitative protocol ends if the patients do not present any deficit, and normal activity is permitted.

Toe-to-Hand Transfers for Posttraumatic and Congenital Reconstruction in Children: Indications and Surgical Technique

31

Neil Jones and Chiara Parolo

Abstract

Miraculous improvement in hand function can be achieved by microsurgical toe-to-hand transfers, either for children who have sustained severe trauma resulting in amputations of their thumb or fingers or for children with congenital absent digits, due to symbrachydactyly, congenital constriction ring syndrome, or transverse and longitudinal deficiencies. From the first experimental microsurgical toe-to-hand transfer performed by Buncke et al. (Br J Plast Surg 19:332–337, 1966), the procedure has subsequently evolved to minimize the harvest of tissues from the foot and to customize the appearance of the great toe similar to that of the thumb. Great toe and second toe transfers for posttraumatic reconstruction of amputations of the thumb, and single second toe, simultaneous double second toe transfers (O'Brien, Hand 10:232–240, 1978; Coskunfirat et al., Plast Reconstr Surg 115:1064–1069, 2005), and combined second and third toe transfers (Wei et al., Plast Reconstr Surg 84:651–661, 1989) for posttraumatic reconstruction of multiple digital amputations have subsequently evolved for specific indications. Indications for posttraumatic microsurgical reconstruction of the thumb and fingers in children may be classified exactly similar to the classification of congenital absent digits (Jones and Kaplan, Hand 7:391–399, 2012; Jones and Clune, Hand 11:77, 2016). The optimal age for performing a toe transfer to reconstruct a congenital hand difference has not been defined. Generally, the earlier that a toe transfer is performed, the better the chance of cortical integration. Preoperative counseling of the parents with the opportunity to meet and speak with other families and children who have undergone a toe transfer is absolutely vital.

Keywords

Toe-to-hand transfer · Microsurgical toe transfer · Congenital absent digit · Finger amputation · Hand trauma · Hand reconstruction

31.1 Introduction

Miraculous improvement in hand function can be achieved by microsurgical toe-to-hand transfers, either for children who have sustained severe trauma resulting in amputations of their thumb or fingers or for children with congenital absent digits, due to symbrachydactyly, congenital constriction ring syndrome, or transverse and longitudinal deficiencies.

N. Jonesn
e-mail: nfjones@uci.edu

C. Parolo (✉)
Department of Hand Surgery and Rehabilitation, San Giuseppe Hospital IRCCS MultiMedica, Milan University, Milan, Italy
e-mail: chiara.parolo@multimedica.it

G. Pajardi (ed.), *Pediatric Hand Surgery*, https://doi.org/10.1007/978-3-031-30984-7_31

Buncke [1] performed the first experimental microsurgical toe-to-hand transfer in a monkey in 1964, and this was followed by the first microsurgical second toe-to-thumb transfer in a human by Yang in 1966 [2]. Cobbett [3] performed the first great toe-to-thumb transfer based on the plantar arterial system, and Buncke et al. [4] performed the first great toe-to-thumb transfer based on the first dorsal metatarsal artery system. Great toe transfers have subsequently evolved to minimize the harvest of tissues from the foot and to customize the appearance of the great toe similar to that of the thumb, using the Morrison "wrap-around" flap [5] and the "trimmed toe" transfer [6, 7]. Great toe and second toe transfers for posttraumatic reconstruction of amputations of the thumb and single second toe, simultaneous double second toe transfers [8, 9], and combined second and third toe transfers [10] for posttraumatic reconstruction of multiple digital amputations have subsequently evolved for specific indications.

31.2 Conventional Reconstruction of Amputations in Children

Fortunately, severe amputations of the thumb and fingers are relatively rare in children. For sharp amputations, replantation should be attempted if at all possible, if necessary using vein grafts (performed on a back table) from the dorsal radial artery or even from the brachial artery at the elbow. Ectopic replantation in the groin or axilla may be considered in very unusual circumstances such as gross contamination. Conventional reconstruction of amputations or failed replantations includes pollicization of a normal or injured finger for thumb reconstruction [11, 12] and distraction lengthening for thumb and finger reconstruction [13–17].

31.3 Toe-to-Hand Transfers After Trauma in Children

Microsurgical toe-to-hand transfers have revolutionized posttraumatic reconstruction in adults after amputation of the thumb and/or fingers. Toe transfers should now be considered as the optimal technique for reconstruction of amputated fingers and thumbs in children, just as in adults. It is a single stage procedure that provides greater length and maintains the potential for growth [18, 19], compared with distraction lengthening. For thumb reconstruction, it preserves all four fingers or the remaining fingers compared with pollicization.

The second toe is always used for finger reconstruction and is preferred for thumb reconstruction in younger children. The second toe also provides the most inconspicuous donor site in the foot and is preferred by cultures requiring the use of sandal footwear. The great toe and its variations are preferred for thumb reconstruction in older children, when the appearance of the new "thumb" becomes more important and also when multiple fingers are also amputated since the great toe has a greater area of sensate pulp. The Morrison wraparound [5] and "trimmed great toe" [6, 7] variations of a great toe transfer minimize the harvest of tissues from the foot and provide the most normal appearance of the reconstructed thumb. The "trimmed toe" technique allows the potential for growth in children, but the Morrison wrap-around does not.

Amputation stumps previously covered with skin grafts may need to be replaced using a groin flap or a reverse radial forearm flap, prior to toe transfers. Similarly, severe thumb-index finger web space contractures may need to be released before performing a toe-to-thumb transfer, utilizing a groin flap, reverse radial forearm flap, or reverse posterior interosseous artery flap. Alternatively, the toe-to-thumb transfer and thumb-index finger web-space release can be performed simultaneously, using a small dorsalis pedis artery skin flap based on the same arterial pedicle or by using a reverse radial forearm flap to cover the web space and the proximal radial artery to provide arterial inflow to the toe transfer [20].

Several small series of toe-to-thumb and toe-to-finger transfers have been reported for posttraumatic reconstruction of children's hands with success rates comparable to adults [21–32].

31.4 Indications for Toe-to-Hand Transfers After Trauma in Children

Indications for posttraumatic microsurgical reconstruction of the thumb and fingers in children may be classified exactly similar to the classification of congenital absent digits [22, 33]. Of the 15 different phenotypes of digital amputations, only 6 are potential candidates for microsurgical reconstruction with toe-to-hand transfers—R1, R2, R3, R4, R5, and U4R1—with a further three potential relative indications: U3R2, C2R2U1, and C3R1U1.

The indications for toe-to-thumb transfers after trauma in children include the following:

1. **Isolated amputations of the thumb, from distal to the CMC joint out to the accepted critical functional level at the midpoint of the proximal phalanx** (**R1** classification). Very rarely, an emergency toe transfer may be indicated for reconstruction of a degloved thumb with an intact bony skeleton and tendons.
2. **Amputations of the thumb and several other fingers** (**R2, R3**, and **R4** classification).
3. **Amputation of all five digits**—the "metacarpal hand" [27, 34] or **R5** hand [22].

Indications for toe-to-hand transfers for finger reconstruction after trauma in children include the following:

1. **Complete or partial amputation of multiple or all four fingers, but with an intact thumb** (**U4R1** classification)
2. **Amputation of all five digits**: the "metacarpal hand" [27, 34] or **R5** hand [22]

31.5 Conventional Reconstruction of Congenital Hand Differences

Conventional non-microsurgical reconstruction of congenital absent digits usually involves pollicization of the index finger for children born with a hypoplastic or absent thumb [35, 36] and nonvascularized toe phalangeal bone grafting [37–45] and distraction lengthening of hypoplastic digits due to symbrachydactyly, cleft hand, or congenital constriction ring syndrome [13–17, 46–50].

31.6 Toe-to-Hand Transfers for Congenital Hand Differences

The first microsurgical toe transfer to reconstruct a congenital hand difference was performed by O'Brien et al. [51] in 1977 who successfully transferred a great toe to reconstruct a hypoplastic thumb in two children. Yoshimura [30, 31] performed second toe transfers in two children with congenital differences. May [52] reported bilateral great toe-to-thumb transfers to reconstruct a nine-year-old boy with bilateral aplasia of his thumb, index, and middle fingers. After other case reports [53, 54], several surgeons have reported larger series of microsurgical toe-to-hand transfers to reconstruct various congenital differences of the hand [23, 24, 55–65].

31.7 Indications for Toe-to-Hand Transfers for Congenital Hand Differences

Microsurgical toe-to-hand transfers for reconstruction of congenital hand differences have not evolved to a similar extent as toe transfers for reconstruction after trauma and still remain controversial. Firstly, surgeons may be reluctant to risk the small but potential loss of a toe transfer in children who are already missing one or more digits in their hands. Secondly, some pediatric hand surgeons still maintain that children with unilateral absence of one or more digits adapt to their impairment as they grow or can be helped with a static or functional prosthesis. Finally, parents may be reluctant to accept a very complicated reconstructive procedure that carries a small risk of ending up with a missing great or second toe as well as more scars on the hand to show for the failed endeavor.

Very little has been published on the specific indications for microsurgical reconstruction of congenital absent digits. Most pediatricians and even some hand surgeons do not understand which children should be considered for microsurgical reconstruction. Previous reports of toe transfers for congenital hand differences have all been based primarily on the specific embryological diagnoses, according to the classification of the International Federation of Societies for Surgery of the Hand [66]. However, it is the authors' contention that specific indications for toe transfers are more logically defined by the anatomy of the hand difference itself, a concept that is also much more easily understood by referring pediatricians and surgeons [33]. From an analysis of 235 hands in 204 children born with congenital absent digits over a 15-year period, Jones and Kaplan [33] developed a simple documentation system, which allows hand surgeons to describe the morphological or radiographic appearance or the functional status of a child's hand with congenital absent digits, based on which digits are missing and their level of absence. Each hand can be described by three letters R (radial), C (central), and U (ulnar) as well as five numbers. The first letter and number designate which rays are missing and the second and third letters and numbers designate which rays are present. Consequently, an absent thumb would be designated as R1U4, a hand with a thumb but absent fingers would be designated as U4R1, and complete absence of all five digits would be designated as R5. The spectrum of radial deficiencies includes R1U4, R2U3, R3U2, and R4U1. There are 15 morphological phenotypes of congenital absent digits—the three most common phenotypes being U4R1 (thumb but absence of all four fingers corresponding to the monodactylous type III symbrachydactyly), R1U4 (absent thumb), and R5 (aplastic hand). Unlike most other classifications, this documentation system not only facilitates communication between hand surgeons but also incorporates all the previous subclassification systems that have attempted to describe congenital absent digits in radial, central, and ulnar deficiencies, symbrachydactyly, and congenital constriction ring syndrome. However, most importantly, it has allowed the development of an algorithm which predicts whether conventional or microsurgical reconstruction is indicated for each specific phenotype. Of the 15 phenotypes, only 7 phenotypes are potential indications for microsurgical reconstruction with toe-to-hand transfers: R1U4, R2U3, R3U2, R4U1, R5, U4R1, and occasionally C3R1U1. For a child missing a thumb but with four relatively normal fingers (R1U4), it is intuitive to reconstruct a thumb to oppose to these fingers, either by pollicization of the index finger or by a toe-to-thumb transfer. Similarly for a child missing all four fingers (U4R1), it is logical to reconstruct one or two fingers to allow pinch and grasp to the normal thumb, either by distraction lengthening or by toe-to-hand transfers.

The following are four indications for considering microsurgical reconstruction of an absent thumb [60]:

1. **Isolated absence of the thumb with four normal or relatively normal fingers, in which the carpometacarpal joint and base of the thumb metacarpal and thenar muscles are preserved (R1U4).** This is usually seen in congenital constriction ring syndrome or occasionally transverse failure. Reconstruction of these thumbs with a toe transfer is superior to index finger pollicization, distraction lengthening, or nonvascularized toe phalangeal bone grafting, because it provides greater length and the potential for growth and preserves the full complement of fingers. A second toe transfer in a 2–3-year-old child will provide almost 5 cm length of the bone and soft tissue compared with only 13–17 mm length of a nonvascularized toe phalangeal bone graft or 3 cm that can be achieved by distraction lengthening, albeit with a secondary bone graft procedure. If the thenar muscles are poorly developed, an

opposition tendon transfer using the flexor digitorum sublimis from the ring finger can be performed at a secondary procedure.

However, if there is an isolated absence of the thumb and four relatively normal fingers, but the carpometacarpal joint is absent, pollicization of the index finger remains the gold standard of reconstruction [36], although there are two reports of toe transfers for reconstruction of Blauth type IV and V hypoplastic thumbs [67, 68].

2. **Absence of the thumb as well as the index, middle, and ring fingers, but with one or two fingers remaining on the ulnar side of the hand (R2U3, R3U2, and R4U1)**. This is usually seen with severe radial longitudinal deficiencies or the monodactylous type III atypical cleft hand variant of symbrachydactyly [69]. A second toe can be transferred to reconstruct the absent thumb with minimal donor site morbidity, but the modified "wrap-around" [5] or trimmed great toe [6, 7] techniques can occasionally be considered in older children to provide both an excellent functional result and a "thumb" very similar in appearance to the contralateral normal thumb. If the carpometacarpal joint is absent in these severe radial deficiency phenotypes, the second toe metatarsal can be fixed to the scaphoid or spliced into the radial styloid as described by Vilkki [25] and by Yu [32]. Very rarely, a similar morphological deformity also occurs in one or both feet (cleft hand and cleft feet), and the abnormal great toe is sometimes amputated to facilitate the fitting of shoes. In these situations, the abnormal great toe is a "free spare part" that can be transferred to reconstruct the absent thumb [18, 19].
3. **Unilateral (or extremely rarely bilateral) absence of the thumb and all four fingers (R5).** This is usually seen with the adactylic type IV symbrachydactyly [69] or with transverse failure of formation.
4. Finally, there are very rare cases in which the thumb or radial side of the hand becomes totally enveloped by a rapidly growing vascular malformation which is unresponsive to embolization or sclerotherapy or by progressive macrodactyly. This situation can potentially be salvaged by radical resection of the thumb but preserving the carpometacarpal joint and base of the thumb metacarpal and thenar muscles, followed immediately by a second toe transfer [56, 70].

The following are two indications for considering toe transfers to reconstruct absent fingers [60]:

1. **Absence of all four fingers (from the carpus out to the base of the middle phalanges), but with a normal thumb (U4R1).** This is usually seen with the monodactylous type III symbrachydactyly, transverse failure of formation, congenital constriction ring syndrome, or severe ulnar longitudinal deficiency. The location into which the toe transfer is positioned depends on the anatomy. Microsurgical reconstruction of a finger can be accomplished by a single second toe transfer into the middle, ring, or small finger position (Figs. 31.1 and 31.2). Placement of the toe transfer on the ulnar side of the hand allows both grasp of large objects and tip-to-tip pinch. An alternative option, if the parents are agreeable, is to transfer two second toes, either simultaneously or sequentially, into the middle and

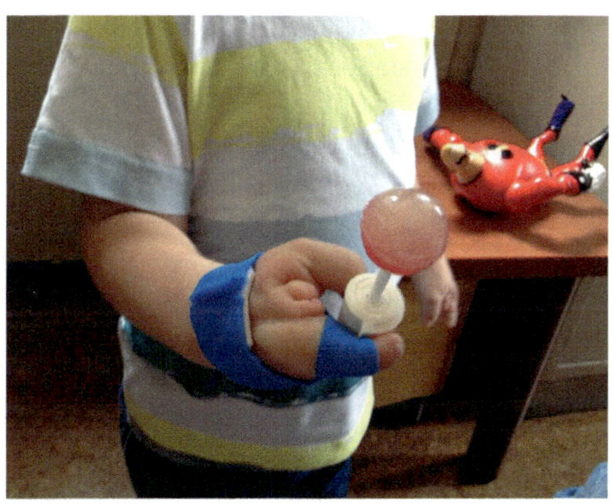

Fig. 31.1 Toe transfer in U4R1 hand Post op

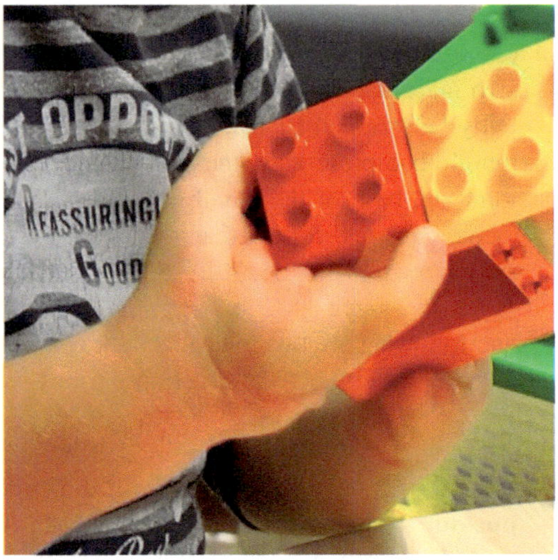

Fig. 31.2 Toe transfer in U4R1 hand Post op

small finger positions to allow three-point pinch. Rarely, if the parents are willing to accept the appearance of the donor foot, combined second and third toes can be transferred into the middle—ring or ring—small finger positions. The range of motion of a toe transfer used for reconstruction of a finger depends on whether there is an existing metacarpophalangeal (MCP) joint in the hand. If the proximal phalanx of a toe transfer can be fixed to a remnant of the proximal phalanx of a finger, excellent motion can be expected at the existing metacarpophalangeal joint, whereas if the metatarsal of the toe transfer has to be fixed to a metacarpal in the hand, the motion achieved at the metatarsophalangeal and proximal interphalangeal joints is significantly less.

2. **Complete absence of all five digits (R5).** This is usually seen in the adactylic type IV symbrachydactyly [69] or transverse failure of formation. Reconstruction may be accomplished using two second toe transfers into the thumb and ring or small finger positions to provide grasp and tip-to-tip pinch. This can be performed simultaneously but is probably better performed sequentially, so that positioning of the second transfer into a finger position can be adjusted to the position and mobility of the first transfer into the thumb position (Fig. 31.3).

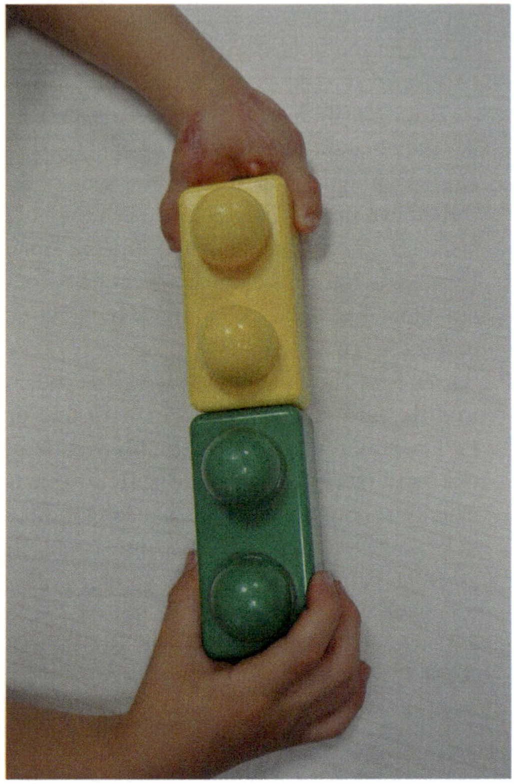

Fig. 31.3 Double Toe transfer in R5 hand Post op

31.8 Timing of Toe Transfers for Congenital Hand Differences

The optimal age for performing a toe transfer to reconstruct a congenital hand difference has not been defined. Generally, the earlier that a toe transfer is performed, the better the chance of cortical integration. Children with a unilateral congenital hand difference should probably be reconstructed at an earlier age, before the use of the contralateral normal hand dominates. However, the real limiting factor in pediatric toe transfers is the size of the donor and recipient vessels, which must be of adequate size to facilitate the microsurgical anastomoses. Gilbert [57, 58] and Lister [62] have performed toe transfers in children as young as 6–12 months of age, but toe transfers have also been successful in older children between 11 and 17 years of age [71]. The author usually performs toe transfers between two and three years of age.

31.9 Evaluation of a Child for a Toe-to-Hand Transfer

After a traumatic injury to a child's hand, there is always some blame, either attached to or accepted by one of the parents. The parental response to a child born with a congenital hand difference resembles the bereavement response. Each parent must deal with their own sense of loss, as well as the obligation to direct the treatment of their child. Listening to the child's parents and allowing them to express their understanding of their child's condition and their hopes and expectations for reconstruction are vitally important. Some surgeons have recommended that the parents and child meet with a clinical psychologist prior to considering a toe-to-hand transfer, and it has been documented that psychological counseling may play an integral role in decision-making in pediatric hand surgery [72].

Rather than just showing pre- and postoperative photographs or videos or fabricating moulages, the author's practice is to arrange for prospective parents to meet the parents of a child with a similar congenital hand difference who has previously undergone a toe transfer, so that the parents can see for themselves the potential function and appearance of the reconstructed hand and speak with the other parents about their concerns [60].

The parents should be prepared psychologically for the significant amount of time and energy that will be required during the pre- and postoperative period. In addition, they must understand and accept the fact that a toe transfer can fail, leaving the child with the same deficit in the hand but also, now, missing a toe in the foot. If the parents and/or child cannot accept the time commitment and the potential risk of failure, toe-to-hand surgery should not be considered.

The child with a congenital hand difference will usually have been examined by a pediatrician for other congenital anomalies and possibly even by a geneticist to exclude a syndromic association. A detailed examination of the involved upper extremity should be performed, or if the child is very young, he/she should be observed while playing. More proximal shoulder or elbow abnormalities should be excluded such as Poland's syndrome or radioulnar synostosis. The presence or absence of a radiocarpal joint as well as the number and length of any metacarpal bones should be determined. The presence or absence of a thumb and whether there is a thumb carpometacarpal joint is important if a toe-to-thumb transfer is being considered. Dimpling of the skin in symbrachydactyly may indicate the presence of flexor tendons in the vicinity of the nubbins.

One or other of the child's feet may be positioned close enough to the affected hand, so that the parents and/or child can visualize what the transferred toe might look like. Occasionally, congenital differences of the lower extremities may co-exist with upper extremity differences and especially with bilateral congenital hand differences; the availability of donor toes may be limited because of associated foot abnormalities.

Plain radiographs of both hands and both feet should be obtained to determine the presence of metacarpals and whether a carpometacarpal joint of the thumb is present or absent. In children where the carpal or metacarpal bones have not yet ossified, an MRI scan may occasionally be considered.

The necessity for preoperative angiography of either the upper or lower extremity remains controversial. Greenberg [73] found a preoperative lateral angiogram of the foot to be helpful in identifying the location and size of the first dorsal metatarsal artery (FDMA) and first plantar metatarsal artery (FPMA). The author no longer obtains angiograms but listens to the dorsalis pedis and first dorsal metatarsal artery in both feet with a handheld Doppler probe. The dorsalis pedis artery can be traced distally into the first dorsal metatarsal artery lying between the great toe and second toe metatarsals using an 8 mHz pencil Doppler ultrasound probe. The dominance of the FDMA can be assessed from the presence or absence of a Doppler signal, and the potential depth of the FDMA (superficial, within or deep to the interosseous muscles) can be assessed from the intensity of the signal.

31.10 Anatomy of the Great Toe and Second Toe

The arterial anatomy of both the great toe and the second toe is based on either the first dorsal metatarsal artery (FDMA), a continuation of the dorsalis pedis artery, or the first plantar metatarsal artery (FPMA) [74]. Superficial veins drain to the medial side of the dorsum of the foot and then into the greater saphenous vein. Sensibility to the plantar surface of the great toe or second toe is provided by the tibial (medial) and fibular (lateral) digital nerves and to the dorsal surface by the deep peroneal nerve.

31.11 Surgical Technique

The child is positioned supine with the arm and hand on a hand table and the donor foot at the end of the operating table. General anesthesia is occasionally supplemented with an axillary block or continuous brachial plexus infusion. A Foley catheter is used to monitor urine output and fluid status, but central venous catheters are not used routinely. A regular tourniquet is applied to the upper arm, and a sterile tourniquet is applied to the thigh, since a skin graft may need to be harvested later from the thigh or groin.

Two surgical teams are utilized to dissect the hand and foot simultaneously, but dissection should usually start with the hand in congenital cases to confirm that recipient tendons and nerves are available. If only one team is available, the dissection usually commences with the hand to confirm that the specific tendons and digital nerves are available for subsequent tendon and nerve repairs.

31.11.1 Dissection of the Donor Foot

Preoperatively, the 8 mHz Doppler ultrasound probe is used to mark the location of the dorsalis pedis artery and/or the posterior tibial artery, depending on the local anatomy and the needs of the recipient hand. The location of suitable dorsal veins may be marked by inflating the thigh tourniquet to 100 mmHg after the draping but prior to the start of the surgery. The leg is then elevated but not exsanguinated in order to leave some blood within the venous system. A racquet-shaped incision is used to harvest the great toe. A V-shaped incision is used to harvest the second toe. The midpoint of the web space between the great toe and the second toe and the midpoint of the web space between the second and third toes are marked, and dorsal and plantar triangular flaps are designed from these two points proximally to their apex at the level of the metatarsophalangeal joint. The dorsal incision is extended proximally in either a longitudinal fashion or a lazy S-shape to the level of the extensor retinaculum. Draining veins from the apex of the dorsal flap are dissected in a distal-to-proximal direction to a dominant dorsal vein, which is dissected further proximally to its origin from the greater saphenous vein at the level of the extensor retinaculum.

Either the extensor hallucis longus (EHL) tendon to the great toe or the extensor digitorum communis tendon (EDC) to the second toe is dissected in a distal-to-proximal direction and transected at the level of the extensor retinaculum.

The deep peroneal nerve is identified proximally by dividing the extensor hallucis brevis tendon and traced in a proximal-to-distal direction to the proximal margin of the V-shaped dorsal flap. The fascicles supplying either the great toe or the second toe are divided from the main trunk of the deep peroneal nerve.

In the original technique of harvesting a toe transfer, the dorsalis pedis artery was identified proximally and dissected in a proximal-to-distal direction into the first dorsal metatarsal artery (FDMA). However, it is faster to identify the FDMA distally in the web space between the great toe and second toe [75]. The FDMA may lie in a superficial dorsal, intramuscular, or plantar position in relation to the interosseous muscles. A communicating branch between the FDMA and the first plantar metatarsal artery (FPMA) may be visualized passing over and distal to the intermetatarsal ligament. The ligament is divided and the FPMA may be dissected further proximally through the plantar incision. If the second toe is being transferred, the fibular digital artery to the great toe is ligated and divided. If the great toe is being transferred, the tibial digital artery to the second toe is ligated and divided. The surgeon can then decide whether the dorsal or plantar arterial system is dominant. If the FDMA is considered to be large enough and in a superficial position, the FDMA is dissected in a distal-to-proximal direction to its origin from the dorsalis pedis artery, which is itself dissected further proximally to the level of the extensor retinaculum by dividing the extensor hallucis brevis tendon. If the FDMA is very small in caliber or lies deeply intramuscularly, the FPMA is chosen as the dominant arterial system but has to be extended with an interposition vein graft, anastomosed on a back table [76]. If both the FDMA and FPMA are absent or hypoplastic, the great toe may still be transferred using the medial plantar arterial system [77]. In children with congenital cleft feet, the great toe is usually transferred on the posterior tibial artery pedicle which can be traced distally to the medial plantar arterial system.

The flexor hallucis longus tendon to the great toe or the flexor digitorum longus and flexor digitorum brevis tendons to the second toe are identified through the plantar incision and are divided as far proximally as possible. The flexor tendons may be difficult to harvest without creating a long incision on the plantar surface of the foot. In order to gain more length, the flexor tendons may be divided through the dorsal incision after the metatarsal osteotomy.

The tibial and fibular plantar digital nerves are traced proximally to their bifurcation from the common digital nerves. The common digital nerves to the great toe-second toe web space and the second-third toe web space are split more proximally using micro-forceps and microscissors before transecting the tibial and fibular digital nerves to either the great toe or second toe. Each nerve is tagged with a small micro clip to facilitate later identification.

Harvest of a second toe transfer is completed by osteotomy of the second toe metatarsal at the level of the metaphyseal flare with a short, thin, narrow oscillating saw blade. The great toe is usually harvested at the level of the base of the proximal phalanx, as a more proximal osteotomy through the metatarsal head may interfere with gait. The tourniquet is then deflated and the vascular pedicles irrigated with 1:20 papaverine solution to relieve any vasospasm, and the foot is wrapped in a laparotomy pad bathed with warm irrigating solution.

Prior to transfer to the hand, the toe transfer should be pink with normal capillary refill and should have an excellent Doppler signal. The toe transfer should be allowed to reperfuse for at least 20 min before reinflating the tourniquet on the leg. The arterial and venous pedicles to the toe are ligated with 4-0 silk ties and reinforced with small micro-clips. The toe transfer is wrapped in a moist laparotomy pad and handed to the surgical team operating on the hand.

31.11.2 Dissection of the Recipient Hand

This may be performed simultaneously with the foot dissection if two teams are available or primarily before the foot is dissected, especially in congenital cases to ensure that there are adequate nerves and tendons present in the hand. Even though the external morphological appearance and a plain radiograph of the hand are reliable indications for consideration of a toe-to-hand transfer, they do not imply availability of internal recipient structures. In general, the anatomic structures (tendons and nerves) are more developed in children with congenital constriction ring syndrome compared to those children with symbrachydactyly, hypoplasia, and transverse deficiency. Several authors [56–58, 60, 61, 78] have observed that tendons and nerves are more likely to be normal proximal to a constriction ring compared with symbrachydactyly. However, with increasing experience of the surgeon, the lack of suitable recipient tendons and nerves, which may be encountered in symbrachydactyly, can be circumvented by using tendon grafts or tendon transfers and nerve grafts or nerve transfers.

The dorsal aspect of the hand is explored first, either through a transverse incision at the level of the wrist or through a longitudinal incision extending proximally from the proposed metacarpal stump. The extensor tendons in a congenital hand are almost universally present, and a recipient extensor tendon is selected which has satisfactory gliding and excursion. A large dorsal vein is identified and tagged with vessel loops. A branch of the superficial radial nerve is also identified for later coaptation to the deep peroneal nerve or as a nerve transfer to the plantar digital nerves of the toe transfer. For a toe-to-thumb transfer, the dorsal branch of the radial artery passing through the anatomical snuff box is dissected and tagged with vessel loops.

The palmar aspect of the hand is explored through a Bruner zigzag incision. Either the median or ulnar nerve is identified at the level of the wrist and dissected in a proximal-to-distal direction to identify common digital nerves or proper digital nerves for later coaptation to the plantar digital nerves of the toe transfer. The flexor tendons are dissected either proximal or distal to the transverse carpal ligament, but a portion of the transverse carpal ligament should always be left intact to prevent bowstringing. One flexor tendon should be selected which has satisfactory gliding and excursion. For a toe-to-finger transfer, the ulnar artery is dissected through Guyon's canal and tagged with vessel loops. The periosteum over the stump of the selected metacarpal is elevated, and dorsal-palmar and radial-ulnar drill holes are made with a 0.035 inch K-wire for subsequent 90–90 interosseous wiring. The incisions in the hand are temporarily closed with staples to prevent excessive swelling and the tourniquet deflated.

31.11.3 Transfer of the Toe to the Hand

Before reinflating the arm tourniquet, the relevant structures in the toe transfer are reidentified—the dorsal vein, extensor tendon, deep peroneal nerve, flexor tendons, and tibial and fibular digital nerves—and either the dorsalis pedis artery, FDMA or the FPMA system. The position and length of the toe transfer are then determined by placing the base of the metatarsal of a second toe or the proximal phalanx of a great toe at the proposed site of osteosynthesis with the selected metacarpal, checking the length and relationship of the toe transfer to the remaining digits in the hand or to the proposed location of a future additional toe transfer. Excess length of the metatarsal of a second toe transfer is removed with an oscillating saw. Dorsal-palmar and radial-ulnar drill holes are made in the metatarsal or proximal phalanx of the toe transfer using a 0.035 inch K-wire, and osteosynthesis between the toe metatarsal or proximal phalanx and the recipient metacarpal or proximal phalanx is accomplished using 90–90 interosseous wiring with 26 gauge stainless steel dental wire. Alternatively, osteosynthesis can be accomplished using crossed K-wires or a longitudinal K-wire or even a small plate and screws. Any propensity for hyperextension at the metatarsophalangeal joint of the toe transfer is prevented by suturing the volar plate more proximally to soft tissues or to the metatarsal itself to limit extension to a neutral 0°.

The extensor hallucis longus tendon of a great toe transfer or the extensor digitorum communis tendon of a second toe transfer is repaired to the selected extensor tendon in the hand. The toe transfer is positioned in full extension at the MCP (metacarpophalangeal) and interphalangeal joints and the selected recipient tendon at its resting tension. The extensor tendon repair is performed with multiple 4-0 clear nylon mattress sutures and a running locked suture to allow early motion. If a toe-to-thumb reconstruction is being performed, the extensor indicis proprius (EIP) tendon to the index finger may need to be transferred as a donor tendon transfer. When reconstructing a finger, the "quadriga" effect, due to tethering of adjacent extensor tendons with a common muscle belly to the absent digits, must be prevented by releasing adjacent extensor tendons.

Usually only one flexor tendon, the flexor hallucis longus of a great toe transfer or the flexor digitorum longus tendon of a second toe transfer, is repaired to the selected recipient flexor tendon in the hand or at the wrist level. The flexor tendon repair is accomplished using several 4-0 nylon mattress sutures supplemented with a running locked suture. To prevent any "quadriga" effect, adjacent flexor tendons that may tether the newly reconstructed flexor tendon to the toe transfer are divided. Occasionally, an interposition flexor tendon graft may be necessary to make up for any discrepancy in length between the flexor tendon of the toe transfer and the selected flexor tendon at the wrist. If a flexor tendon with adequate excursion cannot be identified, a primary tendon transfer may be required.

Neurorrhaphies of the tibial and fibular digital nerves of the toe transfer to recipient common or proper digital nerves in the hand are performed using an end-to-end epineurial technique with 10-0 nylon microsutures under the operating microscope. Digital nerve neurorrhaphies can occasionally be facilitated using fibrin glue. Neurorrhaphy of a branch of the deep peroneal nerve of the toe transfer to a branch of the superficial radial nerve in the hand is similarly performed. If there is a gap between the digital nerves of the toe transfer and recipient nerves in the hand, interposition nerve grafts may be necessary, using either the superficial or deep peroneal nerves harvested as a nerve graft from the donor foot. If recipient digital nerves are unavailable in a toe-to-thumb transfer, end-to-side neurorrhaphies may be required, or a nerve transfer can be performed using a branch of the superficial radial nerve coapted to the ulnar digital nerve of the toe transfer.

Osteosynthesis, extensor and flexor tendon repairs, and neurorrhaphies of the digital nerves and deep peroneal nerve should hopefully be performed within a 2 h period of tourniquet inflation. The tourniquet is then deflated for the arterial and venous anastomoses. The venous anastomosis is usually performed first before the arterial anastomosis. The draining vein of the toe transfer is anastomosed end to end under the operating microscope using standard microsurgical techniques using 10-0 nylon microsutures to the selected vein on the dorsal aspect of the wrist. The recipient vein is then occluded just proximal to the anastomosis with a small microvascular clamp. The site of the arterial anastomosis depends on whether the dorsal or plantar arterial system of the toe transfer has been harvested and the location of the recipient radial or ulnar artery. If a "long" dorsalis pedis—FDMA arterial pedicle—has been harvested, end-to-end or end-to-side anastomosis to the ulnar artery at the wrist or the dorsal branch of the radial artery in the anatomical snuff box can be performed. If the "short" FPMA pedicle has been harvested, it can occasionally be anastomosed to the superficial palmar arch or to a common digital artery, but it is usually better to elongate the FPMA with an interposition vein graft anastomosed on a back table prior to osteosynthesis [76]. The vein graft can then be anastomosed end to end to the dorsal branch of the radial artery in the anatomical snuff box or the ulnar artery at the wrist. After completion of the arterial anastomosis, the double approximator clamp is removed, but the single microvascular clamp on the proximal side of the venous anastomosis is maintained to create a high-pressure column of blood flowing through the toe transfer to expand any collapsed vessels due to vasospasm. The anastomoses are irrigated with 1:20 papaverine solution. The toe transfer should rapidly turn pink and have excellent capillary refill. After removal of the microvascular clamp from the proximal side of the venous anastomosis, the patency of the arterial and venous anastomoses can be confirmed by the Acland "milking test."

The incisions are loosely closed with interrupted 4-0 or 5-0 chromic sutures. Split thickness or full thickness skin grafts are liberally used to prevent any tension on the underlying anastomoses. A sterile pulse oximeter probe is applied to the nail plate of the toe transfer before the dressings are applied for continuous postoperative monitoring of the patency of the arterial and venous anastomoses [79]. The pulse rate of the toe transfer should correspond exactly to the pulse oximeter on the opposite hand and monitors the patency of the arterial anastomosis. Any decrease in the pulse rate compared to the systemic heart rate may indicate that the arterial anastomosis is compromised. The oxygen saturation (SaO_2) monitors the patency of the venous anastomosis, and any decrease in the oxygen saturation for an extended period of time when compared to the systemic oxygen saturation may indicate thrombosis of the venous anastomosis. The incisions are covered with antibiotic ointment and nonadherent gauze dressings and the hand, wrist, forearm, and elbow immobilized in a loose plaster of Paris sugar-tong splint.

31.11.4 Closure of the Donor Foot

The thigh tourniquet is deflated and hemostasis achieved in the donor foot. If necessary, a small Jackson-Pratt drain is placed. After harvesting the second toe, the gap between the great toe and the third toe is closed by repairing the intermetatarsal ligament using 2-0 or 3-0 Ethibond sutures. The skin is loosely closed with interrupted 4-0 or 5-0 chromic sutures. After harvesting the great toe, the dorsal and plantar skin can usually be approximated or the remaining defect covered with a skin graft. After harvesting the Morrison "wraparound" or "trimmed toe" variations of a great toe transfer, the proximal-based flap on the medial aspect of the foot is used to cover any remnant of the proximal phalanx of the great toe, and any remaining soft tissue defect is covered with a skin graft. The donor foot is immobilized in a posterior plaster of Paris splint with the foot in neutral position.

31.12 Postoperative Care

Both the hand and foot are elevated and the hand kept warm with a heating blanket. The child is monitored in a pediatric intensive care unit for up to three days postoperatively. The child is kept sedated using opiates and benzodiazepines as necessary, and a first-generation cephalosporin is administered intravenously for 5–7 days postoperatively. Anticoagulation with dextran 40 (0.36 ml/kg/h) is continued for five days, and low-dose aspirin 81mg is started on the first postoperative day and continued for four weeks. The dextran infusion is reduced to half on postoperative day 6 and discontinued on day 7. If the clinical appearance of the toe transfer or the differential pulse oximetry monitoring indicates compromised perfusion to the toe transfer, the child should be returned to the operating room immediately for exploration and possible revision of the microsurgical anastomoses.

The splints on the hand and foot are removed 10–14 days postoperatively and the "take" of any skin graft is assessed. The child can then begin to ambulate with a bulky sock in a slipper or sneaker. The hand is protected with a removable thermoplast splint for two more weeks when passive and active range of motion exercises of the toe transfer are begun.

These children may require secondary tenolyses, tendon transfers, bone grafting, arthrodeses, osteotomies, or scar revisions to reach their optimal functional and aesthetic outcome.

31.13 Conclusions

Microsurgical toe-to-hand transfers for posttraumatic reconstruction in children and for reconstruction of congenital hand differences will hopefully continue to evolve to become accepted into the armamentarium of pediatric hand surgeons, although it will continue to remain a technical challenge requiring a high level of microsurgical skill on the part of the hand surgeon and the ultimate trust of the child's parents. Preoperative counseling of the parents with the opportunity to meet and speak with other families and children who have undergone a toe transfer is absolutely vital. Most importantly, the parents should fully understand the small potential for failure of the procedure with consequent loss of the toe transfer. While the indications for toe transfers are now better defined [60], the optimal age for toe transfers remains unknown. Just like other congenital hand surgeries, most experienced surgeons believe that toe transfers between two and three years of age have the best chance of cortical integration, although toe transfers have been successfully reported in older children between the ages of 11 and 17 years [71].

It will always be very difficult to prove conclusively that microsurgical reconstruction of congenital hand differences is superior to either no surgical intervention or conventional reconstruction, but a child who is able to write his/her name for the first time, or who can pick up a cup singlehandedly and hold an utensil or who can now ride a bicycle, provides the hand surgeon with far greater confirmation than the most sophisticated outcome instruments. In the future, parental assessment of their child's functional outcome and even the child's own assessment will be important validation of these techniques [80, 81].

References

1. Buncke HJ, Buncke CM, Schultz WP. Immediate Nicoladoni procedure in the Rhesus monkey, or hallux-to-hand transplantation, utilizing microminiature vascular anastomoses. Br J Plast Surg. 1966;19:332–7.
2. Yang DY. Thumb reconstruction by free second toe transplantation. Report of 40 cases. CJS. 1977;15:13.
3. Cobbett JR. Free digital transfer: report of a case of transfer of a great toe to replace an amputated thumb. J Bone Joint Surg. 1969;51:677–9.
4. Buncke HJ, McLean DH, Geroge PT, Creech BJ, Chater NL, Commons GW. Thumb replacement: great toe transplantation by microvascular anastomosis. Br J Plast Surg. 1973;26:194–201.

5. Morrison WA, O'Brien BM, MacLeod AM. Thumb reconstruction with a free neurovascular wrap-around flap from the big toe. J Hand Surg. 1980;5:575–83.
6. Littler JW, Upton J. Microsurgical thumb reconstruction with toe transfer: selection of various techniques: discussion. Plast Reconstr Surg. 1994;93:352–7.
7. Wei FC, Chen HC, Chuang CC, Noordhoff MS. Reconstruction of the thumb with a trimmed-toe transfer technique. Plast Reconstr Surg. 1988;82:506–15.
8. Coskunfirat OK, Wei FC, Lin CH, Chen HC, Lin YT. Simultaneous double second toe transfer for reconstruction of adjacent fingers. Plast Reconstr Surg. 2005;115:1064–9.
9. O'Brien BM. Simultaneous double toe transfer for severely disabled hands. Hand. 1978;10:232–40.
10. Wei FC, Colony LH, Chen HC, Chuang CC, Nordhoff MS. Combined second and third toe transfer. Plast Reconstr Surg. 1989;84:651–61.
11. May JW, Donelan MB, Toth BA, Wall J. Thumb reconstruction in the burned hand by advancement pollicization of the second ray remnant. J Hand Surg. 1984;9A:484–9.
12. Ward JW, Pensler JM, Parry SW. Pollicization for thumb reconstruction in severe pediatric hand burns. Plast Reconstr Surg. 1985;76:927–32.
13. Dhalla R, Strecker W, Manske PR. A comparison of two techniques for digital distraction lengthening in skeletally immature patients. J Hand Surg. 2001;26A:603–10.
14. Kessler I, Baruch A, Hecht O. Experience with distraction lengthening of digital rays in congenital anomalies. J Hand Surg. 1977;2A:394–401.
15. Matev IB. Thumb reconstruction after amputation at the metacarpophalangeal joint by bone lengthening. J Bone Joint Surg. 1970;52A:957–65.
16. Pensler JM, Carroll NC, Cheng LF. Distraction osteogenesis in the hand. Plast Reconstr Surg. 1998;102:92–5.
17. Seitz WH, Shimko P, Patterson RW. Long-term results of callus distraction-lengthening in the hand and upper extremity for traumatic and congenital skeletal deficiencies. J Bone Joint Surg. 2010;92A:47–58.
18. Chang J, Jones NF. Simultaneous toe-to-hand transfer and lower extremity amputations for severe upper and lower limb defects: the use of spare parts. J Hand Surg. 2002;27:219–23.
19. Chang J, Jones NF. Radiographic analysis of growth in pediatric microsurgical toe-to-hand transfers. Plast Reconstr Surg. 2002;109:576–82.
20. Kim JH, Yoon AP, Jones NF. Reverse radial forearm flap to provide arterial inflow to a toe transfer. Hand. 2017;12:154–61.
21. Cooney WP, Wood WB. Microvascular reconstruction of congenital anomalies and post-traumatic lesions in children. Hand Clin. 1992;8:131.
22. Jones NF, Clune J. Thumb amputations in children. Hand. 2016;11:77.
23. Kay SP, Wiberg M, Bellew M, Webb F. Toe to hand transfer in children. Part 2: functional and psychological aspects. J Hand Surg. 1996;21B:735–45.
24. Shvedovchenko IV. Toe-to-hand transfers in children. Ann Plast Surg. 1993;31:251–4.
25. Vilkki SK. Grip reconstruction with toe to antebrachial stump transfer. In: Landi A, editor. Reconstruction of the thumb. London: Chapman and Hall Medical; 1989. p. 233–41.
26. Wei FC, El-Gammal TA, Chen HC, Chuang DCC, Chiang YC, Chen SHT. Toe-to-hand transfer for traumatic digital amputations in children and adolescents. Plast Reconstr Surg. 1997;100:605–9.
27. Wei FC, El-Gammal T, Lin CH, Chuang CC, Chen HC, Chen S. Metacarpal hand: classification and guidelines for microsurgical reconstruction with toe transfers. Plast Reconstr Surg. 1997;99:122–8.
28. Wei FC, Mardini S. Revaluation of the technique of toe-to-hand transfer for traumatic digital amputations in children and adolescents. Plast Reconstr Surg. 2003;112:1870–4.
29. Wolff G, Posso C. Second-toe transfer for traumatic thumb amputation in children under 5 years: bone and soft tissue growth. Tech Hand Upper Extrem Surg. 2014;18:175–80.
30. Yoshimura M. Toe-to-hand transfer. Plast Reconstr Surg. 1980;66:74–83.
31. Yoshimura M. Toe-to-hand transfer. Plast Reconstr Surg. 1984;73:851–2.
32. Yu ZJ, Huang YC, Yu S, Sui SP. Thumb reconstruction in a bilateral upper extremity amputee: an alternative to the Krukenberg procedure. J Hand Surg. 1999;24A:194–7.
33. Jones NF, Kaplan J. A new documentation system for congenital absent digits. Hand. 2012;7:391–9.
34. Wei FC, Lutz B, Cheng SL, Chuang CC. Reconstruction of bilateral metacarpal hands with multiple-toe transplantation. Plast Reconstr Surg. 1999;104:1698–704.
35. Buck-Gramcko D. Pollicization of the index finger: method and results in aplasia and hypoplasia of the thumb. J Bone Joint Surg. 1971;53:1605–17.
36. Manske PR, McCarroll HR, James M. Type III-A hypoplastic thumb. J Hand Surg. 1995;20A:246–53.
37. Buck-Gramcko D, Pereira JA. Proximal toe phalanx transplantation for bony stabilization and lengthening of partially aplastic digits. Ann Chir Main Memb Super. 1990;9:107–18.
38. Carroll RE, Green DP. J Bone Joint Surg Am. 1975;57:727.
39. Cavallo AV, Smith PJ, Morley S, Morsi AW. Non-vascularized free toe phalanx transfers in congenital hand deformities–the Great Ormond Street experience. J Hand Surg. 2003;28B:520–7.
40. Entin MA. Reconstruction of congenital abnormalities of the upper extremities. J Bone Joint Surg Am. 1959;41:681–701.
41. Gohla T, Metz C, Lanz U. Non-vascularized free toe phalanx transplantation in the treatment of symbrachydactyly and constriction ring syndrome. J Hand Surg. 2005;30B:446–51.
42. Goldberg NH, Watson HK. Composite toe (phalanx and epiphysis) transfers in the reconstruction of the aphalangic hand. J Hand Surg. 1982;7A:454–9.
43. Jones NF. Nonvascularized toe phalangeal bone grafts for congenital anomalies of the hand. J Am Soc Surg Hand. 2004;4:27–34.

44. Radocha RF, Netscher D, Kleinert HE. Toe phalangeal grafts in congenital hand anomalies. J Hand Surg. 1993;18A:833–41.
45. Unglaub F, Lanz U, Hahn P. Outcome analysis, including patient and parental satisfaction, regarding nonvascularized free toe phalanx transfer in congenital hand deformities. Ann Plast Surg. 2006;56:87–92.
46. Hülsbergen-Krüger S, Preisser P, Partecke BD. Ilizarov distraction-lengthening in congenital anomalies of the upper limb. J Hand Surg. 1998;23B:192–5.
47. Matsuno T, Ishida O, Sunagawa T, Ichikawa M, Ikuta Y, Ochi M. Bone lengthening for congenital differences of the hands and digits in children. J Hand Surg. 2004;29A:712–9.
48. Miyawaki T, Masuzawa G, Hirakawa M, Kurihara K. Bone-lengthening for symbrachydactyly of the hand with the technique of callus distraction. J Bone Joint Surg. 2002;84A:986–91.
49. Ogino T, Kato H, Ishii S, Usui M. Digital lengthening in congenital hand deformities. J Hand Surg. 1994;19B:120–9.
50. Seitz WH, Froimson AI. Callotasis lengthening in the upper extremity: indications, techniques, and pitfalls. J Hand Surg. 1991;16A:932–9.
51. O'Brien BM, Black MJ, Morrison WA, Macleod AM. Microvascular great toe transfer for congenital absence of the thumb. Hand. 1978;10:113–24.
52. May J, Smith RJ, Peimer C. Toe-to-hand free tissue transfer for thumb construction with multiple digit aplasia. Plast Reconstr Surg. 1981;67:205–13.
53. Meals RA, Lesavoy MA. Hallux-to-hand transfer during ankle disarticulation for multiple limb anomalies. JAMA. 1983;249:72–3.
54. Nyarady JP, Szekeres, Vilmos Z. Toe-to-thumb transfer in congenital grade III thumb hypoplasia. J Hand Surg. 1983;8:898–901.
55. Eaton CJ, Lister GD. Toe transfer for congenital hand defects. Microsurgery. 1991;12:186–95.
56. Foucher G, Medina J, Navarro R, Nagel D. Toe transfer in congenital hand malformations. J Reconstr Microsurg. 2001;17:1–7.
57. Gilbert A. Toe transfers for congenital hand defects. J Hand Surg. 1982;7A:118–24.
58. Gilbert A. Reconstruction of congenital hand defects with microvascular toe transfers. Hand Clin. 1985;1:351–60.
59. Jones NF, Hansen SL, Bates SJ. Toe-to-hand transfers for congenital anomalies of the hand. Hand Clin. 2007;23:129–36.
60. Jones NF, Kaplan J. Indications for microsurgical reconstruction of congenital hand anomalies by toe-to-hand transfers. Hand. 2013;8:367–74.
61. Kay S, McGuiness C. Microsurgical reconstruction in abnormalities of children's hands. Hand Clin. 1999;15:563–83.
62. Lister G. Microsurgical transfer of the second toe for congenital deficiency of the thumb. Plast Reconstr Surg. 1988;82:658–65.
63. Richardson PWF, Johnstone BR, Coombs CJ. Toe-to-hand transfer in symbrachydactyly. Hand Surg. 2004;9:11–8.
64. Van Holder C, Giele H, Gilbert A. Double second toe transfer in congenital hand anomalies. J Hand Surg. 1999;24B:471–5.
65. Vilkki SK. Advances in microsurgical reconstruction of the congenitally adactylous hand. Clin Orthop Relat Res. 1995;314:45–58.
66. Swanson AB. A classification for congenital limb malformations. J Hand Surg. 1976;1A:8–22.
67. Harashina T, Inoue T, Fujino T, Uchinishi K, Itoh Y. Reconstruction of a floating thumb with an excess big toe. J Reconstr Microsurg. 1994;10:11–5.
68. Tu YK, Yeh WL, Sananpanich K, Ueng SWN, Chou YC, Ma CH, Lee ZL. Microsurgical second toe-metatarsal bone transfer for reconstructing congenital radial deficiency with hypoplastic thumb. J Reconstr Microsurg. 2004;20:215–25.
69. Blauth W, Gekeler J. Morphology and classification of symbrachydactyly. Handchirurgie. 1971;3:123–8.
70. Carlsen B, Jones NF. Radical resection of a massive venous malformation of the thumb and immediate reconstruction with a microsurgical toe transfer. J Hand Surg. 2007;32A:1587–91.
71. Spokevicius S, Radzevicius D. Late toe-to-hand transfer for the reconstruction of congenital defects of the long fingers. Scand J Plast Reconstr Surg Hand Surg. 1997;31:345–50.
72. Bradbury ET, Kay SPJ, Hewison J. The psychological impact of microvascular free toe transfer for children and their parents. J Hand Surg. 1994;19:689–95.
73. Greenberg B, May J. Great toe-to-hand transfer: role of the preoperative lateral angiogram of foot. J Hand Surg. 1988;13A:411–4.
74. Villen G, Julve G. The arterial system of the first intermetatarsal space and its influence in toe-to-hand transfer: a report of 53 long-pedicle transfers. J Hand Surg. 2002;27B:73–7.
75. Wei FC, Silverman R, Hsu WM. Retrograde dissection of the vascular pedicle in toe harvest. Plast Reconstr Surg. 1995;96:1211–4.
76. Brown EE, Chang WT, Jones NF. Temporary arteriovenous loop between the saphenous vein and first plantar metatarsal artery in toe-to-hand transfers. J Hand Surg. 2006;31:1543–5.
77. Koman LA, Weiland A, Moore JR. Toe-to-hand transfer based on the medial plantar artery. J Hand Surg. 1985;10A:561–6.
78. Kay SP, Wiberg M. Toe to hand transfer in children. Part 1: technical aspects. J Hand Surg. 1996;21B:723–34.
79. Jones NF, Gupta R. Postoperative monitoring of pediatric toe-to-hand transfers with differential pulse oximetry. J Hand Surg. 2001;26A:525–9.
80. Bellew M, Haworth J, Kay SP. Toe transfer in children: ten year followup of psychosocial aspects. J Plast Reconstr Aesthet Surg. 2011;64:766–75.
81. Kaplan JD, Jones NF. Outcome measures of microsurgical toe transfers for reconstruction of congenital and traumatic hand anomalies. J Pediatr Orthop. 2014;34:362–8.

32 Compartment Syndromes (CS) and Volkmann's and Upper Limb Vascular Pathology in the Peri- and Neonatal Period

Antonio Landi, Giuesppe Caserta, Andrea Giorgini, Silvana Sartini, and Scott Oishi

Abstract

The borderline between perinatal compartment syndrome (CS), Volkmann's contracture and vascular lesion appears to be very subtle.

As regards CS, a new pathophysiological classification has been introduced. Location, clinical symptoms and complementary investigations vary significantly from adults. The overlying area of skin necrosis, "the sentinel lesion", usually accompanies the intrauterine and CS and Volkmann's syndrome.

Treatment consists of early fasciotomy which has exceptionally carried out as the newborn already presents at birth with an established Volkmann's contracture.

Ideal treatment consists of early escharotomy followed by skin grafting, early removal of the scar and neurolysis of the main nerves. Tendon or free muscle transfer will be subsequently performed according to the severity of the lesion.

Vascular lesions in the newborn are also very rare but must be distinguished from CS and Volkmann's syndrome as treatment must be urgently addressed due to the fact that thrombosis of the main vessels might lead to necrosis followed by amputation of the upper limb. During the growing phase, residual problems such as joint stiffness, first web contracture and bone non-union should be dealt with. Surprising in spite of significant residual limb discrepancy, favourable long-term outcomes might be obtained.

Keywords

Perinatal compartment syndrome
Volkmann's classification · Fasciotomy
Tendon transfer · Free muscle transfer · Limb discrepancy · Perinatal vascular lesion
Sentinel lesion

32.1 Introduction

The pathology of CS and of Volkmann's syndrome, especially in relation to the associated skin lesion of the upper limb in the peri- and neonatal period, was initially confined within the

A. Landi (✉)
Hand Unit Casa di Cura Toniolo, Bologna, Italy
e-mail: landi_antonio@virgilio.it

G. Caserta
Hand Surgery Unit, Policlinico di Modena, Modena, Italy

A. Giorgini
Orthopaedic and Traumathology Unit, Policlinico di Modena, Modena, Italy

S. Sartini
Hand Rehabilitation Service, Policlinico di Modena, Modena, Italy
e-mail: ssartini@gruppociemme.it

S. Oishi
Department of Upper Extremity and Microsurgery, Scottish Rite Hospital for Children, Dallas, TX, USA
e-mail: Scott.Oishi@tsrh.org

G. Pajardi (ed.), *Pediatric Hand Surgery*, https://doi.org/10.1007/978-3-031-30984-7_32

internal medicine domain, especially among dermatologists [1–4] or specialists of intensive care units [5, 6]. From the prevailing literature, it is clear that this particular topic has been visited mainly by hand surgeons, plastic surgeons, orthopaedic surgeons and paediatric surgeons [1, 7–14] or by personnel of general surgery departments where there is an afference of paediatric surgery [6] and specialized centres dedicated to the treatment of congenital malformations of the upper limb, equipped with personnel possessing specific microsurgical expertise [4, 15–21].

The definition of Volkmann's syndrome refers to the first description by the author of a 14-year-old boy subjected to an excessively rigid immobilization for a spontaneous effusion of the knee [22].

The great merit of this pioneer is to have identified cause and effect of the syndrome but not the underlying pathogenetic process that will only be elucidated when the knowledge of the microcirculation will allow to define the key parameters of function and survival of the muscles contained in the muscle compartments.

The values of compartmental pressure in the normotensive adult are nowadays recorded routinely. When the pressure is maintained continuously for 4–6 h beyond 30 mmHg, muscle survival can be severely compromised. Just as with the heart muscle, muscle insult can evolve into scarring (ischaemic retraction) or colliquative necrosis. The two processes often coexist in the skeletal muscle, and the muscle infarction remains confined in the central hypoperfused area, while scarring usually affects the peripheral muscle tissue. It is also known that in hypotensive patients, the risk of ischaemic lesions is already present with a compartment pressure of about 20 mmHg [15].

Volkmann's syndrome therefore represents the natural outcome of an unrecognized and therefore not promptly treated compartment syndrome, in which increased tissue pressure within a limited space compromises the circulation, function and potentially the viability of the contents of the affected area and thus of the main vessels and nerves [1].

As far as vascular lesions are concerned, these can be linked to a lesion of a main vessel upstream, both venous and arterial, which, despite the increased resistance of the epidermis to ischaemia, lead to massive necrosis and consequent debridement or amputations at various levels of the upper limb.

32.2 Affected Locations and Pathophysiological and Aetiological Classification

Volkmann's syndrome is rarely seen in adults and children today and should be considered an exceptional event in the perinatal period.

In this chapter, we will focus on the substantial differences between age groups with regard to aetiological factors, sites of onset, clinical symptoms and the different uses of complementary investigations for diagnostic purposes.

The entire upper limb in its various muscle compartments is a potential site of compartment syndrome, and this can be evidenced in clinical practice [23, 24]. At the shoulder level, there are essentially two compartments: scapular and deltoid. In 1932, Comolli was the first to describe a clinical picture of the compartment syndrome at the level of the scapula in association with a fracture [25].

So far in literature, compartment syndrome has only been described in adults [12]. Furthermore, the area of the deltoid is almost exclusively the prerogative of adulthood and is established in patients who are habitually alcoholics and drug addicts who develop pressure sores in the deltoid area during long periods of unconsciousness. There is no description of this in the perinatal period [16] but only in the paediatric age, usually following injections of medication or vaccines in the deltoid area [26].

Even at the level of the upper limb, the adult's CS is often associated with natural catastrophic events such as earthquakes and road accidents that take form in the Crush syndrome [15, 21, 27].

There are two main muscle compartments in the forearm: the anterior and the postero-lateral. The forearm represents the most frequent site of CS in association with supracondylar elbow fractures, closed and compound fractures of the forearm [4, 8, 10, 18, 21, 28]. This site also represents the most frequent location of Volkmann's syndrome and peri- and neonatal CS [1, 4, 11, 17, 21, 29, 30].

As regard the hand, the compartments are formed by the interosseous of the thenar and hypothenar intrinsic muscles. CS can develop in this location both in the peri- and in the neonatal phase but especially in the paediatric age. Fingers can also be considered non-muscular compartments where the boundaries between the skin of the dorsum and palm are formed by the ligaments of Grayson and Cleland with the neurovascular bundles between them. Fingers can therefore be the site of a CS in burns and high-pressure injection injuries in adults, while in the paediatric phase, they are the most frequent location of amniotic bands that can generate venous and lymphatic stasis up to perfusion defect which compromises survival [31].

The present classification based on pathophysiological criteria follows Perricone and Holden's classification modified by Landi [17] in Table 32.1. Group I includes lesions of a main proximal arterial vessel [15], revascularization syndrome and subtotal occlusion of the venous circulation (type ID). In type II, CS is the result of exclusively local multifactorial pathology (type IIA) or in association with aggravating systemic factors (type IIB). In type III, CS might spread all over the body and are linked to systemic diseases that can entail acute permeability of the capillary network, as observed in the Leak syndrome (Table 32.1) [32]. In the peri- and neonatal phase, the etiopathological classification differs substantially. Group I, similar to the adult, includes pathologies of the main proximal vessels both on the arterial and venous sides; however, they are caused by completely different aetiological agents (Table 32.2). In group IIA, CS may occur as a result of a hypothetical compression of the upper limb during the intrauterine phase of prolonged labour. In group IIB, the possible aggravating factors should be differentiated into maternal (chickenpox, gestational diabetes, etc.) or foetal (clotting disorders, dehydration, etc.). In group III, the systemic factors causing multiple CS include meningococcal septicaemia [34] and severe foetal dehydration [6]. Especially in the infant, the boundaries between CS, Volkmann's syndrome and vascular lesions appear subtle [36].

Table 32.1 Etiological and physiopatological classification of C.S. in adults

	Type I	Type II	Type III
A	Major artery lesion proximal to the ischaemic muscle region	Compartmental syndrome due to multifactorial and exclusively local causes	Systemic disease inducing multiple CS: 1. Leak syndrome (acute increased capillary permeability) [32] 2. Local myotoxicity in various muscular compartments (heroin overdose, theophylline or alcohol abuse) 3. Adrenal massive haemorrhage (Waterhouse-Friderichsen syndrome) [33]
B	Late revascularization syndrome	Local disease associated with systemic factors (haemophilia, patient in treatment with anticoagulant and antiplatelet drugs, blood tumors: leukemias)	
C	Isolated lesion of the vascular peduncular in type I muscle (with only one vascular pedicle)		
D	Complete occlusion of the venous circle (phlegmasia cerulea dolens)		

Table 32.2 Etiological and physiopathological classification of C.S. in the peri- and neonatal period

	Type I	Type II	Type III
A	Major artery lesion proximal to ischaemic muscle region (phlegmasia alba dolens)	Compartmental syndrome due to multifactorial but exclusively local causes (intrauterine compression) 1. Oligohydramnios 2. Amniotic band 3. Prolonged pressure against sacrum	Systemic diseases inducing multiple CS: 1. Dehydration [6] 2. *Meningococcal septicaemia* [34] 3. *S. epidermidis septicaemia* [35] 4. Malignant hyperthermia [5]
B	Complete occlusion of the venous circulation: hypercoagulability in the newborn of diabetic mother	Local disease associated with maternal factors or foetal systemic factors 1. Smallpox 2. Maternal diabetes 3. Mother and fetus coagulation disorders	

For simplification purposes, peri- and neonatal vascular lesions could include all the pathologies for which, once a vascular obstruction has been diagnosed, an anticoagulant therapy or microsurgical exploration and repair of the vessels by microvascular technique should be carried out. This group usually includes extensive skin necrosis requiring serial debridement or proximal and distal amputations of the upper limb.

32.3 Aetiological Factors in Atypical Upper Limb CS: Differences Between the Newborn and the Adult

Perinatal CS should certainly be included among atypical CS both for their incidence and pattern of occurrence [1, 11, 18, 21, 24, 28]. According to Bae [18] in fact, out of 33 patients, 26 (76%) of the child's CS occur in the setting of fractures, most frequently in the upper limb. On the other hand, we consider radial head fractures to be rare and atypical as well as aspiration of the upper limb during the emptying of a pool, the primary tumour pathology such as leukaemia, promyelocytic leukaemia where the surgical treatment of CS is absolutely contraindicated and the extravasation of anti-rejection drugs in organ transplants in the paediatric age group (Fig. 32.11). An atypical aetiology is also represented by the intraosseous infusion in infant, a technique for administration of fluid to a child who is in a state of haemodynamic collapse and for whom the access through conventional means has not been successful. This method is used in the child from three months to three years. The best sites for intraosseous infusion are the distal metaphysis of the femur and the proximal and distal metaphysis of the tibia. Displacement of the needle might be responsible of a CS at the lower limb. Therefore, in this group, the upper limb is usually spared [37].

32.4 Upper Limb Intrauterine Compartment Syndrome

32.4.1 General Aspects

Perinatal CS appears to be restricted to the upper limb [7] and it is included predominantly within groups IIA, B and III in our classification (Table 32.2).

In the subgroup IIB (Table 32.2), the predisposing factors can be found both on the maternal and on the foetal sides [29]. On the maternal side, there is often an association with chickenpox infection, gestational diabetes or pre-existing insulin dependence. There is a risk of partial thrombosis during childbirth or immediately before, due to placental rupture and related insufficiency. A pre-eclamptic condition also plays a negative role in this.

Simultaneous dehydration or infection can play a decisive role on the foetal side. Coagulation disorders of the foetus represent an aggravating systemic factor in type IIB compartment syndromes (Table 32.2), but they are more frequently associated with neonatal gangrene of the upper limb.

Among the loco-regional factors contributing to the development of a CS of the upper limb, we must consider the oligohydramnios which can cause the compression of the limb, in particular the right one, against the sacrum or the maternal lumbar spine [8, 29, 38]. The foetus is in fact most vulnerable to compression after the 37th week of gestation, when the amniotic fluid begins to decrease [9]. The amniotic bands, especially at the finger level and in the presence of a swollen and sub-cyanotic segment, represent the only rare cases that require, when promptly diagnosed, decompression in the first hours of life [31, 39].

32.4.2 Clinical Symptoms

Acute CS of the upper limb should be diagnosed before it evolves into established Volkmann's syndrome. However, this scenario occurs very rarely, and so far, there are only two cases in literature where fasciotomy was performed urgently soon after birth [8, 40] followed by a complete recovery. Only in the case where the pathology of amniotic bands belongs to group IIA of our classification (Table 32.2), the preconditions of an emergency decompression are met. This evidence can also be found in other animal species where a case of amniotic band syndrome (ABS), caused by a stenosis from the maternal fur, in the front leg of a baby rabbit has been observed. We proceeded with a circumferential removal of the causal agent and the skin band, as suggested by Buck-Gramcko and described by Habenicht [39]. The removal of the band was done in full respect of the periosteal and peritendinous vascularization with complete restoration of the normal vascularization of the paw (Fig. 32.1).

In the clinical setting, we were able to perform a similar operation only in one case 2 h after the

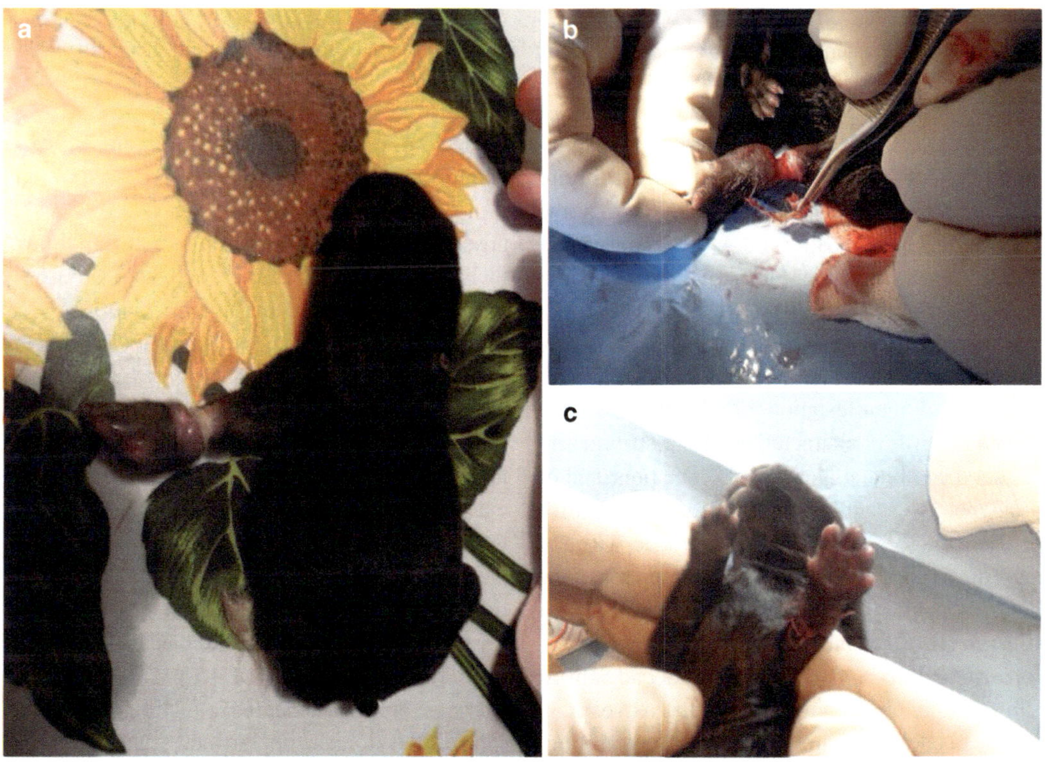

Fig. 32.1 (**a**) Amniotic band syndrome caused by the constriction of the maternal fur in a baby rabbit. (**b**) The constriction ring has been removed. (**c**) Closure of the gap by multiple Z plasties

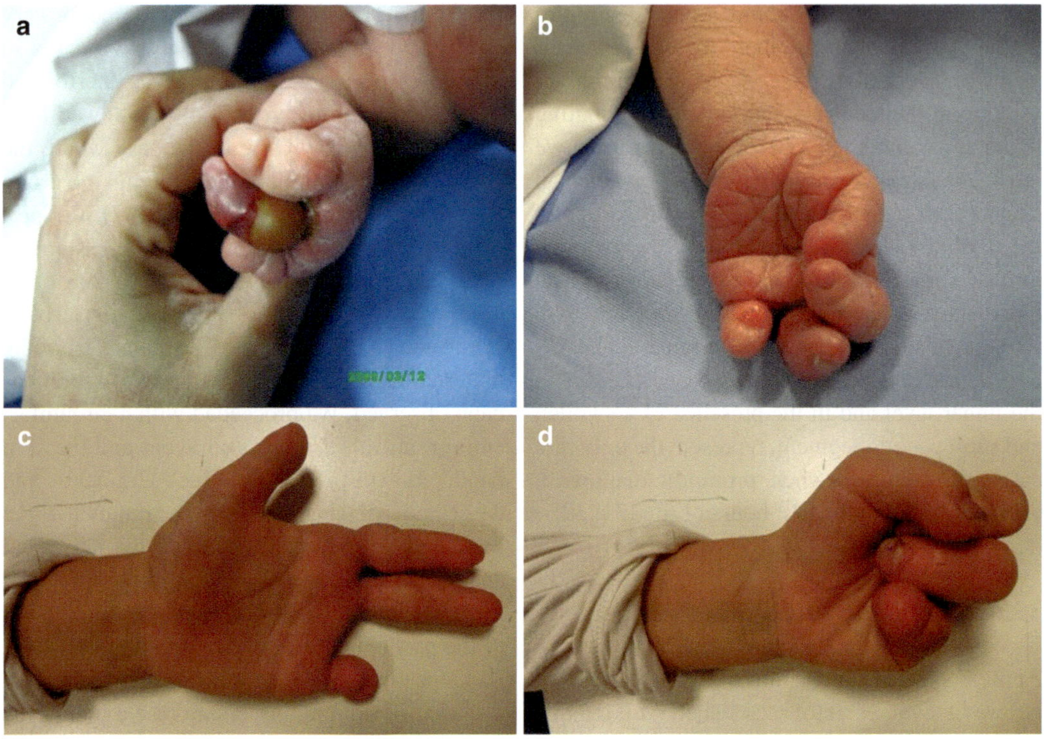

Fig. 32.2 (**a**) Amniotic band syndrome associated with swelling and vascular impairment of the middle finger associated with intrauterine amputation of the ring finger. (**b**) Decompression of the finger 2 h after birth by removal of the constriction and skin closure. (**c**) Return of normal vascular feeding of the finger. (**d**) Long-term follow-up showing a normal aspect and good function of the middle finger

birth of a premature baby who presented a digital amniotic band and who was treated according to the described technique (Fig. 32.2) [39].

32.4.3 Stabilized Peri- and Neonatal Volkmann's Syndrome

The typical manifestation of Volkmann's syndrome at birth is characterized by a sufficiently stereotyped clinical picture [41]. The presence of a cutaneous eschar (sentinel lesion) is almost a constant [8, 29, 42] and could coincide with the site of a greater intrauterine compression or depend on an underlying thrombo-embolic event (Fig. 32.3). Oedema is often widespread in the forearm and in the hand and it is associated with sub-cyanotic phenomena. The eschar as such can be traced back to the intrauterine phase and not to perinatal adverse factors. The eschar may also be present in association with caesarean sections`, and the peripheral pulses appear even in the event of a significant oedema [41, 42]. Of the 11 cases reported by Cham [43], the most frequent clinical picture corresponds to the adult with deformity of the hand in flexion and ulnar deviation.

However, when the eschar is located at the lateral-external surface, the position at birth is in wrist extension, and it is often associated with stiffness of the MPJ (metacarpal-phalangeal joint). The retraction of the muscles of the latero-external compartment is therefore at the basis of the deformity in extension of the wrist which is not passively correctable [43]. The wrist retraction in extension is also reported in 2 out of 4 of the cases of Rombouts [9] and can also be seen in our clinical experience of 15 cases where in 7 cases we found ischaemic retraction of the muscles of the dorsal compartment, in some cases associated with stiffness of the MPJ [11].

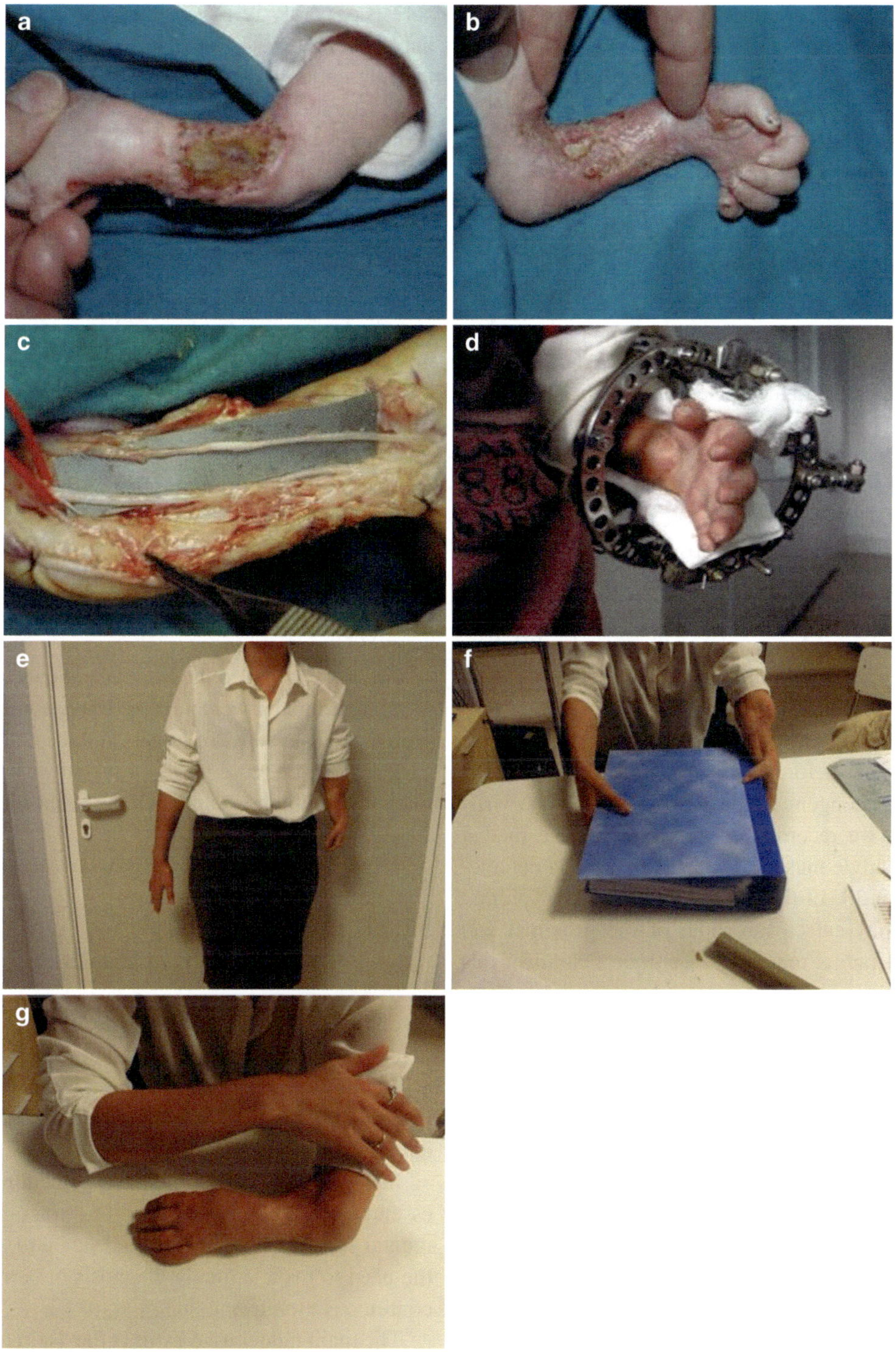

Fig. 32.3 (**a**, **b**) Skin defect after removal of the sentinel lesion performed one week after birth. The defect was covered shortly with a skin graft. (**c**) Early neurolysis and superficial dislocation of the median and ulnar nerve three months after birth. Tenotomy of the wrist flexors and of FPL. (**d**) Latissimus dorsi free muscle transfer performed at the age of four years. The Ilizarov apparatus was implemented to overcome the irreducible wrist flexor contracture. (**e**–**g**) Follow-up at 23 years: obvious limb discrepancy but good elbow flexion. No impairment on DLA and bimanual activities

The skin lesion is to be considered pathognomonic of a prenatal Volkmann's syndrome, especially since it is present in 20 out of 24 cases reported by Ragland [8] who defines it as "the sentinel lesion", and is confirmed by many other studies [4, 6, 15–17, 21].

32.4.4 Clinical Picture

The association of the skin lesion and the underlying compartment syndrome is often missed and fasciotomy in emergency rarely performed. The possible cause of the condition might be related to an associated intrinsic pathology. The relationship between the skin lesion, the underlying muscles ischaemia and the late effects on angular deformity and physeal closure of the radius distal to the lesion in the proximal forearm might be related to the concept of the angiosome and the arterial vascular supply of the muscles [8]. The overlying areas of the skin and underlying physis of the radius might benefit the same vascular supply [44]. In one of our cases, where the proximal Volkmann's forearm contracture was associated with a congenital constriction ring at the wrist level, we recorded a contracture of the medial epicondyle muscles leading to a flexion contracture of 30° of the elbow. The underlying premature physeal closure both of the proximal and distal radius represents a unique feature in this pathology.

In conclusion, the substantial difference between paediatric and adult Volkmann's syndromes lies in the almost constant presence of the sentinel skin lesion at the forearm level.

32.4.5 Clinical Symptoms

Only in the paediatric age group it is easy to discriminate the clinical symptoms of CS to those of the adult. In a retrospective report of 33 children with diagnosis of CS of the Boston Children's Hospital [45], it appeared that the traditional 5 P symptoms (pressure increased in the compartment, pain with stretch, paresis or anaesthesia, paresis or paralysis, pulses intact) [24] was unreliable in children [7, 18]. The AA recommended that the children at risk of CS should be monitored with the 3 As (increasing analgesic requirement, anxiety and agitation) [7, 21].

The muscle involvement has been taken into account and we classified our patients into four clinical groups as suggested by Ragland [8].

Group I that included patients who had skin involvement without compartment ischaemia or muscle dysfunction but late evidence of compromised skeletal development of the distal radius on a vascular basis (none of our patients).

Group II comprised seven patients of our series who had a skin lesion with late extrinsic contracture only of the muscles of the dorsolateral compartment.

Group III comprised five patients of our series who had a skin lesion associated with either a complete flexor or extensor compartment involvement [17].

Group IV included the residual patients where all compartments were involved and associated with distal tissue loss of fingers and the hand.

We have three cases of this kind but we believe that they should be included in the subheading of vascular lesion.

32.4.6 Complementary Investigations in the Adult

To complete the clinical diagnosis, the role of an objective examination plays a crucial aspect, especially in the case of complex diagnostics, in patients with acute disorders of the state of consciousness.

In acute cases, where the time element has an essential role, the measurement of intracompartmental pressure is in fact the gold standard, given the need to make a timely diagnosis or carry out continuous monitoring.

The main model used by us is the "split" catheter consisting of a hollow tube, the terminal of which has a series of fissurations, connectable to a small pocket-sized detection unit with a silicon transducer (STIC Catheter) or the Camino

Catheter; this contains a local detection microsensor that must be connected to an external control unit equipped with a monitor [45, 46] that enables evaluation of the variations of the PC over time [47].

CT in established Volkmann's contracture in forearm muscles was introduced in 1989 [48] and enabled identification of the muscle infarct which corresponds to a sharp area of hypodensity (10,2 Hounsfield Unit (HU) compared to 50–60 HU in contralateral normal muscles). The extent of the muscle damage within the muscle compartment and involvement of different compartments might positively influence the choice of the most appropriate surgical treatment. CT as MRI imaging has so far been utilized exclusively in adults [48, 49].

32.4.7 Complementary Investigations in the Child

Compartmental pressure in children has been measured by some authors with the same technique used in adults [15]. Normal resting compartment pressure in children has been described in the lower limb and reported to be higher (13.3 mmHg and 16.6 mmHg) compared with adults (5.2 mmHg and 9.7 mmHg). Generally intracompartmental pressure over 30 mmHg [16] or 40 mmHg, which corresponds quite accurately to the infant's diastolic blood pressure, should be considered as a threshold for fasciotomy. In any case, apprehension, poor cooperation and difficulties with communication in the conscious child [28] complicate the evaluation by any needle device. We never resorted to it as the majority of our cases presented as an already established Volkmann's contracture.

Near-infrared spectroscopy has been introduced as a noninvasive technique to overcome this problem [7]. Based on the same principle, FRIR (Fourier transform infrared spectrophotometer), a smartphone thermal imaging which consents the detection of perforator for free flaps and monitoring even at a physical distance from the operator, has been used in recent years [19, 20, 50, 51].

X-rays are mandatory as the radiological findings are similar in these children: forearm bone shortening and widening of the distal epiphysis [10].

Ultrasound sonography remains the most straightforward method for a rapid assessment of the extent of residual muscle mass in the various compartments.

In conjunction with the evaluation of compartmental pressure or the use of near-infrared spectroscopy, the echo-Doppler for the study of the main and deep arterial and venous circulation, especially when the distal pulses are not detected during the clinical examination, is mandatory.

Angiography and MR angiography represent techniques used in malformative and iatropathic pathologies of main vessels [15, 43].

EMG studies are not easily tolerated by the paediatric population and are not routinely administered. Surprisingly in two cases of the established perinatal Volkmann's contracture in children with the age of six and eight years, SEPs were comparable to the values recorded in the unaffected site in spite of the overt damage of the median and ulnar nerve observed at surgery (unpublished data).

32.5 Surgical Treatment in Perinatal Volkmann's Contracture

32.5.1 General Aspects

The overall experience of the Institute of Orthopedics of University of Modena for the period 1999–2013 was of 175 operated cases of Volkmann's contracture, including the upper and lower limbs (Table 32.3). The incidence of perinatal Volkmann's contracture has been of 8%, and this significant value might be related to the presence of a dedicated congenital deformities of outpatient clinic.

The complexity of cases and difficult family context sometimes leads parents to adopt an attitude of abstention when faced with a proposal of multiple complex surgeries from the medical team.

Table 32.3 1998–2013 upper and lower limb Volkmann's syndrome

Site	Aetiology	Cases
Upper limb Volkmann's syndrome		
Proximal humerus	Fracture + axillary artery lesion	4
Distal humerus	Supracondylar	15
Elbow	Fracture	3
Forearm	Fracture	19
Forearm	Crush syndrome	9
Forearm	Radio ulnar synostosis (osteotomy)	2
Forearm	Perinatal Volkmann	15
Forearm	Others (iatropathic)	8
Hand (intrinsic muscles)	Miscellaneous (mainly posttraumatic)	12
Leak syndrome		2
Waterhouse-Friderichsen syndrome		1
	Total	90
Lower limb Volkmann's syndrome		
Clinica Ortopedica, Modena		71
Hesperia Hospital, Modena		14
	Total	85
	Total cases	175

The natural history of the syndrome has not been reported in literature and has been monitored and illustrated in detail as in the case of our series (Fig. 32.4) [17]. In the adolescent phase, this patient encountered alternating problems of social integration, eventually entering a community and maintaining a pertinent use of the dysmetric limb in its remaining potential.

The priority of treatment is represented by removal of the skin eschar of variable dimensions, which in itself might herald underlying CS, which can be solved (Fig. 32.3) by simple escharotomy. The exposed skin areas must then be resurfaced by simple skin grafts. The second priority is represented by the need to displace nerves of the forearm, median ulnar and radial, out of the scarred bed, so they should be superficialized when the skin problem is solved (Figs. 32.3 and 32.5), considering that the necrotic and therefore removable muscle is already easily recognizable after three weeks [11].

32.5.2 Surgical Techniques

The surgical techniques are adopted according to the well-established grade of severity of the syndrome [21].

The substantial difference between newborn and adult is that newborn severity of involvement can vary significantly, ranging from no muscle ischaemia to complete flexor and extensor compartment loss. In the newborn if acute (fresh), extensive skin lesions are noted over the flexor and/or extensor surfaces; emergent fasciotomy is recommended, especially if distal cyanosis is present. Timing is critical as the compartments must be released before ischaemia and muscle death occurs. If the skin lesions appear to be older (i.e. partially healing), waiting to explore and debride the involved muscle and performing neurolysis are warranted. When the infant is stabilized, formal exploration and debridement of the dead muscle and neurolysis are warranted to prevent fixed contracture. Importantly, if the FDP (flexor digitorum profundus)/ FPL (flexor pollicis longus) muscles are debrided, the stumps of the tendons should be secured in the forearm to the radius to prevent retraction into the carpal tunnel, which makes secondary reconstruction much more difficult. Also, the anterior interosseous nerve should be tagged for easier identification at the time of reconstructive surgery. In these severe cases, free functional muscle transfer can restore reasonable function for the patient. In the adult and paediatric population, the main involvement is located at the anterior surface, where the following treatment guidelines are usually suggested, based on the classification of the extent of damage according to Tsuge [21]:

- Mild localized type extensor compartment, scar tissue removal and planning for palliative surgery
- Mild localized type deep flexor compartment: muscle sliding operation
- Moderate type deep and superficial flexor compartment + neurological deficit: flexor sliding with neurolysis median and ulnar nerve

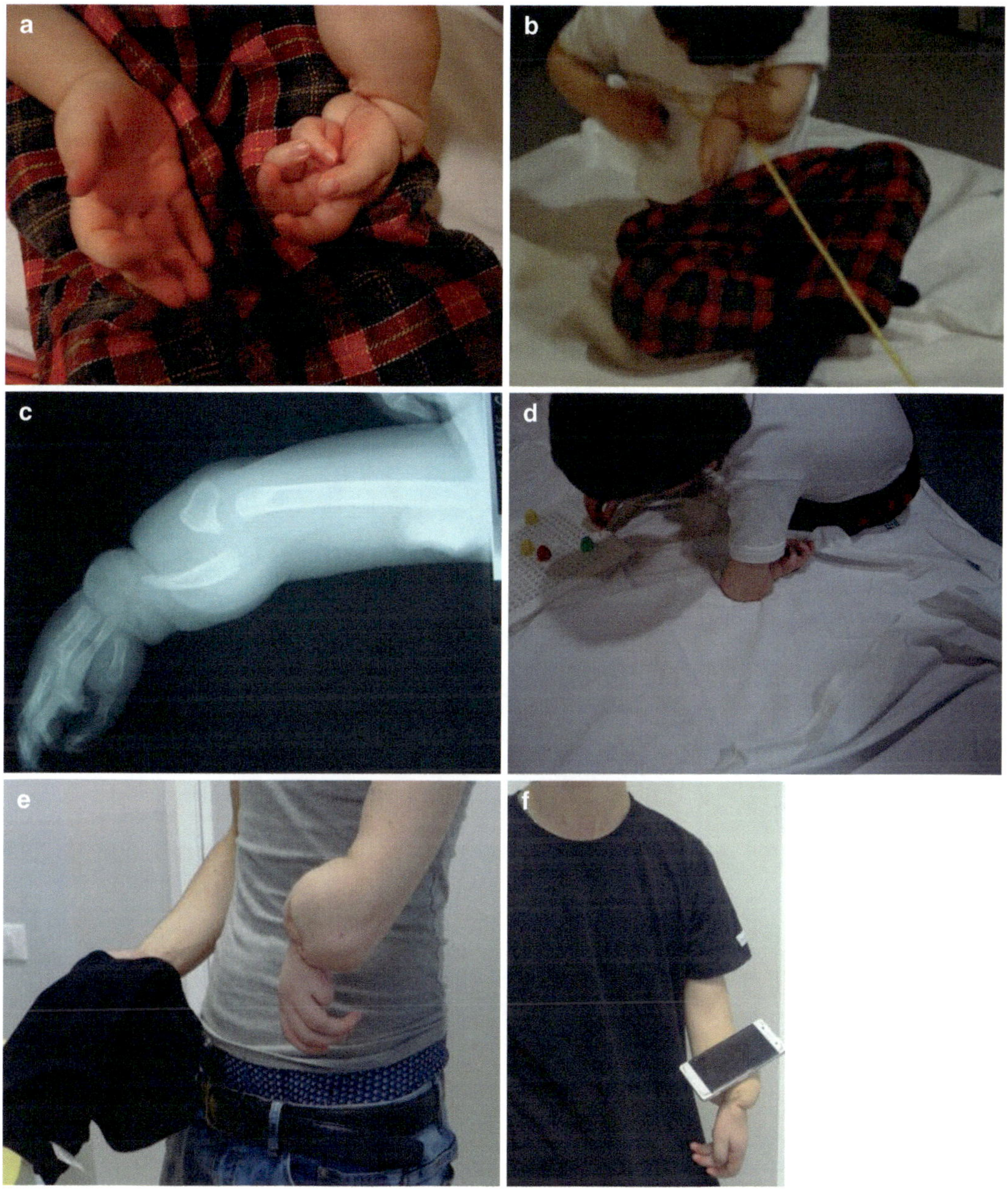

Fig. 32.4 (**a**) Severe outcome of a deep amniotic band and at the forearm. (**b**) Coping strategies by holding objects between the trunk and the affected limb (**c**) X-rays show discontinuity of the radius and ulna caused by the amniotic band. (**d**) Possibility to support the body at the site of pseudarthrosis of the forearm. (**e**) Follow-up at 18 years. The adopting parents have not consented to stabilize of the forearm bones early in life. (**f**) Patient is bimanual in virtue of the normal function of the elbow joint and in spite of the significant limb discrepancy

- Severe type superficial and deep flexor compartments + extensor compartment: single [52] or double free muscle transfer [13, 14]

In the newborn, normally the extensor muscles of the wrist are spared and scarring is limited to the EDC (extensor digitorum communis). We

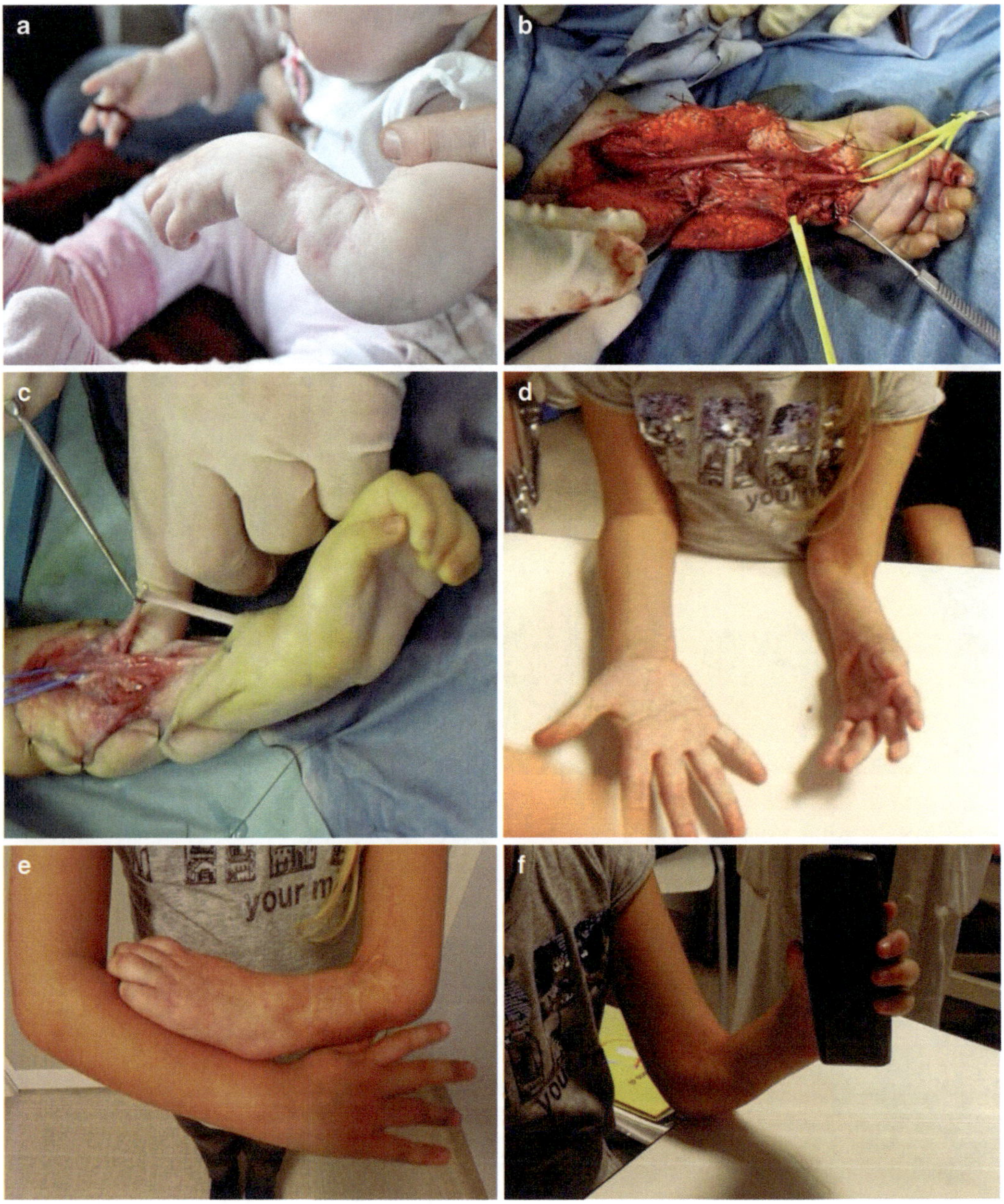

Fig. 32.5 (**a**) The sequela of the skin scar at the posterolateral compartment. (**b**, **c**) At one-year neurolysis, of the median and ulnar nerve, transfers of BR to wrist extensors were carried out. (**d**–**f**) Follow-up at six years: good range of motion at the elbow associated with active wrist extension. Grip strength measured by Jamar reduced to one-third compared to the unaffected side

believe that scar excision and palliative surgery should be postponed to an age where one can rely on the understanding and collaboration of the young patient (Fig. 32.6). In severe injuries, the most affected compartment is usually the volar one where often free muscle transplantation should be carried out, while in the dorsal compartment, there is often the possibility of pallia-

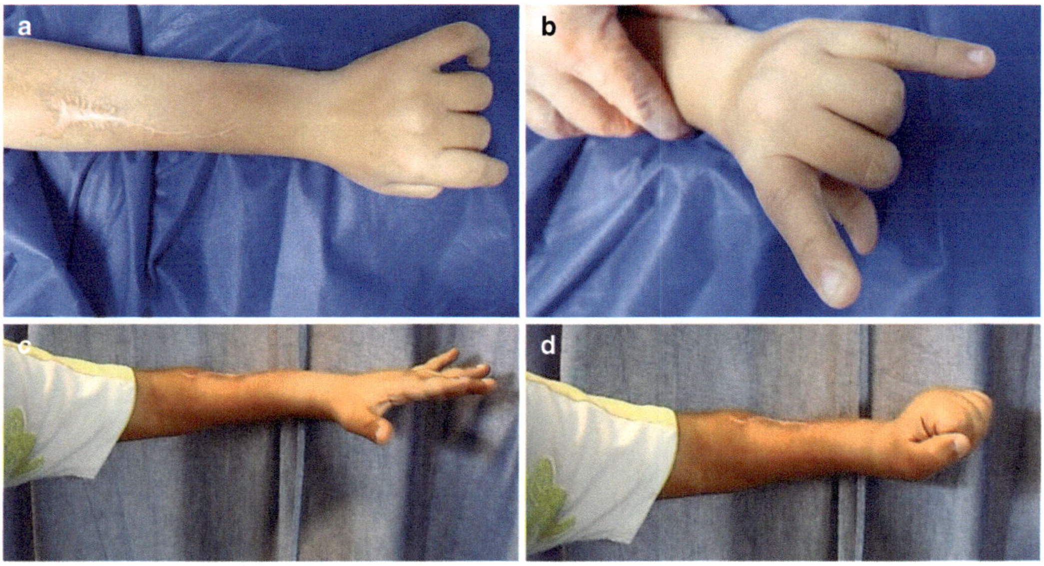

Fig. 32.6 (**a**) The scar sequela of a sentinel lesion with the underlining Volkmann's contraction of the muscle of the postero-lateral compartment. (**b**) No active contraction of the EDC while EIP and EDM are normal. FCU was transferred early in life to EDC leading, during growth, to a gradual dorsal contracture of the wrist. (**c**, **d**) Long-term follow-up after tenolysis of the tendon transfer and dorsal capsulotomy of the wrist. Normal function of EDC. AROM at the wrist improved from −70° fixed in extension to +20° of active flexion

tive surgery preceded by excision of the scar tissue. In the severe Volkmann's retraction of both compartments, similar to the adult, there is no alternative to the double free muscle transplant [21].

In the infant who suffered severe neonatal compartment syndrome leading to both volar and dorsal compartment muscle losses, a staged approach is warranted. Exploration with debridement of nonviable muscle as well as neurolysis is important, as this prevents fixed contractures and assists with re-gaining hand sensation and intrinsic muscle function. This should be performed within the first few months of life if the patient is medically stable. It is important to suture the ends of the FDP tendons to the radius in the forearm to prevent retraction into the carpal tunnel, which can make secondary reconstruction much more difficult. In addition, tagging of the ends of the future donor nerves, most commonly anterior and posterior interosseous nerves, can be very helpful when performing the secondary functioning muscle transfer. Occupational therapy is also an imperative adjunct in these patients to obtain full passive range-of-motion and prevent fixed contracture. This allows secondary free functioning muscle transfer to be performed when the patient is older, 1–3 years of age, and structures are larger. Usually, the flexor compartment is first to be reconstructed, followed by the extensor compartment 1–2 years later (Fig. 32.7) contrary to Chuang who performed by first reconstructing the muscles of the extensor group followed by the free transplant in the flexor group when the first ones displayed signs of reinnervation [11]. Permanent nerve injuries can be prevented when they are superficialized at an early stage. Otherwise, the repair will be proportional to their severity: neurolysis, nerve grafts or implementation of the Strange technique [53, 54].

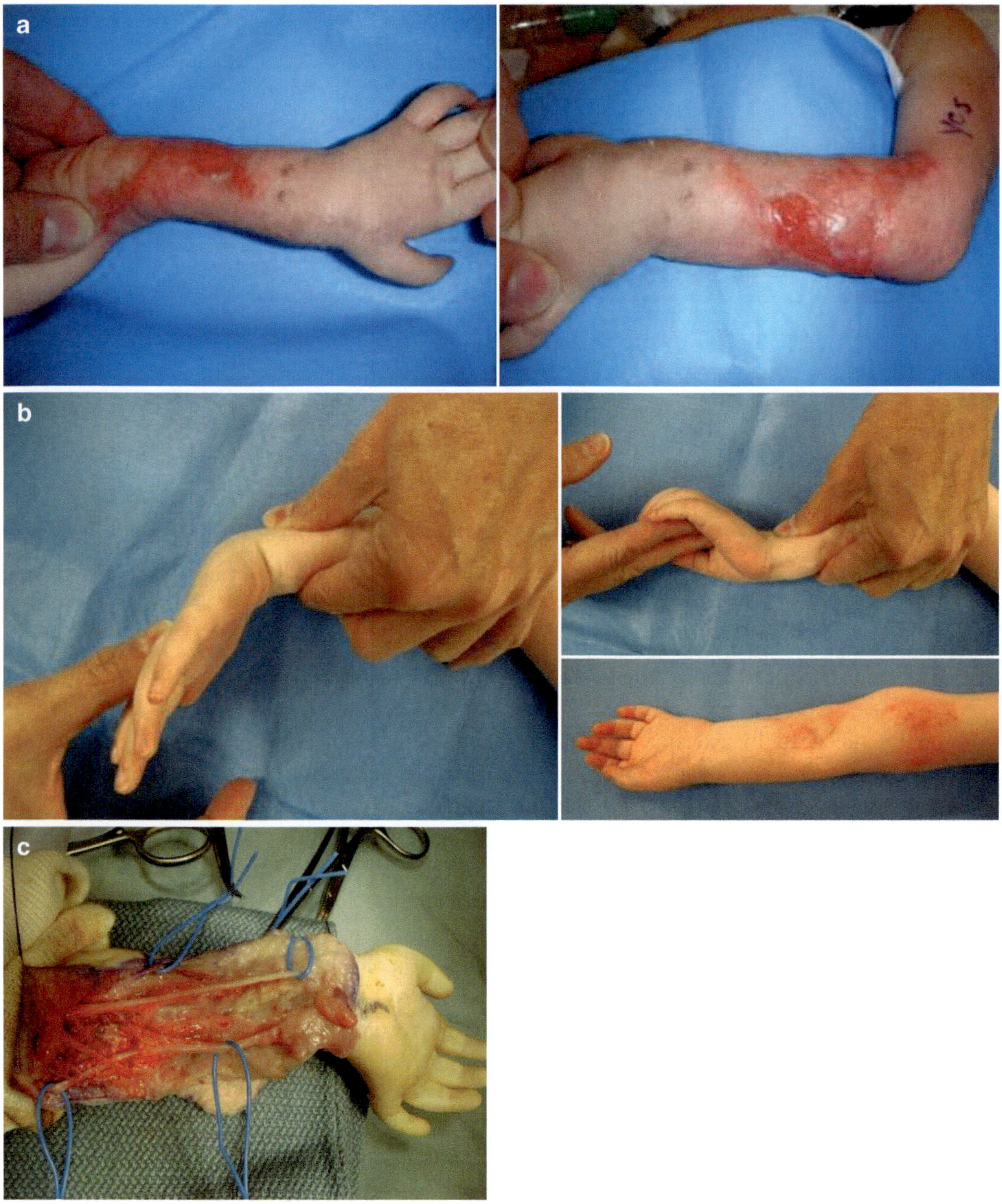

Fig. 32.7 (**a**) Initial presentation two weeks after birth. (**b**) After debridement and therapy, prior to free functioning muscle transfer. (**c**) Intra-operative debridement surgery. (**d**) Postoperative gracilis transfer to volar and dorsal compartment

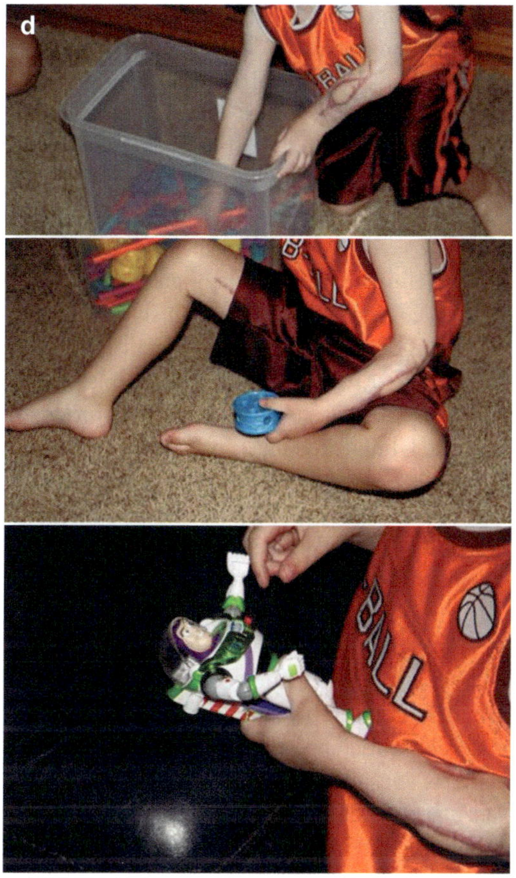

Fig. 32.7 (continued)

32.6 Vascular Lesions

32.6.1 Spontaneous Vascular Lesions

Neonatal ischaemia of the upper limb represents a rare occurrence, and to distinguish it from the compartment and Volkmann's syndromes described in the previous section, it can be simply assumed that for its treatment, a decompression of the affected muscle compartments is not sufficient, whereas a substantial medical or surgical intervention on the arterial or venous system is indispensable [55].

A fasciotomy should be considered a complementary measure, but the gangrene of the newborn (Figs. 32.8 and 32.9) can only be prevented by intervening directly on the major vascular axes.

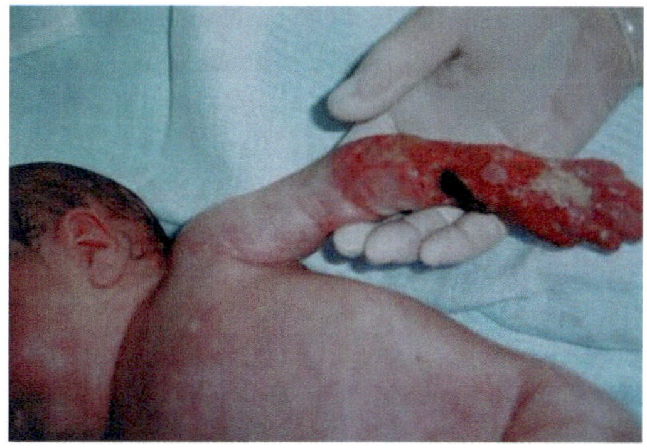

Fig. 32.8 Vascular lesion of a newborn left upper limb where multiple debridements were carried out. The whole area covered by granulation tissue ready for skin grafting

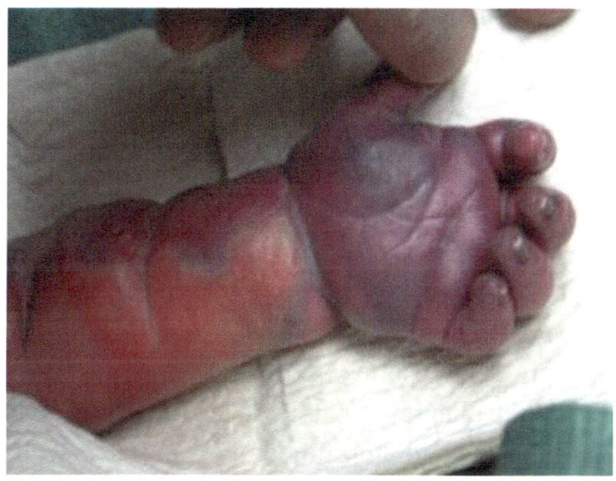

Fig. 32.9 Clinical picture of a severe ischaemia of the left upper limb

When this is not feasible for technical reasons (avulsion of iliac vessels) or general health of the newborn (coexisting hyaline membrane diseases), the residual survival of the limb is entrusted to the establishment of collateral circulation.

The experience on which this chapter is based refers to the 32 cases already reported by GEOP (Paediatric Orthopedic Group) collected in France, Canada, Portugal and Belgium [29] in addition to 3 cases, treated by the Modena Hand Surgery Unit, for a total of 35 cases.

Vascular lesions of the upper limbs in the perinatal period are quite rare: it should be considered that less than 100 cases of ischaemia of the limbs (upper and lower) at birth or in the first hours of life are reported in the literature [38].

Vascular lesions may be spontaneous and often generated as a result of renal vein thrombosis where the presence of calcific thrombus stands for an intrauterine genesis [56].

Vascular lesions may fall into group I (Table 32.2) due to impairment of a large arterial vessel (phlegmasia alba dolens) or venous vessel (phlegmasia cerulea dolens) or group III where pre-existing systemic factors (meningococcal septicaemia, epidermidis staphylococcal septicaemia, dehydration, etc.) are to be considered responsible for the involvement of several limbs with consequent necrosis of small and large segments.

In utero ischaemia of the limb may be associated with necrosis of the ipsilateral hemiface generated by a placental thrombus likely migrated through the oval foramen destined to the brachiocephalic arterial trunk [35].

Limb ischaemia manifests itself at birth or within a few hours after birth. Several conditions can cause ischaemic episodes: thromboembolism could be a cause and be associated with maternal diabetes, gestational hypertension (eclampsia and pre-eclampsia), oligohydramnios and pressure of maternal pelvic structures. Venous thrombosis and thromboembolism are well-known complications in infants of diabetic mothers. Oppenheimer and Esterley, in their 4000 newborn autopsies, describe 45 cases of venous thrombosis, 13 of which from diabetic mothers [57]. Renal and adrenal veins are usually more frequently involved.

Vallerame [58] published the first case of peripheral gangrene in a newborn from a diabetic mother in 1972, hypothesizing that the adrenal vein was the probable starting point of the embolus occluding the right brachial artery, which it reached through the patent foramen ovale.

Carr [41] hypothesized that the emboli resulting from a placental infarction could be transported in the right ulnar artery and in the right internal carotid artery of the newborn through the same foramen.

Extremity gangrene is a very likely complication of neonatal infections in the presence of severe dehydration [6, 35] or meningococcal [34] (Fig. 32.10) or staphylococcus epidermidis septicaemia (Table 32.2). There is also the sector of multiple gangrene with self-amputation in association with severe dehydration, even in the absence of occlusive vascular phenomena. The most frequent cause is related to adverse underlying conditions, such as illiteracy and tribal practices, which for the treatment of mild intestinal disorders resort to herbal enemas that also have a cytotoxic effect on the kidney and liver. Herbal enemas can have a phlebo-occlusive effect and the vaso-constrictive effects typical of the alkaloids of ergot [6]. The clinical picture is characterized by dehydration, acidosis, hyperuricemia and renal failure. Gangrene can affect all four limbs, the tip of the nose, ears or perineum as in case of meningococcal septicaemia.

On the neonatal side, the immaturity of the coagulation systems and the presence of congenital thrombophilia play a relevant role [38]. Moreover, in the cardiovascular pathology, anatomical anomaly situations can be at the basis of a paradoxical embolism that starting from the maternal or foetal periphery (placental embolism or renal and adrenal veins) is distributed to the vascular district of the upper limb (an axillary or humeral) and/or to the cerebral circulation becoming responsible for the porencephalic degeneration found in 9 of the 32 cases reported by Romaña [29]. The most frequent cardiovascular malformations associated with upper limb abnormalities are atrioventricular defects (atrial septal defect (ASD) and ventricular septal defect (VSD)), Fallot's tetralogy, large vessel transposition and the presence of the common arterial trunk [55, 59], but especially emboli that can spread from the closing arterial duct.

32.6.2 Iatropathic Causes

The most frequent etiopathogenesis of vascular lesions of the upper limb, however, is iatropathic, linked to the more aggressive attitude in the treatment of infants at risk in intensive care units, and it might include a false aneurysm caused by the perforation of the lower third of the humeral artery that required excision and microsurgical repair [60].

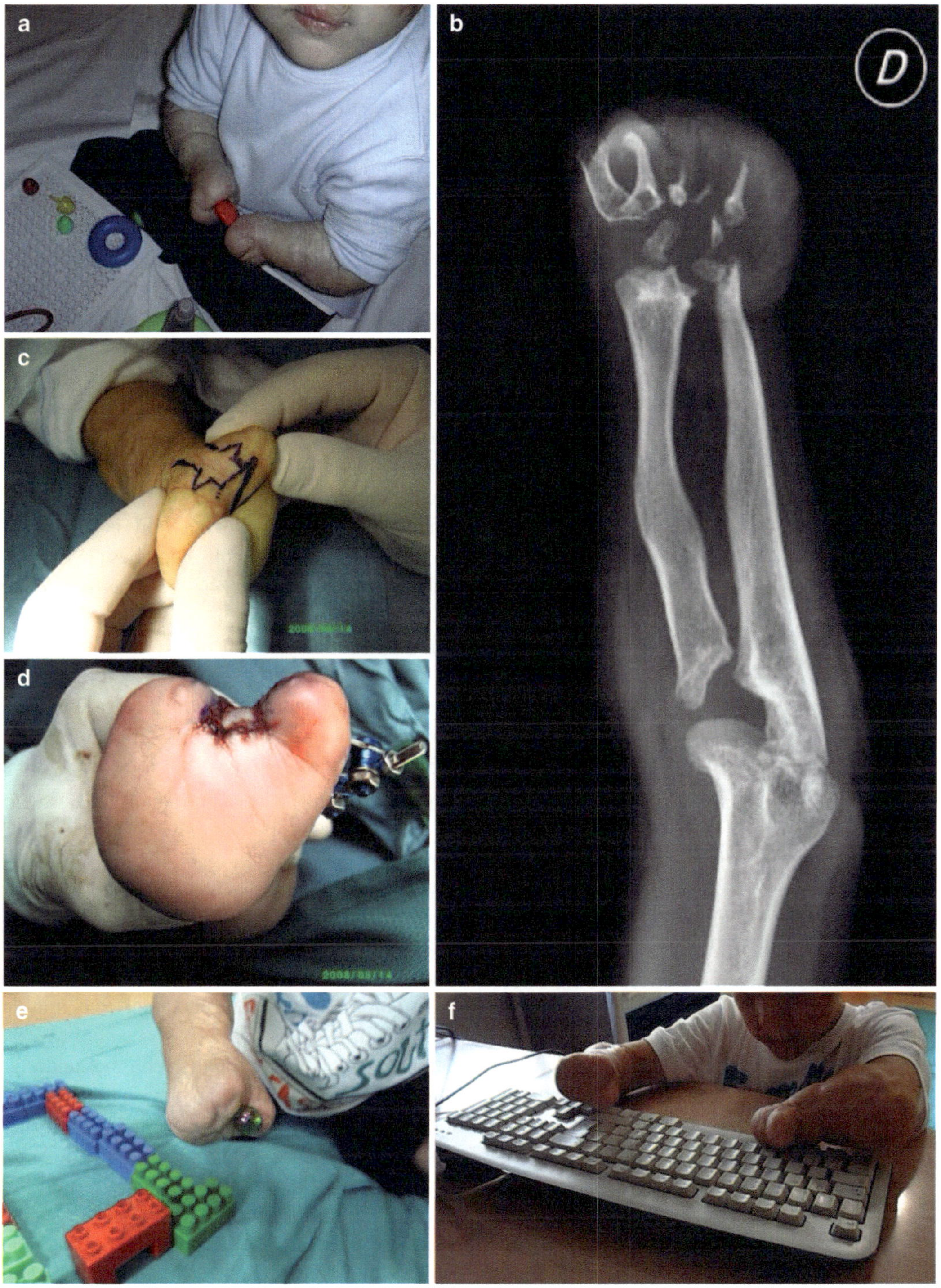

Fig. 32.10 (**a**) Four-limb amputation as consequence of a meningococcal septicemia occurred after birth. Residual trans-metacarpal amputation on the right side with minimal function. (**b**) Corresponding X-rays. (**c-d**) Deepening of the first web by a local plasty according to the Ostrowsky technique. (**e**) Functional opening of the web. (**f**) Possibility of performing bimanual activities

In a seemingly inexplicable way, even the injection of an unknown substance, in a newborn suffering from gastroenteritis into the anterior belly of the deltoid muscle, resulted in severe vascular suffering followed by an amputation of the middle third of the arm [61].

Regarding the use of central venous catheters (CVC), the access can be superficial or deep: among the superficial access routes, it is worth mentioning the cephalic, the basilic and the external jugular veins and among the deep ones, the internal jugular and the subclavian veins.

Venous embolisms can pass to the arterial circle, always through the oval foramen, causing peripheral ischaemia of the limbs.

Data from the Canadian Registry showed an incidence of 3.5 events of thromboembolism related to the presence of CVC for every 100,000 admitted patients. According to the same authors, the placement of a central route, used for the administration of liquids, drugs, parenteral nutrition or chemotherapy, would be responsible for about 90% of DVT (deep vein thrombosis) and pulmonary embolisms in the first year of life [38].

The indication to use arterial catheters is based on the need to perform frequent blood tests or to continuously monitor blood pressure. In the neonatal age, within the first 24–48 h of life, arterial cannulation can be performed through the umbilical arteries.

In case of failure of the umbilical access or in case of infants over 48 h of life, the radial artery stands for the most used access; the criteria of choice towards this artery are represented by its superficial anatomical path and good secondary circulation (validated by Allen's test). The permanence of the catheter in the artery must not exceed 72–96 h.

Ischaemia is not the only complication that can occur after radial catheterization: there can also be a bacterial infection. The most frequently identified germs are staphylococcus and streptococcus, which are usually non-pathogenic but might become so in the presence of debilitated patients or those with an underdeveloped immune system like the newborn.

32.6.3 Complications in Stabilized Outcomes

CS and Volkmann's perinatal pathology are peculiar conditions connoted by scanty report and unavailable long-term outcome studies.

There are substantial differences in the timing of execution of fasciotomy, especially between the newborn and adult. In the adult, fasciotomy may sometimes be useless if performed for a suprafascial oedema mainly in burns carrying the side effects such as lack of strength at the hand and fatigue in walking [15].

Late fasciotomy is often subject to bacterial colonization, and when incomplete, it can be accompanied by the fibrous evolution of the non-decompressed myotendinous components, whereas late paediatric fasciotomy is not necessarily related to irreversible outcomes [18, 21]. In traumatology, fasciotomy has been performed for up to 88 h [7] 7 days [62] with an almost always complete recovery of function [63].

This observation is confirmed by a retrospective analysis conducted at the Mayo Clinic by Eichler and Lipscop [64]. This observation suggests that in these circumstances, there might be a subliminal muscle circulation or early neoangiogenesis in children that guarantees their survival or that the muscles in the perinatal age group have a greater tolerance to ischaemia than in adulthood.

In the surgical treatment of Volkmann's contracture, the possible complications are liaised to flexor origin sliding or functional free muscle transfer. In this last scenario, the complications can be categorized as acute or chronic: underlying flap loss (either skin paddle or partial muscle loss). Long-term complications include scarring and tendon attenuation at the repair site [5, 21].

In paediatric patients, bone growth may be more rapid compared to the transferred muscle, to which the following coercive aspects to the surrounding scarring retractions can be added, which can lead to joint contracture and tendon adhesions despite excellent muscle contraction [13, 21]:

- The slowly increasing tenodesis effect of a premature tendon transfer, which might lead during growth to an extension contracture of the wrist.
- Ulnar deviation of the wrist usually occurs when muscle sliding has been associated with carpal tunnel decompression leading to a volar dislocation of flexor tendons which implies that the tunnel should be repaired in the first instance.
- Joint stiffness mainly at the MPJ and wrist level which can assume aspects of severity that can only be encountered in arthrogryposis and may require first row carpectomy.
- Pseudoarthrosis, retracting scars and contracture of the first web space (Fig. 32.11) may be present both in Volkmann's outcomes and in vascular lesions of the perinatal period [17].

32.6.4 Differential Diagnosis

The almost constant skin lesion is the one that has certainly aroused the most interest in the various medical disciplines. Effectively, this area of the skin with the subcutaneous tissue with an inflammatory reaction can occur in different fields. This description coincides with the one given by R. Lightwood [2] and by Haymann [3] where three cases of infants who had fat necrosis were reported above the elbow were suggestive of compression syndrome of the radial nerve in the region of the spiral groove. C.V Feldmann [65] also reported four cases, one of which was a bilateral paresis of the radial nerve highlighted three days after birth associated with fat necrosis of the lateral surface. Function of both wrists was fully restored after three months. A similar experience is reported by Rombouts [9].

Sclerema neonatorum is a systemic form which manifests itself with a hardening of the skin that suddenly appears in the third or fourth day of life, often in malnourished, dehydrated, hypotensive, hyponatremic or hypoglycaemic infants. The thickening often starts from the lower limbs and spreads to the trunk and cheeks. Sclerema is probably the result of an enzymatic neonatal dysfunction involved in the conversion of saturated palmitic and stearic acid into unsaturated oleic acid [66].

Aplasia cutis represents a group of congenital skin lesions ranging from the absence of skin to small achromic scars. The preferred location of these lesions, however, is the scalp but the forearm is also frequent. The classical pathogenetic theory of aplasia cutis hypothesized an adhesion between lesions affecting the teguments of the foetus and amnion. It could also be a genetically determined skin malformation because more than 50% of cases are associated with trisomy 13 [3, 17].

Analysing all the reported cases, the neural damage, when present, is framed by a temporal paralysis of the radial nerve that recovers spontaneously and is therefore easily distinguishable from the muscle contracture associated with a Volkmann's syndrome of the lateral-external compartment.

Moreover, the congenital deformity in flexion of long fingers might be connected to an aberrant origin to flexor digitorum profundus [67], a condition that belongs to the field of congenital malformations.

32.6.5 Long-Term Outcomes

As expected, long-term outcome following neonatal compartment syndrome is largely dependent on the severity of involvement. In cases with a skin lesion but no muscle dysfunction or compartment ischaemia, near full function can be expected although abnormal forearm growth is still the norm and should be discussed with the parents. This is in sharp contrast to the patient that has flexor and extensor compartment involvement who did not undergo emergent fasciotomy at birth. Depending on the time delay until exploration, these patients may have severe joint and skin contractures along with severe neurologic deficits in the hand that must be addressed. Even with debridement, neurolysis +/- nerve grafting and free muscle transfer hand function may be limited. However, if timely staged reconstruction is performed, good to excellent results can occur even in the severely involved patient. As dis-

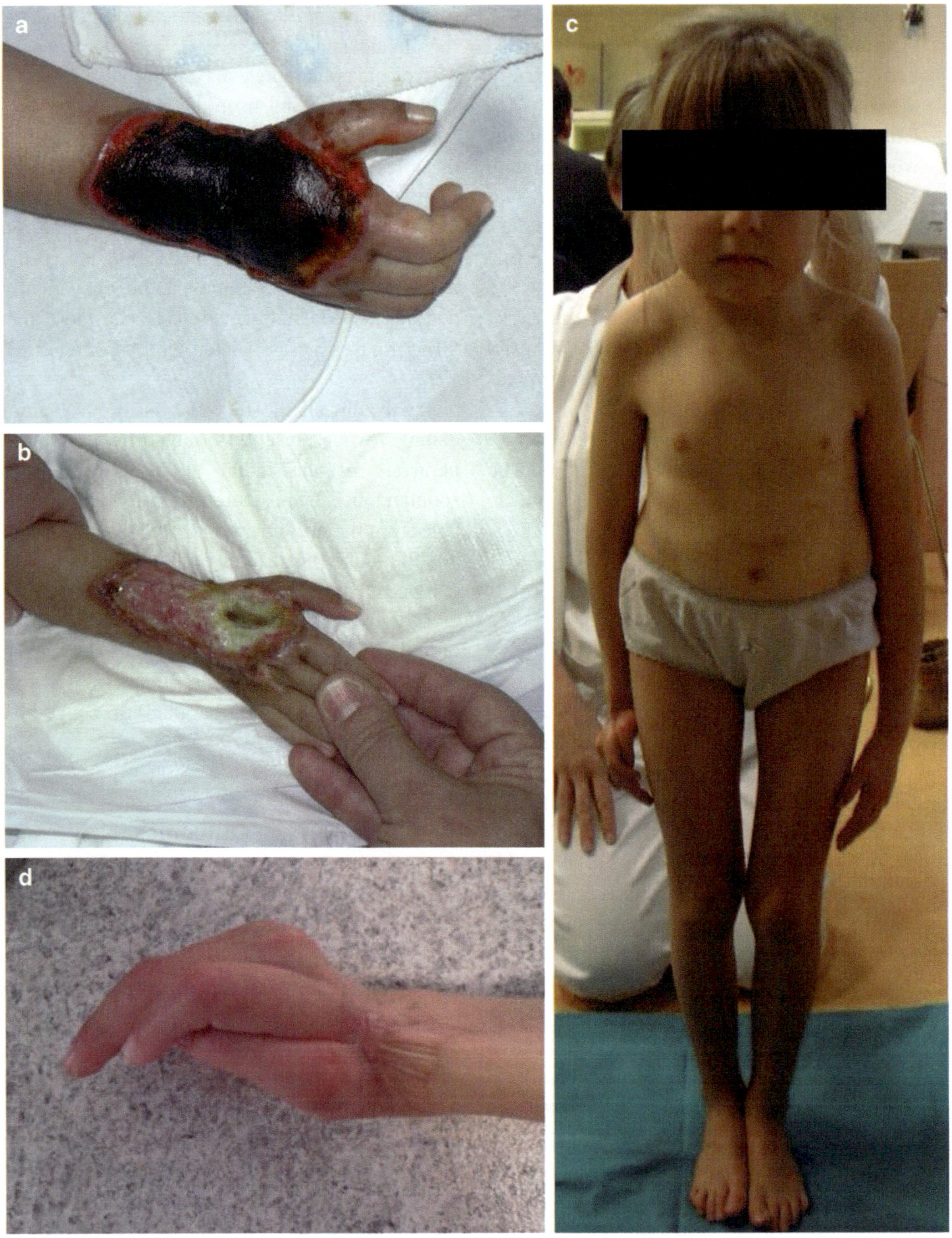

Fig. 32.11 (**a**) Skin necrosis at the dorsal aspect of the wrist following extravasation of antirejection drug administration following a renal transplantation in the first year of life. (**b**) Surgical debridement and resurfacing by dermal graft. (**c**) Clinical appearance a still unclassified syndromic pattern. (**d**) Severe first web contracture. (**e**) Resurfacing by dermal graft. (**f**) Clinical result following release of the first web space initially caused by the Volkmann's contracture of the intrinsic muscle. (**g**) Functional opening of the wrist web consenting a useful key-pinch

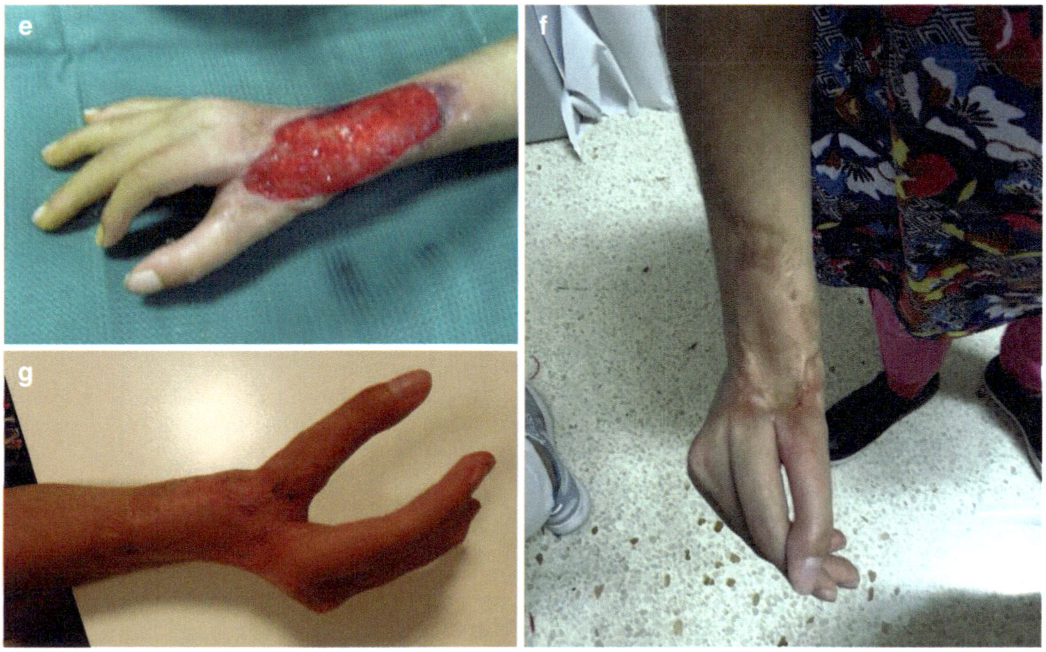

Fig. 32.11 (continued)

cussed earlier, less involved cases can undergo expectant management depending on the clinical progression of deformity.

32.7 Prevention

In the majority of cases, the newborn will be affected by an irreversible established Volkmann's contracture. Therefore, it would be reasonable to check if any preventive fetoscopic surgery could be possibly undertaken during the intra-uterine phase. Mentioning of this possibility is made only for amniotic band syndrome to prevent amputation caused by the attachment or entanglement of amniotic membrane remnants to the foetus. The median gestational week at diagnosis was 22 weeks/5 days [68]. A literature review included a group of patients who had the fetoscopic release of the amniotic bands using a laser (16 cases), scissors (6 cases) or both (5 cases) in a series of 27 cases. In only one case, the hand and fingers were affected; some of his fingers were amputated. In the majority of cases, a single entry was made and a functional limb was acquired in 71.4%. Foetal morbidity was mainly linked to the consequences of premature rupture of the membranes (57.1%) and preterm birth (28.5%). The AA concluded that fetoscopic band release was encouraging in cases of ABS in the limbs [69].

32.8 Conclusions

The borderline between perinatal CS and Volkmann's contracture in the newborn and in the vascular lesion appears to be very subtle; this is the reason why these topics have been assembled in this chapter [23].

For the purpose of the classification of the pathophysiological aspects, we relied on the Holden classification, already described in 1958 by Perricone, to which we made added significant modifications [16]. Group A concerning the lesion of a proximal major vessel, which we divided into arterial and venous components including also the distal pathology, is related to the vascular compromise of a muscle with a single vascular supply (Table 32.1).

Group II was also divided into group IIA where CS occurs in muscle groups only for local causes ranging from hypothetical intrauterine compression to group IIB where this condition is associated with systemic aggravating factors that can be differentiated into maternal or foetal factors (Table 32.2). Finally, we introduced a group III where CS are multiple and are associated with systemic diseases [32, 33] completely different from those of the adult (Tables 32.1 and 32.2). In the different parallelism between children and adults, the clinical symptomatology should also be understood: if the adult still maintains the value of the five Ps, the symptoms in the paediatric group are often inductive and are represented by the three As (anxiety, greater demand for analgesics, etc.). Volkmann's syndrome has a specific clinical connotation in the perinatal period due to the almost constant association of the sentinel skin lesion overlying the affected muscle compartments.

The surgical treatment must be performed promptly and consists of a fasciotomy in the first few hours after birth.

The subsequent stages of treatment require an early repair of the skin defect. After healing, the main nerves of the forearm should be superficialized. Subsequent reconstructive procedures should be postponed to the pre-school period in cases of intermediate severity and in Volkmann's syndrome of the postero-lateral compartment, through scarring excision and the use of palliative surgery. In the presence of irreversible damage in both compartments, there is no choice but to resort to free muscle transplantation. Nevertheless, a lesion as complex as Volkmann's syndrome often requires interventions that have to be planned at a later age.

The natural history of the disease is objectively unfavourable, but young patients know how to use unimaginable coping strategies. The evaluation of the long-term surgical results must be made using both objective and subjective assessment tools to verify whether the overall medical case has ultimately positively influenced the social integration of the young patient and his life in its wholeness [70].

In newborns presenting with forearm skin lesions, prompt, accurate diagnosis is imperative as a subgroup of them can undergo emergent fasciotomy with resultant normal or almost normal hand function. In less involved patients, timing and type of surgical intervention varies widely but is important to optimize the ultimate function of the upper extremity.

Acknowledgements Dr. Della Rosa for the documentation concerning the case of amniotic band treated in the first hours after birth.

Dr. Grazia Salimbeni for the collaboration on the surgical treatment and on the follow-up of the patience described in Fig. 32.3.

Terri Beckwith, MPH, CCRP, Clinical Research Manager-Hand and Hip Divisions and Scottish Rite Hospital for Children for revising the manuscript.

References

1. Matsen FA, Veith RG. Compartmental syndromes in children. J Pediatr Orthop. 1981;1:33–41.
2. Lightwood R. Radial nerve palsy associated with localized subcutaneous fat necrosis in the newborn. Arch Dis Child. 1951;26(129):436–7.
3. Hayman M, Roland EH, Hill A. Newborn radial nerve palsy: Report of four cases and review of published reports. Pediatr Neurol. 1999;21(3):648–51.
4. Romana MC, Barthelemy R, Goubier JN. Ischemia neonatale degli arti superiori. In: Landi A, Bernasconi S, editors. L'arto superiore nell'ambito della patologia perinatale. Fidenza: Mattioli; 2003. p. 72–6.
5. O'Donnel CJ, Beck DH, Taylor BL, Smith GB. Upper limb compartment syndromes: a complication of malignant hyperthermia in a patient with ill-defined myopathy. Br J Anesth. 1995;74:343–4.
6. Mokoena T, Hadley GP. Surgical management of multiple limb gangrene following dehydration in children. S Afr Med J. 1991;80:185–8.
7. Hosseinzadeh P, Hayes CB. Compartment syndrome in children. Orthop Clin N Am. 2016;47(3):579–87.
8. Ragland R, Moukoko D, Ezaki M, Carter PR, Mills J. Forearm compartment syndrome in the newborn: report of 24 cases. J Hand Surg. 2005;30(5):997–1003.
9. Rombouts JJ, Debauche C, Verellen G, Lyon G. Paralysies congenitales par compression. Ann Chir Main. 1993;12(1):39–44.
10. Caouette-Laberge L, Bortoluzzi P, Egeszegi EP, Marton D. Neonatal Volkmann's ischemic contracture of the forearm: a report of five cases. Plast Reconstr Surg. 1992;90:621–8.
11. Chuang DCC, Carver N, Wei FC. A new strategy to prevent the sequelae of severe Volkmann's ischemia. Plast Reconstr Surg. 1996;98:1023–31.

12. Landi A, Schoenhuber R, Funicello R, Rasio G, Esposito M. Compartment syndrome of the scapula. Ann Hand Surg. 1992;11(5):383–8.
13. Zuker RM, Egerszegi EP, Manktelow RT, McLeod A, Candlish S. Volkmann's ischemic contracture in children: the results of free vascularized muscle transplantation. Microsurgery. 1991;12:341.
14. Zuker RM, Bezuhly M, Manktelow RT. Selective fascicular coaptation of free functioning gracilis transfer for restoration of independent thumb and finger flexion following Volkmann ischemic Contracture. J Reconstr Microsurg. 2011;27:439–44.
15. Esposito M, Busa R, Landi A. Sindromi compartimentali: acute, croniche, atipiche. In: Landi A, Catalano F, Luchetti R, editors. Trattato di chirurgia della mano. Roma: Verduci; 2007. p. 319–36.
16. Landi A, Caserta G, Saracino A, Esposito M. Atypical compartment syndromes of the upper limb. In: Copeland SA, Gschwend N, Landi A, Saffar P, editors. Joint stiffness of the upper limb. London: Martin Dunitz; 1997. p. 335–79.
17. Landi A, Romana C, Abate M. Sindromi compartimentali (S.C.), di Volkmann e patologia vascolare dell'arto superiore nel periodo perinatale. In: Landi A, Catalano F, Luchetti R, editors. Trattato di chirurgia della mano. Roma: Verduci; 2007. p. 937–48.
18. Bae DS, Kadiyala RK, Waters PM. Acute compartment syndrome in children: contemporary diagnosis, treatment, and outcome. J Ped Orthop. 2001;21:680–8.
19. Pereira N, Valenzuela D, Mangelsdorff G, Kufeke M, Roa R. Detection of perforators for free flap planning using smartphone thermal imaging: a concordance study with computed tomographic angiography in 120 perforators. Plast Reconstr Surg. 2018;141:787–92.
20. Hardwicke JT, Osmani O, Skillman JM. Detection of perforators using smartphone thermal imaging. Plast Reconstr Surg. 2016;137:39–41.
21. Stevanovic MV, Sharpe F. Compartment syndrome and Volkmann ischemic contracture. In: Wolfe S, Pederson W, Kozin SH, Cohen M, editors. Green's operative hand surgery. Elsevier: Amsterdam; 2017. p. 1763–87.
22. Volkmann R. Die ischaemic muskellahmungen und kontrakturen. Zbl Chir. 1881;8:801–3.
23. Mubarak SJ, Hargens AR. Compartment syndromes and Volkmann's contracture. London: WB Saunders; 1981.
24. Mubarak SJ, Carrol NC. Volkmann's contracture in children: aetiology and prevention. J Bone Joint Surg. 1979;61:285–93.
25. Comolli A. Uber ein deutliches Zeichen bei geswissen schulterbruchen. Zbl Chir. 1932;15:937–40.
26. Knappe DM, Truumes E. Posterior arm and deltoid compartment syndrome after vitamin B12 injection. Orthopedics. 2004;27(5):520–1.
27. Gulgonen A. Invited review article: surgery for Volkmann's ischaemic contracture. J Hand Surg. 2001;26B:283–96.
28. Grottkau BE, Epps HR, Di Scala C. Compartment syndrome in children and adolescents. J Pediatr Surg. 2004;40:678–82.
29. Romana MC, Bartelemy R, Goubier JN. Ischemia neonatale degli arti superiori. Soc Ital Chirur Mano. 2003;5:73–6.
30. Moazzam A, Riaz M, Brennen MD. Neonatal gangrene in an extremity of an infant of a diabetic mother. Int J Obs Gynaecol. 2003;110:74–6.
31. Gilbert A. Sindrome da costrizione da fibre amniotiche. In: Landi A, Bernasconi S, editors. L'arto superiore nell'ambito della patologia perinatale. Fidenza: Mattioli; 2003. p. 72–6.
32. Bozzini MA, Milani GP, Bianchetti MG, Fossali EF, Lava SAG. Idiopathic systemic capillary leak syndrome (Clarkson syndrome) in childhood: systemic literature review. Eur J Pediatr. 2018;177(8):1149–54.
33. Varon J, Chen K, Sternbach GL. Rupert Waterhouse and Carl Friderichsen: adrenal apoplexy. J Emerg Med. 1998;16:643–7.
34. Miedema A, Stubenitsky BM, Jansen NJ, van der Molen AB, van Vught AJ. Improving outcome in meningococcal disease: don't forget compartment syndrome! Pediatr Crit Care Med. 2008;9(3):e20–2.
35. Dakourè PWH, Beogo R, Barro D, Somè DA, Cessouma R, Kambou T. Ischemie in utero du membre superior et de l'hèmiface droits: à propos d'une observation. Chir Main. 2010;29:121–4.
36. Martin B, Treharne L. Neonatal compartment syndrome. Ann R Coll Surg Engl. 2016;98:e111–3.
37. Burke T, Kehl D. Intraosseus infusion in infants. J Bone Joint Surg. 1993;75A:428–9.
38. D'addato M, Testi M, Ferri M, Gentili A, Freyrie A, Baroncini S. Le lesioni vascolari perinatali dell'arto superiore. Soc Ital Chir Mano. 2003;5:98–104.
39. Habenicht R, Hülsemann W, Lohmeyer JA, Mann M. Ten-year experience with one-step correction of constriction rings by complete circular resection and linear circumferential skin closure. J Plast Reconstr Aesthet Surg. 2013;66(8):1117–22.
40. Engel J, Heim M, Tsur H. Late complications of neonatal Volkmann's ischemia. Hand. 1982;14:162–3.
41. Carr MM, et al. Extremity gangrene in utero. J Hand Surg. 1996;21(5):652–5.
42. Isshiki H, et al. Ischemic contracture in an infant's forearm-a case report. J Hand Surg. 2004;29(5):510–3.
43. Cham PMH, et al. Congenital Volkmann ischaemic contracture: a case report and review. Br J Dermatol. 2004;150:357–63.
44. Taylor GI, Palmer JH. The vascular territories (angiosomes) of the body: experimental study and clinical applications. Br J Plast Surg. 1995;34:81–3.
45. Rowland AR. The treatment of compartment syndrome. In: Green DP, Hotchkiss RN, Pederson WC, editors. Green's operative hand surgery, vol. 1. Philadelphia: Churchill Livingstone; 1998. p. 689–710.
46. Esposito M, Caserta G, Saracino A, et al. La misurazione della pressione compartimentale nella sindrome

compartimentale acuta. In: Le sindromi compartimentali della gamba e del piede, vol. 5. Bologna: Aulo Gaggi; 1996. p. 55–62.
47. Guyton AC. A concept of interstitial negative pressure based on pressures in implanted perforated capsules. Circ Res. 1963;12:339–414.
48. Landi A, De Santis G, Torricelli P, Colombo A, Bedeschi P. CT in established Volkmann's contracture in forearm muscles. J Hand Surg. 1989;14B:49–52.
49. Tominaga A, Shimada K, Temporin K, Noguchi R. Post-exertional MRI is useful as a tool for diagnosis and treatment evaluation for chronic exertional compartment syndrome of forearms. J Hand Surg Asian Pac. 2019;24(3):311–6.
50. Ko WS, Chiu T. Detection of perforators using smartphone thermal imaging. Plast Reconstr Surg. 2016;138(2):380.
51. Tattersal GJ. Infrared thermography: a non-invasive window into thermal physiology. Comp Biochem Physiol. 2016;2016:1–21.
52. Innocenti M, Ceruso M, Angeloni R, Lauri G, Nigi M, Beltrami G, Bufalini C. Reinnervated free gracilis muscle transplantation in the treatment of Volkmann's syndrome of the forearm. Chir Organi Mov. 1996;81:287–93.
53. Strange FGSC. An operation for nerve pedicle grafting. Br J Surg. 1947;34(136):423–5.
54. Greenberg BM, Cuadros CL, Panda M, May JW. St. Claire strange procedure indications, technique, and long-term evaluation. J Hand Surg. 1988;13(6):928–35.
55. Friedman J, et al. Treatment of acute neonatal vascular injuries. The utility of multiple interventions. J Pediatr Surg. 1999;34(6):940–5.
56. Nazer H, Abu Rajab A, Qaryouti S, Tarawneh M, Hamzeh Y, Arda H, et al. Neonatal limb gangrene and renal vein thrombosis. Eur J Pediatr. 1987;146:429–31.
57. Oppenheimer EH, Esterly JR. Thrombosis in the newborn: comparison between infants of diabetic and nondiabetic mothers. J Pediatr. 1965;67(4):549–56.
58. Vallerame E, et al. Peripheral gangrene in a newborn infant associated with renal and adrenal vein thrombosis. J Pediatr. 1972;80:101–3.
59. Marcelletti CF, et al. La patologia cardiovascolare. Soc Ital Chir Mano. 2003;5:45–50.
60. Duteille F, Costargent A, Perrot P, Pannier M. False aneurism of a brachial artery in a very premature newborn. J Reconstr Microsurg. 2008;24:147–50.
61. Dhar A, Bagga D, Taneja SB. Extremity gangrene following intramuscular injection. Indian Pediatr. 1988;25(12):1209–11.
62. Choi PD, Melikian R, Skaggs DL. Risk factors for vascular repair and compartment syndrome in the pulseless supracondylar humerus fracture in children. J Pediatr Orthop. 2010;30(1):50–6.
63. Tsur H, Yaffe B, Engel Y. Impending Volkmann's contracture in a newborn. Ann Plast Surg. 1980;5:317–20.
64. Eichler GR, Lipscomb PR. The changing treatment of Volkmann's ischemic contractures from 1955 to 1965 at the Mayo Clinic. Clin Orthop Relat Res. 1967;50:215–23.
65. Feldman GV. Radial nerve palsy in the newborn. Arch Dis Child. 1957;32(165):469–71.
66. Zeb A, Darmstadt GL. Sclerema neonatorum: a review of nomenclature, clinical presentation, histological features, differential diagnoses and management. J Perinatol. 2008;28(7):453–60.
67. Xiong G, Sun Y, Wang S. Congenital flexion deformity of the long, ring, and little fingers with an aberrant origin of the flexor digitorum profundus: case report. J Hand Surg Am. 2008;33(8):1358–61.
68. Quintero RA, Morales WJ, Phillips J, et al. In utero lysis of amniotic bands. Ultrasound Obstet. 1997;10:316–20.
69. Dogru S, Acar A. Fetoscopic surgery for amniotic band syndrome: case series. Congenit Anom. 2023;63(1):4–8.
70. Chaudhry S. Upper extremity care for children: unique medical and psychosocial aspects. J Hand Surg Am. 2019;44(7):606–9.

Postoperative Dressings and Care

33

Ellen Kroin and Terry R. Light

Abstract

The postoperative management following pediatric hand surgery depends upon a secure dressing that provides immobilization, protection, compression, and absorption of wound fluids. The dressing should be simple to remove and should minimize the child's pain and anxiety in the removal process. We present the author's approach to applying and managing pediatric postoperative dressings. Several additional strategies which may also consistently achieve these goal are presented.

Keywords

Pediatric dressing · Postoperative care

33.1 Introduction

David Green's *Basic Principles* introductory chapter in his eponymous text states: "In no other field of surgery does the post-operative management of the patient play so critical role as it does in hand surgery" [1]. This is particularly true in the young child. The ideal pediatric dressing should be flexible enough to protect and immobilize the small squirming hand. By compressing the hand, edema is reduced and hemostasis is facilitated. The dressing should absorb any bleeding and should facilitate adsorption of medications applied to the wound. The appearance should also be attractive to families.

The pediatric hand dressing is an essential element of postoperative care. The dressing must protect soft tissue reconstruction, tendon transfers, and pin fixation, and it must limit motion of skin grafts. In other children, tendon repairs or tendon transfers are protected by the immobilization with the postoperative dressing. It is imperative that the pediatric hand dressing be reliably maintained during the postoperative period [2]. As Kleinman and Bowers observed, "Young children have an enormous predisposition to either destroy or wiggle out of their immobilization. In the absence of internal fixation, standard casting techniques used in adults are often ineffective in children" [3]. Because the dressing is by design confining, children may persist in their attempts to wiggle out of splints, casts, or other forms of immobilization. The goal is to create a dressing that stays in place, in spite of the best efforts of our young patients.

Several elements contribute to the effectiveness of the hand dressing. The dressing must protect the surgical wound during initial healing. To provide stable immobilization, the dressing may incorporate a plaster splint or be surrounded by a cast. The portion of the dressing that is in direct

E. Kroin (✉)
Northwestern Medical Group, Lake Forest, IL, USA

T. R. Light
Department Orthopaedic Surgery, Loyola Stritch School of Medicine, Maywood, IL, USA
e-mail: tlight@lumc.edu

G. Pajardi (ed.), *Pediatric Hand Surgery*, https://doi.org/10.1007/978-3-031-30984-7_33

contact with the wound will act to absorb postoperative fluid drainage. When medication such as bacitracin or silvadene is applied directly to the wound, the dressing facilitates their adsorption. A conforming compressive dressing provides uniform pressure on the hand to minimize capillary oozing and thus provide hemostasis.

The appearance of the dressing is important, since it is the first visible evidence of the surgery seen by the patient and family. It should appear neat, without blood or other fluid staining.

Repeated uncomfortable dressing changes are unnecessary if the initial dressing is carefully and thoughtfully applied to the child's hand. We find it unnecessary to change the pediatric dressing during the first week following surgery and yet recognize that parents are anxious to see the operated part as soon as possible. Repeated dressing changes are uncomfortable and may be distressing for the child, as well as for the parents and surgeon. Developing a comfortable dressing routine can minimize the stress experienced by the child. In addition, developing rapport with the child while removing the dressing can help ease the distress to the child. It is essential that the parents understand the importance of the dressing and its role in postoperative care [4]. If the dressing is applied and maintained properly, it can be left in place for several weeks.

33.2 Authors' Preferred Method

Our technique of applying the postoperative dressing has proven adaptable and durable in young children. We build the dressing to include three independent components, each layer will separately resist the young child's efforts to remove the dressing. The dressing is best placed while the child is asleep. Communication with the anesthesiologist is essential to keep the child soundly asleep while the final elements of the dressing are being secured behind the child's neck. If the child starts to awaken while one is applying the dressing, it is best to ask that the child be reanesthetized so that a secure dressing may be placed. A hastily applied dressing may be easily dislodged. The time spent properly placing the dressing on a fully anesthetized child is a worthwhile investment of time to maximize the result of the just completed surgical procedure. The inner dressing is held in place by a Kling wrap secured about the ipsilateral wrist; the second element is a plaster splint crossing the flexed ipsilateral elbow, while the outer layer is a Velpeau sleeve secured to the contralateral shoulder and axilla.

The first or inner dressing includes Xeroform and 4 × 4 sterile mesh gauze in sufficient quantity to create even compression as a Kling bandage is wrapped around the hand. The Kling is wrapped circumferentially around the gauze pads and around the wrist in order to secure the dressing to the hand (Fig. 33.1). After syndactyly release, we place saline-soaked cotton balls over the skin

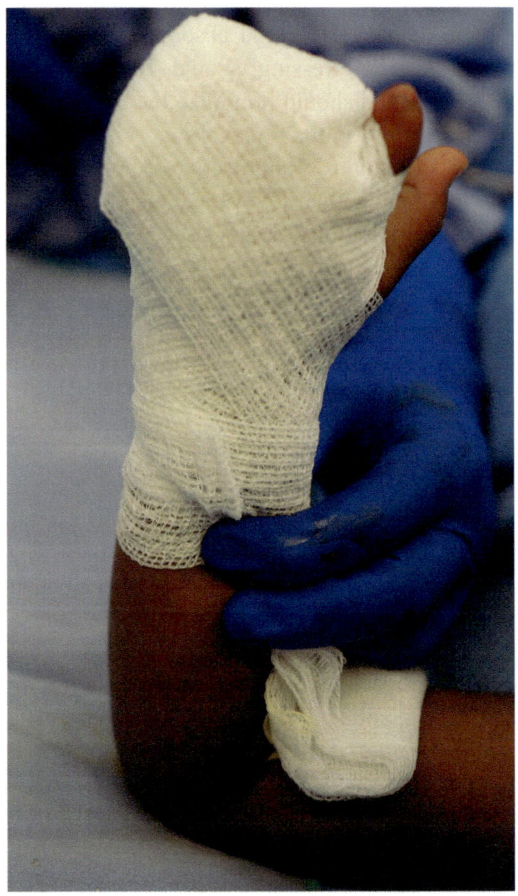

Fig. 33.1 The hand is wrapped circumferentially with Kling around the gauze pads and the wrist securing the dressing to the hand

grafts to compress the grafts and to hold the fingers apart. Oozing of fluids from the incisions and grafted sites will cause the dressing to adhere to the wound. Two weeks after syndactyly surgery, the fingers are soaked in saline freeing the cotton balls from the healing fingers. Any residual open area is covered with a simple Band-Aid.

The second component, a sugar-tong plaster splint, is extended to cover the operative site and any protruding pins. The splint extends above the elbow and positions the elbow in flexion (Fig. 33.2). We apply the splint while the child is under anesthesia to assure proper elbow positioning. The plaster splint wraps around the elbow in a sugar-tong fashion while also covering the wrist and hand. It is important to ensure that the plaster splint sits anterior to the axis of the elbow. The extremity is maintained with the wrist in neutral position, the forearm in mid-rotation, and the elbow at 100° of flexion. A bias-cut stockinette is wrapped circumferentially around the plaster and secured with tape. Additional tape reinforces the flexed position of the elbow (Fig. 33.3).

The third component of the pediatric postoperative dressing is the Velpeau stockinette sling depicted in Fig. 33.4a–c. This sleeve secures the hand, forearm, and arm close to the body with the hand elevated. The sleeve is created from a length of 3- or 4-inch-wide stockinette cut to approximately one and a half times the height of the child. The sling has three components: the sleeve, the back, and the ties (Fig. 33.4a). The hand dressing is slipped into the cut stockinette sleeve. The stockinette is then passed behind the back and neck from the ipsilateral axilla to the contralateral axilla (Fig. 33.4b). One of two ties is passed up through the contralateral axilla while the other tie is passed over the shoulder. The two ties are secured to one another with a knot tied over the contralateral shoulder (Fig. 33.4c). The dressing is then secured through to the contralateral shoulder. A hole in the stockinette adjacent to the hand allows the two ties to be tied together with a bow (Figs. 33.4d and 33.5). The knot should not be disturbed. The family is instructed that they may temporarily untie the bow to change the child's clothes or to provide a sponge bath.

The Velpeau stockinette and plaster splint are usually removed one or two weeks postoperatively. For the dressing changes, young children

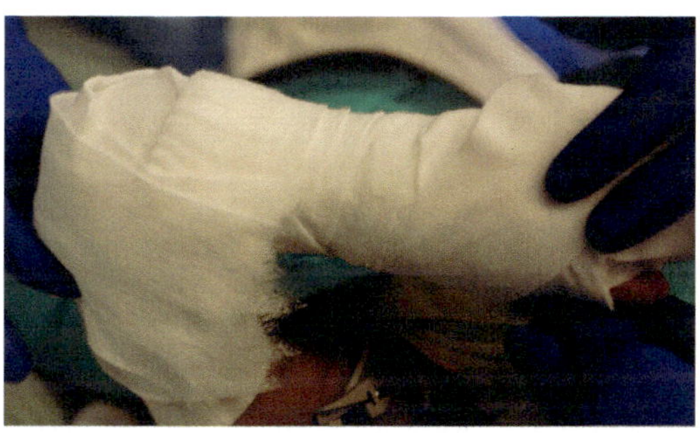

Fig. 33.2 Cast padding is applied extending the dressing above the elbow and positioning the elbow in greater than 90° of flexion prior to applying the plaster sugar-tong splint

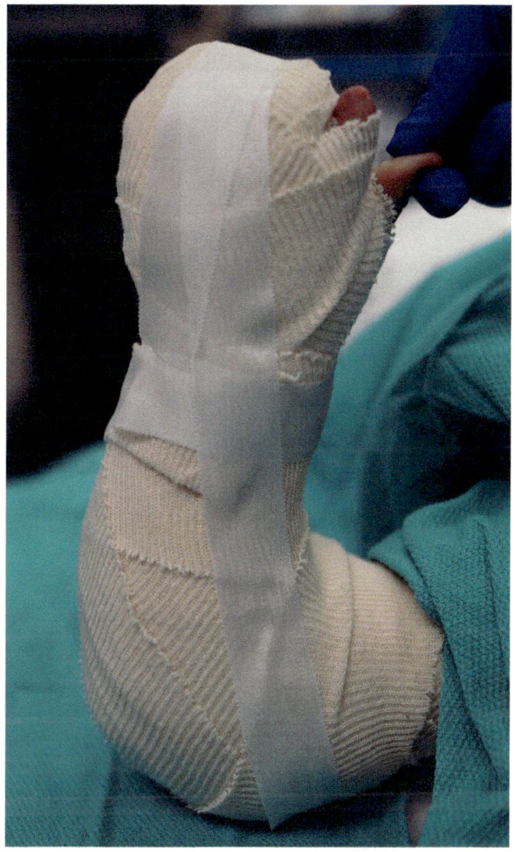

Fig. 33.3 A bias-cut stockinette is wrapped circumferentially around the plaster component. This is secured down with cloth tape crossing the flexed elbow

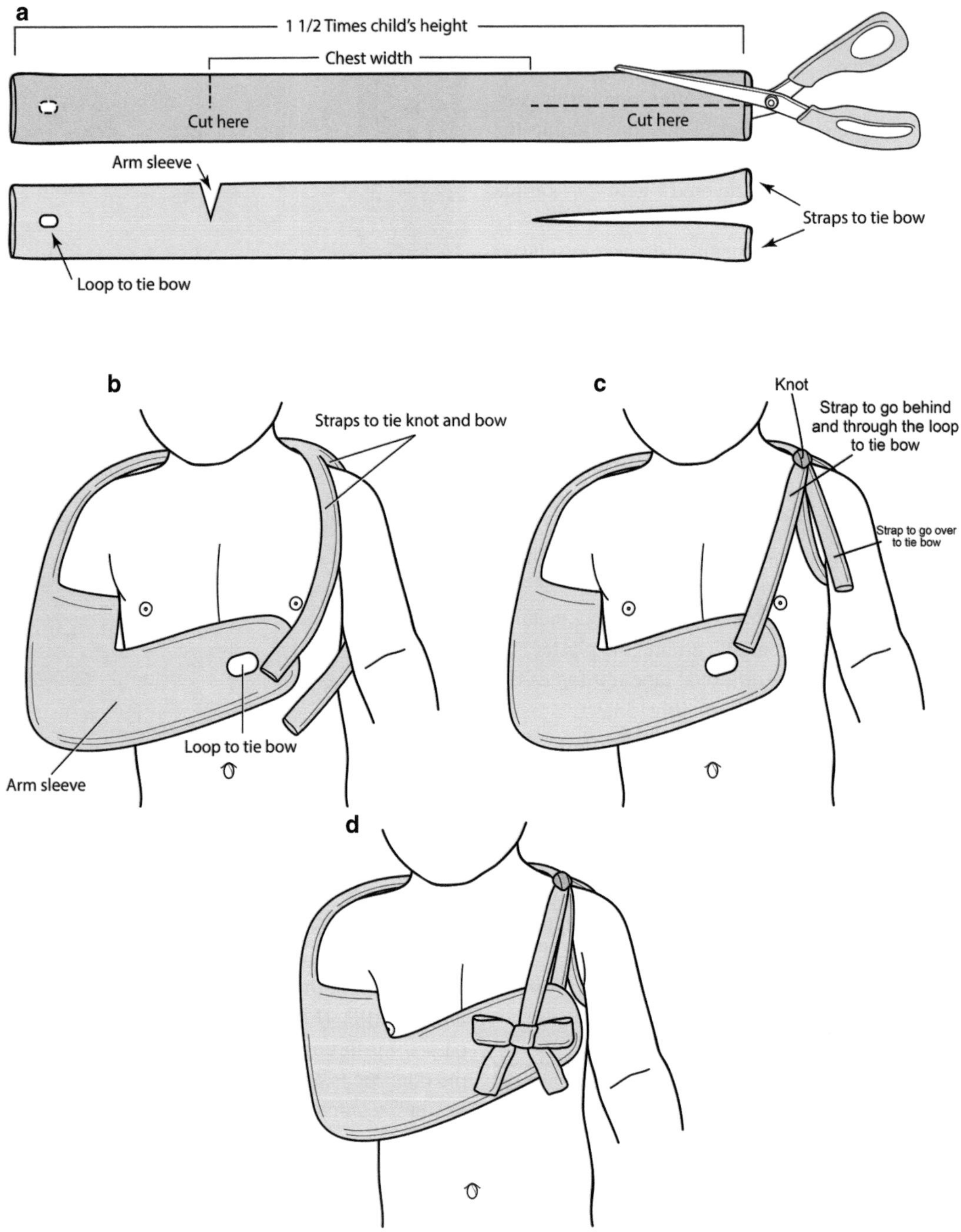

Fig. 33.4 (**a**) A 3- or 4-inch-wide stockinette is cut to approximately to one and a half times the height of the child. The three components of the sling are the arm sleeve, the back portion, which is the width of the chest wall, and the two straps used to tie the knot and bow. (**b**) The dressed hand is slipped into the cut stockinette arm sleeve. The stockinette back portion is passed behind the back and neck from the ipsilateral axilla to the contralateral axilla. (**c**) One of two ties is passed up and around the contralateral axilla while the other tie is passed over the shoulder. The two ties are secured to one another with a knot tied over the top of the contralateral shoulder. This creates straps of unequal length. (**d**) The operative hand is secured to the contralateral shoulder by tying a bow through the hole in the stockinette adjacent to the hand. The longer strap is passed from behind to the front of the hole where it is then tied to the shorter strap with a bow

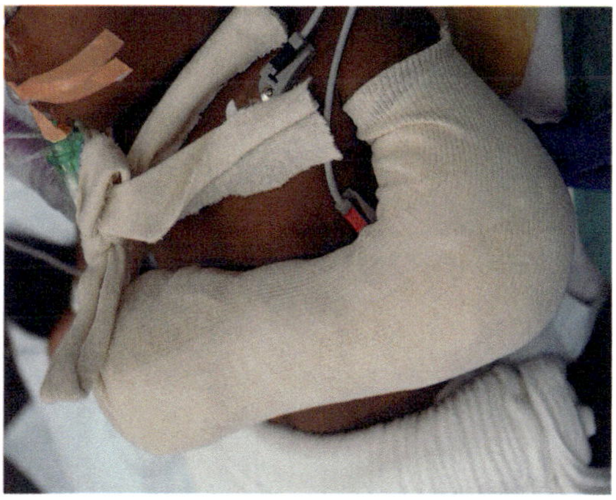

Fig. 33.5 The Velpeau stockinette sling is slipped on the arm and anchored to the opposite shoulder with a knot and a bow

sit in their seated parents' lap. The person removing the dressing is also seated to avoid hovering over the apprehensive child. Dressing change is facilitated by sequentially removing each of the three layers. The stockinette is simply divided at both axilla and slid off. The sugar-tong plaster splint is then removed. The inner dressing may be partially removed and a new Kling can be wrapped about the hand and wrist.

Our hand therapist then fabricates a protective thermoplastic splint. We retain the inner dressings compressing the skin grafts for two weeks after syndactyly release. In thumb duplication cases, if K-wires are used, the pin is retained in place for 5–6 weeks and protected and immobilized during that time. We have the luxury of having a hand therapist available at each of our outpatient sessions who will make a thermoplastic u-shaped splint to protect the underlying dressings and/or pins. The advantages of the thermoplastic splint over plaster include direct access to the wound, easy reapplication, simple modification, minimal bulk, and greater durability [5]. Removal and reapplication are made easier with the use of Velcro straps. This strategy also avoids the noise and terror involved with fiberglass cast removal.

We employ a simple soft dressing following trigger thumb release, which is removed in a week. If the child removes it earlier, we advise the family to cover it with a Band-Aid.

The dressing removal is performed in a quiet room in the office. The child is held in the parent's arms. No cast saw is necessary. The three segments of the dressing are removed separately.

33.3 Alternative Approaches

There are many effective postoperative dressing strategies. Several American pediatric hand surgeons were queried about the specifics of their dressing protocols for four common procedures. Table 33.1 lists hand surgeons' protocols that are based on procedure type.

The main difference between the protocols is the use of a cast or plaster splint for several weeks for immobilization and protection. Many surgeons use a circumferential cast made of fiberglass material applied in the operating room. Some immobilize the entire limb in a long arm cast for five or six weeks. All surgeons queried use a thermoplastic splint constructed by a hand therapist for protection after cast removal.

Dr. Douglas Hutchinson describes his technique with the use of a tape cast (Fig. 33.6a–c). This consists of plaster, layered tape, and Coban wrapped over the tape. The plaster is only used on the hand over the surgical areas. This leaves the wrist and elbow flexible while the digits are protected. It allows improved ease of use of the arm while caring for the child. The Coban is used as a protective layer and can be replaced by the family if it gets soiled. The child is also usually hesitant to pull tape off their own skin; thus the tape cast is able to stay in place for a full 4–5 weeks. The Coban is then removed and the family is asked to soak the tape cast in warm water before the child comes into clinic. This loosens the tape and minimizes the discomfort of pulling it off. Overall, this eliminates multiple dressing changes and does not require a loud saw and child's fear when removing [6].

Table 33.1 Pediatric hand surgeons' postoperative dressing and care protocols

		Thumb duplication—18 months	Pollicization—18 months	Syndactyly release—18 months	Trigger Thumb—36 months
Dr. Charles Goldfarb—Washington University St. Louis	Materials	• Soft dressing mitten • Long arm fiberglass cast	• Soft dressing mitten • Long arm fiberglass cast	• Soft dressing mitten • Long arm fiberglass cast	• Soft dressing • Coban wrap
	Timing of postoperative dressing change	• Remove long arm cast at five weeks • Thermoplastic splint	• Remove long arm cast at three weeks • Thermoplastic splint	• Remove long arm cast at three weeks • Thermoplastic splint	• Family removes on day 7 at home • Band-Aid for five days
Dr. Ann Van Heest—University of Minnesota	Materials	• Soft dressing • Long arm cast if ligament reconstructed	• Soft dressing • Long arm cast	• Wet cotton balls in web space • Soft dressing • Long arm cast	• Soft dressing • Coban
	Timing of postoperative dressing change	• Remove long arm cast at one month	• Remove long arm cast at one month • Thermoplastic splint	• Remove long arm cast at one month	• Removed at day 7 at home • Band-Aid until sutures dissolve
Dr. Douglas Hutchinson—University of Utah	Materials	• Soft dressing • Small conform • Above-elbow tape cast if ligament reconstruction required	• Soft dressing • Small conform • Above-elbow tape cast	• Cotton balls soaked in mineral oil • Loose gauze • Above-elbow tape cast	• Soft dressing • Coban
	Timing of postoperative dressing change	• Remove dressing at 4–5 weeks by soaking in bathtub before clinic • Thermoplastic splint for two months if ligament reconstruction	• Removed at 4–5 weeks by soaking in bathtub before clinic visit • Thermoplastic splint for three months	• Removed at 4–5 weeks by soaking in bathtub before clinic	• Removed 5–7 days postop • Band-Aid
Dr. Joseph Upton—Beth Israel Deaconess Medical Center	Materials		• Wet gauze • Soft dressing • Bivalved long arm cast (plaster or fiberglass)	• Wet gauze • Soft dressing • Bivalved long arm cast (plaster or fiberglass optional)	
	Timing of postoperative dressing change		• Cast removed at 2.5–3 weeks • Thermoplastic splint	• Cast removed at 2.5–3 weeks • Thermoplastic splint	

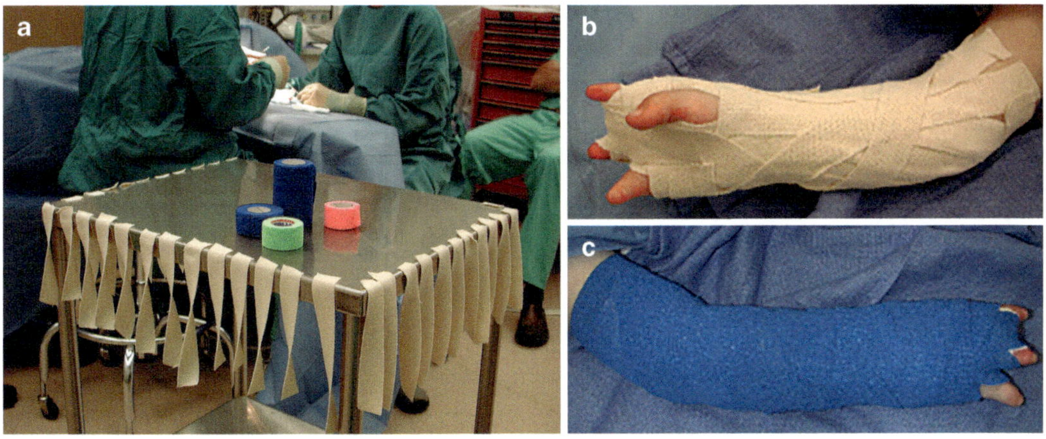

Fig. 33.6 (a–c) Dr. Hutchinson's tape cast technique consists of plaster covering the surgical site, layered tape, and Coban wrapped over the tape. The colored Coban is used as a protective layer and can be replaced by the family if it gets soiled

33.4 Summary

The postoperative management following pediatric hand surgery depends upon a secure dressing that provides immobilization, protection, compression, and absorption of wound fluids. The dressing should be simple to remove and should minimize trauma to the child in the removal process. Several different strategies may consistently achieve this goal.

References

1. Green DP. General principles. In: Green DP, editor. Operative hand surgery. 3rd ed. New York: Churchill Livingstone; 1993. p. 15–9.
2. Cooney WP III, Dobyns JH. Pediatric hand dressing: technical report. J Hand Surg. 2005;13:1009–13.
3. Kleinman WB, Bowers WH. Fractures, ligamentous injuries to the hand. In: Bora FW, editor. The pediatric upper extremity: diagnosis and management. Philadelphia: WB Saunders; 1986. p. 150–76.
4. Dobyns JH, Wood VE, Bayne LG. Congenital hand deformities. In: Green DP, editor. Operative hand surgery. 3rd ed. New York: Churchill Livingstone; 1993. p. 251–548.
5. Osterhout BM. Postoperative splinting of the pediatric upper extremity. Hand Clin. 1990;6(4):693–5.
6. Hutchinson DT, Frenzen SW. Digital syndactyly release. In: Jupiter J, editor. Techniques in hand and upper extremity surgery. Philadelphia: Lippincott Williams & Wilkins; 2010. p. 33–7.

34 Rehabilitation in Congenital Hand and Forearm Defects: Rehabilitation of the Child's Hand—General Aspects

Elena M. Mancon, Luigi Bartolomeo, Elisa Ceccarelli, Sara Cesaroni, Claudia Corsi, Greta Culicchia, Ambra Gelatti, Roberta Genova, Antonella Guerriero, Sara Longhi, Claudia Maiolino, Carmen Meloni, Silvia Minoia, Marta Nobilia, Rossella Pagliaro, Stefania Paparo, Valeria L. Petrillo, Michela Ramella, Federica Suriano, Patrizia Rossi, Francesca Tolosa, and Simona Vecchi

Abstract

Patients affected by radial club hand present different aspects all involving the general use of the entire upper limb: shorter forearm, radial deviation, low to severe dysfunction of the thumb or in the most severe stages, its absence and reduced AROM (active range of motion) of long fingers.

The major problem during the growth of those patients is the frequent recurrence of relapses that may occur despite the kind of surgery performed: this can be due to different causes linked both to intrinsic factors such as the impossibility of releasing radial soft tissues completely or extrinsic elements such as the poor use of a proper splint and the frequent stimulus to the radial deviation due to functional gestures like bringing the hand to the mouth. Unfortunately, the clinical situation can be considered stabilized only with the end of physiological bone growth.

The rehabilitation programme begins taking charge of the patient after the first visit with the surgeon. It is divided in two different approaches:

- Conservative treatment: it starts immediately after the visit and lasts in the preoperative time.
- Post-surgery treatment: it starts after the surgery.

In both, the treatment is endorsed by the surgical team, the therapist and the patient's family, who becomes both a receiver and an active participant in the rehabilitation process.

E. M. Mancon · L. Bartolomeo · E. Ceccarelli
S. Cesaroni · C. Corsi · G. Culicchia · A. Gelatti
R. Genova · A. Guerriero · S. Longhi · C. Maiolino
C. Meloni · S. Minoia (✉) · M. Nobilia · R. Pagliaro
S. Paparo · V. L. Petrillo · M. Ramella · F. Suriano
P. Rossi · F. Tolosa · S. Vecchi
Department of Hand Surgery and Rehabilitation, San Giuseppe Hospital IRCCS MultiMedica, Milan University, Milan, Italy

Milan, Italy
e-mail: elenamarta.mancon@multimedica.it

G. Pajardi (ed.), *Pediatric Hand Surgery*, https://doi.org/10.1007/978-3-031-30984-7_34

Keywords

Radial club hand · Hand malformations Children's hands · Rehabilitation in paediatric hand malformations · Thumb dysfunction Trigger finger · Thumb · Rehabilitation Conservative · Splint · Congenital malformation · Syndactyly · Finger · Hand malformation · Congenital hand rehabilitation Polydactyly · Radial polydactyly · Ulnar polydactyly · Central polydactyly · Amniotic band syndrome · Hand · Blood circulation Constriction · Thumb hypoplasia Opponensplasty · Pollicization · Pinch · Club hand · Splinting · Manipulation · Children Psychomotor · Therapy · Body · Mind Congenital hand malformation

Children are our present and future, so they need the most specialized and prepared equipe as little patients.

When they get to the hospital to be visited, they normally do not understand why their parents took them to that strange and new place, especially if they are very young as it normally is.

That is why the equipe as big team needs to make children feel at home, through different tools.

34.1 Setting

In the pediatric field more than every other medical fields, the setting is very important to catch the attention of the little patient and the parents too. They need to have around them a familiar atmosphere when possible with bright colors, and different rooms for the rehabilitation of different ages of children.

Normally in pediatric rehabilitation departments, therapists need more than one single room to work in.

They will need a room with a kettle/heater and a table to make splints. To make splints you need different types of thermoplastic materials, velcros, scissors, a riveter, a stripper (?), padding, etc.

Then therapists will need a sanitary cot for children younger than 3 months of age as putting them on the ground and also on soft carpets can be uncomfortable for parents and the therapists themselves.

Another room can be structured with soft carpets on the ground and pillows; this room can be suitable for children from 4/5 months until about 18/24 months. In this way children can be protected from falls and can be comfortable in sitting, lying, or side position.

At last but not least, it is important to have a small table with chairs for 20/36 months old children.

Children normally are a little worried at first during physiotherapy but they love to play and during rehabilitation there is a lot of fun too. Talking about setting, we have to underline the importance of closets. Children normally like to change toys and games more often than they should so it is appropriate to have closets to store toys; in this way the child can choose with the therapist one game at the time.

Children older than 4 years of age need a proper table and proper chairs too.

We have to admit that these are the most appropriate spaces that we can suggest, but it is not always possible to have all these rooms, if it is not the therapists have to do their very best with the space that they have, putting the safety of the child at the first place (Images 34.1–34.4).

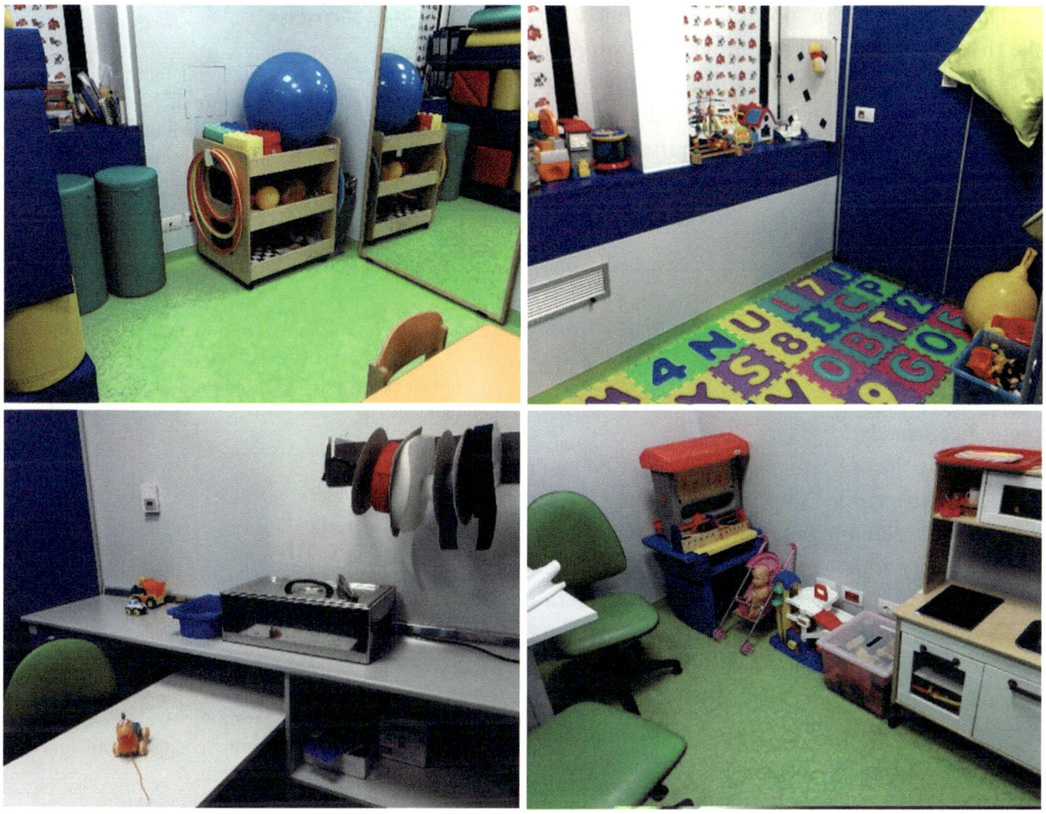

Images 34.1–34.4 The setting

34.2 Rehabilitative Program

When a child and his family come to our attention it is for sure after a surgical visit. The surgeon may suggest rehabilitation before or after a surgical operation.

Either if is before surgery or after it is very important to schedule with the family and in agreement with the doctor the length and the frequency of the rehabilitation that should change from a little patient to the other to follow their necessities.

In a conservative treatment normally, especially if the child is very young we do rehabilitation sessions ones a week, or maximum twice a week at the beginning. This allows the parents to understand what they are supposed to do with their children as home exercise, and the therapist can control the growth and the improvements of the little patient. Splint checks are required during rehabilitation too, when the child grows up the splint needs to be replaced.

After surgery the patient can keep the immobilization or the dressing for 3/4 weeks and then they normally suggest daily physiotherapy, and in some cases twice a day. There are some cases in which rehabilitation is immediate.

Daily physiotherapy is useful at the beginning because the child has to get used to the "new situation" of the hand; proper stimulation and manipulation are essential. The parents are supposed to exercise very often at home too, so they participate in the session to learn how to help their children. After a few weeks the sessions can be normally reduced, three times a week and then two times, then one and so on.

The rehabilitation program is defined by the therapist in collaboration with the surgeon and parents and has to be followed precisely by all the members of the equipe; obviously it can be changed later on if required by the situation.

34.3 Assessment

In pediatric rehabilitation, assessment of the child is very important to set up the rehabilitation program correctly.

Basically the assessment should be based on a double approach. First the child as a young infant needs to be valued in his psychomotor complexity. It is very important for children to respect psychomotor stages, as any other child; the therapist's task is to check them during their growth. Second the therapist should evaluate the use of the upper limbs, their functionality, and the different grips and pinches the child is capable of doing. Furthermore, it is important to analyze if the limb difference affects the activity of daily living or the quality of life of the child and family.

To understand if the child is respecting the physiological psychomotor steps, it is necessary that all the health workers who deal with little patients know them well. That is why we decided to produce some tables that could summarize the most important ones, divided in ages.

34.3.1 0–3 Months

Motor skills	Median line
	Antigrait control of the head
	Upper limb +
	Lower limb –
Manual skills	Eye-hand-mouth
	Tactile exploration
Interpersonal skills	Attachment to parents
	Consolability
Communication and language	Cry
	Smile/pout
Independence	X

34.3.2 3–6 Months

Motor skills	Antigrait control of the head-trunk
	Prone position with upper limb support
	Beginning of rolling
Manual skills	Eye-object-hand-mouth
	Catch
Interpersonal skills	Beginning of separation from adults
	Follows auditory and visual stimuli
Communication and language	Babbling
Independence	X

34.3.3 6–9 Months

Motor skills	Independent sitting position (parachute)
	Pivoting
	Lie down position to sitting position
	Sitting position to all-fours position
	Creep and crawl
Manual skills	Inferior pinch (abduction of the thumb)
	Extended wrist in the grips
	Voluntary release
Interpersonal skills	Permanence of the object
	Search of people and objects
Communication and language	Comprehension of verbal language +
Independence	Play
	Feeding

34.3.4 9–12/18 Months

Motor skills	Standing with support
	Side steps
	Be able to fall
	Standing alone
	Autonomous walking
Manual skills	Superior pinch
	Point
	Small objects
Interpersonal skills	Permanence of the adult
	Problem-solving
	Imitation

Communication and language	Words Simple verbal commands
Independence	Feeding Sleep

34.3.5 18–24 Months

Motor skills	Run Jump Overcomes obstacles
Manual skills	Fine dexterity Bimanuality
Interpersonal skills	Symbolic games Sense of themselves Emotional variability
Communication and language	Proper vocabulary
Independence	Meals Beginning of sphincteric control

34.3.6 24–36 Months

Motor skills	Stairs Ride
Manual skills	Fine dexterity + dominant side, hand
Interpersonal skills	Rules Socialization
Communication and language	Vocabulary + sentences
Independence	Eat with cutlery Sphincteric control Personal care

These tables can be useful in daily practice to understand quickly if a child is respecting his psychomotor growth or not, and this can also help the therapist to focus the rehabilitation program on that single patient.

A comprehensive evaluation may include range of motion measurements, sensory testing, strength and functional testing, self-care and playing skills, and developmental assessments.

There are also validated scales to use, if necessary (about the children development), like the "Griffiths mental development scale" or the "Bayley scales of infant and toddler development," in its third edition. The positive aspects of using a validated scale is that the result can even be diagnostic and used also in collaboration with a neuropsychiatrist, particularly of syndromic patients. On the negative side we have that it is necessary to attend a long and expansive course to be able to administer them, and specific tools are needed too.

It is possible, however, to find some easier charts about children developmental screening such as "Ages and Stages Questionnaires (ASQ-3)," the "Ireton's chart," "Denver developmental screening test (DDST)," "Battelle developmental inventory (BDI-2)," and "Pediatric evaluation of disability inventory (PEDI)."

It is globally recognized that it is important to focus on the child's abilities and not on its disabilities, as reported in the International Classification of Functioning Disability and Health (ICF-CY) and psychomotor development milestones as described also by the World Health Organization (WHO Motor Milestones).

New studies have been conducted about a global assessment that can include grips, complex use of the upper limb, and quality of life adaptable also to child with limb differences like our little patients. However this international and multicentric studies are not currently completed and it is still not possible to use them in daily practice.

The Pediatric Outcome Data Collection Instrument (PODCI) is a commonly used assessment tool to evaluate the outcome and function in pediatric orthopedic population. There are also other key performance indicators for evaluating the health system in a global way, like the Patient Reported Outcomes Measures (PROMs). They can provide validated evidence of health from the point of view of the little patient. Some studies underlined that a child is able to self-report his well-being and function only after he is between 5 and 8 years old. Unfortunately it is really difficult to find a scale that can be perfect for our children. In fact hands can be very different one from the other and it is barely impossible to make comparisons. It is also very hard to have one single scale for children of different ages, because obviously each age has specific skills.

Most scales suitable for children and upper limbs are made for neurologic patients, and this is for sure a limit, like the "Abilhand Kids," "Bimanual Motor Function Classification (BFMF)," "Gross Motor Functional Classification System (GMFCS)," and "Mini-Manual Ability Classification System (Mini-MACS)."

However is still possible to measure the range of motion (with goniometers), and the strength of the pinch and grasp, also through new electronic devices (Exergames).

There are lots of scales that can assess the quality of life of young infants like the "PedsQL."

Without having the possibility to administer a single scale per patient, the therapist's observation, records, joints measurements, strength measurements, pictures, and videos are essential to understand and recognize our little patient's improvements.

All these different assessment tools remind us of the importance of the difference between what children are able to do (function) and how they feel about it (well-being).

34.4 Splinting

Splinting is for sure one of the most important tools that we, as hand therapist, have for children with hand malformations.

Indication of splinting can be given from the surgeon after an operation in order to protect the limb, can be chosen to protect the hand after a period of immobilization, or can be chosen by the therapist to obtain a determined position.

There are endless possibilities of splints for children: different materials, thickness, elasticity, sizes, but the major subdivision is between fixed splint and removable ones. With "fixed splints" we mean splints that cannot be removed, they can be suggested after surgery or after fractures, normally in children splints need to be particularly resistant and are a little bit wider that in adults to allow children to play and go to school with the immobilization without risks. Removable splints can be worn or taken off, and this is allowed by Velcro. The posology of the splint is decided by the therapist and the surgeon.

There is no age limit for splinting; in our experience we did splints also on a 7-day-old child, and the younger is the child the most the splint need to be correctly padded. For extremely young children sometimes the Velcro is too stiff, and splints are fixed to the limb with soft bandages. Very stiff material is not needed for smaller hands, also if the position of the hand, fingers, or elbows has to be correct a semi-rigid material can be enough (Images 34.5–34.7).

For children that are more than 6/7 months of age some tougher material can be used.

Another very big subdivision between types of splints is between static, dynamic, or static progressive splints. A static splint keeps a position that the segment can reach, a dynamic splint

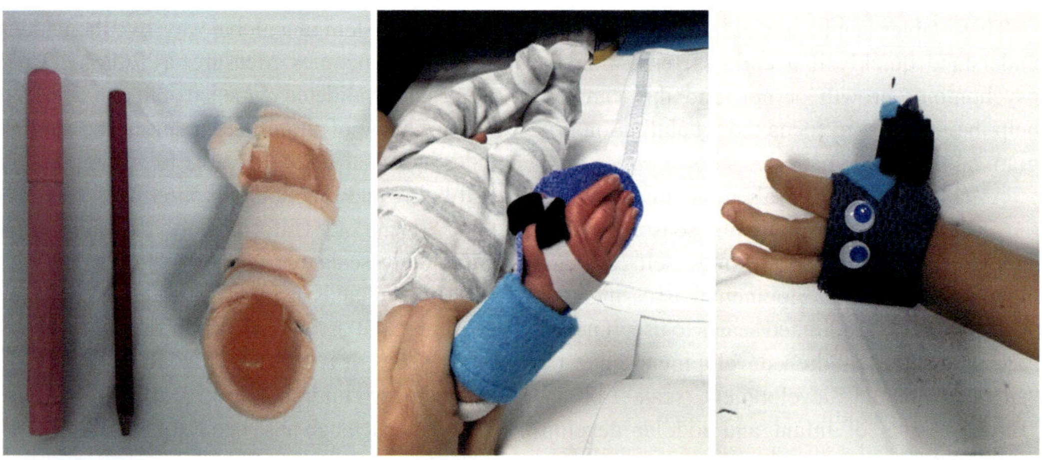

Images 34.5–34.7 Splints

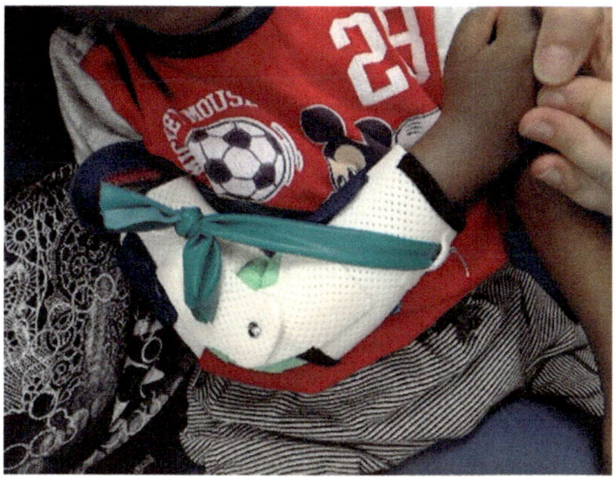

Image 34.8 Dynamic splint with elastic for elbow

has a dynamic traction to beat a stiffness (caused by joint stiffness or scar stiffness for example), and a static progressive splint has a static traction that can be regulated by the parent or the therapist. For dynamic splints the therapist needs also leather (more comfortable than Velcro on the skin), fishing wire, and different kind of elastics (Image 34.8).

It is very important to choose the correct type of material and splint for a single little patient: if a fixed splint is made with a soft material it cannot be protective enough, if a stiff thermoplastic material is chosen for a very young patient it can be dangerous for the skin, if a dynamic splint is not correctly padded it can be harmful for the child. So choosing the correct splint and correct material is very important, but respecting the anatomical point (punti di repere) is essential, for example a splint that blocks the wrist and one ray lets the long fingers free to move have to be under the line of the heads of the metacarpal heads.

Thermoplastic material is washable with cold water, and this is very important for children; an extra portion of padding is given to the parents so they can change it if necessary.

34.5 Scar Management

34.5.1 Introduction

Any surgery or skin lesion produces a scar. It may be normal, atrophic, hypertrophic, or keloid. The hypertrophic and keloid scars are

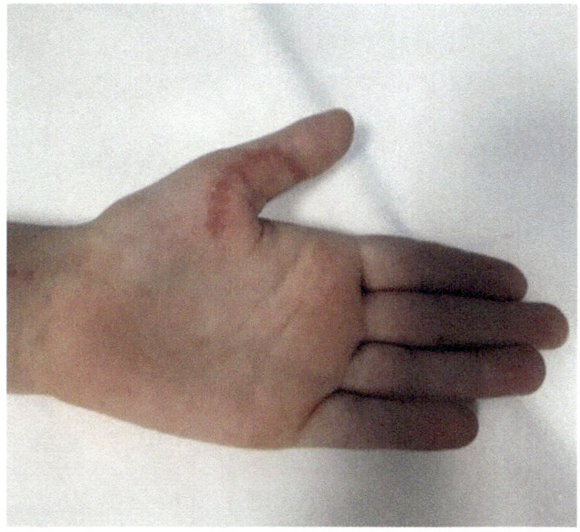

Image 34.9 Example of pediatric scar

formed as a result of the process of abnormal wound healing, causing aesthetic and functional deficits, discomfort, and disturbances in the normal growth of children. In hand rehabilitation departments, most of the treated scars are surgical, but often there are also traumatic scars due to cutting injuries, crushing, or burns. However, any wound can have complications due to intrinsic (patient) or extrinsic factors (type of intervention, technique, medications used, etc.) (Image 34.9).

34.5.2 Evaluation

An appropriate classification of scars is a significant element because the differences in their clinical types determine the type of therapeutic approach. The evaluation of a scar must examine three important aspects: physical characteristics, aesthetic aspect, and the patient's symptoms. For the physical characteristics, it is fundamental to analyze the thickness, the relief that is the height of the scar which is variable according to the scar maturation, the flexibility that represent the extensibility, elasticity, and stiffness of the scar. In fact, a scar lacking flexibility can contribute to the loss of movement and therefore represents an important evaluation index. For the aesthetic aspect, it is important to observe the color of the scar, which is due to both vascularization and pigmentation. The

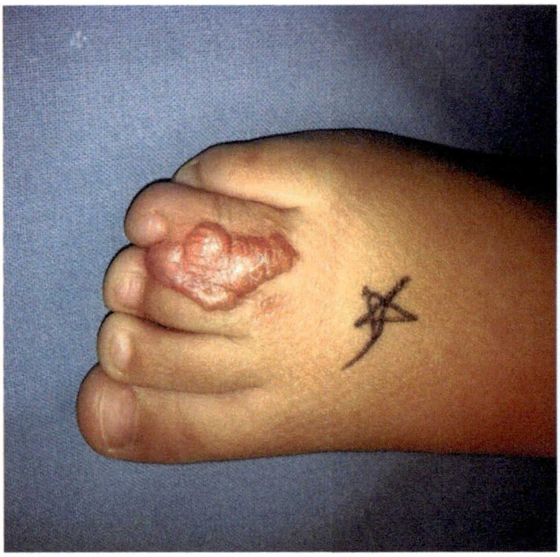
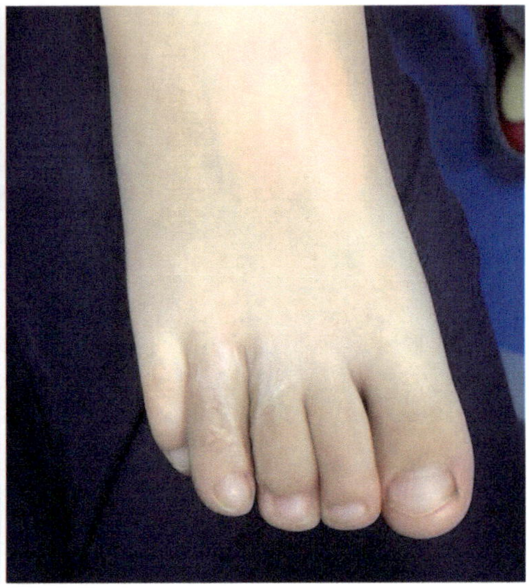

Images 34.10 and 34.11 Example of scars

degree of vascularization is connected to the wound healing phase; in fact, the active scars have a greater blood supply and therefore will appear reddened. Patient symptoms are also essential: pain and itching are the most common. In the literature there are scales that allow to evaluate and monitor the progress of the scar during treatment. Among these are the Vancouver Scar Scale, Hamilton Scale, and Patient and Observer Scar Assessment Scale (P.O.S.A.S). Unfortunately, children's scars are hardly measurable due to growth. Therefore, an objective evaluation is often used by observing color through visual evaluation or photography, analyzing movement of joint with regard to flexibility, or using the measurement in centimeters for thickness (Images 34.10 and 34.11).

34.5.3 Treatment

Scarring is a dynamic process with marked activity in the first 18 months. Knowing the factors that influence this process, prevention of the formation of keloid or hypertrophic scars is more effective than their subsequent treatment. Therefore, the entire treatment of post-surgical wounds is subject to a single objective, that is the reduction of the risk of developing pathological scarring, in order to guarantee the best possible aesthetic and functional result. In our hand rehabilitation department, post-surgical scars of children with different congenital malformations are often treated: syndactyly, symbrachydactyly, camptodactyly, clinodactyly, hypoplasia and thumb agenesis, arthrogryposis, polydactyly, amniotic reins syndrome, trigger finger. After the surgery, the scar treatment is started only when the wound is completely healed, which usually occurs around 21 days. The scar must be elastic, non-hypertrophic, non-adherent, non-hypersensitive, and non-painful. It is necessary to remove any necrotic material through good cleansing or with warm baths. The massage is the first approach used. It improves skin hydration, reduces itching and pain, and also helps the little patient to accept the scar and his hand. The therapist explains to parents the importance of massage and the need to perform it independently at home. Parents are instructed on the correct technique of massage, which must be done in a rotational sense, without rubbing but lifting the scar from the deeper levels, using an emollient cream. It must be performed at least 4 times a day for about 10 min. Parental constancy in massage and scar treatment is essential for successful treatment. Furthermore, continuous monitoring by the therapist is necessary, which allows to intervene in case of excessive inflammatory reaction to the treatment. If the scar appears hypertrophic, silicone sheets are applied to the scar overnight, until it is improved. They improve scar hydration, color, and reduce height and volume. Alternatively, the elastomer (silicone polymer) is made, the advantage of which is to be modeled directly on the patient's skin. Also, it could be used as an evaluation tool. In fact, by modeling it on the skin, the negative mold of the scar remains so as to be able to evaluate its evolution over time. If the scar is adherent to the underlying tissues, vacuum therapy is used. To allow home use, the "succhiaveleno syringe" is recommended, a syringe without a needle that produces negative pressure by lifting the superficial tissues. The application of k-tape can help to maintain rehabilitation control. It can be applied both with 50% voltage and without voltage. If the scars are in the commissure of the hand (pathologies such as syndactyly, Simbrachidattilia) a static "saddle" splint is made to be worn during the night, to allow a prolonged compression on the commissure scar. It also helps to keep scars stretched for a long time. Another aspect to consider is the hypersensitivity that affects the scar tissue, which can represent a limit in the daily use of the hand. In these cases, a desensitization program is carried out through sensory stimulation with different types of objects or tissues of increasing discomfort, in order to bring the scar area back to a normo-sensitivity. The rehabilitative treatment described above is not always sufficient for definitive resolution. If the scars become retractable, causing a functional deficit, a surgical correction will be performed.

34.6 Trigger Finger

Trigger finger of the thumb and long fingers in children must be evaluated by a hand specialist. After the diagnosis, a conservative or surgical management is started, both including an appropriate rehabilitation protocol.

In some cases a conservative treatment can be started even if surgical approach is the surgeon's choice, to reduce stiffness and pain before surgery.

The collaboration between the hand therapist and the surgeon is very important in order to apply the correct rehabilitation protocol.

34.6.1 Conservative Treatment

Short-term aims:

- Improving PROM/AROM
- Reducing stiffness
- Reducing pain
- Tendon sliding

Long-term aims:

- Complete PROM/AROM with no pain and stiffness
- Recovering complete use of the hand

The hand therapist has several tools and strategies: it is very important to involve parents and caregivers in the rehabilitation protocol to obtain better results.

34.6.2 Splinting

It is very important for the little patient to have a tailor-made splint created by a hand therapist. When the trigger finger is the thumb, the splint puts the IF joint of the thumb in extension. It can be a static splint if the IF joints reaches 0° of extension with no stiffness and pain, while it must be a dynamic splint when the IF presents more stiffness or it is not possible to put it at 0°. In some painful cases the therapist can provide a static splint in the beginning and then convert it into a dynamic splint when pain is reduced and the child gets used to wearing thermoplastic splints.

The static splint is made of thermoplastic, and it is anti-brachiometacarpal with a dorsal component for the thumb that puts in extension both MCP and IF joints (Image 34.12).

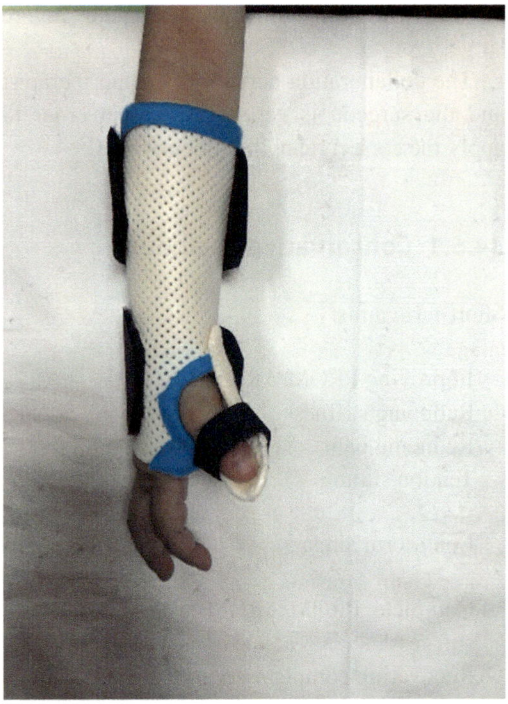

Image 34.12 Static splint for thumb

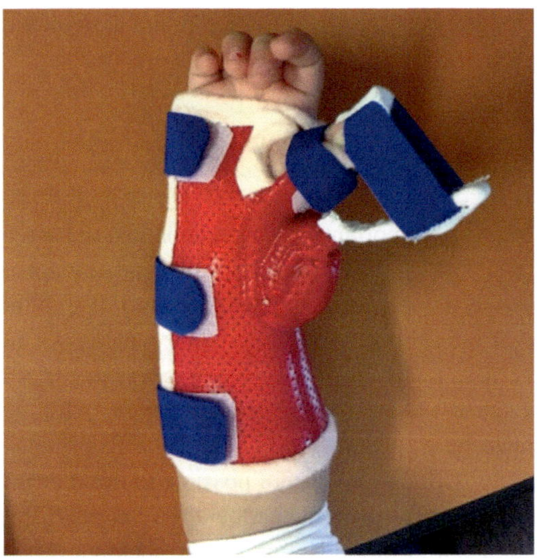

Image 34.13 Dynamic splint for thumb

The dynamic splint has an elastic traction for the IF joint, made with an elastic band: it is important to create a gentle traction that can be tolerated for a long time, more than a strong traction that the child cannot stand for more than a few minutes (Image 34.13).

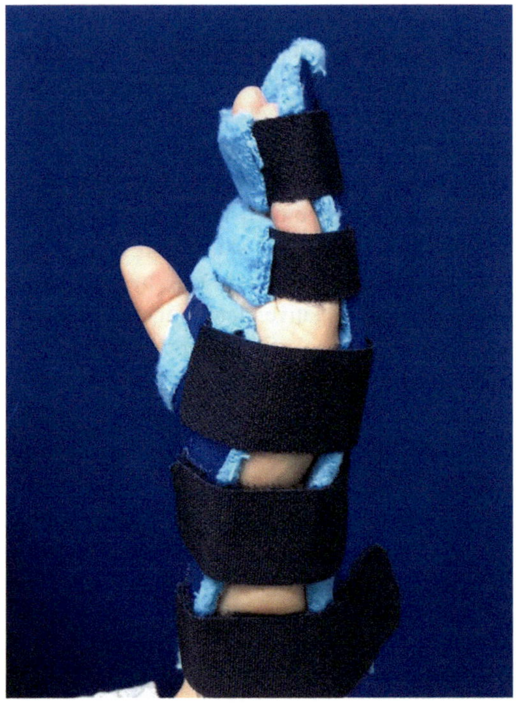

Image 34.14 Static splint for long fingers

When a long finger is affected, the conservative splint puts in the best extension the involved structures: neutral wrist, extension of MCP, PIP, and DIP joint (Image 34.14).

In our experience splints are more effective and if the wrist is included and put into a neutral position, they are more stable especially for the younger patients.

Splint must be worn during the night and during the afternoon nap; it is more effective if it is worn for at least 8 h: day by day parents are recommended to increase the time of wearing.

34.6.2.1 Passive Mobilization and Stretching

MCP and IF joints must be mobilized to reduce stiffness. It is important to prevent stiffness and deformities to allow a better tendon sliding and to improve PROM/AROM.

Stretching in extension for MCP and IF joints is useful to reduce contraction in flexion of the involved joints, to improve tissues elasticity and tendon gliding.

The therapist does it during the rehabilitation session and teaches parents how to do it at home often during the day.

34.6.2.2 Tendon Gliding

The therapist creates exercise and activities to improve flexor tendons gliding and to stimulate extensor tendons. When long fingers are involved, the complete flexion is not recommended.

34.6.3 Taping

Kinesio taping could improve extensor tendons work in order to reduce flexion contraction. Children can wear it all day long during their daily activities.

The conservative treatment must be periodically evaluated and reviewed by the surgeon and therapist, the splint in fact has to be checked, the stiffness can decrease, and the growth of the hand can change the tractions.

34.6.4 Rehabilitation After Surgical Treatment

Rehabilitation program must be started immediately after surgery to reduce edema and pain and further complications.

Short-term aims:

- Reduce edema
- Reduce pain
- Promote global activity of the hand
- Improve AROM/PROM
- Improve tendon gliding
- Correct scar healing

Long-term aims:

- Maintain and improve AROM/PROM
- Improve dexterity
- Improve scar tissue elasticity
- Maintain and improve tendon gliding

34.6.4.1 Edema and Pain Management

After surgery children are allowed to move and use their hand without pain. The day after surgery the therapist must check the bandage and in case of important edema it is important to change it, to allow a correct healing. Global active and passive exercises can be taught and elastic bandage or kinesio taping can be used to reduce edema, where necessary. Every exercise and activity must be done without pain. Ice and rest position can be useful to reduce pain, in alternation to active moments.

34.6.4.2 Active Mobilization and Tendon Gliding

Simple active exercise can be requested to the child to evaluate and improve hand use. Selective tendon gliding exercises are very important to prevent tendons adhesion while the scar is healing and will be started immediately (Image 34.15). Gradually exercises will be increased to improve dexterity and strength.

Passive Mobilization and Stretching

Reducing stiffness of the involved joints is important to allow a better active motion and a better tendon gliding. Stretching must be gentle and gradually more intensive for the involved joints and tendons (Images 34.16 and 34.17).

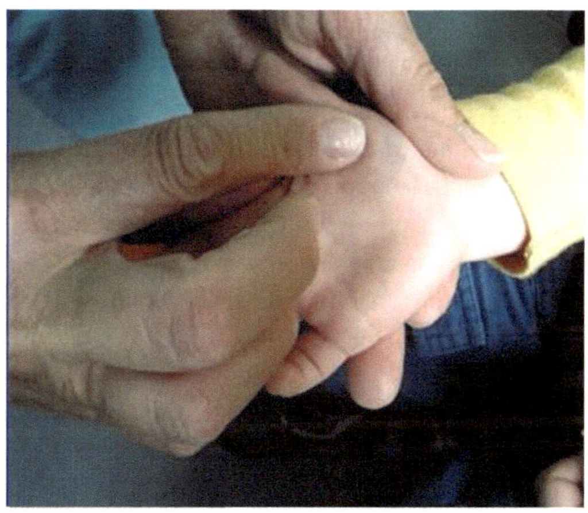

Image 34.15 Scar treatment

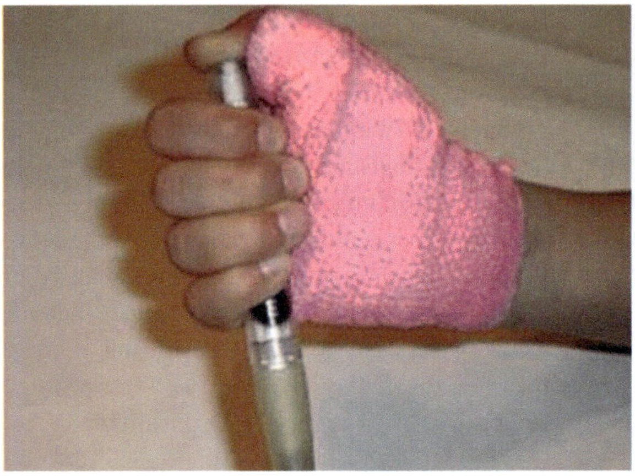

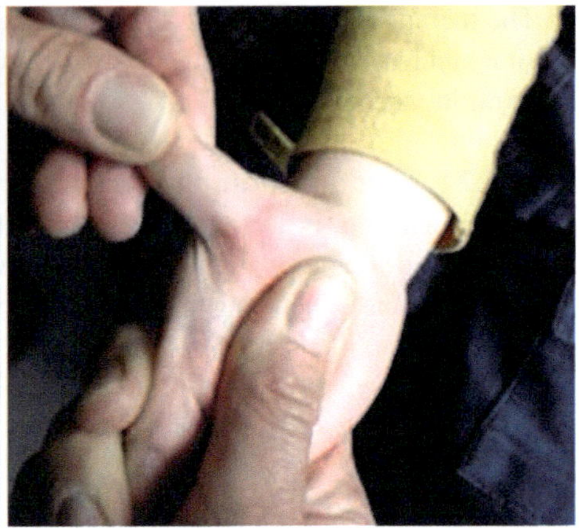

Images 34.16 and 34.17 FLP gliding and stretching

34.6.4.3 Scar Management

Scar massage must be started when the healing is complete. It is very important to manipulate the scar many times a day to have soft and elastic tissue. Stretching also increases skin elasticity. During the night a silicon band can be put on the scar to improve the scar healing. Kinesio taping and compressive elastic bandage can be used for a few hours a day to maintain the scar flat and elastic. Sensitive rehabilitation is started after skin healing to prevent sensibility defects.

34.7 Syndactyly

34.7.1 Post-surgery Treatment

Syndactyly is one of the most heterogeneous congenital malformations described in literature.

This malformation can be isolated or one of the signs in a more complex syndrome, but the surgical approach is the only one suggested. This means that the rehabilitative approach is for post-surgery, and it begins the day of the surgery.

34.7.1.1 Time 0

Immediately after surgery the hand therapist has to protect the structures that underwent surgery, the fingers have to be separated, and the new webs have to be protected but maintained deep during the healing process. In the most severe cases the therapist can provide a splint in thermoplastic material on the dressing to wear during the night, or also during the day if the bones were involved too (Image 34.18).

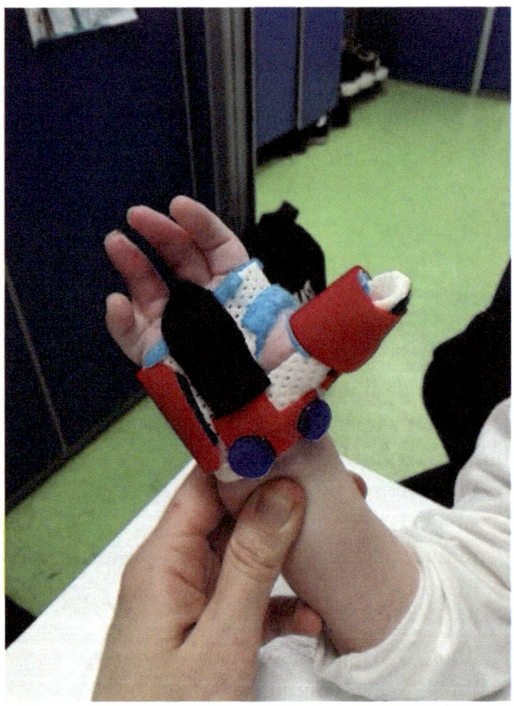

Image 34.18 Splint for syndactyly

Active movement will be promoted from the very beginning, especially for the non-involved structures, such as flexion and extension of the fingers.

The dressing will be constantly checked; if the hand presents edema it will be replaced, like the splint if there is one in order to optimize the results obtained with the surgery.

34.7.1.2 From the Third Week On

When the wound is completely healed the splint has to be adapted to the new size, a smaller one. The deeper part of the new web space that has been created through surgery has to be pressed properly to keep it wide and low; to do it on the splint the therapist puts elastic bands like neoprene bands or thermoplastic saddle. The same aim will be obtained also through a deep and compressive massage with a cream or oil; this massage will be taught by the therapist to the parents or caregivers during the rehabilitative sessions. The parents must massage the scars at home for a few minutes but very often during the day, to prevent the thickening of the scar and most of all to prevent the web to become higher. In addition, during the night, the use of silicon sheets or elastomer is suggested under the splint, to guarantee a good hydration that means a better elasticity and a better movement of the involved structures.

For the first web a special saddle has to be done by the therapist; in this case it helps to widen the web, and to keep it low, normally during the rehabilitative sessions the saddle needs to be modified.

In both cases, first web or others, the little patients will be involved in play activities to involve the whole upper limb, the single segments to have a full recovery.

Taping (like kinesio-tape) can be useful to correct the single digit or more of them if needed; elastic compressive bandages can be used to increase the width of the web or to compress hypertrophic scars.

In case of slight stiffness in flexion of the fingers it is possible to create static splint to promote extension. In most severe cases a dynamic splint can be suggested, with a more precise, strong perpendicular traction on the finger.

The child during the therapy will use both hands or only the operated one to easily adapt to the new situation; obviously the activity that the therapist proposes will be different from a child to another, considering the age and what the patient likes most.

It is important to underline that parents or caregivers must engage time at home to go on with the therapy, the massage of the scars must be done at least 4–5 times a day (avoiding "rubbing" the scar), the splint needs to be worn every night for at least 3–4 months, and daily the child has to be encouraged in the use of the single hand and of both of them during ADL and games. Only in this way the child is able to corticalize the "new hand" and its new possibilities.

34.8 Symbrachydactyly

34.8.1 Introduction

Patients affected by symbrachydactyly can present different phenotypes; Blauth's classification, modified by Foucher, provides a valid guidance for treatment.

In stage I therapeutic indication is to separate any possible syndactylies with consequent lowering of the interdigital webs (see the introduction).

In stage II therapeutic indication is to stabilize digital segments with bone hypoplasia with free phalanx transfer from the foot.

In stage III therapeutic indication is, where possible, phalanx transfer from the foot or toe-to-hand transfer; in the monodactylous type it can also be necessary to improve the position of the first finger with web correction or bone lengthening.

In stage IV there are no specific therapeutic indications.

34.8.2 Phalanx Transfer

The little patients affected by symbrachydactyly phenotypes 2a, 2b, and 2c have surgery indication of free phalanx transfer.

After surgery, the child has a cast immobilization for 4 weeks: it includes the wrist and the operated fingers up to the tip.

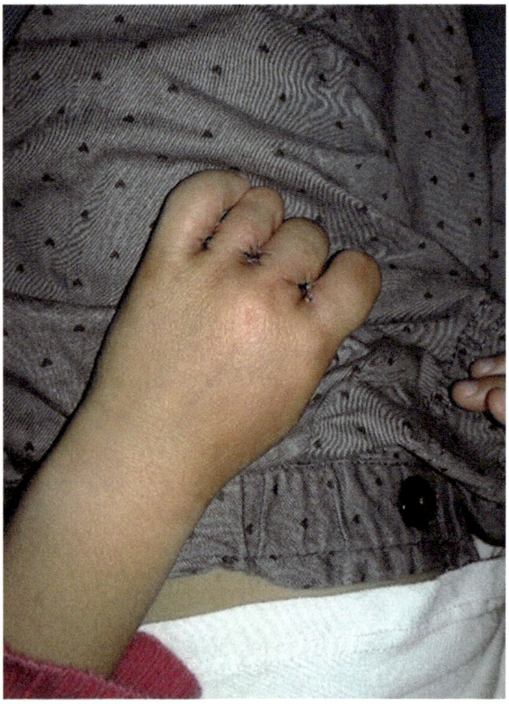

Image 34.19 Scar treatment

After 4 weeks the patient has a change of dressing under anesthesia and the cast is removed. At this stage the therapist makes a handmade removal splint with thermoplastic material that includes the wrist and with a protection above the toes that had surgery.

From week 4 the therapist can start working on bimanual grip stimulus through games to include the operated hand and stimulate active mobilization via the grip of objects of different shape, dimension, and texture.

Also it is important to do the scar massage to prevent scar adhesions (Image 34.19).

It is essential to maintain long-term follow-up to monitor bone growth by surgeons; quite often it is necessary to do a web lowering.

34.8.3 Rehabilitation After Toe-to-Hand Transfer

The pediatric hand therapist will follow the little patient during all the therapeutic period and will teach the parents how to manage and rehab both the hand and foot at home.

The therapist has to give the child the correct stimuli to increase both bimanual grip and the pinch with the operated hand; so we focus on preventing the exclusion of the operated hand and, if an opposable segment is present, we stimulate it to increase its functionality.

It is important to work with objects with different shapes, dimensions, textures, and material surfaces to arouse sensibility of the transferred toes. Whether the patient had already developed an autonomous path prior to surgery, it is also important to do a walking training to balance the weight distribution and to re-establish the biomechanics of the step; otherwise it is advisable to follow the patient during the development of motor skills which involve passing to the standing position and then to the path.

Rehabilitation goals after toe-to-hand transfer are divided in short-medium term and long-term goals.

- Short-medium term goals: 0–8 weeks after surgery
  - Vitality of the transferred toe
  - Edema control
  - Integration of the limb and the transferred toe
  - Increased active and passive range of motion
  - Sensibility development
  - Corticalization progress
  - Correct weight distribution and walking path
- Long-term goals: over 8 weeks from surgery
  - Transferred toe integration during daily life activities
  - Increased active and passive range of motion
  - Sensibility enhancement
  - Strength increase
  - Corticalization progress
  - Autonomous path

Early rehabilitation program:

- Day 0–3: immobilization
  - Child is hospitalized.
  - Cast immobilization.
  - Constant vascular check by surgeon.

- Day 3–7:
  - The child is still hospitalized.
  - Constant vascular check by surgeon.
  - First approach with the physiotherapy department.
  - Integration of the limb through games with particular attention on the transferred toe.

Our rehabilitation program begins during the first week after surgery, compatible with the vascular check of the transferred toe and preserving bone synthesis, and tendon, nerves, and vessels sutures.

The donor site is immobilized with a cast up to the knee and the load is not allowed to guarantee the healing of the intermetatarsal ligament between the first and the third metatarsal bone, after the removal of the second ray. The upper limb is immobilized with a cast from the elbow to the fingers included, to protect bone synthesis, vessels, tendons, and nerves sutures. The transferred toe tip remains uncovered to monitor its vascularization.

During the week after surgery the child has the first approach with the rehabilitation department and the therapist, in order to know each other and to establish the trust relationship between the therapist, the patient, and, in this case, the patient's parents. Rehabilitation takes place through games and bimanual activities, to avoid limb exclusion and to keep the elbow and the shoulder joints free. If the patient is compliant, it is important to bring since the very beginning the child concentration on the transferred toe to start the integration process. At days 7–10 after surgery, the patient has a change of dressing under anesthesia. Both to the hand and the donor site: the hand cast is removed and replaced by a handmade removal splint in thermoplastic material, with the wrist included and a protection above the transferred toe (Image 34.20).

- Day 7 to week 4: passive mobilization of the PIP and DIP joints, sensory stimulation, active recruitment
  - Bimanual activities
  - Passive mobilization of the PIP and DIP joints
  - Active recruitment both in flexion and extension
  - Sensibility stimulation
  - Walking training with casts
  - Scar treatment, when possible

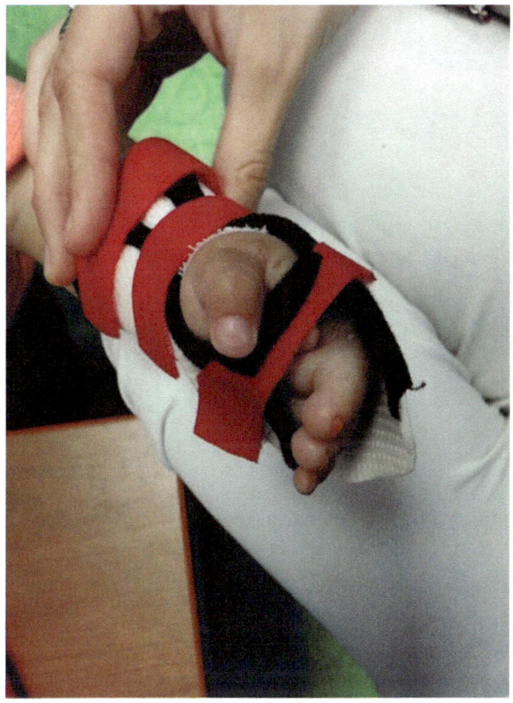

Image 34.20 The post-medication splint

During these weeks the patient has physiotherapy every day. The splint is removed during physiotherapy and at home when the child is under parental control.

To limit the exclusion of the operated limb due to the defensive mechanisms, the therapist has to promote bimanual activities through games. Also, it is important to maintain free shoulder and elbow joints and their muscular mass, in order to limit damages from non-use hypotrophy.

In this stage, the therapist begins passive mobilization of the PIP and DIP joints, as they are distal to the bone synthesis, with the aim of preventing joint stiffness, increasing their passive

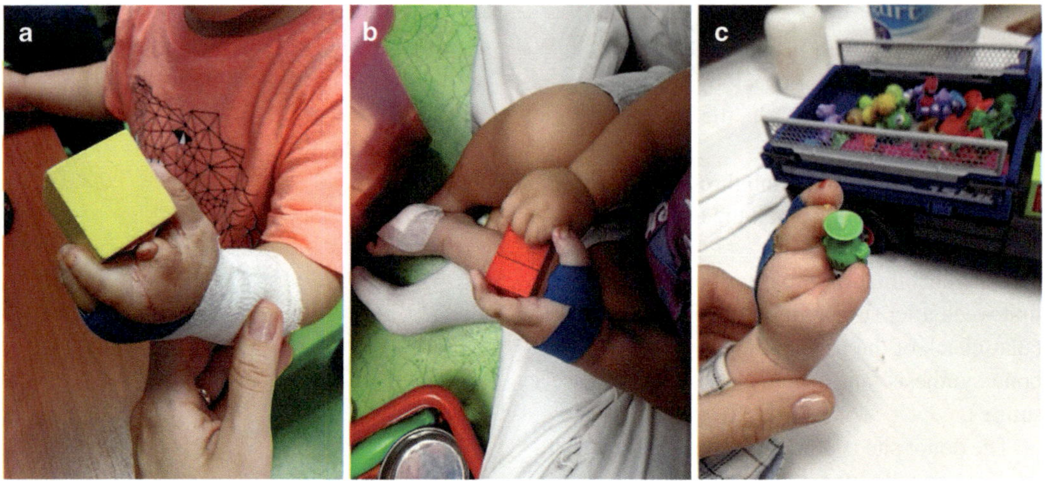

Image 34.21 (**a**–**c**) Active recruitment and stimulation

range of motion and promoting passive tendon sliding.

Moreover, the therapist will stimulate active recruitment both in flexion and in extension, always through games and modulating the rehabilitative requests based on the child's age and his interests and preferences; it gives an initial cortical motor scheme, making the child focused and conscious on his transferred toe (Images 34.21a–c and 34.22a–d).

It is important to introduce a sensibility stimulation program as soon as the skin allows it. In fact it has been demonstrated that foot toes can recover a greater degree of discrimination when transferred, than those that are not transferred. Also, the cortical representation can be modified when receiving peripheral inputs and therefore working on sensibility on early stages led to an earlier and better recovery.

Scars treatment includes compression massages, lifting to prevent adhesions, and silicone patches at night.

The donor site has been immobilized for 4 weeks by a proper splint with a raised part to avoid weight on the forefoot. Therefore the therapist must train the child how to walk with the cast, focusing on the correct weight distribution and the gait pattern, to prevent secondary damage from incorrect walking scheme and non-use (Image 34.23a, b).

From week 4 to K-wire removal: electrostimulation introduction and increase in functional demand

- Bimanual activities
- Passive PIP and DIP joint mobilization
- Active recruitment both in flexion and in extension
- Sensory stimulation
- Scars treatment
- Electrostimulation
- "Exergames"
- Walking training
- Psychomotor therapy

The physiotherapy sessions can now be intensified and we also introduce psychomotor therapy twice a week (see Sect. 34.16).

During physiotherapy we prosecute with passive and active mobilization of synthesis-free joints, as well as sensory stimulation.

As soon as the vascular stability is achieved and the surgeon gives the consent, it is possible to work on the edema control with elastic compressive bandages or with Kinesio Taping®.

The immobilization period of the lower limb lasts for 4 weeks. After this, the therapist has to reeducate the child to the correct load distribution during standing position, then walking, according to the gait biomechanics, and eventually run-

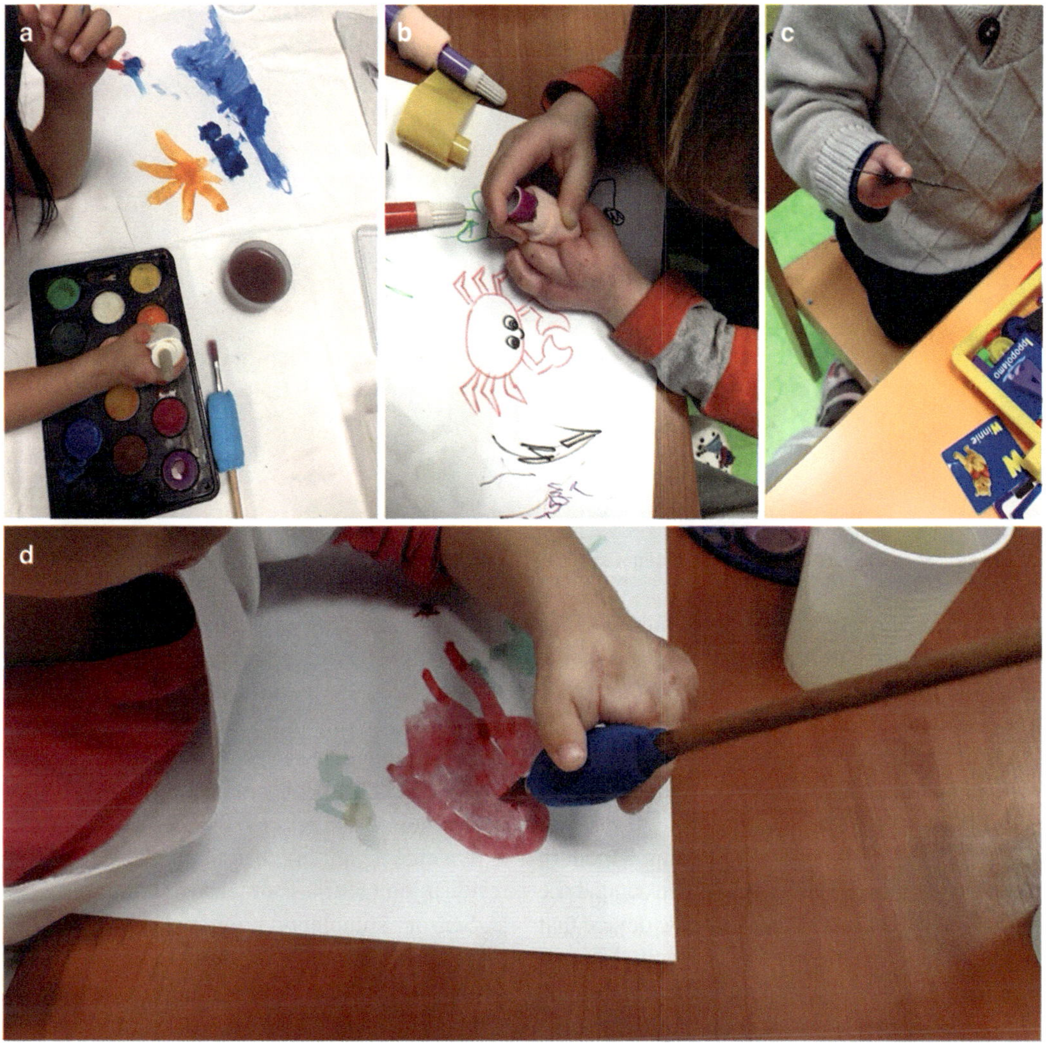

Image 34.22 (**a**–**d**) Activities for hand movement

ning and jumping. On the other hand, if the child in the preoperative period had not yet achieved or completed the motor skills of walking, the therapist should favor the postural steps that lead the child to reach the standing station with the correct weight distribution on the donor foot and then the walking scheme, involving also parents and teaching them how to stimulate the child at home.

Subsequently, variable stimuli for stability and foot support surfaces are provided to increase adaptability, coordination, and balance.

From week 8 the patient will introduce the use of the electrostimulation once a day on the flexor tendons of the transferred toe.

The stimulus is used above all as biofeedback, trying to provide the child the sensation determined by the contraction of the flexor muscles and consequently the movement at the level of the transferred finger to promote corticalization processes.

Moreover, an increase on the intensity of the electrical stimulus will increase muscle strength to obtain a more efficient movement. The thera-

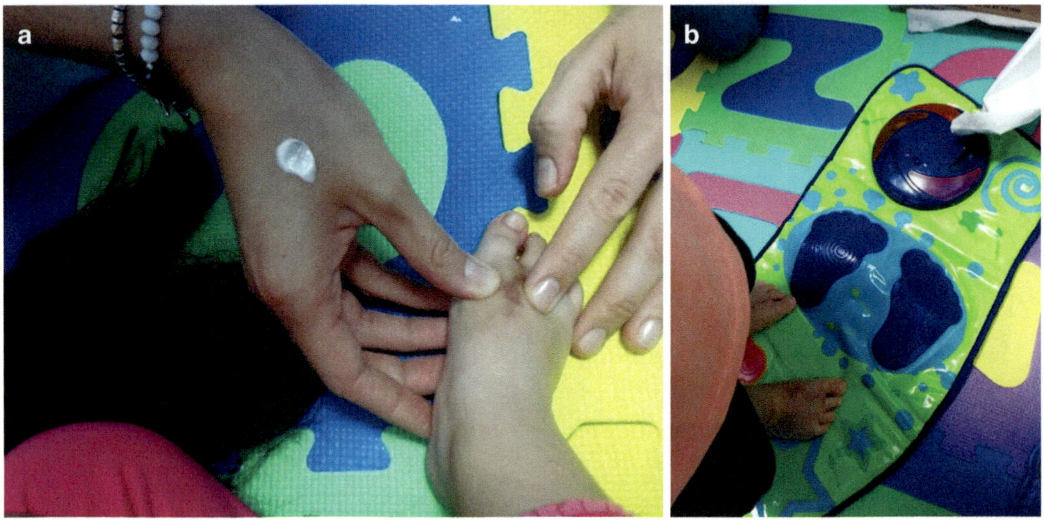

Image 34.23 (**a**, **b**) Scar treatment of the donor site

pist to correctly set the work must talk with the surgeon to have specific indications about the course of the sutured muscles and tendons. Once it is set by the therapist, the patient will perform electrostimulation daily at home.

Rehabilitation requests must always be proposed in the form of play, according to his fantasy and preferences, also using modern technology. In our department we introduced the use of the "Exergames," an electronic device that stimulates coordination and the capacity to modulate pressure intensity and movement wideness. These tools help the corticalization process and facilitate the integration and use of the transferred toe. Nowadays, we can consider them a new endearing rehabilitative experience for our little patients.

- From K-wire removal:
  - Scar treatment
  - AROM and PROM increase (including MP joint)
  - Sensory stimulation
  - Strength training
  - Coordination and dexterity
  - Psychomotor therapy

After X-ray control by the surgeon approximately 8 weeks after surgery, the patient has a change of dressing under anesthesia to remove the Kirschner wire.

After this, the patient will continue physiotherapy and psychomotor therapy regularly.

At this stage, passive and active mobilization has no limits also concerning the metacarpophalangeal joint. If necessary, the therapist can make a dynamic splint to increment flexion due to residual joint stiffness or tendons adhesions.

Sensory stimulation program become increasingly complex and exercises are modulated according to the sensitivity improvement. The patient will continue electrostimulation daily for 3 months from surgery. Rehabilitation will now be focused on implementing coordination, dexterity, and ability in grasping objects with different shape and dimensions.

34.9 Polydactyly

34.9.1 Radial Polydactyly

Radial polydactyly is the form with the largest number of presentation variants ranging from a duplication of the distal phalanx to a triphalangia. With this variable presentation framework, it is necessary to know the type of surgery carried out. If only the supernumerary segment has been

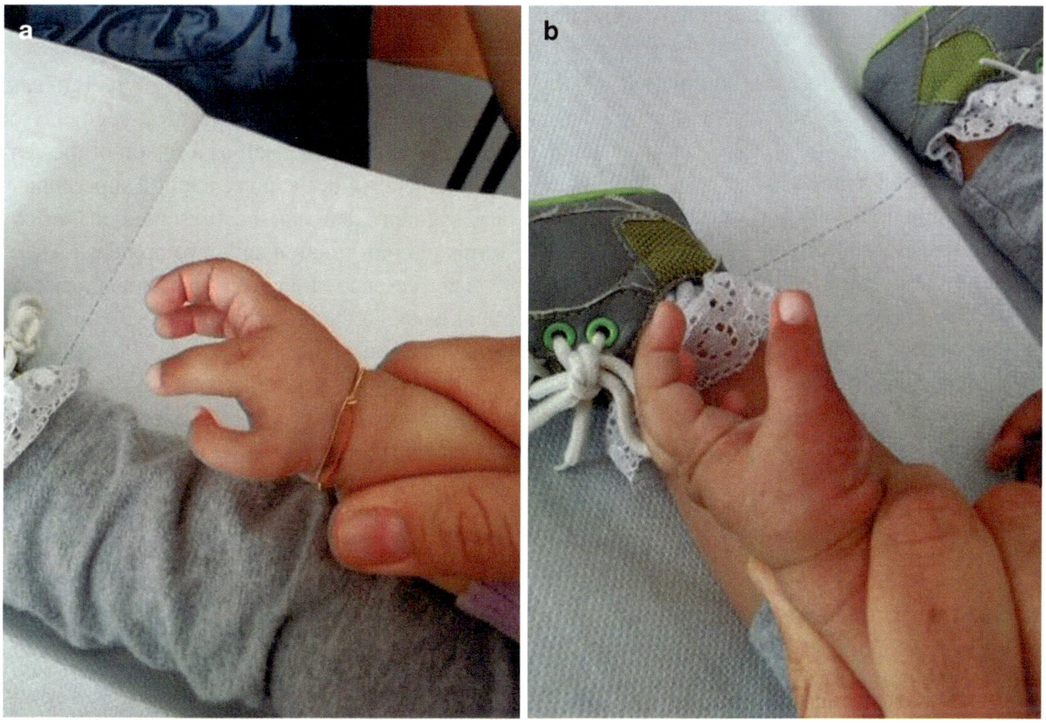

Image 34.24 (**a**, **b**) Radial polydactyly in bilateral case: pre- and post-surgery

removed, if a ligament reconstruction has been performed, if the patient has been subjected to tendon disruptions and shifts or cuneiform osteotomies. The primary objective in the immediate postoperative phase is to protect the structures involved in the surgery through a child-tailored splint. Subsequently, a protected mobilization protocol will be started to resume the mobility of the first finger and reeducate it for use in gaming activities (Image 34.24a, b).

Below we describe the rehabilitation phases.

34.9.1.1 0–4 Weeks

- Immobilization with a splint in opposition and abduction of the thumb.
- At the end of the fourth week the dressing is performed and an anti-brachiometacarpal splint is packaged with long fingers free and the first ray positioned in opposition.

34.9.1.2 4–6 Weeks

- The splint is converted in a removable one that will be removed in a first phase only for the physiotherapy and in safe situations. The splint will slowly be weaned during the day. In the case in which in the surgery a ligament reconstruction has been performed, the operated segment will be protected for another 2 weeks.
- Mobilization of the interphalangeal and metacarpophalangeal articulations in flexion and extension paying attention to deviations. It is also important to stretch the first web and work to open it to encourage the opposition. It is crucial to teach the parents how to do those exercises at home.
- Scar treatment with the application of silicon patches on the same during the night under the splint. It is possible also to package a saddle splint for the opening of the first web in order to avoid the formation of an hypertrophic or retracting scar that could severely restrict the free movement of the first ray, in particular in grip activities.
- Prevention and correction of any deviation through the use of splints or the application of

Kinesio Tape® with functional correction technique.
- Game activities for the stimulation of the bimanual grip.

34.9.1.3 6–8 Weeks

- The splint is abandoned during the day and maintained for the night. It is still important to value the position of the finger and the scar trophism before taking any decision.
- Proposal of various recreational activities to stimulate the grip between the thumb and long fingers (pinch and tridigital grip) such as drawing and the use of constructions or puzzles.

34.9.1.4 8 Weeks

- If there is stiffness of the MCP's joint due to the scar a pro-flexion dynamic splint can be packaged (Image 34.25).

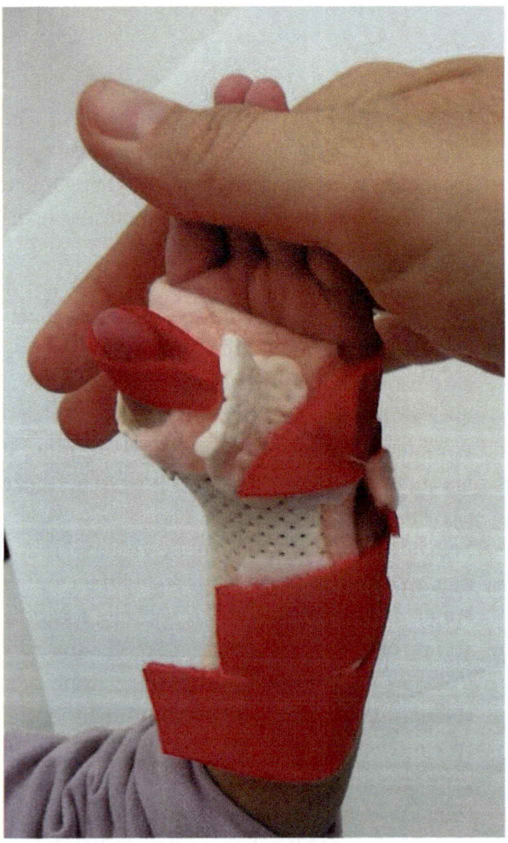

Image 34.25 Dynamic splint for MCP flexion

34.9.2 Central Polydactyly

Central polydactyly, or synpolydactyly, is a hand malformation affecting the central segments of the hand. It presents itself as a fusion of the central elements with the presence of a supernumerary segment that can be presented in various forms of conformation and development.

The presence of a central supernumerary segment leads, in the majority of cases, to an alteration of the adjacent joints. Postoperative rehabilitation following surgical removal of the segment therefore has, as its primary objective, the recovery of the articular excursion of all the joints of the hand and the stimulation of the use of the hand and especially of the grip.

Below we describe the rehabilitation phases.

34.9.2.1 0–4 Weeks

- Immobilization with a compressive dressing and pinstripe valve.

34.9.2.2 4–6/8 Weeks

- A protection splint is packaged to protect the operated structures allowing the mobilization of the not involved segments. The splint is used during the night and for not-safe activities for the first period and then is weaned gradually.
- Treatment of edema, in particular with Coban dressing.
- Scar treatment to prevent the formation of hypertrophic scar that will reduce the opening of the web creating a limitation of articular mobility. As soon as the wound is cured, an elastic component is applied on the splint that can allow a compression on the scar and an opening stretching of the web (Image 34.26).
- Mobilization of the various articulation involved and instruction of the parents to perform it at home.
- Proposal of recreational activities that allow global hand mobility, encouraging movements of long fingers and manipulation activities to stimulate grip development.
- Diurnal syndactyly between the operated finger and one of the adjacent fingers to avoid any deviations and the exclusion of the oper-

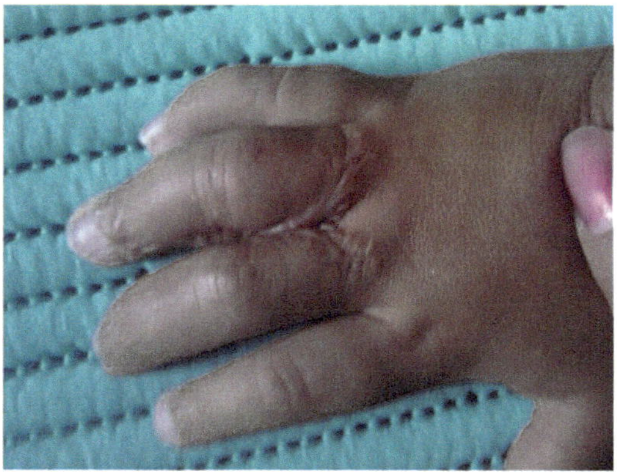

Image 34.26 Scar

ated finger encouraging an harmonious movement.

- On reaching the eighth after surgery week in the case there remained an extension rigidity a dynamic splint for the flexion of the interphalangeal joints can be packaged.

34.9.3 Ulnar Polydactyly

Ulnar or post-axial polydactyly is characterized by the presence of a supernumerary portion that may be a small floating appendage or a complete normal finger formed on the ulnar side of the hand. Surgical treatment of choice consists in the removal of the supernumerary segment with variable techniques based on the presentation. The rehabilitative treatment in ulnar polydactyly has as a short-term objective the protection of the operated structures while in the long term it is necessary to work on the recovery of the global mobility of the hand, in particular of the ulnar segments (Images 34.27 and 34.28).

Below we describe the rehabilitation phases.

34.9.3.1 0–4 Weeks

- Immobilization with a compressive dressing and mobilization of the free segments.

34.9.3.2 4–6/8 Weeks

- Scar treatment with silicon patches and any splint to open the space between the fingers and maintain longitudinal axis of the finger (Image 34.29).
- Long fingers mobilization, in particular of the ulnar segments.
- Game activities that stimulate the child to use the hand with particular attention to the integration of the last two fingers in the grips of large objects and general dexterity.

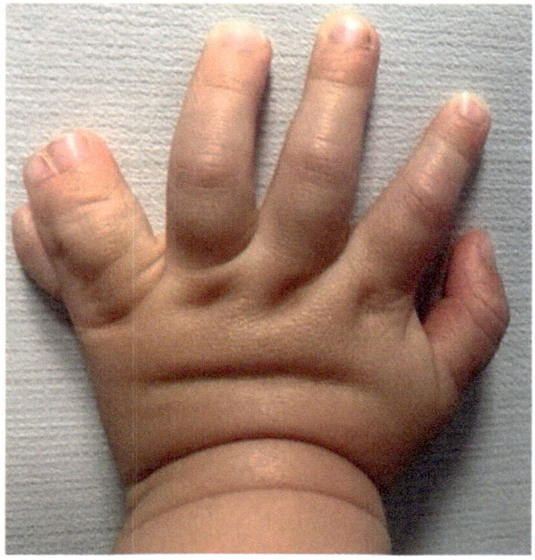

Image 34.27 Ulnar polydactyly

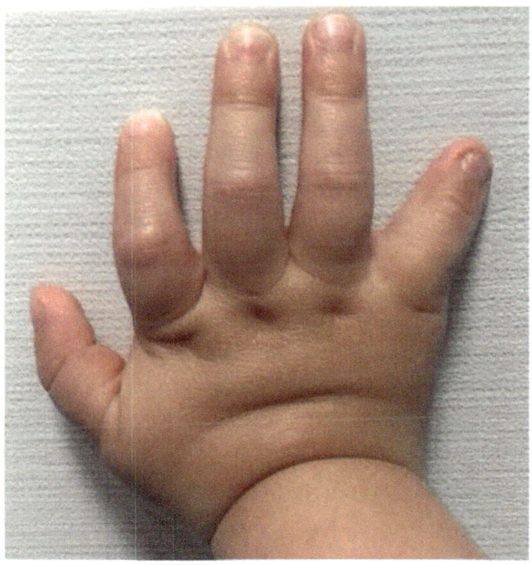

Image 34.28 Picture post ulnar polydactyly surgery

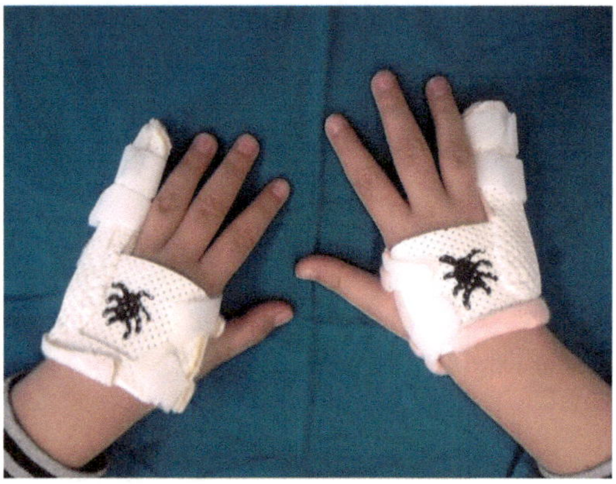

Image 34.29 Removable splint in ulnar polydactyly

- If necessary a syndactyly can be used to avoid the exclusion and stimulate the integration of the finger in grip movements.

34.10 Arthrogryposis

Arthrogryposis is a malformation present at birth.

The stiffened joint is the major problem for this little patient.

It always affects the upper arm and the pathology could be distal or proximal; this malformation could affect also the spine and the legs.

The diffuse stiffness and the strength reduction prevent both the movement and the functionality of the arms. Usually the stiffness is bilateral (Image 34.30).

There are rarely problems related to the development and the sensibility.

The conservative treatment should start as soon as possible and it should be carried on during his entire childhood.

Unfortunately some of the patients arrive in our unit at school age.

The origin of this pathology is uncertain and the manifestation is different depending on the case.

The typical stiffness of the upper arm is:

- Shoulder: adducted and intrarotated
- Elbow: extended and stiffened
- Wrist: flexed and deviated ulnarly

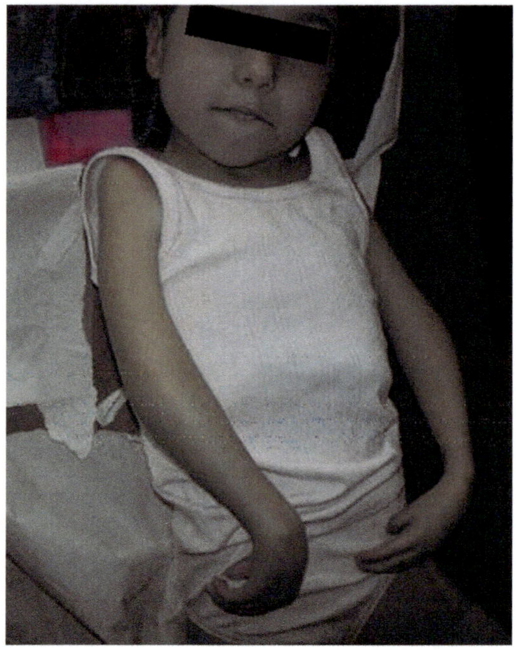

Image 34.30 Bilateral stiffness of the upper limb

- Fingers: extended, deviated ulnarly, and camptodactilous
- Thumb: flexed adducted and in palm (Images 34.31–34.33)

The objective of the conservative treatment is to achieve the best mobility of the stiffened articulation and improve PROM and AROM of the shoulder, elbow, wrist, and fingers to maximize the grip that is important for touching and exploring the environment to optimize the grip.

It is important to recuperate these specific joints:

- The shoulder controls the arm orientation.
- The elbow is responsible for feeding, touching, and personal care.
- The wrist is responsible for stabilizing the arm during the grasp.
- The fingers are responsible for touching and playing.
- The thumb is responsible for the fine pinch.

The mobilization in the correct position is the first thing to do, and then we prepare the splint to

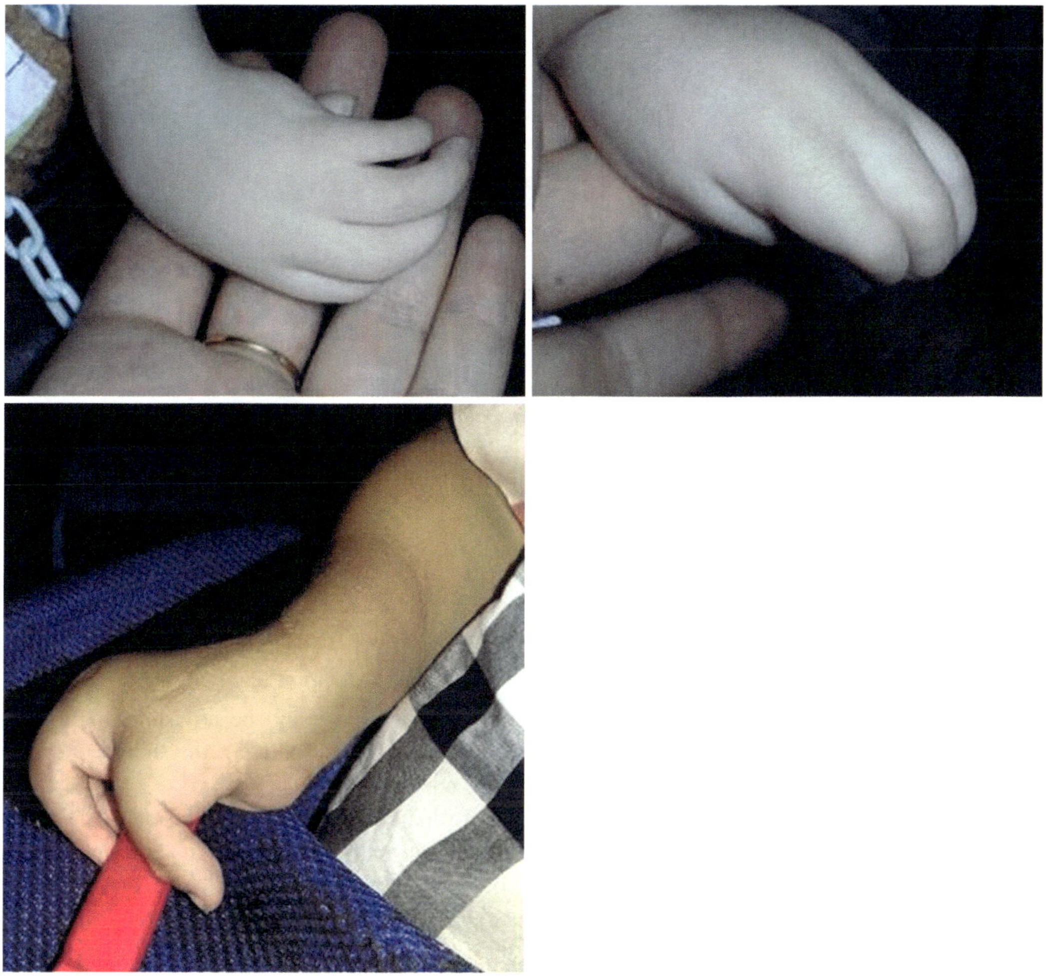

Images 34.31–34.33 Hand and wrist position

maintain the achieved position. The little patient wears the splint in the night and during the day; it depends on the age and the conditions.

Play is the best tool for the reeducation.

With the active and passive mobilizations we obtain the best position for the arm. The mobilization consists of passive stretching and pressing the baby to play for cognitive development.

The splint is prepared as soon as possible, sometimes as early as 20 days after birth; it can be as small as a pen (Image 34.34a–c).

It is made by thermoplastic material modeled with warm water. The splint substitutes the old serial cast.

At the start we do manipulation and stretching and then using the splint we maintain the ROM.

The splint also increases the ROM.

It is removable and it must be controlled frequently because of the baby development.

At the beginning the baby must always wear the splint and it should be removed only for the bath.

Then when the ROM is achieved it is possible to wear it only during the night.

The splints are also useful for playing or eating without problem to keep the toy or the spoon (Image 34.35).

But if we also have the problem with the wrist and the fingers in flexion and deviation, it is possible to prepare a splint for the wrist and finger to be joined together.

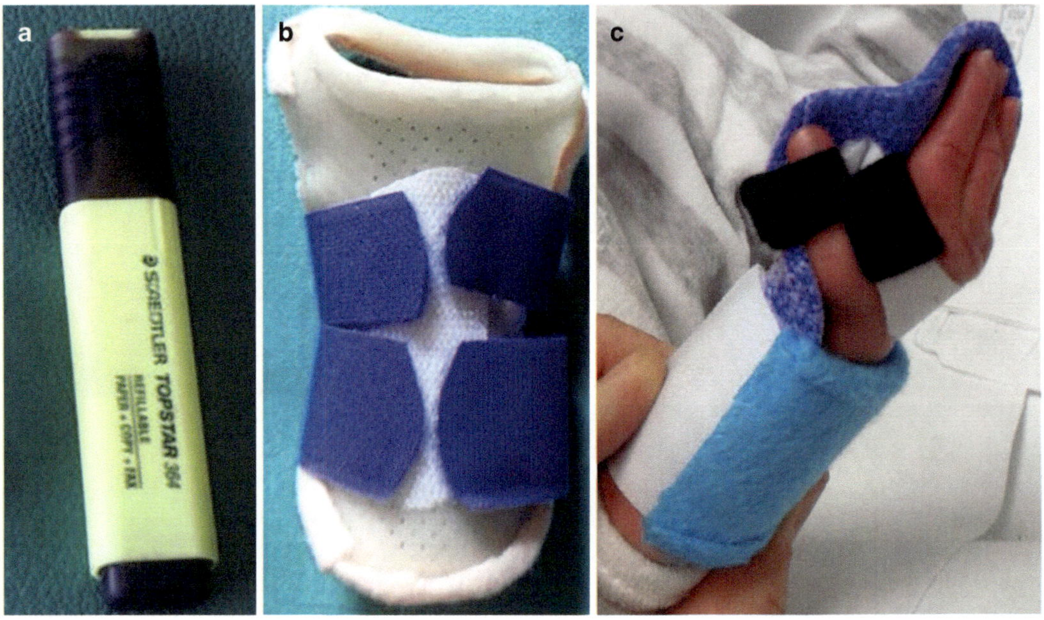

Image 34.34 (**a**–**c**) Example of splint

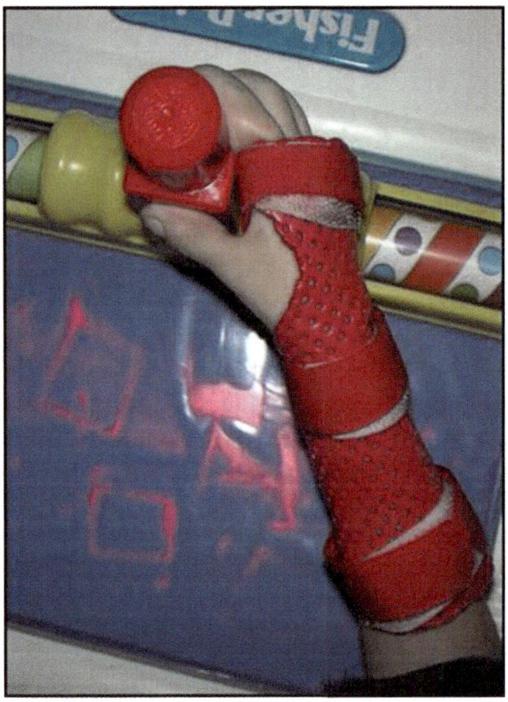

Image 34.35 Functional splint for the wrist

Sometimes it could be advisable to make a dynamic splint to maintain the thumb open for the activities.

To maintain the correct position of the wrist the thumb and the finger are a great problem for a baby with arthrogryposis.

We use also the k-tape for the thumb for the best outcome. Taping provides immediate senso-motor feedback regarding functional abilities. The k-tape is elastic, latex-free, very thin, and stretches in the longitudinal plane.

It has been suggested to provide proprioceptive input.

Pressing the baby to play is the first means available to stimulate and mobilize.

It is important to remember that the activities are selected depending on the age and the development of the baby.

In conclusion we must remember that the conservative treatment should start as soon as possible and be "aggressive"; we have to monitor the splint very closely in the first 2–3 years based on a tailor-made strategy and involving the parents.

34.11 Amniotic Band Syndrome (ABS)

Amniotic Band Syndrome (ABS) can involve the upper limbs at different levels: forearm, arm, hand, or fingers.

Some cases require immediate surgery; in fact a very strict band can compromise blood circulation and the tissues survival. Little patients can undergo surgery very few hours after birth if necessary to save the whole upper limb or a single segment.

After surgery, rehabilitation protocol is started as soon as possible. Surgery could require an immobilization period to ensure a correct scar healing. The immobilization's length is decided by the surgeon, and it depends on the structures involved. If necessary, a static thermoplastic splint is made on the bandage to keep the arm and fingers in the right position.

Sometimes surgery can be necessary but needs to be delayed because of other medical needs of the baby; in this case a preoperative period of rehabilitation can be suggested to evaluate the baby's motricity, to stimulate motorial abilities, and to stretch soft tissues where necessary.

Each case must be analyzed both by the surgeon and therapist in order to study the better treatment for the baby. Evaluation is important to find the structures involved or limited by ABS: vessels, bones, tendons, muscles, and nerves. Parents will be taught by the therapist to do rehabilitation sessions at home: parents and caregivers collaboration is always fundamental to achieve better results.

34.11.1 Postoperative Rehabilitation

34.11.1.1 Splint

Thermoplastic splint is tailor-made on the child's hand. It must be done respecting the structures involved in surgery and putting the body segments involved into a safe position. If necessary it can be unremovable in the first healing period and after that a removable one is done by the therapist. Parents will be taught to put it on and off during the night and the day.

34.11.1.2 Active Mobilization

Adequate stimulation, based on patient's age, is important to improve active motricity and abilities to pick up objects and explore the surrounding environment. Taping helps to improve active motion: it can be used to stimulate or reduce muscles activation or to stabilize segments in order to have a better and correct active motion.

34.11.1.3 Passive Mobilization

Compatible with surgery and time of healing, passive mobilization is important to improve joints' range of motion (ROM). During mobilization the little patient should not feel any pain; this kind of mobilization prepares structures and joints to a better active motion.

34.11.1.4 Scar Treatment

As soon as the scar healing is complete, it is important to massage it in order to have soft scar tissue. Scars need compression made by silicon sheets or elastomer put under a splint worn during the night or sleeping time of the baby. Sensitive stimulation is important to gain a good sensibility in the area of the scar.

34.11.1.5 Edema Treatment

After surgery and eventually immobilization, edema could be present and could limit active and passive motion. Scars or the remaining part of the amniotic band can make it difficult to resolve it but through massage, bandage, and taping the scar can become elastic enough to allow all the movements needed.

34.11.2 Preoperative Treatment

34.11.2.1 Splint

After an adequate evaluation, a removable thermoplastic splint can be done to stretch soft tissues and to put in a safe and correct position the segments involved in the ABS. Splint is usually worn during the night or the sleeping time of the baby.

34.11.2.2 Passive Mobilization

Stretching soft tissues and mobilizing joints involved is extremely important to have a better active motion, like important to arriving at the surgery time in the better condition as possible, in order to have an easier postoperative rehabilitation.

34.11.2.3 Active Mobilization

As every kind of rehabilitation, stimulation must be adequate at child's age in order to maintain and improve active abilities. Taping can help muscles activation and can be useful to improve active motion and complete recovery.

34.12 Epidermolysis Bullosa

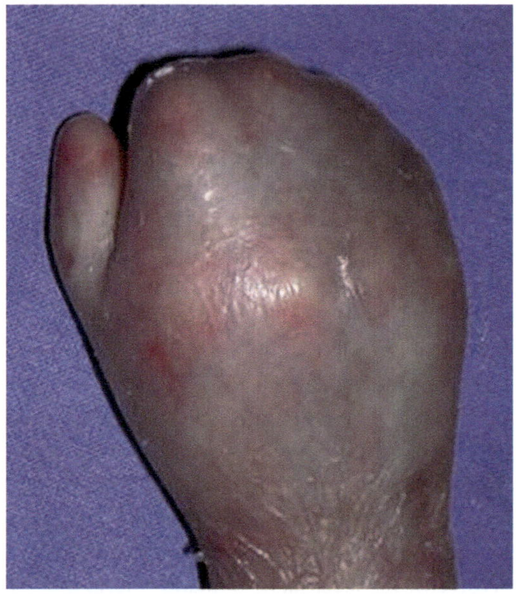

Image 34.36 Hand with EB

Epidermolysis bullosa (EB) is, as we described in the previous chapter, a rare and disabling genetic disease that causes boils and lesions on the skin and in the inner mucosa, symptoms that can occur spontaneously or because of the slightest friction. It is also known as "butterfly children's syndrome," referring to the fragility of patients in common with the proverbial of the wings of a butterfly. The tissues involved are those underlying the basal lamina; therefore the healing of the lesions involves the formation of scars and this is of particular interest in the treatment of the upper limb and even more the hand.

The treatment of these young patients will be at 360° on the various systemic problems, focusing on all aspects of the pathology in the various localization of onset.

The most affected areas to the formation of lesions and bubbles are the parts most exposed to friction, therefore the hands and feet, often ulcerated with loss of skin annexes.

In the first months and years of life, the repeated small traumas to the hands and the consequent injuries, followed by the cicatrization phase, imply the formation of more or less tight syndactyls, until the hand remains closed in a fist with the long fingers flexed and the thumb adducted (Image 34.36). This position, if maintained for a long time, can cause serious injuries up to the loss of the nails and sometimes the last phalanx and almost always marked and significant retraction of the first web, with notable and serious repercussions on both the functional and the morphological levels.

The main goal in these patients is to preserve, recover, and maintain the functionality as long as possible to give the patient autonomy in the management of the daily life activities.

The approach on this pathology, that is extremely disabling and recessive, is for most of the cases surgical; rehabilitation is a very important tool to optimize and maintain the results that have been obtained through surgery and can also delay the relapse that, unfortunately, always occurs. In the dystrophic-recessive EB the majority of literature agrees about the surgical treatment that consists in a degloving of the fingers and a widening and opening of the first web.

Rehabilitation starts early with a good medication and splint with a good position of fingers and wrist. Each finger is abducted and extended as much as possible to guarantee a better healing and elasticity of the skin.

The dressing will be cleaned up and done if necessary in the surgery room to optimize the results but most of all to respect the pain on our little patients; it is very important to keep the hand as open as possible until the complete healing (Image 34.37a–c).

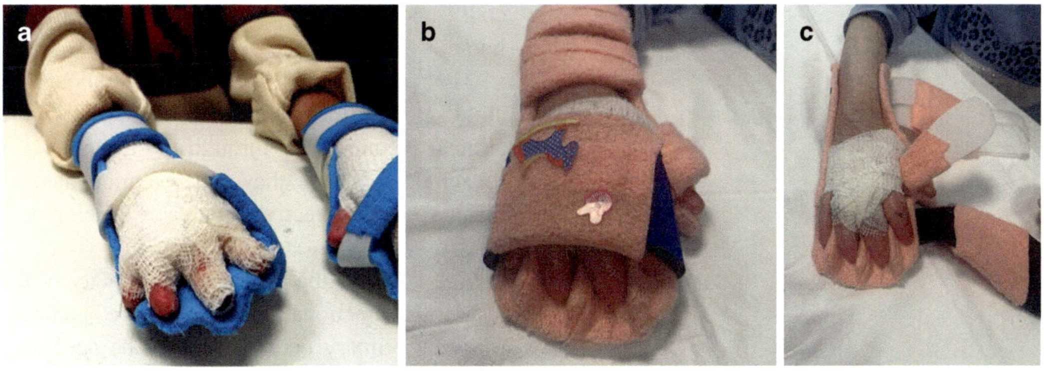

Image 34.37 (**a**–**c**) The post medication splint

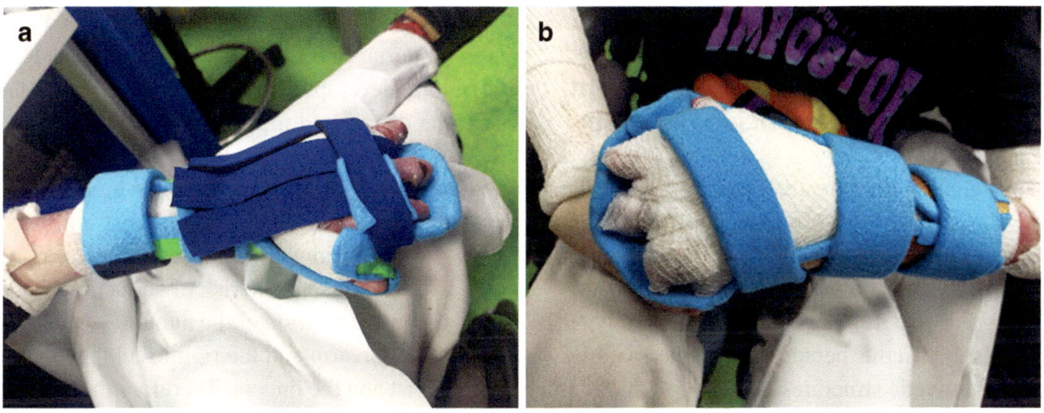

Image 34.38 (**a**, **b**) Splint

When the wounds are completely healed the splint will be removed and it will be possible to start with rehabilitation. The mobilization will be active at first and playing will be encouraged, of course in different ways for different ages. The sessions have to be associated with a tailor-made "shell" splint: in this splint the digits are abducted and the webs are compressed with paddings.

As we wrote in the introduction making a pediatric splint requires a great ability and a high experience and this is for all the children, however we can say that splints for EB are the most difficult ever. This is because every little pressure or every small part of the splint without padding can cause a rubbing on the skin and this means excoriation and wounds that can take a lot of time for healing. This problem can also speed up the relapse. A great attention has to be made on paddings and the choice of materials, often splints for EB patients need to be covered and protected also externally to avoid rubbing on the face or on other parts of the body (Image 34.38a, b).

Every exercise or game has the aim of opening the hand as much as possible, especially for the widening of the first web to promote its independence.

Because of the skin fragility in those patients the scar massage and the use of silicon patches are not suggested, to avoid the occurrence of hypertrophic scars (Image 34.39).

Physically those patients are extremely limited; however it is very important for the therapist to remember that cognitively they are perfectly on time and this is why they need to improve in daily activity as much as possible; an appropriate and individual ergonomic proposal is needed and different for every little patient.

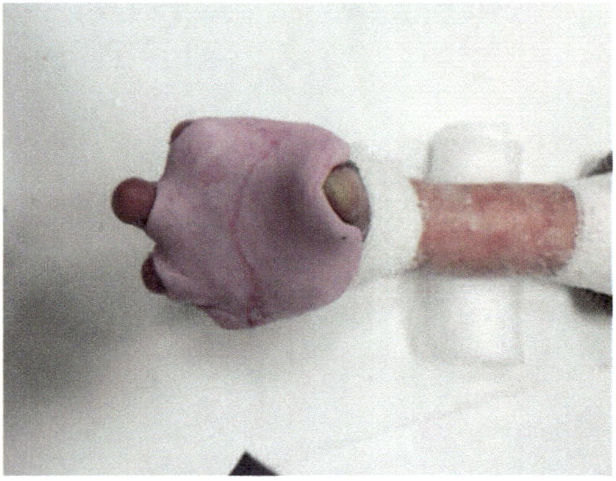

Image 34.39 Silicon patch with elastomer

34.13 The Rehabilitative Treatment of the Obstetrician Paralysis

The rehabilitative treatment of the obstetrician paralysis is a long process that must start with the diagnosis, i.e., since the birth until the end of the growth of the little patient.

To adequately deal with this long way, it is necessary that the therapist knows the anatomy of the involved structures associated with the lesions, the timing of the nervous regeneration, the problems related to the nervous lesion, and the phases of the development of the child's motor and cognitive competences.

Knowledge from all these allows us to elaborate a rehabilitative project whose long-term aims are streamlining of functional recovery and the overtaking of all the psychomotor development phases.

To reach the aims, all the operations adopted by the therapist must have as a primary purpose the prevention of secondary lesions of the musculoskeletal and cutaneous apparatus generated by the nervous lesion, the promotion of the activation of muscle groups under reinnervation, and the facilitation of the development of a correct body scheme that includes the superior limb involved in the nervous lesion.

In order to optimize the treatment results, it is necessary to involve the parents who must be taught about the meaning of their child's pathology, about its correct management, and especially about how to carry out the exercises at home.

The parents must be informed about the child's possibilities based on the evolution of the clinical picture. Only through the awareness of the clinical picture they will be motivated to reach specific objectives for each development phase.

According to the level and the gravity of the lesion, the functional recovery can be spontaneous or a primary operation might be necessary after 3 or 4 months of birth if the biceps action is absent as well as palliative operations to balance out residual motoric deficits at the age of 3 or 4.

In all of these cases a rehabilitation has a primary importance because it allows the prevention of rigidity development as well as joint deformation, the denervated muscle hyperextension, and the neglection of involved limb.

For each lesion level, the superior limb tents to acquire specific faulty attitudes that must be known to be prevented. In case of high lesions (C5, C6, C7), there is the risk of adduction rigidity and internal rotation of the humerus, in pronation of the forearm and the rigidity in the flexion of the wrist and the fingers. Therefore in this type of lesions the passive mobilization must be focused on the maintenance of the external passive complete rotation, on the elevation and abduction of the shoulder.

The rigidities of the inter-rotation are very common and dangerous as they lead to a bone deformity of the humerus head and they promote the posterior sub-dislocation of the humerus head. They are caused by the withdrawing of the shoulder inner-rotation muscles, the front capsule, and the anterior glenohumeral ligament.

The bone deformations of the humerus head do not allow the mechanic rotation of the head itself inside the glenoid cavity of the shoulder blade, and they make impossible the external passive rotation and as a consequence they frustrate any possibility of recovery of the active movement.

The most efficient intervention to lengthen the inner rotator cuff, above all the subscapular one, is the one with abducted humerus and 90° bent elbow. In case of premature rigidities it is recommended to tailor a night tutor which maintains the humerus in abduction and extrarotation, in order to keep the muscles retracted and in extension for many hours.

The second risk in these lesions is the dislocation of the radius head that could happen in case of operations of forced supine position and it could provoke, as a consequence, a rigidity in the flexion of the elbow.

In low lesions (C8 T1) the risk of rigidity is set in the supine position of the forearm and the deformations of the hand are similar to the ones provoked by the lesions of median and ulnar.

In total lesions risks and problems are summed up and they lead to a much more difficult clinical picture.

The mobilization must be carried out by the parents at home many times a day; it must be gentle and complete and it must cover all the involved zones of the lesion.

During the first week of birth, it is suggested to keep the arm at rest through the use of the pin that maintains the humerus close to the chest and the elbow in bent position, to facilitate the reabsorption of the post-traumatic, mostly in case of associated lesions as the collarbone breaking.

At the end of the first week, the program of passive mobilization of all the districts of the superior limb should start; it has to be gently and delicately carried out, without forcing the joint to the maximum grade and by making stable the proximal joint compared to the mobilized one.

During the arrangement of the mobilization program associated possible lesions have to be considered; according to them, timing and procedures of the mobilization and the treatment must be modified. The most frequent lesions are the breaking of the collarbone and the humerus as well as the lesion of the phrenic nerve and, as a consequence, the alteration of the breathing pattern caused by the ipo-validity of a hemidiaphragm.

The parents have to be informed not only on the procedure of mobilization but also on the baby's daily handling, in order to avoid other traumas and tractions of the arm.

Proper strategies have to be taught for the baby's nappy changing moment, for breastfeeding, for the position during sleeping and for the moment in which the baby is awake.

A very useful but practical example, which could seem banal, is to dress up the baby starting from the damaged arm and continuing with the healthy one, and vice versa to undress him.

The little attention allows the parents to reduce at the minimum the arm traumas in the baby's changing moments.

Finally, we have to teach the importance of stimulating the involved arm with surfaces of different consistency, put themselves to the side of the damaged arm, and so on, to facilitate the integration of the arm into the body scheme.

As it is in this very first phase, the use of positional static tutors to obtain the correct alignment of the wrist and the hand is suggested. In case of total lesions it must be produced a tutor in safety position (extended wrist MF bent IF in position zero, thumb in opposite position with the opening of the first space), and in case of high lesions C5, C6, and C7 a tutor in extension of the wrist and, if needed, one tutor to correct the attitude in extension and pronation of the elbow.

The use of tutors is an integrating part of the obstetrician paralysis treatment. They can be static, dynamic, or functional, for the wrist and the hand or for the elbow, according to the different phases and to the baby's clinical case.

In addition to the tutors, another tool at disposal is the functional bandage, used to control the instability of the shoulder blade, to encourage the shoulder movement, or to correct with attitude in pronation of the forearm.

In addition to the passive mobilization, the therapist has to stimulate the active recruitment of the muscular groups in the innervation phase, through postures, games, and movement that call and reinforce those muscular groups.

With the child's birth, games and manual activities have to be proposed to him and sports like swimming and dancing are recommended; they are not only useful as a muscular reinforcement but also as a psychological crossing of the diversity given by the primary lesion.

The most frequent residual deficits in the older children are, in the high lesions, the complication in the active abduction and in the elevation of the shoulder, the asymmetry in the flexion of the elbow, and the deficit in the supine position.

The elevation deficit is due to the weakness of the anterior deltoid and to the hyposthenia of the external rotators, whose activation allows the *greater tuberosity* to turn and pass under the coracoacromial arch.

Therefore in the reinforcement program, the deltoid and the external rotators of the humerus have to be reinforced.

Another particular element is the detachment of the medial border of the scapula during the movement of abduction of the shoulder.

The scapula mobility must be optimal to allow the recovery of scapular-humeral rhythm and, in case of muscular deficit that activates the scapular-humeral one, the movement of the scapular-thoracic allows a better orientation of the humerus into the space.

Associated contractions are another problem. They inhibit the expression of movements functionally valid for the lack of the normal balance between agonist and antagonist muscles.

Co-contractions and hyperactivity of muscular group that prevents to the ipo-valid antagonist to express its strongness (for example the hyperactivity of the triceps that causes a deficit in the flexion of the elbow) can be treated with the use of botulinum toxin. This procedure is under experimentation.

In the obstetrician paralysis treatment the patient's global vision must not be forgotten. With the growth, the imbalances generated by the asymmetry of the superior limbs must be supervised.

Sometimes other problems can occur, like the scoliosis or the lumbar hyperlordosis, which increases the effort of elevation of the arm.

For the complexity of the pathology and for the presence of many factors to be evaluated, the treatment has to be carried out by a multidisciplinary equipe composed of the surgeon, the physiotherapist, the pediatrician, and the psychologist.

The role of the psychologist is fundamental to follow the parents the initial phase and, in the second period, the baby, who in the growth become aware of the problem.

34.13.1 Summary of the Rehabilitative Project of the Obstetrician Paralysis

0–3 months: aims of physiotherapy the muscular-skeletal secondary lesions stimulations sensibility involvement of the damaged limb into the development of the body scheme stimulation active muscular recruitment correct placement and handling.

34.13.1.1 Activation of the Biceps?

YES: carry on with FKT: aim: progressive stimulation of the active muscular contraction and development of the psychomotor scheme.

NO: primary surgery intervention:

0–3/4 weeks: fixed tutor in damping

4 week: begin with the mobilization in damping and the placement in damping since week 5: carry on with the passive mobilization and the progressive muscular recruitment together with the recovery due to the distal reinnervation (see paragraph).

34.13.1.2 3–4 Years Old: Sufficient Functionality for ADL?

YES: carry on with a focused FKT and sport

NO: possible palliative intervention (see paragraph)

34.13.1.3 Supervision of FKT Until the End of the Development

Pay attention to the posture, stimulation for the use in the ADL, sport activity (Images 34.40, 34.41, and 34.42)

34.13.2 Post-surgery Treatment

Surgery for both primary and palliative obstetric paralysis has to be considered a rehabilitative

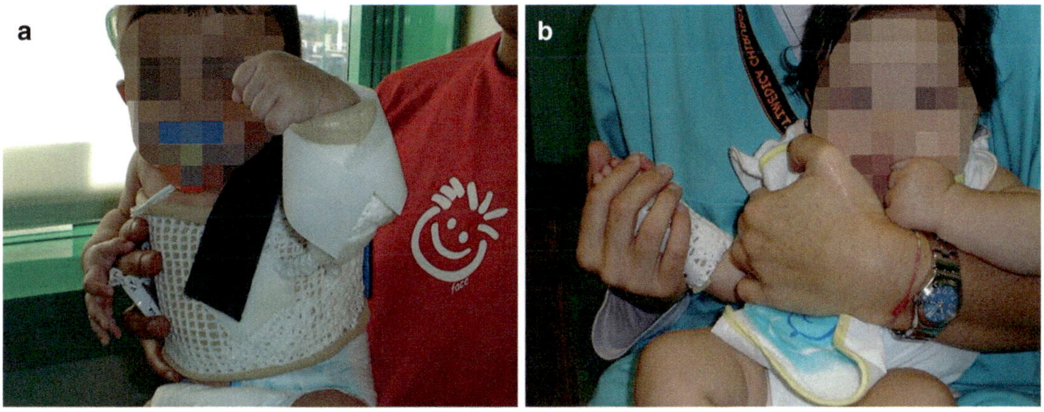

Image 34.40 (**a**, **b**) Splint in abduction and external rotation of the humerus and stretching of the interrotators

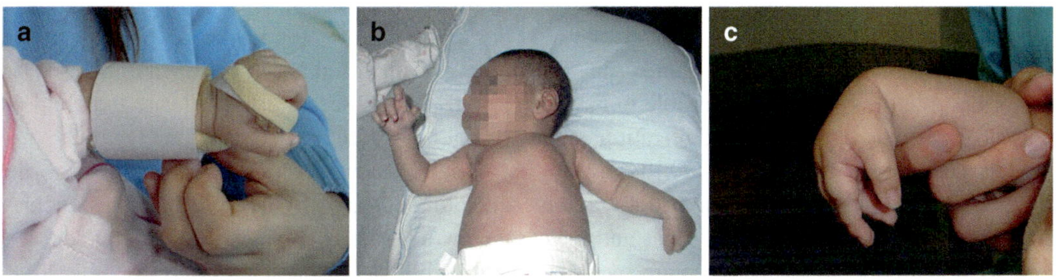

Image 34.41 (**a**–**c**) Tutor in extension of wrist in p.o C5 C6 C7

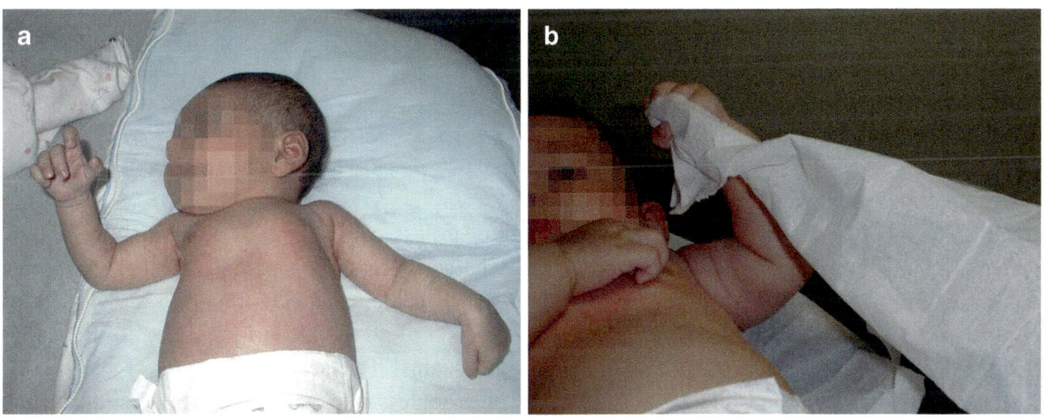

Image 34.42 Appearance of the biceps activity after 3 months after birth. (**a**) At birth. (**b**) After 3 months

moment. As such its aim is to optimize the recovery of the upper limb's mobility.

For some children, recovery is spontaneous. For others surgical intervention is necessary and it is the therapist's job to set the conditions to reach an optimal result.

During this stage it is necessary to educate parents on the desirable objectives of the surgery and on the meaning of each rehabilitative step after the surgery. Parents' collaboration is fundamental to obtain constant mobilization and stimulus for the young patient.

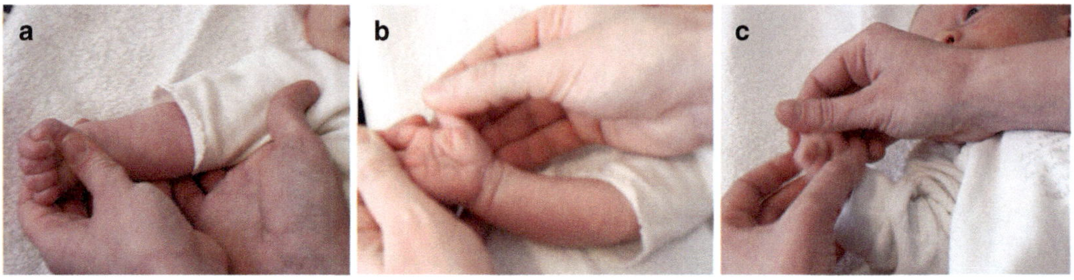

Image 34.43 (**a**–**c**) Passive mobilization

The therapist has to give parents a written and personalized program. This program includes home rehabilitation exercises, the position of the upper limb, and the correct activities for a specific rehabilitative moment and the physical development of the child.

In the rehabilitative program games play an important role. It is in fact not possible to have a classic program based on mobilization and strength exercises. The therapist will have to develop a specific play-based program taking into consideration the child's physical and psychomotor abilities, which can change over the course of the treatment.

All post-surgery treatments have common as well as specific elements based on the surgical technique used. Because of this it is necessary to communicate with the surgeon about the patient's clinical picture and the anatomical structures involved in the surgery, before preparing a program.

Another important element to consider before writing a treatment is the importance of the young patient's evaluation. This evaluation has to be done constantly to verify the evolution of the clinical picture and adjust the objectives of the treatment.

It is hard to evaluate a child as he/she will hardly remain in classical position for muscular evaluation and even harder to comprehend muscles sensitivity. For muscular evaluation the therapist will once again have to use games and activities that allow testing on major muscle groups or once the child is a little older use simple exercises such as bringing a hand over the head or to his/her mouth. As for muscle sensitivity the therapists will use a scale of evaluation by Narakas; this scale evaluates responses to hurtful stimulus on a scale of s0–s5.

Sensitivity is fundamental for functional recovery: an arm that can't feel, can't be used, so it will also be necessary to educate the child on recognizing stimulus from different entities.

The last consideration has to be done to the evolution of the body structure and has to include the involved limb. If not correctly stimulated, the child will likely exclude the limb from this structure. This will limit the possibilities of its functional use, no matter the post-surgery or spontaneous regeneration of nerve tissues (Image 34.43).

34.13.3 General Principles of Post-surgery Treatment

Regardless of the type of surgical intervention, whether primary or palliative, there are some treatment elements in common to be considered.

First of all the idea of protection of the surgical seams. The seams, nervous, or the tendon ones are less resistant and, under stress at an early stage, they can break.

The first aim of every post-surgery intervention is the protection of the seams. The strains that can break the seams, frustrating the surgical intervention, are strains in the hyperextension of the nerve or of the involved mio-tendon unity.

Therefore to protect means to put in damping, i.e., in shortening the involved anatomic element.

It is fundamental to know the anatomy and to communicate with the surgeon to know the timing and procedure of mobilization that will be specific for each surgical intervention.

During the immobilization period, it is important to supervise and to treat the edema, which is an actual physiological glue that, if not treated adequately, leads to retractions of the soft tissues and joint rigidities.

To eliminate the edema, the parents must be informed about the correct placement of the limb that must be kept raised up as much as possible, about the icy applications that must be carried out many times a day for at most 20 min, and about the early mobilization of the joints not involved in the intervention.

Moreover during the period of immobilization, the parents must be taught about the supervision of the plastered device or of the fixed tutor that must not cause reddenings or secondary damages to the skin.

In this period it is suggested that the therapist supervises the baby once a week to verify the correct placement of the fixed tutor as well as its tolerability.

At the removal time, the therapist sews a removable tutor that usually proposes the same position of damping given during the immobilization.

This tutor will be initially removed only for the daily hygiene or for the physiotherapy and it will be gradually left, with specific timing and procedure based on the type of intervention.

During this phase, the scar treatment starts. It is fundamental to prevent adhesions with the underlying tissues and to avoid problems of scarring hypersensibility.

It is important to teach the parents about the scar tissue release massage that must be carried out ¾ times a day with the use of cream for 10 min each. If the scar becomes hypertrophic the use of little sheets of silicone or elastic compressive sheaths is suggested, whereas in case of adhesive scars the negative syringe that plays the function of vacuum therapy is used.

In children, as the cellular hyperproduction, the formation of hypertrophic scars is easy, which must be treated and eliminated as soon as possible.

The treatment of desensitization establishes the use of gradually more rough surfaces that must be rubbed on the whole hypersensible zone in order to bring sensibility threshold back to a normal level.

Besides the scar treatment, a program of protected mobilization takes place, i.e., an analytical joint mobilization which maintains still in damping (in shortening) the involved structures. These structures will be stimulated during the following weeks.

In this case too, timing and procedure of protection change according to the surgery technique.

One important thing to remind is that after the primary intervention, nervous graft of neurotization, and after the period of immobilization, the active motility is overlapped to the previous one before the intervention.

To observe change in the clinical situation, we must wait for the reinnervation period, whereas in case of mio-tendon transfer we could notice the results after the immobilization period, because a functioning muscle has been moved to obtain the missing function. It is fundamental to communicate this to the parents who must not have false hopes after the primary intervention, in order to be motivated in carrying on the treatment.

Another important principle in the recovery of the functional contraction: in case of primary intervention, we must evaluate the different muscle groups that regain their functionality based on the nervous regeneration, whereas after the transfer it is necessary to teach the child how to recruit the muscle that carried out a different function and how to recover the one that was missing before.

In the reinforcement program of the denervated muscle that is gradually reinnervated, we have to remind that at the beginning the muscle will be able to carry out only isometric contractions and only with time isotonic contractions.

All the neuromuscular techniques of facilitation must be used that lead spontaneously or with reflection the active contraction in the involved muscle. Techniques like tapping, the brushing of the muscular stomach, etc. can be carried out, and above all games that allow the baby to recruit the involved muscular groups.

Electrostimulation must be mentioned, but it is very much discussed in literature, in particular in children' treatment.

Regarding the primary intervention, the only possible indication is the use of e.s. with exponential streams, to be applied during sleeping with the only aim of maintaining the trophism of the denervated fibers waiting for the reinnervation. In case of transfer the use of rectangular e.s. is suggested, indeed, in the pre-surgery treatment, with the aim of reinforcing the muscle to move that is going to lack a grade in the scale m0–m05 of strength, once moved.

For the recovery of function besides movement the recovery of sensibility is fundamental. In case of obstetrician lesions, it is more correct to speak of education to sensibility, because the involved parts have never been experimented to have any kind of sensible perceptions.

The treatment considers the brushing of objects and tissues of different consistencies on the on the cutaneous zones involved in the lesion. We must remember that the child's competences evolve with his growth. Indeed, a child learns how to recognize an object at the age of 4–5 and he learns to discriminate due dots at the age of 9.

We have to try to reactivate the sensibilities, reminding that the proprioceptive is supported also by the passive mobilization, which has a double role: maintaining the PROM and sending proprioceptive important information or the integration of the limb in the body scheme during the growth.

In all the post-surgery treatments the use of tutor that plays different functions according to the specific rehabilitative phase is useful.

They can be used in place of the plaster cast during the immobilization period, with the advantage of being light weight, transpiring, and hence much more tolerable by the patient; they can be also used as a prevention tool or to correct rigidities (for example static tutors that maintain the wrist in extension or the hand in safety position in case of total lesions, or in the treatment of the rigidities of the elbow, tutors that flex the elbow gradually that tends to the extension position, to inhibit the activity of the triceps during the period in which the biceps activity is absent or lacking).

Another function of the tutors is helping in the use of the limb involved in the lesion: for example in case of an approximal recovery of the shoulder but not distal of a hand, a tutor for the wrist with an applied Velcro on which anchor games help the child in the use of the damaged superior limb in the bimanual grabs, using the paretic hand as a passive grab, or in case of ipo activity of the triceps, it is possible to tailor a tutor in extension of the elbow to facilitate the quadrupedal stand and so stimulate the child to creeping.

Thanks to this, besides helping the psychomotor development of the child, we stimulate the recruitment of the muscles of the shoulder girdle thanks to the load induced by the superior limb in stand.

In case of untreatable rigidities through passive mobilization, it is suggested to tailor dynamic tutors that keep the retracted pericapsular structures in a gradual traction as well as the tendon structures that are tight to the adjacent tissues.

The tailored tutors for children must be stuffed to avoid cutaneous ulcers and they must be modified over time, according to the child's growth or to development of the clinical situation (Image 34.44).

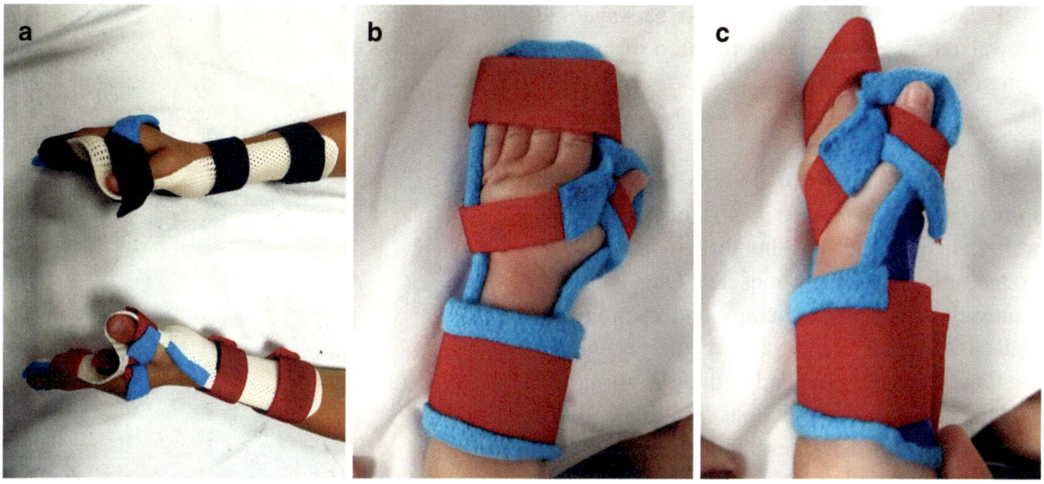

Image 34.44 (a–c) Preventive splints: rest position

34.14 Thumb Hypoplasia and Pollicization

Thumb hypoplasia and thumb agenesis represent at the same time the more compromising malformations for hand usage, but also those with more reconstructive surgery options with good results.

In fact, in several forms the results obtained with the surgery have acceptable morphological and functional aspects.

On the basis of pathology staging and surgical options (see Chap. XX), the rehabilitation program will optimize and improve the results obtained both in terms of aesthetics and mobility.

Therefore, the rehabilitation program will be personalized and adapted to the surgeon indications.

The main goal is to improve and stimulate the integration of the first ray during game and keep the first web wide enough to allow the correct grasping of objects with different dimensions.

The day of surgery the hand therapist made a splint in thermoplastic material.

The day of surgery an immobilization splint is packaged directly in the surgery room either by the surgeon through a pinstriped valve or by the therapist. After the change of dressing, which can take place in deep sedation or in the clinic according to the indications, a removable splint is packaged to allow the start of the mobilization and rehabilitation protocol. The splint may have different characteristics depending on the surgical technique performed, but it will always pursue the objectives such as:

- Protection of the transferred/reconstructed structures
- First web opening
- Comfort and ease of use for our little patient and caregiver

34.14.1 Rehabilitation Protocol Post-surgery in Thumb Hypoplasia

In the case in which surgery has been performed to reinforce the thumb in the malformation of the thumb hypoplasia, such as the tendons transposition interventions like the one according to Huber Littler, the hospital protocol will pursue the following objectives.

In the immediate post-intervention we will have to protect the transferred structures allowing the correct healing in the position given by the surgeon and avoiding stress on the transferred tendons/muscles.

A cast immobilization will be packaged to keep fixed for 3–4 weeks in position of opposition of the first ray.

34.14.1.1 21 Days

Following the change of dressing a removable splint is packaged (Image 34.45) to keep the first web well open and the thumb in opposition to protect the transferred muscle. This splint is removed during physiotherapy and in moments dedicated to the re-education of the gesture, to the functional recovery, and to the grip stimulus.

The rehabilitation sessions will take place every day to teach the parents/caregiver the appropriate stimulation techniques and at the same time the rules for the protection of the transferred muscle. Attention should be given to stress-threatening moments for the transferred muscle, for example during the child's sleep and free play, as well as if the small patient is in the training phase of the walk because of the risk of falling on the hands.

The treatment of the scar through manual massages is very important to mature it elastic and normotrophic. To limit the risk of pathological scarring, saddles in thermoplastic material or tape will be used combined with a silicon patch or elastomer compression able to keep open the first web (Image 34.46).

We will gradually insert exercises to stimulate the grasping of objects of various sizes by taking advantage of games and play activities based on the age and predisposition of the little patient.

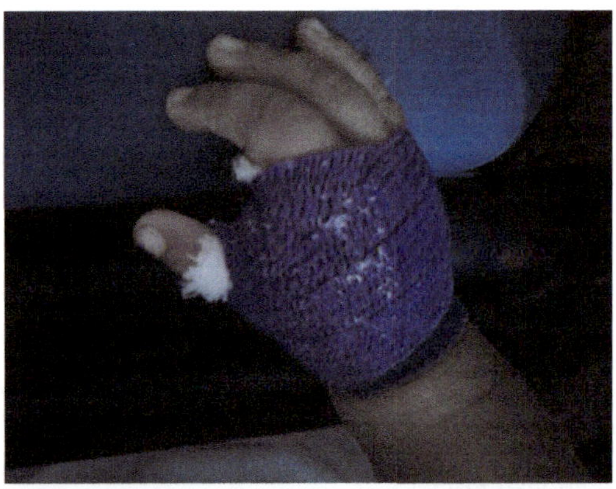

Image 34.45 First dressing

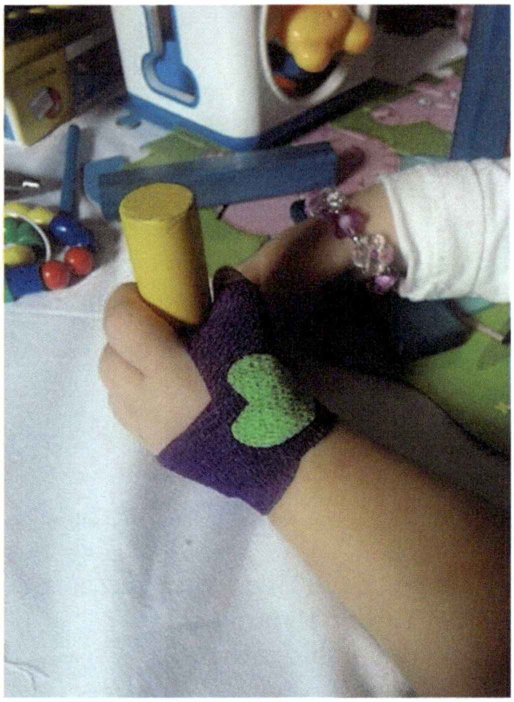

Image 34.46 Dressing with compression and first web opening

We can also use electrostimulators with low-intensity electrical stimulation to be applied to the transferred muscle both as biofeedback to stimulate the corticalization of the gesture and to strengthen the muscle itself that, as we know, once transferred partially loses its strength if the lever of biomechanical action is modified (Image 34.47).

34.14.2 Early Rehabilitation Program After Pollicization

The rehabilitation after pollicization has two main goals: firstly, to protect the "new" thumb and its sutures on tendons, nerves, veins, and arteries and the stabilization on bones; on the other hand, to stimulate active movement, sensibility recovery and its corticalization.

After surgery the patient wears a cast immobilization for 10 days; after this, the patient has a change of dressing under anesthesia and the cast is removed and replaced by a removable hand-

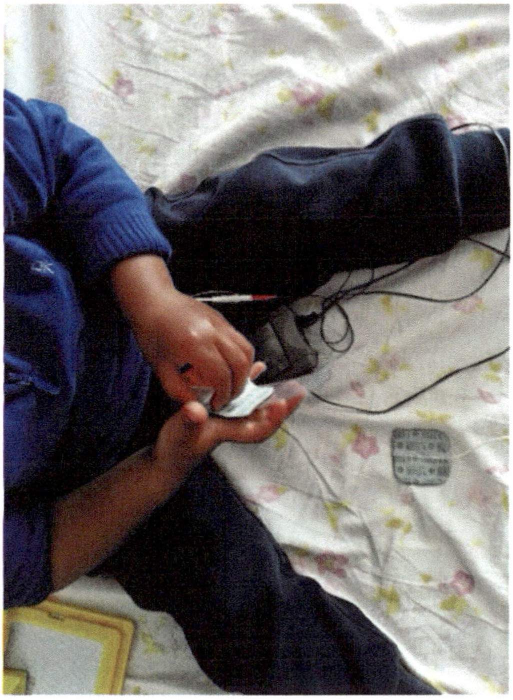

Image 34.47 Electrostimulation

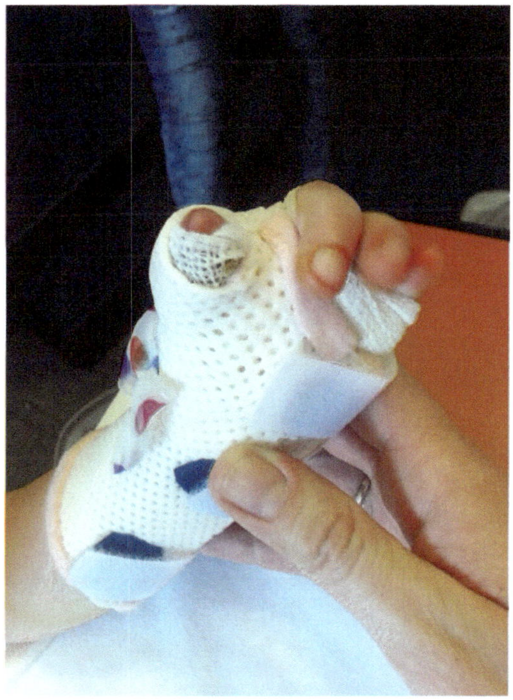

Image 34.48 First splint

made splint in thermoplastic material. The splint includes the wrist, with the MCP joint of the first ray included.

At the beginning the splint will be worn always, except during physiotherapy and home exercises, and it will be progressively abandoned first in the daytime hours.

The rehabilitation program lasts around 8 weeks, with daily sessions and specific exercises at home. After the acute phase, physiotherapy sessions will be complemented by psychomotor sessions, to spur the correct development and involvement of the limb in the pattern of movement of the correct age.

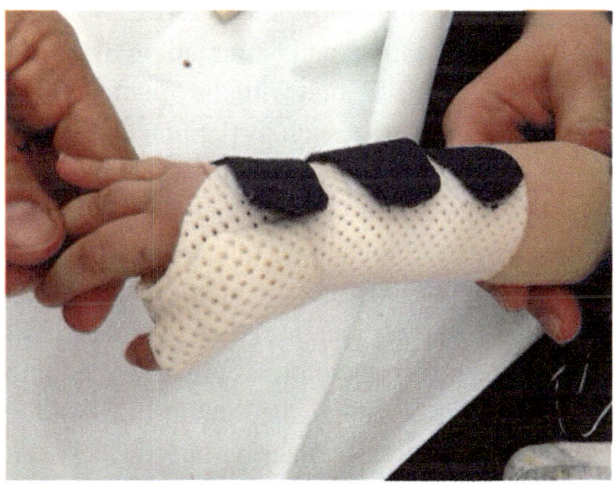

Image 34.49 Removable splint with reduced dressing

34.14.2.1 Days 0–10

Cast/splint immobilization with the wrist included and the thumb in abduction and opposition (Image 34.48).

At day 10 the patient has a change of dressing under anesthesia (to limit trauma for the child), and the cast is removed and replaced by a removable handmade splint in thermoplastic material with the wrist included, the thumb in opposition and abduction and its IP joint free (Image 34.49).

34.14.2.2 Days 10–21

The splint can be removed only for exercises of assisted active mobilization of the first ray, keeping it in an abducted position and avoiding lateral deviation.

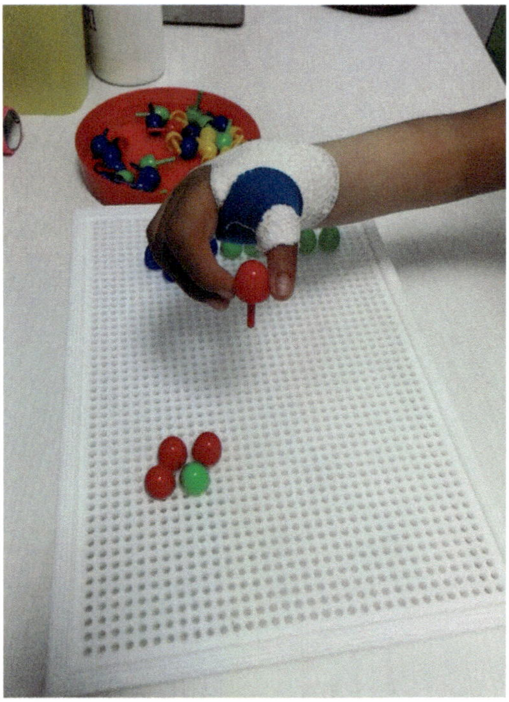

Image 34.50 Games

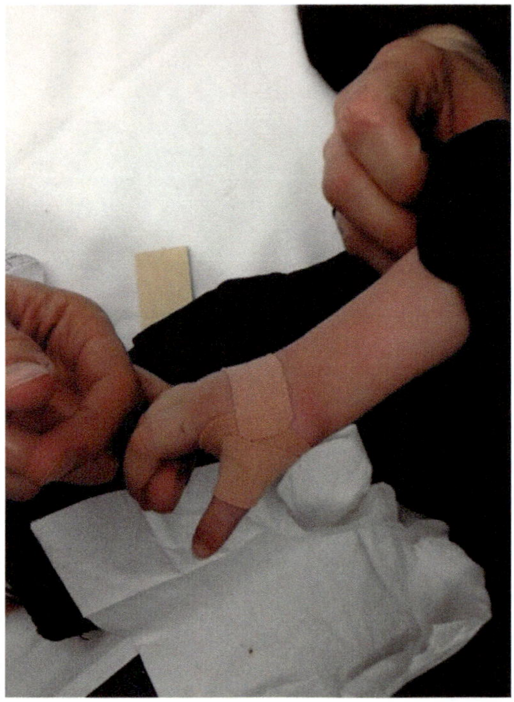

Image 34.51 Taping to stimulate opposition of the new thumb

During physiotherapy sessions we work on passive mobilization and stimulation of active recruitment of the IP joint with the use of targeted recreational activities such as the functional grip of objects of different sizes between the new thumb and the second finger (Image 34.50).

The correct stimulation is fundamental because the brain has to construct the motor image of the neo-thumb (motor imaging) that did not exist before the surgery; therefore it will be essential to avoid since the beginning the establishment of the pathological pattern of interdigital grip between the second and third fingers. The therapist can use a bandage to stimulate and favor the position in opposition of the thumb (Image 34.51).

From day 21 up to the fifth week, physiotherapy will continue with the stimulation of the use of the first ray, favoring the grip of objects of different sizes and shapes, also taking advantage of the bimanual grip. This activity must be progressively increased and meanwhile the splint will be abandoned from daytime also at home by instructing parents or caregivers (Image 34.52a–e).

By the healing of the scars, its treatment begins which involves both manual massage and compression with elastomer and silicone patches at night. At this stage taping can be placed directly on the skin of the new thumb to stimulate through biofeedback the good position in opposition and the wide opening of the first web.

Moreover, the therapist will mobilize globally the new thumb in opposition.

We can also use a functional splint without wrist include (Image 34.53).

From the fifth week the splint can be completely abandoned in protected situations (meals, games in a protected situation, hygiene, etc.) and kept only for protection; it will still be worn at night. Considering the best age for this intervention, between the 12th and the 18th month of age,

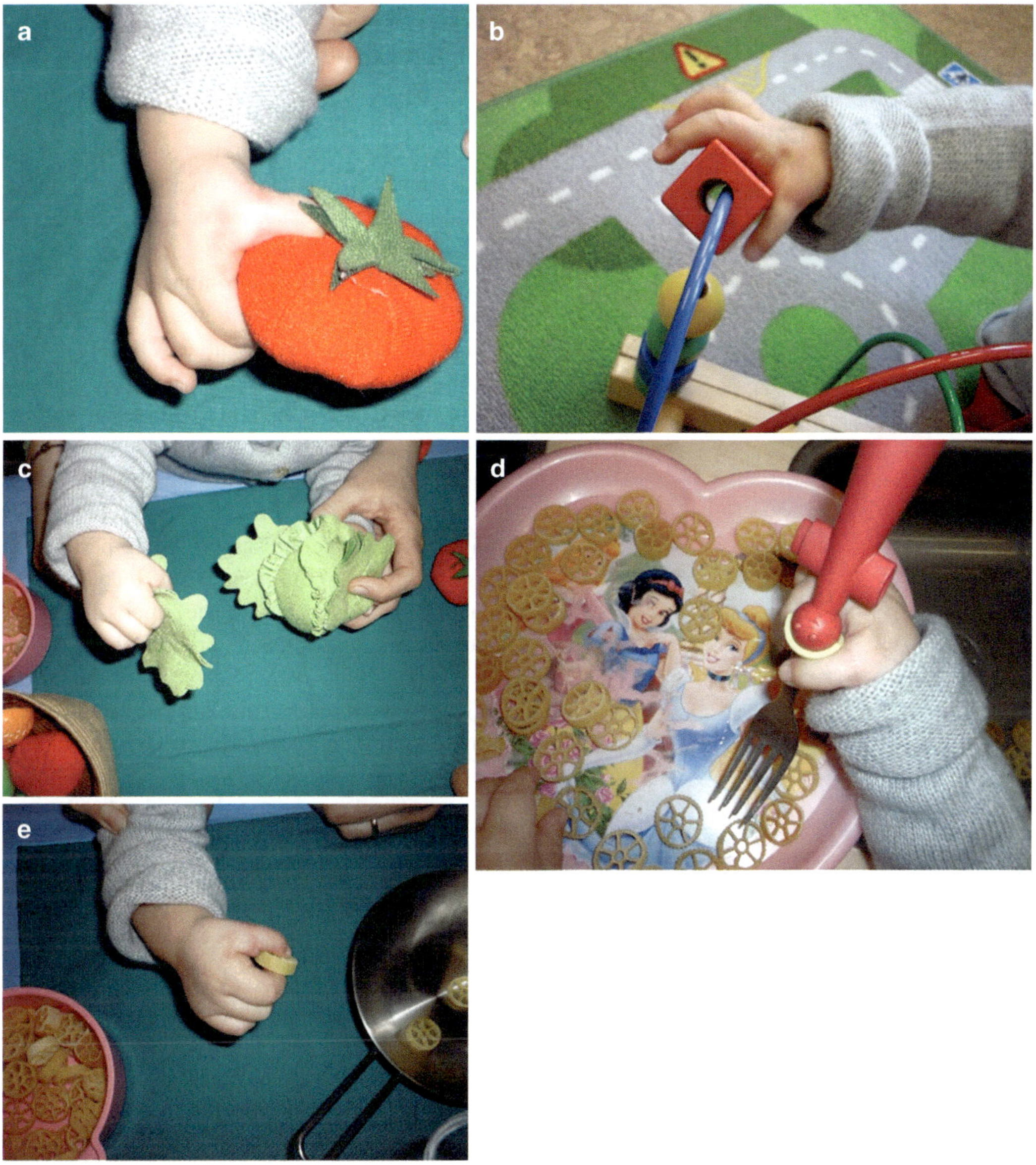

Image 34.52 (**a**–**e**) Examples of games

the moments at risk could be considered the stages of crawling or first steps to avoid excessive trauma to the new thumb.

At this stage, you can also start to selectively mobilize the MP and TM joints as well. From the sixth week it is possible to make a dynamic pro-flexion splint in case of residual stiffness of the MP joint; this is the most frequent event in case of the pollicization of a camptodactyly second finger (Image 34.54). If necessary, the splint can be made to obtain a global flexion of the neo-thumb.

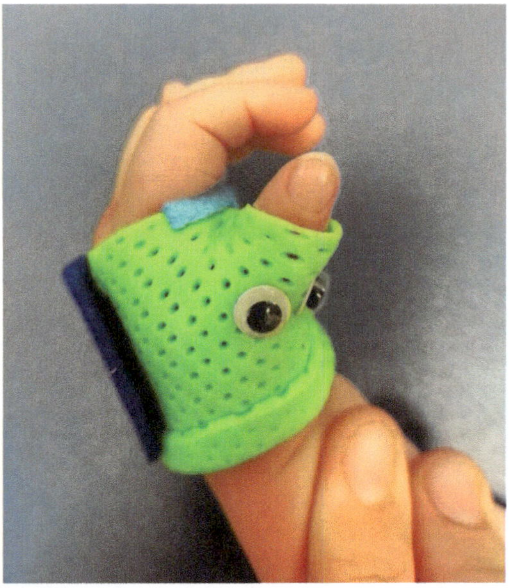

Image 34.53 Functional splint for the day

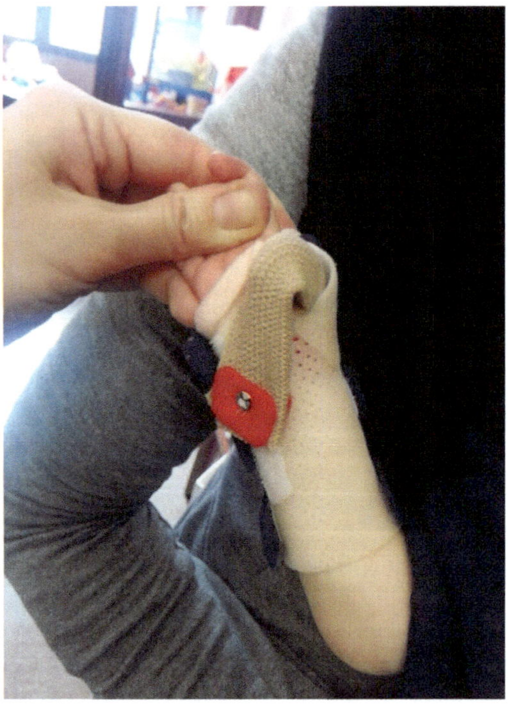

Image 34.54 Dynamic splint

34.15 Radial Cleft Hand: Rehabilitation

Patients affected by radial club hand present different aspects which affect the general use of the entire upper limb: shorter forearm, radial deviation, low to severe dysfunction of the thumb or, in the most severe stages, its absence, reduced long fingers AROM. The concomitance of these problems limits the chance to have a functional grip and consequently it is essential to begin an early rehabilitation program with continuous follow-up to monitor the clinical conditions during the growth.

The major problem during the growth of these patients is the frequent recurrence of relapses that may occur despite the surgery being performed: this can be due to different causes linked both to intrinsic factors such as the impossibility of releasing radial soft tissues completely or extrinsic elements such as the scarce use of the proper splint and the frequent stimulus to the radial deviation due to functional gestures like bringing the hand to the mouth. Unfortunately, the clinical situation can be considered stabilized only with the end of physiological bone growth.

The rehabilitation program begins taking charge of the patient after the first visit with the surgeon. It is divided in two different approaches:

- Conservative treatment: it starts immediately after the visit and lasts in the preoperative time.
- Post-surgery treatment: it starts after the surgery.

In both the approaches the treatment is endorsed by the surgical team, the therapist, and the patient's family, who becomes both a receiver and an active participant in the process.

34.15.1 Conservative Treatment

In this approach the rehabilitation program begins immediately after the first visit with the surgeon: the sooner it occurs, even in the first weeks after birth, the better the chances of obtaining significant results.

The goals are:

- Correct education of the parents concerning the treatment to be performed at home: they become essential to maintain and increase the results obtained during physiotherapy sessions.
- Keep the structures that will undergo surgery soft, to prevent stiffness onset that could affect the surgery itself.
- Keep the wrist, thumb (if present), and long fingers joints mobility free
- Promote the integration of the affected upper limb during daily life activities and games.

The therapist sets up the rehabilitation program together with the parents' child, after an in-depth initial evaluation and considering the surgical timing (if defined and if needed).

It includes:

- Soft tissues manipulation and wrist stretch in ulnar deviation: it needs to be done at least every 2 h.
- Passive mobilization of long fingers and the thumb (if present): it needs to be done at least every 2 h.
- Circular splint with the wrist included must be worn always except during physiotherapy and for hygiene. The splint will be modified gradually according to the achieved results (Image 34.55).
- Stimulation of ulnar active deviation and grasping of different objects through play.

The conservative treatment lasts till the day of surgery or if the functional results achieved can be considered acceptable with no surgery needed.

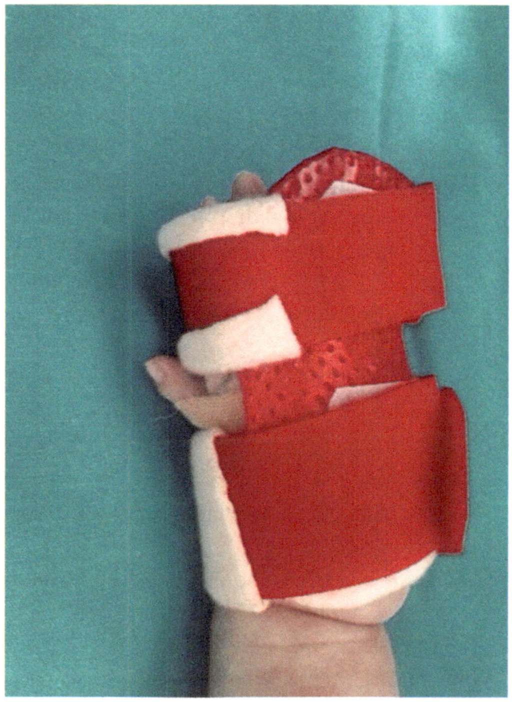

Image 34.55 Circular splint

34.15.2 Post-surgery Treatment

The rehabilitation program begins immediately after surgery. The goals are defined according to the specific indications provided by the surgeon considering the surgical technique.

The short-term goals (0–2 weeks) are:

- Correct parents' education to handle the operated limb.
- Edema control.
- Protection of the structure involved in surgery.
- Maintain or increase long fingers mobility.
- Integration of the limb through games and bimanual activities.

The therapist will pursue these goals through:

- Correct limb placement to favorite edema control, especially during day nap and night.

- Use of a fixed circular splint with the wrist included to maintain the alignment after centralization or a protection in thermoplastic material above the external fixator in case of bone lengthening.
- If necessary, long fingers and thumb (if necessary) stretching both in flexion and in extension.

The mid-long-term goals (2–8 weeks) are:

- Protection of the structure involved in surgery (Image 34.56).
- Maintain the alignment obtained through surgery.
- Prevent scar adhesions that can affect the surgical results.
- Maintain or increase long fingers and thumb (if present) mobility.
- Integration of the limb through games and bimanual activities (Image 34.57).

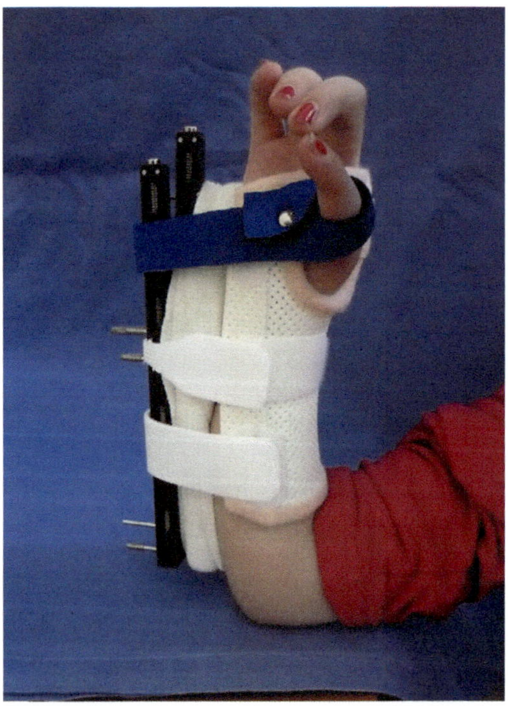

Image 34.56 Protection splint

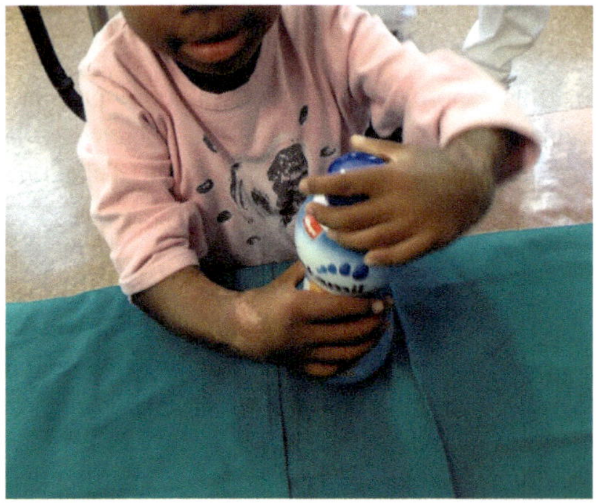

Image 34.57 Integration of the limb through games and bimanual activities

The rehabilitation program is structured as follows:

- Use of a removable circular splint with the wrist included, which will be gradually abandoned, at the beginning during physiotherapy, hygiene, and play. It will be worn at least for 8 weeks, after that only at night time.
- Use of a taping on the ulnar side of the wrist to maintain centralization and as a biofeedback on the wrist movement and muscle stimulation.
- When possible, scar treatment with massage to prevent scar adhesions. During night the patient uses a silicon compressive patch.
- Stretching in ulnar deviation and passive mobilization of long fingers and thumb (if present). In case of severe rigidity of fingers, it is possible to make a dynamic splint to improve MCP joint flexion and a static dorsal splint to be worn during the night to improve extension.
- Stimulus in ulnar deviation and grasping through games.

Rehabilitation in patients affected by radial cleft hand needs specific indications provided by the surgeon according to the surgical technique and so the program must be personalized and well defined.

It is essential to have continuous follow-up during growth and check functional gesture to analyze the results obtained and their evolution over time; in this way it is possible to adapt the splint and the rehabilitation program gradually.

34.16 Psychomotor Therapy

Psychomotor therapy is a rehabilitative discipline useful to rearrange the right balance between motor, psychomotor, emotional, cognitive, and neuropsychological functions, through the privileged use of game and its multiple significances.

The Neurodevelopmental Disorders Therapist takes on the child in all its psychophysics being, using these tools: bodily mediation, motor and symbolic way of playing, tonic dialogue, graphic and physical expression, drama, and music. The rehabilitation enhances the strong points of the child, working on its potentialities to increase its capabilities while understanding its limits.

The psychomotor intervention is directed toward children in their developmental period paying specific attention to those affected by motor delays, coordination problems, spatial disturbances, abnormal movements, disorders of lateral dominance and muscle tone, autistic spectrum problems, psychomotor inhibition, neurological or psychological problems, and so on.

In our Hand Surgery Department, the Neurodevelopmental Disorders Therapist collaborates with the Hand Therapist to rehabilitate children with congenital problems at the upper limbs in their postoperative period. This kind of rehabilitation is beneficial for young patients because it helps reintegrate the operated upper limb into their body schema and their daily activities in a harmonic way.

The rehabilitative session takes place in a specific setting, which changes according to the age and the characteristics of the patient. Before the session begins, the therapist decides the use of tools and toys to reach the target of the therapy.

Psychomotor therapy is a branch of rehabilitative medicine that deals with severe and chronic diseases in youth. It gives value to the entirety of the young patient, considering both the balance and the integration of its functions and competences, and the interaction between the developmental phase and the evolution of the disease. Psychomotor therapy considers the child as an inseparable union between affectivity, motricity, and cognitive structures.

Through strategies based on play, the therapist encourages the harmonic growth of the child's potentialities respecting its age and personality.

In Italy, the Neurodevelopmental Disorders Therapist supports the capabilities of each child by creating specific and individualized plans in an educational-precautionary dimension and in a therapeutic one, by considering both its habilitation and rehabilitation role.

Focusing on the therapeutic aspect, the work of the therapist is part of a complex rehabilitative program that employs a multidisciplinary team. In our Department the Neurodevelopmental Disorders Therapist collaborates with hand surgeons, hand therapists (physiotherapists and occupational therapists), psychologists, pediatric nurses, and anesthetists.

The theoretical frame in which the Neurodevelopmental Disorders Therapist works is represented by the bio-psychosocial model of disability recommended by the World Health Organization.

The Neurodevelopmental Disorders Therapist's intervention area is represented by developmental diseases such as those due to a disease, a disturb or a known impairment, and all other situations in which the patient has got difficulties in performing, participating into, and achieving the Growth Project.

In this Hand Surgery Department psychomotor therapy adapts itself to the children affected by upper limb malformations to promote the use and the participation of the upper limb while playing in the global context.

After a surgical operation, psychomotor therapy is quickly integrated in the treatment protocol respecting the surgical healing. The therapist creates an individualized rehabilitative path based on the problems of the patient.

The Neurodevelopmental Disorders Therapist works with children affected by neuropsychiatric diseases in a preventive and rehabilitative dimension in the areas of neuro-psychomotricity, neuropsychology, and developmental psychopathology. The competence area the therapist can work with is developmental age, from birth up to 18 years of age.

The main domains a Neurodevelopmental Disorders Therapist works on are the following:

- Physical domain: muscle tone, motor coordination (gross motor and fine motor skills), laterality, cooperation between the upper limbs while doing unilateral or bilateral tasks, handwriting planning movements, and spatial and temporal organization;
- Psychological domain: interactive skills, verbal and nonverbal communication, body image, body schema, taking initiatives, body control, space and safety awareness, play level;
- Intellectual domain: praxis domains, cognitive and executive functions, self-care activities.

Referring to what has just been said above, this kind of rehabilitation is useful if the child displays one or more problems in these domains. In this perspective, the pathologies that can be treated by a psychomotor intervention are several and so different from each other that a mere list of pathologies would not be thorough.

The children treated in this Department display upper limb malformations, obstetrical palsies, cerebral palsies, and injuries. These conditions can be isolated or in morbidity with other pathologies and can be the reasons why the child does not use its body correctly or has difficulties with social relationships. It is clear now the complexity of this kind of rehabilitation.

The Neurodevelopmental Disorders Therapist creates an individualized rehabilitative path based on the patient's problems. The objectives are based on the features of the child and the problems shown.

The aim is reached not through a teaching-learning path, but in a communicative context, in which the child and the therapist can exchange and enhance their own resources.

In this Department, the therapist never loses sight of the child's holistic appearance and pays close attention to how the child uses the hand affected by the malformative condition while playing and in the development of the physical abilities suitable for its age. The therapist brings the child to achieve new competences that it will use for the rest of its life.

Starting from the observation and the assessment of the child's global appearance, the therapist makes proposals to reach the child's maximum potential in daily activities (i.e., ADL, self-care activities, school activities such as writing, cutting, and pasting, physical activities such as riding a bicycle or playing sports, and social integration), holding the manipulative function in high regard. The therapist also helps improve attention and focus, self-regulation, sensory processing, and visual perception skills.

The proposals are made by using games and depend on the psychomotor development reached by the patient.

"Setting" means the arrangement of the scene in which the psychomotor takes place. The setting is the place where a person can create new possibilities of connection with the environment where he/she lives thanks to its physical-emotional-informational context.

The therapeutic setting is a reasoned work situation, a combination of specific general conditions that allow to give to the Neurodevelopmental Disorders Therapist's actions the value of therapy.

The setting is a comfortable room that both the therapist and the children can personalize. It must have adequate stimuli, which means that the room must not be bare or chaotic.

This place is unrelated to the medication and it encourages the creation of special connections since in here the therapeutic relation is forged.

In the therapy room nothing is left to chance: the space is set up depending on the age and the characteristics of the patients and the targets to achieve.

There are three kinds of setting: setting as a physical area, setting as a mental space, and setting as a place with rules.

Firstly, the rehabilitative setting is a specific area (the therapy room), the place in which the patient, the family, and the therapist create a rehabilitative-therapeutic contract. Here the therapist can gather every shade of the evolutionary process.

Environmental stability is very important. This stability can be gained through the disposition and proposal of the objects, the safety of the room, light regulation, thermoregulation, and the stability-flexibility of the proposals made.

In this dimension, there is not only the room but also the furniture (little table with chairs, the closet, the wall bars, etc.) and the objects contained inside the room.

This place is characterized by a comfortable and peaceful atmosphere in which the therapist, the patient, and possible observers feel pleasure in staying there.

The space is usually divided into two areas: a wider zone where the patient can test its motor-global coordination and a more defined area where the patient can conduct fine motor activities, play symbolic games, and relax (Image 34.58).

The objects are selected depending on the objective that needs to be reached, the phase of the rehabilitative path, and the capabilities of development of the subject. They can be used with a functional meaning or in a symbolic way.

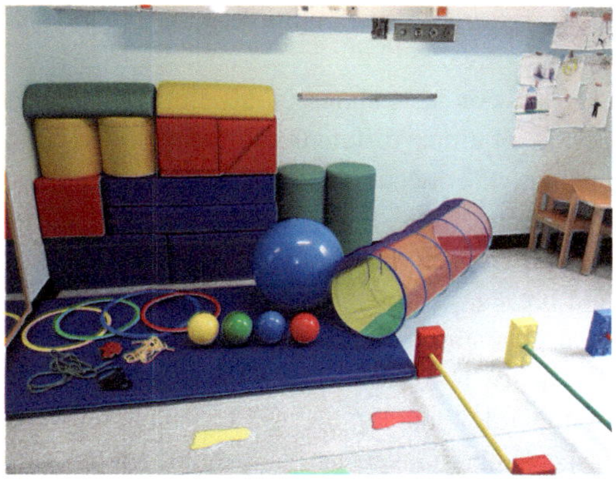

Image 34.58 Setting

There are two main types of objects: de-structured material and structured material.

De-structured objects can be found next to the walls and are always available: cushions, ropes, plastic circles, plastic canes, rubber mats, clothes, and balls are examples of this kind of material. They are objects that assume different functions and aims according to the activity in which they are employed and based on the child's and the therapist's creativity.

Structured material, on the contrary, includes objects that always have a specific function, i.e., puzzles, a small bed, crayons, colored pencils, felt-tips, modeling clay, paint, musical instruments, and assembling bricks like Lego. They are kept in a closet and employed by the therapist only when needed.

Moreover, the setting can be thought as a mental space. The Neurodevelopmental Disorders Therapist creates an empathic kind of relationship with the patient and builds a therapeutic alliance with the family and the caregivers. From this perspective, the setting becomes also a meeting place: the therapist greets the patient's efforts, then gives them back to it in an acceptable form with the aim to overcome the strife.

In addition, in this setting there is a normative dimension, which is represented by all those elements referring to the duration of the session and the rules area.

A session lasts about 45–60 min. During this period of time, different moments follow one another: the meeting in the waiting room, the beginning of the session, the central part of the session characterized by psychomotor activities and breaks, the final part of the session, and the final separation.

Finally, in this dimension there is the respect of the rules and of the roles, which must be respected both inside and outside the room.

Body Every child begins to organize its own individuality through physical experiences: starting from the first days of life, the baby communicates through the senses and the body.

In a first moment through an impulsive and reflexed dimension, then through a practical experimentation on it, the child begins building a conception of an operative itself. The child recognizes its ability to behave and lays the foundations for the future self-awareness.

By growing up, the practical experiences that the child has used so far become the basis to catch the abstract thought (and at last to catch the formal operative thought).

In this branch of rehabilitation, the body and the movement have a central role because they support and promote the global development of the child.

Successfully developing movement, coordination, and cognitive skills is the key to children to overcome their difficulties.

Relationship The quality of the relationship between the patient and the therapist plays an important role in the achievement of good results from the therapeutic path.

Since the leading channel of action in this discipline is represented by movement (not interpreted as gymnastic or sport), the relationship is characterized by a stable balance with the child's physical expression.

The attention paid to the tonic dialogue during the activities permits the therapist to keep in touch with the patient's needs, giving it the chance to build an adequate emotional modulation. This element makes it easier for the children to participate during play activities and the interaction with other people at first during the sessions and then during its lifetime.

Play The child knows the world and grows up while playing. For this reason, play is considered a privileged mediator in the therapeutic relationship and permits the child to test and incentivize its own (real and potential) abilities.

In this perspective, the therapist promotes play activities in its multiple variances (sensorimotor, symbolic, emotional-relational, socialization for instance) adapting it to the individual needs and characteristics of each child.While playing, the child tests its own body and through the movement the child comes into contact with other people and the environment. The play is a spontaneous activity that has the aim to produce pleasure.

Material As explained in the setting section, the therapist uses two kinds of objects: de-structured and structured objects. The therapist offers one or the other with different modalities during the rehabilitative session depending on the target the therapist wants to achieve (Images 34.59 and 34.60).

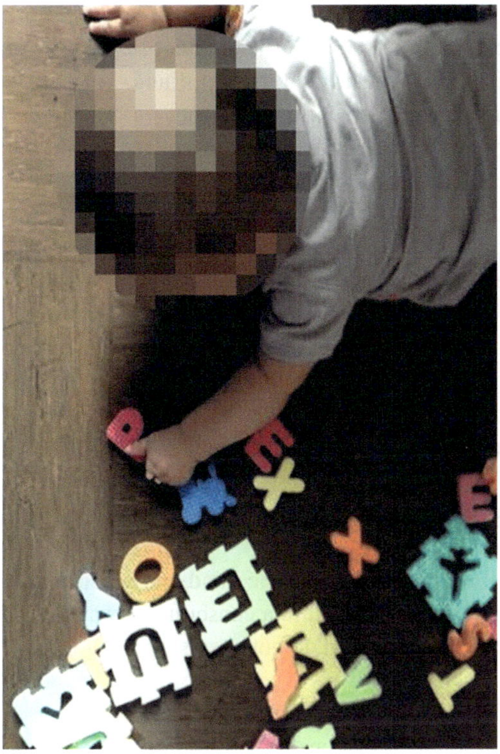

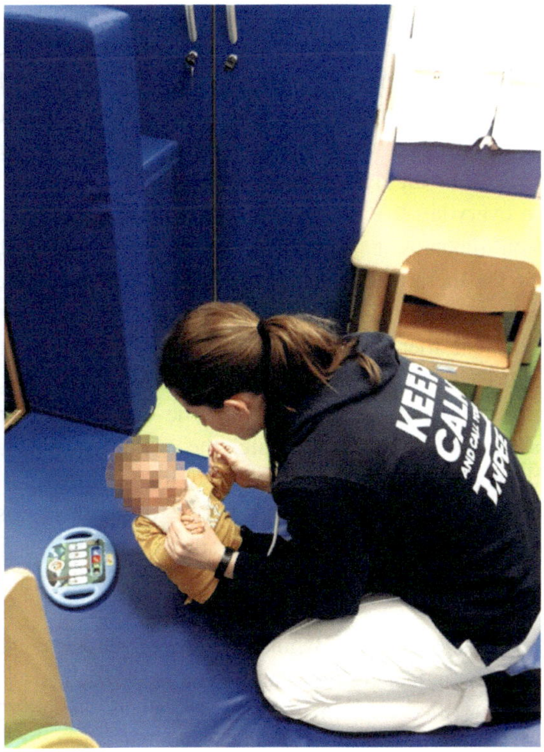

Images 34.59 and 34.60 Therapist's activity

34.17 Pediatric Hand Trauma

A trauma can be for an adult a sudden change of status, the patient is immediately more help from caregivers and the same is for children. Everyday life can change temporarily or definitively, and the child needs help and attention to accept this new status of his/her upper limb.

The trauma often modifies our motor image, and the little patient needs to adapt to this new functional or aesthetic situation and this can be hard for the child and his family. Sometimes children focus on their difference or limitation so much that this aspect becomes the most important feature of their bodies.

Emotionally children are ashamed and desire to hide the hand, they try to put the hand in the pockets, sometimes they do not want to wear T-shirts, or they avoid public situation like school and playground.

One of the first health workers that the family has to deal with is the hand surgeon, for a decision plan of therapy.

A good relationship with the health workers can increase the satisfaction of the patient and of caregivers, and this can be useful and positive also for the psychological aspect of acceptance of the new situation, this also helps to increase the compliance of the patient and of the family.

When is necessary or request a psychological support is given to the child and family, together or separately, this can help both to express the expectations and realize the real possibilities and abilities that the child will have at the end of the surgical treatment and rehabilitation.

After the surgery the limb of the little patient is protected by a bandage; often the dressing covers also some healthy segments, and this can contribute to an inappropriate and miraculous image of the hand. However this is necessary to protect properly the limb after the surgical approach.

The post-surgery period is a lapse of time in which the little patient and family have the chance to deal with anxiety, and loss of the total control of the usual status of heath we all have in everyday life. This is the time of rehabilitation; the patient starts to get used to: be touched by the therapist's hands, to see the injured segment and the whole hand or arm. During the physical therapy it is very important for the patient to have a high compliance, because it plays an important role in it. The aim of the therapist is to rehabilitate the whole limb through games and playing with children. Rehabilitation can be very difficult for pediatric patients, much more than with adults, especially for very traumatic accidents.

It can be very hard to obtain a high level of compliance for the whole section of physical therapy; in fact children can be shy, or worried or even terrified sometimes; this is why the therapist needs to be patient, especially if some particular movements are required for the situation. Often a good observation of the child, respecting the motor milestones and the cognitive growth, can be the key for a good rehabilitation, and also often change games and toys, choosing something appropriate for the aim of the physiotherapy but fun in the meantime is essential.

The younger is the child the easier is for him to adapt to new situations; the same works with neuroplasticity: with a good rehabilitative plan, a good relationship between the little patient and the therapist, the child will be able to regain dexterity and good motor skills, and this means good functionality and quality of life.

34.17.1 Fractures

Over 25% of traumas in pediatrics are fractures: in particular in the early stages of age crushing traumas often occur, and adolescents often injure themselves while they are playing or doing sports.

In crushing traumas distal phalanges and external rays of the hand are often involved. Interphalangeal joint traumas and volar plate lesions are also quite common.

All muscular-skeletal injuries have a different evolution in children compared to the same injury on an adult; in fact the elasticity of the different tissues and the presence of the growth plate need a different therapeutic approach.

Particularly the surgeon will pay attention to the possibility of interfering with the correct growth of the limb or segment, or having distal problems on nerves, or lately with secondary arthritis, stiffness, or chronic pain.

Bones in children can change quite quickly in shape, rotation, and alignment, if they are subjected to stress.

Many fractures of the hand and wrist in children can be treated in a conservative way, with a cast or splint, and do not need surgery.

34.17.1.1 Conservative Treatment

Immobilization needs to be done immediately after the reduction of the fracture, particularly if the little patient is under anesthesia. A cast is probably the better choice for children, casts in fact are very resistant, and often the immobilization is wider than it should be for adults: for example in a very young patient with a fracture of a phalange it is necessary to include the wrist too. If the cast is small or light the risk is that the child can be able to remove it or damage while he plays or sleeps.

In compound fractures normally the treatment is cast immobilization for 3/4 weeks and then a visit after an X-ray, when the cast is taken off a removal splint is made by the therapists. During the following days a specific rehabilitative with a hand therapist begins.

34.17.1.2 Surgical Treatment

Surgery in pediatrics is very different from surgery in adults: the periosteum is thick, growth plates are delicate, so the surgeon has to pay attention during the whole surgical approach.

34.17.2 Apical Traumas: Rehabilitative Part

In pediatrics distal phalangeal traumas are quite common; crushing traumas represent the most of apical traumas, but also hyperflexion or hyperextension.

Crushing can generate lesions of the nail or sub-nail hematoma, or more complex trauma like complete lesion of the nail bed, fracture of the distal phalanx, or a lesion of the flexure or extension tendon.

In case of surgical flap suture also with microfractures after 4 weeks with a fixed digital splint (Image 34.61).

The patient can start the active mobilization with a selective recruitment of the flexor digitorum profundus, exercises for the recruitment of extensor tendons. When the wound will be completely healed, the therapist can begin the treatment of the scar with a hydrating cream and with the use of a silicone elastomer during the night (Image 34.62), associated with a CoBan bandage to give to the finger the correct compression for a proper skin remodeling.

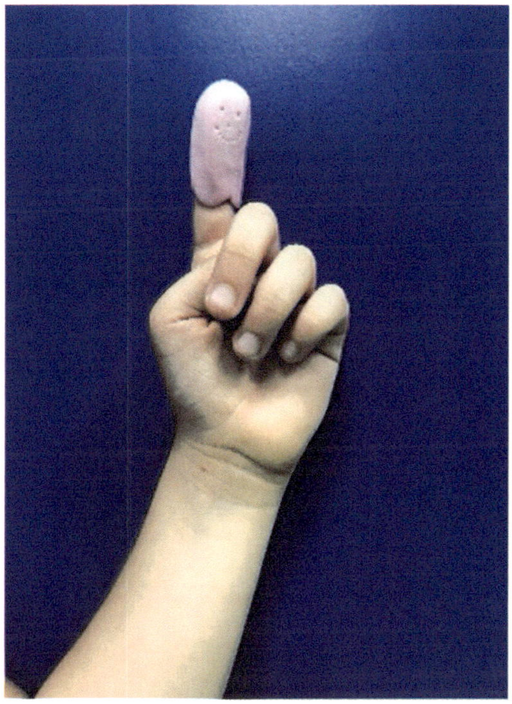

Image 34.62 Compression

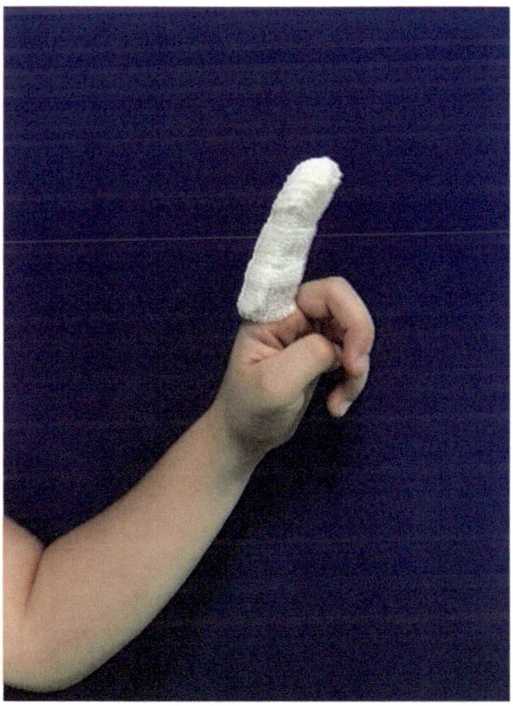

Image 34.61 Digital splint

The therapist will teach the parents how to do exercises for sensibility in order to manage the alteration of sensibility that is completely normal in this situation; this can help a quicker recovery and a quicker corticalization.

A digital and removable splint will be used during the night and in risky situations like schools and playgrounds until 8 weeks from the surgery.

In case of sub-amputation of the distal phalanx the postoperative period will be of immobilization with a digital splint in protection of the amputation stump (Image 34.61).

When all the wounds are completely healed, the hand therapist will make a removable splint in order to protect the stump, the parents will be taught how to massage the scars and the use of silicon sheets will be suggested for the night. Also in this case sensibility has to be stimulated through different tissues. It is very important that the little patient at the end of the therapy is able to

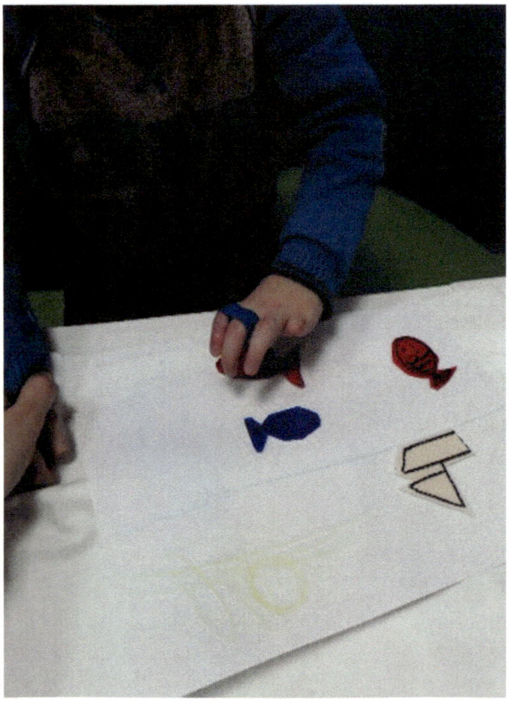

Image 34.63 Example of manual activity

use the fingers involved in the trauma for all the activities of daily living (Image 34.63).

34.17.3 Tendon Lesions in Pediatrics

Tendon lesions in children have a high incidence because they explore the world outside with their little hands often without paying attention. If these lesions are not treated properly they can cause important functional deficits and deficits of growth; the child in fact can learn daily activities with the complete exclusion of the segment or of the whole hand.

However it is very difficult to treat children with this kind of lesions because sometimes they have a very low compliance and little hands and little fingers are very difficult to treat and to splint.

The major difference between the treatment of an adult and a child in this field is that treating a child means a bigger immobilization and bigger splints that can include also did it and joint that are not directly involved in the trauma, with the aim of give more stability and to be safer (Image 34.64a, b).

The time of immobilization is on average longer than in adults; for example in the lesion of flexor tendons we begin physiotherapy at the end of the fourth week keeping the splint that will be made removable, with the wrist extended 0^-20, metacarpal-phalangeal joint at about 30^, and interphalangeal joint extended (Image 34.65a, b).

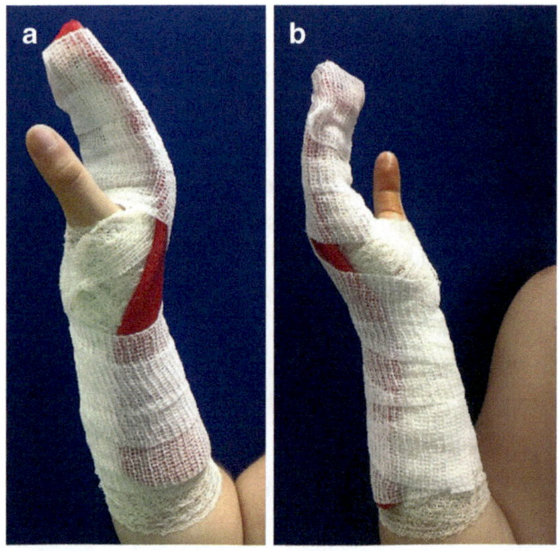

Image 34.64 (**a**, **b**) Immobilization in pediatric tendon lesions

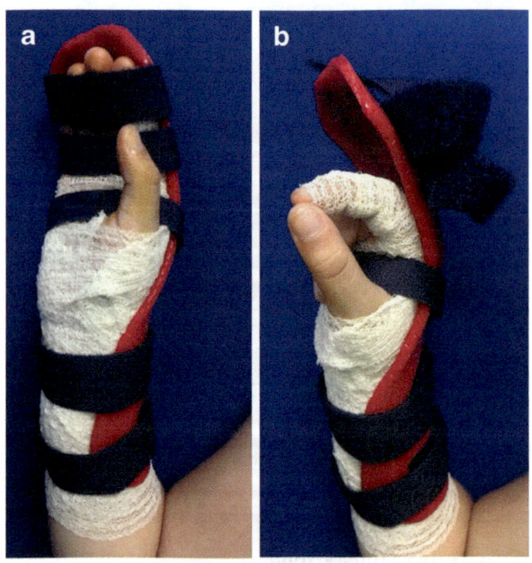

Image 34.65 (**a**, **b**) Removable splint

Disposition is chosen in order to avoid intrinsic muscle retraction.

Sometimes the surgeon chooses the pull-out technique, this can allow immediate mobilization, and the little patient will have of course a limit in the maximum open extension. The splint is going to be removable from the very beginning and will be made in the same position that we explained before in order to protect the suture of the tendon.

The weaning of the splint will take a little bit longer for your patients, especially during the night and in risky situations.

The recovery will be placed basically on playing; the therapist will choose with the little patient games and toys that can be appropriate for the situation and the age.

Fortunately in children the elasticity of the tissues helps to reduce the post-immobilization stiffness.

The massage of the scar will be extremely important and has to be done more than four times a day, not very long but very often during the day. The technique of the massage is to do it slowly with pressure in order to avoid a thickening of the scar and to limit the establishment of adherence in the deep tissues.

Another tool that needs to be associated with the massage is the use of silicon sheets, to wear during the night, that means for at least 8 h per night. It is very important to spend some time during the rehabilitation process paying attention on the recovery of sensibility on the scar and nearby areas; this can be done with the stimulation of the part with different tissues from the softer to the rougher.

In case of stiffness after 8 weeks it will be possible to make dynamic splint to increase the mobility of the single finger or of more of them.

During the tenth week, the therapist can try to use electrostimulation in order to promote the sliding of the tendons and reduce the possibility of adherence, and for biofeedback.

At about 12 weeks if there are no deficits the patient can go back to normal activities and use the whole limb like the other.

Also in extensor tendon lesion the therapeutic approach should be performed cautiously.

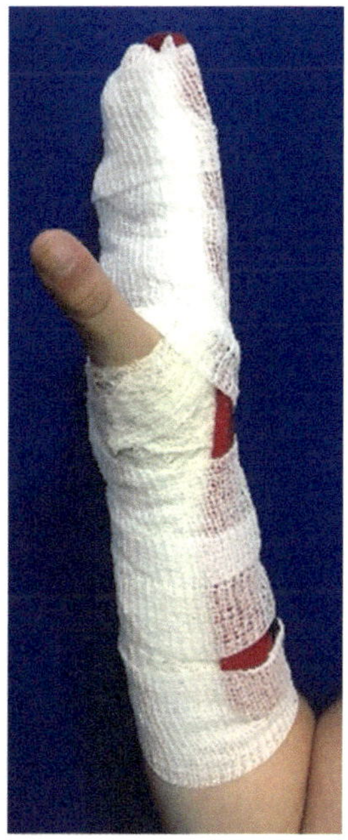

Image 34.66 Splint for extensor lesion

Normally the time of immobilization is of 6 weeks with a splint in extension of the fingers and wrist in a neutral position (Image 34.66).

At the end of the sixth week we start to move the little hand of the child, making a removable splint. The therapist will teach the little patient and parents some exercises for the fingers like the "hook" and the "roof," so gradually as the flexion improves the patient will be able to do a complete fist. To help the patient to understand how to close the hand the therapist will provide some targets, like cylinders from bigger ones to smaller ones. During the rehabilitative session different kinds of grips will be offered to the child in order to recorticalize the correct gesture of the single hand, and of both in bimanual grips.

For sure also in this case the treatment of this scar when healed will be very important, and will follow the rules that we have explained before such as multiple massages during the day and the use of silicon sheets during the night. The extensor tendons slide immediately under the skin; this means that normally a scar has more possibility to do adherence with the next tissues and this can limit the range of motion. This is why the parents need to learn from the therapist how to do dynamic sliding: this means they fix the skin in one way and they asked the child to extend or flex the schools a double effect on the scar and can be very useful. Also in this case during the week if there is stiffness the therapist can make dynamic splint in flexion to increase the range of motion.

At about 12 weeks like for flexor tendons, the rehabilitative protocol ends if the patient do not present any deficit, and normal activity is permitted.

Association to Support Babies and Families

35

Amy Lake, Martina Pajardi, and Elena M. Mancon

Abstract

The concept of therapeutic camps for children with chronic conditions has been around since the 1970s and proven to provide psychosocial interventions to help decrease the burden of disease and provide support, respite, and skill building through recreational activities for diagnoses such as spina bifida, epilepsy, pediatric cardiac conditions, and cancer (Bar et al., J Pediatr Hematol Oncol 32:358–365, 2010; Holbein et al., J Pediatr Psychol 38:412, 2013; Sawin et al., J Neurosci Nurs 33:57–64, 2001; Bultas et al., J Spec Pediatr Nurs 8:320–328, 2013).

Congenital anomalies of the hand and upper limb which can affect function, social interactions, and self-confidence (Lake, Tech Hand Up Extrem Surg 14:78–84, 2010) is a new diagnosis benefiting from the concept of camp. This need was observed by Texas Scottish Rite Hospital, a specialty orthopedic hospital, in 1995. At that time, a Hand Camp model was developed and has evolved and expanded through the years. This model was studied in 2015 which generated a publication. The impact of therapeutic camp on children with congenital hand differences (Lake, Cogent Psychol 8:1, 2021) shows an increase in the areas of self-esteem, physical function, activity participation, and peer relations.

Hand Camp offers children born with a congenital hand difference the opportunity to learn from other peers and counselors with similar hand differences on how to navigate through everyday life. From putting hair up into a pony tail or painting fingernails, to tying shoes and throwing a baseball, each child can learn new skills from individuals with the same exact hand difference. This connection builds self-esteem while also improving physical functioning and ultimately allowing children to be accepted by who they are on the inside instead of defined by what the look like on the outside.

Keywords

Camp · Hand differences · Congenital hand differences · Hand camp · Pediatric hand therapy

The birth of a child brings positive emotions of joy and happiness, but if this event is conjoined with the diagnosis of a congenital malformation

A. Lake (✉)
Department of Upper Extremity and Microsurgery, Scottish Rite Hospital for Children, Dallas, TX, USA

Department of Hand Surgery and Rehabilitation, San Giuseppe Hospital IRCCS MultiMedica, University of Milan, Milan, Italy
e-mail: amy.lake@tsrh.org

M. Pajardi · E. M. Mancon
Department of Hand Surgery and Rehabilitation, San Giuseppe Hospital IRCCS MultiMedica, University of Milan, Milan, Italy
e-mail: elenamarta.mancon@multimedica.it

G. Pajardi (ed.), *Pediatric Hand Surgery*, https://doi.org/10.1007/978-3-031-30984-7_35

sometimes associated with a syndrome, families may live this moment with anxiety, worry, and fear.

The pathologies and malformations involving a child inevitably represent both a familial and social issue, at first micro-social issue referring to the environment surrounding the family's daily life and then tackling the sometimes harsh encounter with society.

The network of relationships that will be created around the newborn will be essential until the rational and conscious social comparisons occur. The newborn will not appreciate that he is special and just born this way initially however will benefit from the invaluable network made up of family, relatives and friends who are able to support the parents and child, who are at the beginning of both an amazing and complicated journey.

The network then expands with the first medical and specialist visits. The medical component provides all-around care, with an entire team dedicated to the patient and his family, and is composed of highly specialized figures: the surgeon, the pediatrician, the pediatric nurse, the pediatric anesthesiologist, the physiotherapist, the neuro- and psychomotility therapist, and the psychologist.

The presence of a supportive network that works as an exchange of information and contacts among the families, can be a positive framework of specialist that can decreased anxiety, confusion and doubts. Today in Italy, there are different associations that are involved with children affected by upper limb malformations. One example is DEBRA Italia Onlus, an association that deals with epidermolysis bullosa congenita, a serious systematic malformation that affects the invalidating limbs, and another example is the Italian Association of POLAND Syndrome, which is concerned with children touched by this syndrome.

Other malformations strictly involve the upper limb or just the hand and therefore are not part of a syndromic picture; in recent times, more associations such as the Macrodactylia National Association founded on 16 December 2017 have been created to unite children affected by macrodactyly and their families.

Other times the malformative frameworks are so rare or diversified that many families find themselves alone when the affected child is born, lacking adequate health information and time guidelines on when to go to specialists and without knowledge about regional permits, reimbursements, or anything else that involves the household. Parents suddenly find themselves in a new life that is inevitably changed, because of the birth of a new child and the added challenges and difficulties that this beautiful moment will bring them.

Most of the children followed by our department present malformation patterns that involve solely the hand or upper limb, without there being signs of a systemic syndrome or of pathologies related to the entire organism. These have evoked such great interest in the past couple of years that an entire association was created to unite and represent them. In 2008, thanks to its President Elisabetta Palleroni Pajardi, the *La Mano del Bambino Association* was founded, an association that helps families share experiences, flashes of daily life, and health information.

"The Child's Hand Association purpose is to create scholarships or financial aid for individuals or organizations that will then begin a specific activity working towards the same goal, and creating regulations to ensure the funding.

It will promote courses or will follow meetings and conferences about the hand and the upper limb, having the ability to range from medical students or similar specialties, to physiotherapists and occupational therapists who are pursuing degrees and courses of various levels and formalities, but whose validity is shown through the structure of the organization and the quality of the speakers and participants. It also works to help and collaborate with professionals of all backgrounds whose work is in synergy to that of the association.

It will work to promote the circulation of information and publicity at every level, journalistic, television, with participation in debates, seminars, and meetings of all kinds both at the associative level and on behalf of the individual components with special reference to occasions that might have wide cognitive emphasis to the user level.

Specifically, its aim is to inform the medical and paramedical field on the one hand, and the population on the other, on what the main pathological events concerning the upper limb may be and the consequent remedies, with particular attention to the preventive moment, as well as traumatic events or arthritic-degenerative pathologies, working to ensure that a more correct social medicine and preventive hygiene can protect the hand as a fundamental organ of family life, work, and relationship."

At the World Conference on Malformations held in Dallas in 2012 and chaired by Elisabeth Ezaki, Professor Pajardi's staff learned about the arrangement of the campus, implemented in that reality and which is discussed in an extremely comprehensive way in the first part of this chapter. Wanting to adapt this initiative to the sensitivity and the Italian mentality, Professor Pajardi, together with his wife Elisabetta, created the first Italian Campus dedicated to the Child's Hand on 22 September 2012. As guests of the Good Shepherd Foundation led by Sister Cristina (Maria Luisa Triulzi), families were given a moment of meeting and confrontation with others that allowed children to live a nonclinical experience of play and entertainment and parents to compare the health journeys that they are going through, deriving benefits and reassurance in a way that is more effective than by solely comparing themselves with the health world.

The campus therefore sees two different moments that take place in parallel throughout the day. During the morning, there are a series of lectures by the surgeon, the anesthesiologist, the rehabilitation therapist, and the psychologist whereas in the afternoon, moments of dialogue and confrontation with families with the "question-answer" approach. In parallel to this, the children are involved in moments of play organized by volunteers and members of the association and the department, in which both the group and individual activities are divided by age group and that are frequently focused on the use of hands. In these moments, there is no distinction between pathologies, and it is wonderful to see how children affected by malformations who are still waiting for treatment compare themselves with others who have already undergone treatment and how they meet and interact with siblings and friends who do not have these problems, perfectly integrated with no reason for difference or marginalization.

Illustrious guests from the sports, art, and social worlds of Milan, who had been treated in the Department of Hand Surgery of the Hospital San Giuseppe Multimedica, always accepted to participate during these moments of celebration and valued the opportunity to get back to their artistic and sports activities. They participated in seven editions: the motorcycle champion Bertolasio Samuele; the Olympic fencing champion Matteo Tagliariol; the marathon runner Luca Zanardini; the Italian basketball champion Luca Fumagalli; the European champions of Judo of the State Forestry Group Luca Ardizio, Aldo Scollo, and Giulio Sacchi; and the musician Alex Battini de Barreiro.

In recent years, the Fire Brigade Corps of the Provincial Command of Milan has been included, thus combining a moment of recreation with one of education, sensitizing children to their duties of social life and relationships.

Starting from the next edition, there will also be a time to meet with the dogs that participated in the Hospital's pet therapy rehabilitation practice.

This is not the only time for family support, though. A similar initiative called "Gazebike - Pedala for La Mano del Bambino" has also been taken in Rome, supported by the Buratti family. Its purpose is to combine cultural experiences such as discovering historical points in Rome through bicycle rides, with times of information and comparison with the population, to sensitize people to the reality and the functional implications, although fortunately often solved, related to children's hands.

The Christmas Market is another activity implemented by the association that serves to unite all families without connotations of pathologies during the festive moment of the wait for Christmas.

Last but not least, the *Mano Del Bambino* Association has been participating in the EA7 Emporio Armani Milano Marathon since 2014, which takes place on the first Sunday of April and sees both marathon runners and relay runners marching through the city with banners of the association, a visible and concrete tool for meet people and talk about this health reality.

The dissemination of news and communication through advertising, mostly social media and websites, is a fundamental element of information and training, two pillars of the *Mano Del Bambino* Association.

It is not a forum or idle chatter but real moments of information that anyone can access from any place in the world, which is in point of fact what animates the network. It should be emphasized that to this day, 80% of children get to the treatment department thanks to information gathered on the internet. Websites are therefore a tool of information and of testimonies that allow those who could not attend courses and events to gather information and to be part of the life of the association (manobambino.org, http://www.lachirurgiadellamano.it/it/news/campus-le-mie-mani-7ed-22-sett-2018).

Even in the digital age, radio- and telecommunication, and printing are of great support. They are instruments related to the time they are released, but that reach us in our home or in our car, without us having to look for them and therefore reaching people who have not had a chance to discover this reality.

It should be stressed that printing is not always sensitive to these problems because speaking by associating the terms children and illness often "annoys" the adult and healthy population who would rather identify themselves with diseases that directly affect them.

Nonetheless, the primary print and television publications have a great social sensitivity for children's problems and validly accept our messages.

The common denominator between the associations and initiatives organized by them is not fund raising, but rather to inform the families who have the opportunity to access care, the health workers potentially involved in the health support of these children, and lastly the people who may interact with those who have these types of problems during school or work life.

The medical and rehabilitative component is helped by the great voluntary support of the associations, especially when it comes to the relational component, as it functions as a container of doubts, confusion, anxiety, and questions. Every single member of this relational network, just like many actors and characters involved in a movie, no matter how different the roles are, will benefit from the association life because the moments of exchange and comparison are moments of growth for everyone.

It has been written that "camp, if it is worthy, is one of the greatest socializing, humanizing, civilizing factors which can enter the life of a boy or girl" [1]. Traditional summer camps are often unable to offer appropriate accommodations in regular camp activities for children with chronic conditions, due to their increased needs in medical care or physical limitations [1, p. 361]. Unfortunately, many children with chronic conditions are not given the opportunity to experience the socialization benefit that attending camp may offer. Research has found that children with chronic illnesses are at a greater risk of experiencing psychological difficulties such as behavior problems, poor self-concept, and social withdrawal [1]. Children with chronic conditions are estimated to have a 1.3–3 times greater risk of psychological or social issues during childhood when compared to a healthy child [1, p. 41]. Furthermore, a child's perception and attitude about their condition may mediate their development of problems, including social adjustments with peers, coping mechanisms, and how they adapt to his/her chronic condition [2].

In the 1970s, the concept of therapeutic camps for children with chronic conditions was created. This camping experience was found to provide psychosocial interventions that helped decrease the burden of disease and provide support, respite, and skill building through recreational activities [1, 3]. Many diagnosis-specific camp models have been established and researched, such as spina bifida, epilepsy, pediatric cardiac conditions, and cancer [4–7]. Among all of these diagnosis-specific camps, there were several common findings and outcomes, such as increased independence with activities of daily living, decreased parent/child anxiety, and increased self-esteem and increased social, emotional, and physical functioning [4–7].

Congenital anomalies of the hand and upper extremity range from mild to severe and can affect function, social interactions, and self-confidence [8]. Reaching maximum functional independence and gaining acceptance of their difference is the most typical goal of children born with a hand difference. Therapy for these children varies from structured outpatient therapy, use of orthoses or prosthetics for specific tasks, surgical intervention, and support groups.

Eileen Bradbury found in her book, *Counseling People with Disfigurement (1996)*, that having a hand difference, or disfigurement, can create social avoidance within individual as well as others surrounding him/her [9]. Additionally, adolescence is naturally a time of considerable change, with a school environment that is more competitive and less protected. The physical changes occurring in adolescence evoke increased self-consciousness, which is intensified in those with a visible difference [9].

Seeing a need within the congenital hand difference community, Texas Scottish Rite Hospital, a specialty orthopedic hospital, developed Hand Camp with the hope to assist this unique pediatric population and attempt to address the concerns of self-image, self-esteem, and confidence. This camp model has expanded and serves children throughout stages of development from early childhood to adolescence. These camps allow patients and families to interact, share concerns, and provide support for one another by engaging in team building activities and programs.

The Camp director's developed a Hand Camp Mission Statement and Objectives to give structure and goal-oriented direction. These objectives were informed by medical expertise, previous research findings, and observation of camp over a 25-year period to define the purpose of camp as well as expected outcomes following the campers' experience.

Hand Camp Mission Statement

Hand Camp is an opportunity for children with upper limb differences to meet others facing similar challenges. The weekend retreat for children ages 10–13 provides a safe environment to share experiences, challenges, fears, and successes. In addition, camp gives children an opportunity to focus on enhancing confidence and self-esteem through team building, exposure to new experiences, and developing leadership skills and to help and encourage each other during goal-directed organized activities.

Hand Camp Objectives

1. Enhance self-esteem and self-confidence.
2. Increase function/participation in activities offered in their home environment.
3. Increase relationships with peers.
4. Increase self-image and acceptance of their hand difference.
5. Increase desire to try new things without being fearful of failure.
6. Increase independence in functional daily activities.
7. Gain confidence in explaining hand difference to others.
8. Acquire coping skills to manage negative reactions from others regarding their hand difference.

Activities offered at Hand Camp consist of high and low rope elements, archery, arts and crafts, team building activities, time for same sex peer-to-peer discussion/activity time, and directed and nondirected time to work on activities of daily living.

Following camp, participants indicated improved skills in interacting with peers, daily physical activities, willingness to try new things, and confidence in explaining hand difference. Meeting these camp objectives combined with increased self-esteem (as seen through utilizing the RSES [10] pre- and post-camp), upper extremity functioning (as seen through utilizing the PROMIS [11–13] both pre- and post-camps), and peer relations (PROMIS) provided useful skills for campers to translate into their everyday life. This suggests that following camp, a child is more apt to participate in extracurricular activities, have higher self-esteem as regards to their hand difference, be more independent in activities of daily living, and manage negative reactions from others regarding the appearance of their hand [14].

Since 1995, Hand Camp has been offered at the Texas Scottish Rite Hospital for Children for children with congenital hand difference and their families to address physical needs as well as psychological needs by incorporating both aspects in the mission and objectives of camp. At camp, kids get the opportunity to learn from other peers and counselors with similar hand differences on how to navigate through everyday life. From putting hair up into a pony tail or painting fingernails to tying shoes and throwing a baseball, each child can learn new skills from individuals with the same exact hand difference. The success that children feel when they accomplish something they thought they would never be able to do all by themselves is uplifting and motivating to the learner and the trainer. Our goal is that kids leave camp with an increased self-esteem and self-confidence, a better body image, and an increased ability to form peer relations. We hope they leave with a greater understanding of their diagnoses and how to explain it to others as well as an increased desire to try new things back home in their communities without being fearful. Ultimately, we hope these kids leave feeling defined by who they are on the inside instead of by what they look like on the outside.

References

1. Barr RD, Silva A, Wong M, et al. A comparative assessment of attendance and nonattendance at camp trillium by children with cancer and their families: including their utilization of health and social services. J Pediatr Hematol Oncol. 2010;32:358–65.
2. Briery BG, Rabian B. Psychosocial changes associated with participation in a pediatric summer camp. J Pediatr Psychol. 1999;24:183–90.
3. Moola FJ, Faulkner GEJ, White L, Kirsh JA. The psychological and social impact of camp for children with chronic illnesses: a systematic review update. Child. 2013;40(5):615–31.
4. Bultas MW, Budhathoki C, Balakas K. Evaluation of child and parent outcomes after a pediatric cardiac camp experience. J Spec Pediatr Nurs. 2013;18:320–8.
5. Holbein CE, Murray CB, Psihogios AM, et al. A camp-based psychosocial intervention to promote independence and social function in individuals with spina bifida: moderators of treatment effectiveness. J Pediatr Psychol. 2013;38:412.
6. Martiniuk A, Silva M, Amylon M, et al. Camp programs for children with cancer and their families: review of research progress over the past decade. Pediatr Blood Cancer. 2014;61:778–87.
7. Sawin KJ, Lannon SL, Austin JK. Camp experiences and attitudes toward epilepsy: a pilot study. J Neurosci Nurs. 2001;33:57–64.
8. Lake A. Hand therapy for children with congenital hand differences. Tech Hand Up Extrem Surg. 2010;14:78–84.
9. Bradbury ET. Counselling people with disfigurement. Leicester: BPS Books; 1996. p. 1–131.
10. Rosenberg M. Society and the adolescent self-image. Princeton: Princeton University Press; 1965. p. 20–252.
11. DeWalt DA, Thissen D, Stucky BD, et al. PROMIS pediatric peer relationships scale: development of a peer relationships item bank as part of social health measurement. Health Psychol. 2013;32:1093–103.
12. Pilkonis PA, Yu L, Dodds NE, et al. Validation of the depression item bank from the patient-reported outcomes measurement information system (PROMIS®) in a three-month observational study. J Psychiatr Res. 2014;56:112–9.
13. Waljee JF, Carlozzi N, Franzblau LE, et al. Applying PROMIS to assess upper extremity function among children with congenital hand differences. Plast Reconstr Surg. 2015;13:200–7.
14. Lake A, Cerza SP, Butler L, Oishi S, Brown A. The Impact of therapeutic camp on children with congenital hand differences. Cog Psychol. 2021;8:1. https://doi.org/10.1080/23311908.2021.1938439.

Index

G. Pajardi (ed.), *Pediatric Hand Surgery*, https://doi.org/10.1007/978-3-031-30984-7

R

S

T

U

V

W

X

GPSR Compliance

The European Union's (EU) General Product Safety Regulation (GPSR) is a set of rules that requires consumer products to be safe and our obligations to ensure this.

If you have any concerns about our products, you can contact us on ProductSafety@springernature.com

In case Publisher is established outside the EU, the EU authorized representative is:

Springer Nature Customer Service Center GmbH
Europaplatz 3
69115 Heidelberg, Germany

Batch number: 10731383

Printed by Printforce, the Netherlands